Vascular Problems in Musculoskeletal Disorders of the Limbs

Vascular Problems in Musculoskeletal Disorders of the Limbs

David I. Abramson

Emeritus Professor of Medicine and of Physical Medicine and Rehabilitation
Abraham Lincoln School of Medicine
University of Illinois College of Medicine

Former Head
Department of Physical Medicine and Rehabilitation
University of Illinois College of Medicine

Donald S. Miller

Clinical Professor of Orthopedic Surgery
University of Health Sciences
Chicago Medical School

Former Chairman
Section of Orthopedic Surgery
University of Health Sciences
Chicago Medical School

With 98 Illustrations

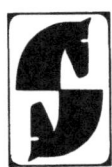

Springer-Verlag
New York   Heidelberg   Berlin

David I. Abramson, M.D., F.A.C.P.
Emeritus Professor of Medicine and of Physical Medicine and Rehabilitation
Abraham Lincoln School of Medicine
University of Illinois College of Medicine
Chicago, Illinois, U.S.A.

Consultant, Veterans Administration Hospital (Hines) and West Side Veterans Administration Hospital

Former Head, Department of Physical Medicine and Rehabilitation, University of Illinois College of Medicine

Donald S. Miller, M.D., Ph.D.
Clinical Professor of Orthopedic Surgery
University of Health Sciences
Chicago Medical School
Chicago, Illinois, U.S.A.

Attending Surgeon, Cook County Hospital and Edgewater Hospital, Chicago, Illinois

Head, Department of Orthopedics, Oak Park Hospital, Oak Park, Illinois

Former Chairman, Section of Orthopedic Surgery, University of Health Sciences, Chicago Medical School, Chicago, Illinois

Former Chairman, Section of Orthopedic Surgery, Cook County Postgraduate School, Chicago, Illinois

Library of Congress Cataloging in Publication Data
Abramson, David Irvin, 1905–
    Vascular problems in musculoskeletal disorders of the limbs.

    Bibliography: p.
    Includes index.
    1. Extremities (Anatomy)—Blood-vessels—Diseases.
2. Musculoskeletal system—Diseases. 3. Peripheral
vascular diseases. I. Miller, Donald Sidney, 1908–
joint author. II. Title. [DNLM: 1. Extremities—
Blood supply. 2. Vascular Diseases. 3. Bone diseases
—Complications. 4. Muscle diseases—Complications.
WE 800 A161v]
RC951.A27   616.7   80–27734

9 8 7 6 5 4 3 2 1

ISBN-13: 978-1-4612-5864-3   e-ISBN-13: 978-1-4612-5862-9
DOI: 10.1007/978-1-4612-5862-9

To Louise

Contents

Preface

That a close relationship exists between the specialties of peripheral vascular diseases and of orthopedic and general surgery has frequently been brought sharply into focus for both of us during many years of clinical experience in our respective fields of endeavor. Frequently, trauma to musculoskeletal structures has also been responsible for the production of a seriously compromised local blood flow, thus requiring a combined therapeutic approach to the solution of the problem. Improper utilization of appliances and conventional surgical procedures for common orthopedic conditions has on occasion likewise been followed by disastrous vascular complications. The fact that these possibilities exist in clinical practice has been the prime motivation for the development of this monograph.

The purpose of the volume is first to make readily available to the orthopedic or the general surgeon information that will allow him to determine whether a limb which he is treating is also suffering from an underlying impairment of arterial, venous, or lymphatic circulation. On the basis of such data, he should be in a better position to institute an appropriate and safe therapeutic program. Second, the subject matter should acquaint him with the necessary steps for early recognition of vascular complications of musculoskeletal disorders produced by trauma, with their differential diagnosis, and with their management. Finally, it should make him aware of the fact that a relatively large number of clinical entities possess both vascular and orthopedic components, and that it is essential to distinguish one from the other.

The monograph is divided into three parts. Section 1 consists of the gross and microscopic anatomy, physiology, pathophysiology, and pharmacology of the circulation in the skin, voluntary muscles, bones, and joints of the limbs. In Section 2 are described both the simple clinical tests of peripheral circulation capable of being carried out in the office or at the bedside and the more complicated laboratory procedures available in a large hospital. Section 3, the last and longest portion of the book, is devoted to discussions of disease states or entities. First, there is a description of clinical findings which are common to both circulatory and orthopedic conditions and then a presentation of vascular symptoms which mimic those of orthopedic origin. The second portion of Section 3 deals with such clinical entities as organic arterial diseases, both chronic and acute, and circulatory complications of musculoskeletal disorders of the limbs produced by trauma; the latter are categorized as injury to main blood vessels, factors responsible for venous thrombosis, clinical aspects of deep venous thrombosis, pulmonary embolism, postphlebitic syndrome, and fat embolism. Vascular and lymphatic tumors and malformation of the limbs are also considered in the volume, since these conditions frequently affect long bones and joints, as well as soft tissues. In addition, the important subject of the possible serious vascular complications of therapeutic procedures utilized in orthopedic disorders is presented in detail, as well as the problems associated with minor or major amputations for the management of gangrene due to ischemia. Because of the current interest in limb replantation, this subject is also discussed. Finally, the medicolegal aspects of vascular difficulties as related to orthopedic disorders are considered.

To consolidate the contents of the volume and to make all data pertaining to a specific subject readily available to the reader, numerous cross references are found interspersed throughout the text. It is realized that such a practice may prove annoying; nevertheless it is believed preferable to repetition of material in different sections of the book. In order to facilitate location of the various items in the contents, each cross reference consists of a capital letter, which refers to a main heading in the chapter, followed by an Arabic number, which identifies a subheading preceded by the same number. The remainder of the cross references consists of the designation of the chapter in which the item is to be found.

If by perusing this monograph the orthopedic surgeon becomes more acutely aware of the role that vascular insufficiency may play in the practice of his specialty, then its purpose will have been achieved. It is hoped, too, that the volume will be of value to the emergency room specialist and to the general surgeon, who must take into consideration the local state of the circulation before undertaking any operative procedure on the limb. For the same reason, it should be useful to the podiatrist when he is contemplating a surgical or even a conservative approach to the treatment of abnormalities of the foot. Finally, it may be helpful to the physiatrist who must deal with the problem of rehabilitation of the injured patient, especially in the chronic stage of disability.

We wish to express our appreciation to Drs. Lee Lichtenberg, Svante O. Rolander, and Irwin Siegel for their painstaking examination of the manuscript and for the very constructive criticisms and suggestions which were then offered. Our thanks also go to Dr. Jack Stevens for making available to us the background material for the chapter on vascular and lymphatic tumors and malformations. We are grateful to Dr. Jiri Linhart for permission to reproduce the angiograms used as figures in the volume. Some of the other photographs have been obtained from the files of the Veterans Administration Hospital, Hines, Illinois, through the courtesy of Mr. Clark Moore. Mr. Abe Krieger of Springer-Verlag very ably and diligently supervised and participated in all the steps involved in the technical production of this volume, for which we are deeply grateful.

David I. Abramson
Donald S. Miller

Section 1

Vascular Beds in the Limbs

Chapter 1

Circulation to the Skin

In this and the subsequent three chapters are discussed the anatomy and physiology of the circulation in the different types of tissues comprising the limbs. Only those points are emphasized which have direct clinical application or are essential for the better understanding of altered structural or functional mechanisms responsible for pathologic changes in the vascular tree. The present chapter is devoted to the circulation to the skin.

A. General Considerations

1. Role of the Cutaneous Circulation

In addition to supplying the skin with oxygen and nutritive substances and removing metabolites arising from tissue activity, the cutaneous circulation has several other functions. Through its many vascular plexuses, capillary and venular beds, and other types of vessels, it acts as a reservoir when there is need for shunting blood to inactive tissues. Moreover, the extensive arteriovenous anastomoses have the capability of allowing large quantities of blood to circumvent the capillary bed and enter directly into the venous system, thus making possible relief from very high levels of blood pressure in the arterial tree. Because the skin is in contact with a wide range of environmental temperatures, the volume of blood that passes through it also plays a significant role in thermoregulation and preservation of a steady body temperature. In fact, under extreme conditions of cold, local metabolic needs may be sacrificed for a long period of time in order to achieve the latter state. Finally, the cutaneous circulation is involved in a number of other homeostatic mechanisms, including the maintenance of the proper relationship between fluid volume and circulating blood volume.

2. Gross Morphologic Divisions of the Skin

The skin of the limbs is made up of a number of different layers. The most superficial one is the avascular epidermis, composed of squamous epithelium which receives its nutrition from the underlying capillaries located in the dermis. The latter structure consists of a thin superficial papillary layer and a deep reticular layer. In the dermis are found the hair follicles and the sweat and sebaceous glands—the appendages of the skin.

B. Anatomy of the Vascular Tree

The types of vascular networks in the skin are determined by the region of the body, the relationship of the skin to the underlying bone or fasciae, and the thickness of the panniculus adiposus. For example, in the fingers there is a very complex and abundant vascularity, beyond the degree necessary to supply nutrition to the comparatively thin epidermis and the small number of adnexal structures found in this site

3

[39]. Here the main function of the circulation is thermoregulation, with satisfaction of metabolic needs playing a secondary role.

1. Arterial and Arteriolar Beds

The vascular tree in the skin is derived from a network of perforating arteries arising in the subcutaneous tissue (Fig. 1.1). These vessels divide into an extensive anastomosing system (the deep arteriolar arcade) located between the deep reticular portion of the dermis and the underlying tissues. Generally vascular interconnections exist at all levels.

The deep arteriolar arcade gives off large numbers of arterioles which pass to sweat glands or hair follicles or supply the adjoining portion of the subcutaneous tissue. Others as-

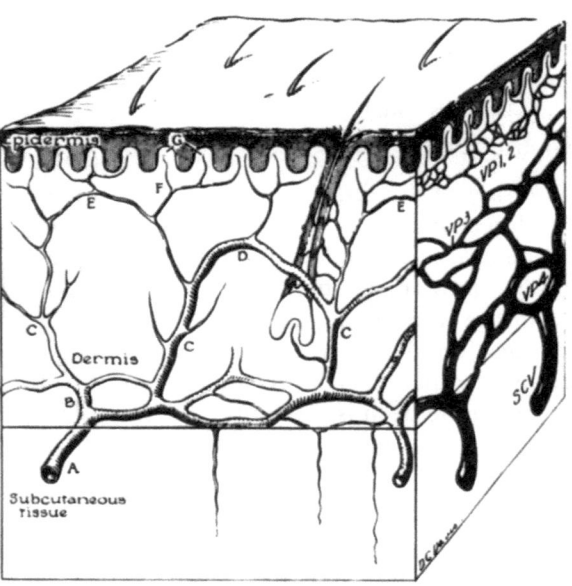

Fig. 1.1. Diagrammatic representation of the arterial and venous systems of the skin. *A*, Perforating artery; *B*, cutaneous plexus; *C*, arteriole (candelabra vessel); *D* and *E*, arched anastomoses—the superficial arcades form the subpapillary arteriolar plexus; *F*, terminal arteriole; *G*, arterial limb of capillary in a papilla. *VP1* and *VP2* form the subpapillary venous plexus. *VP3* and *VP4* form the deeper venous plexuses. *SCV*, Subcutaneous vein. From Moreci AP, Farber EM: In Abramson DI (ed): Blood Vessels and Lymphatics. New York, Academic Press, 1962. Reproduced with permission.

cend through the various layers of the dermis, producing a "candelabrum" type of branching and eventually dividing into nutrient capillaries (Fig. 1.1). The deep arteriolar arcade is also the source of arterioles that spread upward to form a more superficial network (subpapillary arteriolar plexus), which is located in the upper layer of the dermis, below the epidermis (Fig. 1.1).

2. Arteriovenous Anastomoses (Shunts)

Arteriovenous anastomoses are highly organized, short channels, approximately 220 μm in diameter, which establish direct communication between the arterial and venous trees above the level of the capillary bed (Fig. 1.2). They arise from small arteries and end in small veins and are found in the stratum reticulare of the skin of the hands and feet, the greatest number being present in the nail bed of the finger and toe (as many as 500 per square centimeter). The fingertips, finger pad, palmar aspects of the fingers, sole of the foot, and thenar and hypothenar eminences of the hand contain somewhat fewer but still a large number of these structures.

The coiled, thick-walled afferent artery or arteriole, the connecting loop (arteriovenous anastomosis), the neuroreticular and vascular structures around the canal, and the efferent vein, collectively, are termed the glomus (Fig. 1.2B). Distal to this globular organ, the artery divides into smaller branches that ultimately terminate in the capillary bed.

The arteriovenous anastomosis possesses a small lumen (about 20 μm in diameter) and a thick muscular wall devoid of an internal elastic membrane. In the contractile layer are found the characteristic glomus cells, epithelioid in appearance. The arteriovenous anastomosis is enclosed in loose, finely fibrillar collagenous tissue containing a rich network of unmyelinated sympathetic and myelinated nerve filaments.

3. Capillary Bed

The capillaries in the skin are relatively few in number (16 to 65 per square millimeter [37], as compared with 1000 to 2000 per square millimeter in underlying muscle [24]). They originate from a succession of arterioles and do not anastomose freely; instead they form separate loops supplying the dermis and the basal layer of the epidermis. At the base of the nail and dorsum of the finger, the loops are hairpin-shaped, consisting of a shorter, narrower limb, the arteriolar portion, and a thicker, larger limb, the venous portion; the two are joined by a short communicating segment (Fig. 1.3B and D). The capillary loops vary from 0.15 to 0.3 mm in length and, when dilated, are up to 10 μm in diameter at the arteriolar end and up to 15 μm at the venular end. There is an apparent relationship between the number of capillary loops and degree of development of the rete ridges; with age the latter structures tend to flatten and the capillary loops tend to become less in number and smaller in size. In places the capillaries are contorted and spiral, changes which have been interpreted as a means of preventing vessel rupture when the skin moves laterally [28].

4. Venular and Venous Beds

The cutaneous venules consist of four layers of vessels which run parallel to each other and to the surface of the skin and are found at different levels of the dermis, forming a candelabrum system of channels (Fig. 1.1). Those which drain the papillary loops merge to form the most superficial plexus located just below the papillae. The network beneath this one is in close association with the subpapillary arteriolar plexus. Blood from both venular beds (combined subpapillary venous plexus) (Fig. 1.3A and C) is collected into a third one which is located approximately in the middle portion of the dermis. The fourth and deepest venular network is situated between the dermis and the subcutaneous tissue, near the cutaneous arterial plexus (Fig. 1.1). It receives blood from the sweat glands and adipose tissue and empties into large subcutaneous veins and the deep venous system accompanying the arteries. There is marked looping of the venules in the different networks, thus allowing for mobility of the skin without rupture of these vessels.

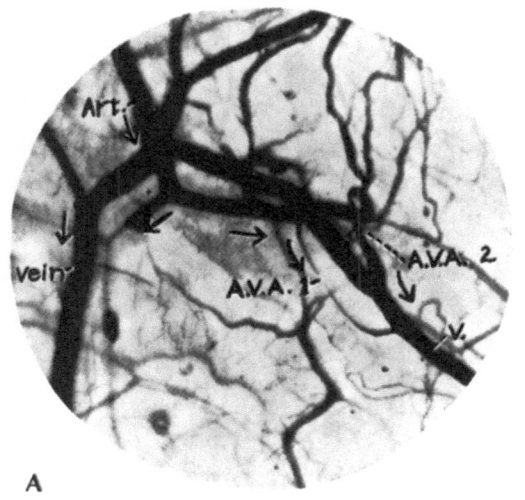

A

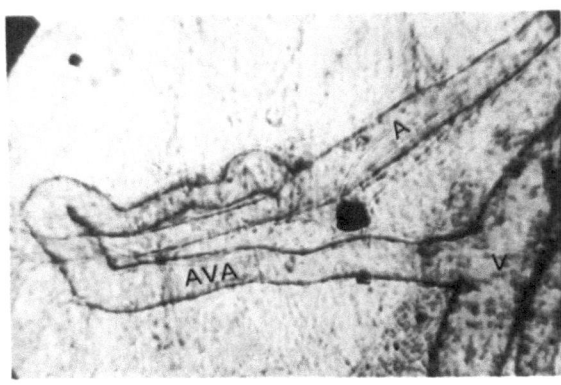

B

Fig. 1.2. Arteriovenous anastomoses. **A** Photomicrograph of a small area of living vessels in the rabbit's ear viewed through a stable preformed tissue chamber installed 1 month previously. Two arteriovenous anastomoses are seen, one straight *(A.V.A.1)* and one coiled *(A.V.A.2)*, both arising from the same artery and emptying into the same vein *(V)*. Arrows indicate direction of flow of blood in arteries. × 32. From Clark ER, Clark EL: Observations on living arteriovenous anastomoses as seen in transparent chambers introduced into the rabbit's ear. Am J Anat 54:229, 1934. Reproduced with the permission of the American Journal of Anatomy. **B** Injected and cleared specimen obtained from the external ear of the rabbit. *AVA,* arteriovenous anastomosis arising from an artery *(A)* and emptying into a vein *(V)*. The continuation of the artery subdivides *(left)*, its branches eventually ending in a capillary bed. From Abramson DI: Pathophysiology of arteriovenous shunts in the extremities. J Cardiovasc Surg 7 (Suppl):217, 1966. Reproduced with the permission of the Journal of Cardiovascular Surgery.

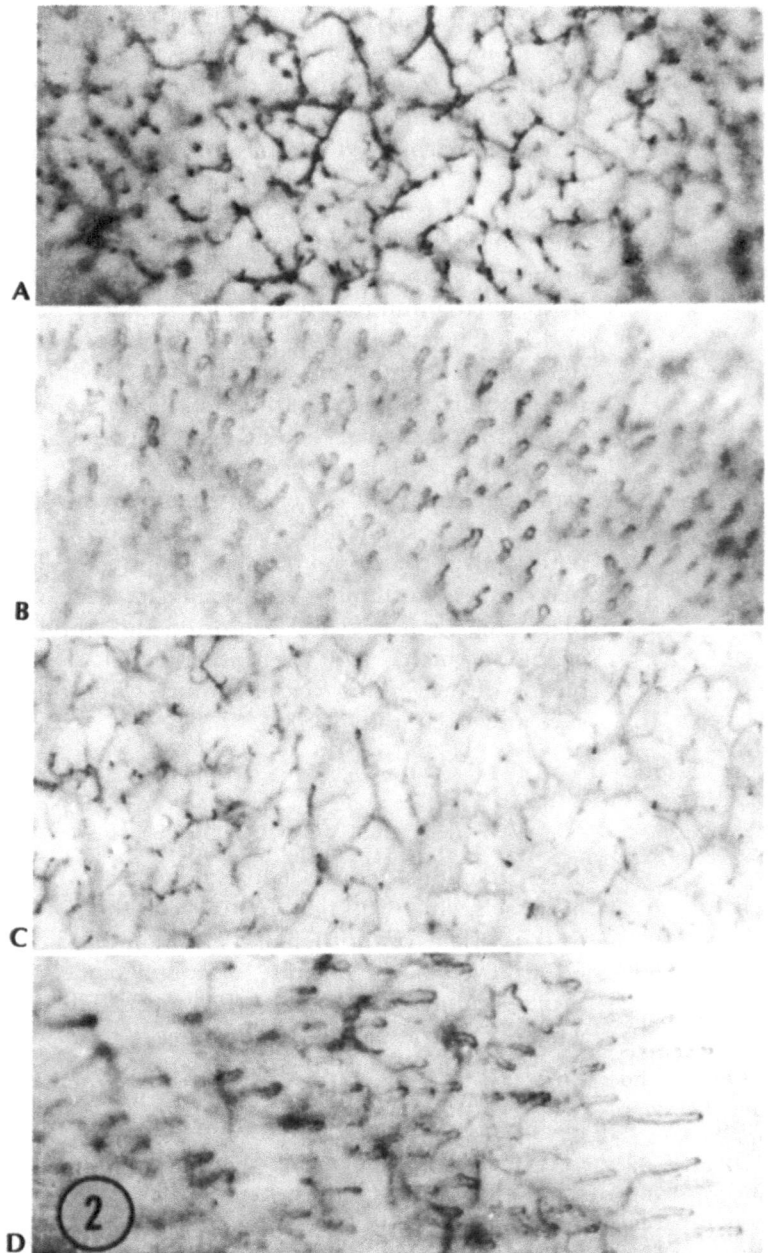

Fig. 1.3. Examination of cutaneous microcirculation in the human hand. **A** Capillaries and subpapillary venous plexus in skin of hand, as seen after removal of keratinized layers. **B** Normal capillary bed of dorsum of finger demonstrating capillary loops. Subpapillary venous plexus not well visualized. **C** Normal capillary bed of dorsum of hand. Subpapillary venous plexus clearly visualized. **D** Nailfold capillaries of finger. Marked sludging of blood noted in end capillaries as indicated by deformity of normal smooth axial stream. From Davis MJ, Lawler JC: In Montagna W, Ellis RA (eds): Advances in Biology of the Skin. New York, Pergamon Press, 1961. Reproduced with permission.

5. Vascular Supply to Appendages

Hair follicles receive their blood supply from branches of the candelabrum system of arteries. From the branches arises an elaborate plexus of capillaries which surrounds the individual hair follicle (Fig. 1.1). In the lower third of the follicle the vessels run parallel to this structure, being interconnected by numerous cross shunts [19] and running straight down to the core of the papilla.

The eccrine sweat glands receive their blood supply partly from the candelabrum system of arteries and partly from the cutaneous arterial plexus. Each gland is surrounded by capillary loops which follow the different contours of the tubule and give off branches that connect vessels that run along adjacent structures [19].

The blood supply to the apocrine sweat glands is from capillaries that have their origin in arterioles located at the junction of the hypodermis and dermis. The microcirculation forms plexuses of loops and intercommunicating branches and cross shunts around the tubules of the gland.

6. Innervation of Blood Vessels

From their origin in the vasomotor center in the medulla oblongata, the sympathetic preganglionic fibers pass down the intermediolateral cell columns of the spinal cord and leave the cord at intervals to make synapse in the paravertebral sympathetic ganglia with the postganglionic fibers. The latter run in somatic nerves to reach the peripheral blood vessels where they terminate in the alpha-receptor nerve endings in the vascular smooth-muscle cells (Fig. 1.4). Many alpha receptors are found in cutaneous vessels, whereas beta receptors are absent, this being the reverse of the situation present in muscle vessels.

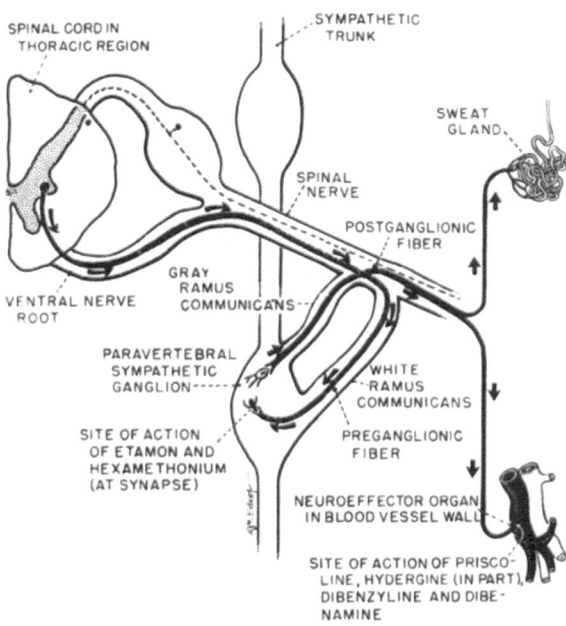

Fig. 1.4. Schematic representation of peripheral sympathetic pathways. From Abramson DI: Peripheral arterial vascular disorders. In Zimmerman LM, Levine R (eds): Physiologic Principles of Surgery. Philadelphia, Saunders, 1957. Reproduced with permission.

As already indicated, the arteriovenous anastomoses possess a rich innervation of sympathetic nerve fibrils. Although the latter enter the adventitia and smooth muscle cells forming the outer layers of the vessel walls, they do not appear to penetrate deeply into the centrally situated mass of epithelioid cells [30].

With regard to the sympathetic supply to venules and veins, the evidence is fragmentary, although the general impression is that these vessels are sparsely innervated by adrenergic fibers. This is of interest in view of the fact that veins have been noted to have rather active contraction and relaxation phases.

C. Physiology of the Vascular Tree

1. Laboratory Methods for the Study of Cutaneous Blood Flow

The cutaneous circulation in the limbs of man has been subjected to extensive physiologic study, due, in great part, to the fact that it is readily accessible to different methods of investigation, particularly in the case of the hand.

Microcirculation. The capillary circulation in the skin has generally been studied in the nailfolds of the fingers, using a capillary microscope (Fig. 1.3D). The vessels in these sites run parallel to the dorsal surface of the digit. In other portions of the limbs, it is necessary first to remove the keratin layer by blistering or by repeated applications of cellulose tape (Fig. 1.3).

Venous occlusion plethysmography. This method has been used in many experimental investigations, generally in the study of the hand which is made up primarily of skin if nonvascular tissues are disregarded. If the forearm (which contains a large quantity of muscle) is being investigated, it is necessary to utilize an equation derived from the average volume of skin in this segment of limb, as determined by dissection of cadavers, to obtain readings which represent the contribution solely of the cutaneous circulation [15].

2. Rate of Cutaneous Blood Flow

It is important at the outset to call attention to the fact that caution must be observed in any attempt to correlate total cutaneous blood flow measurements with the nutritional needs of the skin, since the vascular supply to this tissue also plays a very significant role in thermoregulation (see C-4, below). It has been estimated that as small an amount as 0.8 ml/min per 100 ml of tissue is sufficient to meet normal metabolic requirements of skin. Still, in the fingers, the resting circulation under physiologic conditions has been found to be as high as 15 to 40 ml and the rate may even rise to 90 ml with full dilatation [13]. Under the latter circumstances, most of the increase in blood flow is mediated through arteriovenous anastomoses and does not represent nutritional blood flow. In the forearm, resting cutaneous circulation under physiologic conditions ranges from 0 to 6 ml/min per 100 ml of skin [15]. Such wide fluctuations in local cutaneous circulation in different portions of the limbs and in different functional states reflect the multiple roles of cutaneous blood flow in physiologic processes of the body as a whole.

3. Nervous Regulation of the Cutaneous Circulation

In the skin the sympathetic nervous system plays a very important part in regulating blood flow, whereas inherent myogenic tone is poorly developed. Such a situation is probably related to the significant role that the cutaneous circulation plays in thermoregulation (see C-4, below).

Central control. Nervous regulation of the peripheral vessels resides in the vasomotor center in the reticular formation of the medulla oblongata where vasoconstrictor impulses originate (pressor areas). In addition, there are regions in which inhibitory impulses arise that exert influence on vasoconstrictor outflow (depressor areas). Very little evidence exists to indicate that there is a distinct and separate vasodilator center.

The rate of formation of vasoconstrictor impulses in the vasomotor center is modified by the action of higher centers in the subcortical areas, the hypothalamus (temperature regulating center), and the cerebral cortex. An extensive autonomic representation is found in the latter structure, especially in its motor area, the orbital surface of the frontal lobe, the rhinencephalon, and the temporal lobe. As a result of a very complex arrangement of neuron pools supplying vascular circuits, a differentiated central vasomotor regulation is established which has been characterized as a multilevel control [29].

Vasoconstrictor nerves. Sympathetic vasoconstrictor activity is the most important mechanism available for rapid adjustment of blood flow through the cutaneous vascular bed. As already indicated (see B-2 and B-6, above), the arterioles and arteriovenous anastomoses in the skin are richly supplied by a network of sympathetic adrenergic fibers, stimulation of which causes vasoconstriction at the alpha-receptor sites (neuroeffector end organs). The actual mechanism initiating the response is the release of a neurotransmitter, norepinephrine, at the adrenergic receptor site. This hormone is rapidly formed and liberated, thus permitting a swift and sustained reaction to it. Only very small amounts of norepinephrine escape into the bloodstream by the slower process of diffusion. The rate of discharge of vasoconstrictor impulses is low, not exceeding 1 or 2 per second even under conditions of marked activation [20].

Vasomotor control is particularly marked in the distal portions of the limbs, the fingers and toes. Although there is no question that regulation of the arterioles and arteriovenous anastomoses in these sites is accomplished primarily through adrenergic nerves, there is some suggestive experimental evidence supporting the view that the digital arteriovenous anastomoses also possess a cholinergic innervation which is responsible for vasodilatation [23,27]. In the more proximal portions of the limb, vasomotor control over the cutaneous circulation is much less marked than in the distal segments.

Vasodilator nerves. Although it is generally agreed that vasodilatation in the cutaneous circulation is elicited primarily by inhibition of vasoconstrictor tone or by some locally induced autoregulatory mechanism, some data have been presented in favor of the hypothesis that this state may also be produced actively through sympathetic cholinergic vasodilator nerves [18,34]. According to this concept, impulses passing over these structures stimulate gamma receptors through the production of acetylcholine. However, such a view has not been universally accepted because of conflicting evidence. The only conclusions that can be reached at present are that the functional activity of vasodilator nerves in the hand or foot under normal conditions has not been established [21,36] and that if such structures do exist, their physiologic significance must be very limited [8,35].

4. Role of Cutaneous Circulation in Thermoregulation

Of primary importance in the function of thermoregulation are the arteriovenous anastomoses, particularly those in the hands. When there is need for heat dissipation, these structures dilate and allow large quantities of blood to enter and flood the superficial veins without the need to traverse the cutaneous capillary bed, thus facilitating loss of body heat to the environment. When body heat must be conserved, as with exposure of a large surface area to cold, the arteriovenous anastomoses close entirely. Hence, all of the blood reaching the extremities must now pass through the minute vessels of the capillary bed which are also constricted by the same stimulus. As a consequence, the amount of blood entering the superficial veins is markedly reduced, with the great proportion of circulating blood volume being diverted to the internal organs where loss of heat is minimal. If exposure to cold is prolonged, the arteriovenous anastomoses and capillaries will eventually open intermittently, thus flooding the cutaneous venules with oxygenated blood and temporarily coloring the skin red (cold erythema). Subsequently cyanosis will intervene.

The marked influence that the sympathetic nervous system exerts on the arteriovenous anastomoses permits ready lability in the mechanism of dilatation and constriction of these vessels, in accordance with body requirements. In this function the arteriovenous anastomoses

supplement the action of the capillaries which are limited in their capacity to cope with extremes of environmental temperature because of their relative paucity in the skin.

5. Hormonal Control of the Cutaneous Circulation

Under normal conditions, blood-borne vasoconstrictor substances, like epinephrine, norepinephrine, and serotonin, are of negligible importance in regulating cutaneous blood flow, the vasomotor control being dominated by neural vasoconstriction via the peripheral sympathetic nervous system (see C-3, above). Only when there is a massive sympathetic activation do vasoconstrictor hormones play a role in reinforcing the direct action of sympathetic innervation [14].

Epinephrine causes marked blanching of the skin, due to strong constriction of the cutaneous blood vessels, including the arterioles, precapillary sphincters, and muscular venules; the evidence is lacking for a similar response in the capillary bed.

Norepinephrine also produces vasoconstriction of muscle-containing blood vessels in the skin, but the effect is not as marked as with epinephrine. The action of this hormone, as in the case of epinephrine, is through stimulation of alpha (constrictor) receptors in the blood vessel wall.

In regard to serotonin (5-hydroxytryptamine), the evidence is not as clear-cut. However, most of the experimental work appears to favor the view that this agent produces constriction of resistance vessels and dilatation of the microcirculation in the skin [33]. It may also have a direct vasoconstrictor effect on cutaneous and subcutaneous veins [16,26,31]. Commonly, with intradermal injection of serotonin, erythema and a flare result.

6. Vascular Changes Produced by Physical Agents

Direct heat. The topical application of such a stimulus causes a marked increase in cutaneous blood flow [6,7]. The vasodilatation is due to a very potent direct effect on cutaneous arteries and arterioles and is not related to inhibition of vasomotor tone, the same type of response also being noted in the sympathectomized limb [2]. At the same time, there is a significant rise in tissue temperature (Fig. 2.2A) [6] and a resulting increase in metabolic needs. Under normal conditions, the latter is readily satisfied through the associated marked augmentation in blood flow, which also acts as an efficient cooling system for the removal of heat from the exposed area. As a consequence, the augmentation in tissue temperature and metabolic needs is tempered and reduced.

The situation in the presence of occlusive arterial disease is entirely different. Heat is incapable of effectively dilating vessels that are organically partially occluded and hence the increase in local blood flow produced by this agent is much smaller than normal. As a result, the efficiency of the cooling mechanism supplied by the movement of blood through the tissues is impaired. Consequently, the tissue temperature will begin to approximate the level of the applied heat, thus causing a very great rise in metabolic needs of the exposed tissues. Since under the circumstances no effective means are available to satisfy such extreme requirements, necrosis of skin and underlying structures will inevitably occur. It is for this reason that no form of physical therapeutic procedure which develops heat in the tissues (e.g., short-wave diathermy, infrared lamp, ultrasound, ultraviolet light, topical wet or dry heat, paraffin bath, hot packs, heating pad) should ever be prescribed without first ascertaining that the local arterial circulation is normal.

Indirect heating.   The application of heat to distant portions of the body to produce reflex or indirect vasodilatation in the hands or feet is an effective means of increasing local cutaneous blood flow without any of the risks associated with direct heating (see above). However, the vasodilator response, which is due to inhibition of vasomotor tonus, is never as great as that initiated by the direct application of the agent [1].

The mechanism responsible for the increase in cutaneous blood flow is as follows: The temperature of the blood passing through the heated portions of the body is raised, with the result that after 30 min of exposure, the body temperature is also elevated, provided heat is prevented from being lost to the environment by covering the subject with blankets. The heated blood, on perfusing through the temperature regulating center in the hypothalamus, stimulates this structure and, as a result, impulses originating there pass down to the vasomotor center where they act to inhibit discharges of vasoconstrictor impulses. Such a situation permits the cutaneous arterioles, normally under the control of the vasomotor center, to dilate passively, thus increasing blood flow to the skin, particularly of the fingers and toes.

Since there is only a slight elevation in tissue temperature with indirect vasodilatation (resulting from the more rapid blood flow through the skin) [3], the rise in metabolic needs is minimal. Hence, the procedure is entirely innocuous, even in the presence of a marked compromise of the local arterial circulation. For example, if the vessels are unable to dilate on removal of vasomotor tone because of organic disease, then even the minimal rise in skin temperature will not occur because of the resulting small increase in cutaneous blood flow, and so there will be no change in metabolic needs.

Electric modalities.   Short-wave diathermy has very little vasodilating effect on cutaneous circulation, its greatest response being on underlying tissues [5]. However, the infrared lamp appears to exert a moderate vasodilating action on the skin vessels. Ultrasound is ineffective in this regard [4].

Direct cold.   Topical application of this agent produces marked vasoconstriction of the cutaneous circulation. The response is due to a direct effect on the vessels themselves, particularly the arterioles, without the mediation of sympathetic vasoconstrictor nerves.

7.   Vascular Responses to Drugs

The cutaneous circulation is altered by a large number of vasodilator or vasoconstrictor drugs.

Vasodilator agents. Augmentation of cutaneous circulation can be achieved through several different mechanisms. Normal or abnormal vasomotor tone can be eliminated by means of sympathetic blocking agents which act by competitive inhibition at the alpha-receptor endings (neuroeffector junctions) in the blood vessel wall. Among such drugs are tolazoline (Priscoline), phentolamine (Regitine), derivatives of ergotoxine (Hydergine), and phenoxybenzamine hydrochloride (Dibenzyline). Reserpine (Serpasil) is of value in antagonizing the effects of circulating epinephrine and norepinephrine and in impairing catecholamine retention in tissues, with subsequent loss in physiologic effectiveness by degradation [25]. The drug also appears to abolish the ability of the sympathetic nerves to bind norepinephrine, followed by inactivation of the latter by oxidative deamination. Ganglionic blocking agents, like tetraethylammonium chloride, act temporarily to destroy the continuity of the sympathetic nervous system by blocking vasoconstrictor impulses at the level of the paravertebral sympathetic ganglia. Whiskey and other alcoholic beverages cause cutaneous vasodilatation by depressing the rate of formation of vasoconstrictor impulses in the vasomotor center in the medulla.

Another group of drugs which causes vasodilatation in the skin is the myovascular relaxants, agents which have a direct paralyzing action on the smooth muscle of the cutaneous blood vessels. In this category are oral nicotinic acid, oral cyclandelate (Cyclospasmol), 2 percent nitroglycerin ointment (Nitrol ointment) by topical application, histamine hydrochloride by ion transfer, papaverine hydrochloride by intraarterial injection, and procaine hydrochloride by direct contact with the vessel.

8. Effect of Sympathetic Denervation on Cutaneous Blood Flow

Removal of sympathetic control over normal cutaneous blood vessels, as by sympathetic blocking agents, paravertebral or stellate ganglionic block, peripheral nerve block, or sympathectomy, immediately produces signs of an increase in blood flow through the skin. These consist of a significant rise in cutaneous temperature, rubor of the skin, and bounding pulses, associated with anhydrosis. Blood pressure in the small cutaneous vessels increases.

The changes are most marked in the distal portion of the limbs, the digits, a finding which can be correlated with the relative anatomic distribution of sympathetic vasomotor nerve fibers. The intensity of the response becomes less and less as the proximal portion of the limb is approached. Even in the hand and foot, the rise in cutaneous temperature is almost limited to the digits, with changes elsewhere being of much smaller magnitude. Removal of sympathetic control has been reported to have a paradoxical effect: a decrease in tone of the arterioles and an increase in tone of the capillaries [12]. There is also some suggestive evidence that marked vasodilatation occurs in the arteriovenous anastomoses [32], which could explain the finding that the greatest increase in cutaneous temperature following sympathectomy occurs in the digits, the site of the highest concentration of these vascular structures.

Considerable experimental evidence exists to indicate that the augmentation of cutaneous circulation produced by sympathectomy is transient [9,11,17,22,38]. The return of blood flow to nearly preoperative levels occurs several weeks after surgery. The response appears to be due to reestablishment of vascular tone, although the explanation for such a phenomenon is not clear [9].

D. Pathology of the Vascular Tree

Because of its location, the cutaneous circulation is affected by external factors (such as extremes of temperature, exposure to roentgen rays and ultraviolet light, physical trauma, and chemical injury) to a much greater degree than are similar vessels in internal organs or even in the subcutaneous tissue. As a result, pathologic changes are not uncommon in this vascular bed. Among other abnormalities or states affecting the cutaneous circulation are hereditary defects, systemic disorders, and alterations in vasomotor control. For example, in severe Raynaud's disease, most of the capillaries appear enlarged. In schizophrenia and neurocirculatory asthenia, they may be reduced in number, as well as demonstrating irregularities in size and shape. Changes in capillary structure may also be seen in such disorders as scleroderma and acrocyanosis, the alterations taking the form of unusually shaped loops, minute aneurysms, or saccular enlargements. Also, abnormal periodicity of flow may be noted in the microcirculation. In polycythemia and hyperthyroidism, the number of open capillary loops are significantly increased, individual vessels are more dilated than normally, and the total cross section of capillary bed is enlarged. In thromboangiitis obliterans and arthritis, the capillaries are fairly normal in caliber and tonus [12]. (For discussion of other specific disorders in which there are pathologic changes in the cutaneous circulation, see pp. 116, 130, 152, and 320.)

References

1. Abramson DI: Vascular Responses in the Extremities of Man in Health and Disease. Chicago, Univ Chicago Press, 1944, p 380
2. Abramson DI: Circulation in the Extremities. New York, Academic Press, 1967, p 245
3. Abramson DI, Bell Y, Tuck S Jr, et al: Changes in blood flow, oxygen uptake, and tissue temperatures produced by therapeutic physical agents. III. Effect of indirect or reflex vasodilatation. Am J Phys Med 40:5, 1961
4. Abramson DI, Burnett C, Bell Y, et al: Changes in blood flow, oxygen uptake, and tissue temperatures produced by therapeutic physical agents. I. Effect of ultrasound. Am J Phys Med 39:51, 1960
5. Abramson DI, Harris AJ, Beaconsfield P: Changes in peripheral blood flow produced by short-wave diathermy. Arch Phys Med Rehabil 38:369, 1957
6. Abramson DI, Kahn A, Tuck S Jr, et al: Relationship between a range of tissue temperature and local oxygen uptake in the human forearm. I. Changes observed under resting conditions. J Clin Invest 37:1031, 1958
7. Abramson DI, Zazeela H, Marrus J: Plethysmographic studies of peripheral blood flow in man. II. Physiologic factors affecting resting blood flow in the extremities. Am Heart J 17:206, 1939
8. Arnott WM, Macfie JM: Effect of ulnar nerve block on blood flow in the reflexly vasodilated digit. J Physiol (Lond) 107:233, 1948
9. Barcroft H, Swan HJC: Sympathetic Control of Human Blood Vessels. London, Arnold, 1953, p 66
10. Barcroft H, Walker AJ: Return of tone in blood vessels of the upper limb after sympathectomy. Lancet 1:1035, 1949
11. Beaconsfield P: Veins after sympathectomy. Surgery 36:771, 1954
12. Brown GE: Observations on the surface capillaries in man following cervicothoracic sympathetic ganglionectomy. J Clin Invest 9:115, 1930
13. Burton AC: The range and variability of the blood flow in the human fingers and the vasomotor regulation of body temperature. Am J Physiol 127:437, 1939
14. Celander O: The range of control exercised by the sympathico-adrenal system. Quantitative study on blood vessels and other smooth muscle effectors in the cat. Acta Physiol Scand 32:1 (Suppl 116), 1954
15. Cooper KE, Edholm OG, Mottram RF: The blood flow in skin and muscle of the human forearm. J Physiol (Lond) 128:258, 1955
16. Demis DJ, Davis MJ, Lawler JC: A study of the cutaneous effects of serotonin. J Invest Dermatol 34:43, 1960
17. Duff RS: Circulatory changes in the forearm following sympathectomy. Clin Sci 10:529, 1951
18. Edholm OG, Fox RH, MacPherson RK: Vasomotor control of the cutaneous blood vessels in the human forearm. J Physiol (Lond) 139:455, 1957
19. Ellis RA: Vascular patterns of the skin. In Montagna W and Ellis RA (eds): Advances in Biology of Skin, Vol II. New York, Pergamon Press, 1961, p 20
20. Folkow B: Impulse frequency in sympathetic vasomotor fibres correlated to the release and elimination of the transmitter. Acta Physiol Scand 25:49, 1952
21. Gaskell P: Are there sympathetic vasodilator nerves to the vessels of the hands? J Physiol (Lond) 131:647, 1956
22. Grant RT, Pearson RSB: The blood circulation in the human limb: Observations on the difference between the proximal and distal parts and remarks on the regulation of body temperature. Clin Sci 3:119, 1938
23. Hurley HJ Jr, Mescon H: Cholinergic innervation of the digital arteriovenous anastomoses of human skin: A histochemical localization of cholinesterase. J Appl Physiol 9:82, 1956
24. Krogh A: The Anatomy and Physiology of Capillaries, rev. ed. New Haven, Yale Univ Press, 1929
25. Lindmar R, Muscholl E: Die Wirkung von Pharmaka auf die Elimination von Noradrenalin aus der Perfusionsflüssigkeit und die Noradrenalinaufnahme in das isolierte Herz. Naunyn Schmiedebergs Arch Exp Pathol 247:469, 1964
26. Lorincz AL, Pearson RW: Studies on axon re-

flex vasodilatation and cholinergic urticaria. J Invest Dermatol 32:429, 1959

27. Mescon H, Hurley HJ Jr, Moretti G: The anatomy and histochemistry of the arteriovenous anastomosis in human digital skin. J Invest Dermatol 27:133, 1956

28. Nelms JD: Functional anatomy of skin related to temperature regulation. Fed Proc 22:933, 1963

29. Peiss CN: Concepts of cardiovascular regulation: past, present, and future. In Randall WC (ed): Nervous Control of the Heart. Baltimore, Williams & Wilkins, 1965

30. Pritchard MML, Daniel PM: Arteriovenous anastomoses in the tongue of the dog. Am J Anat 95:203, 1954

31. Reid G: Circulatory effects of 5-hydroxytryptamine. J Physiol (Lond) 118:435, 1952

32. Richards RL: Some observations on vasodilation after sympathectomy. Glasgow Med J 34:245, 1953

33. Roddie IC, Shepherd JT, Whelan RF: The action of 5-hydroxytryptamine on the blood vessels of the human hand and forearm. Br J Pharmacol 10:445, 1955

34. Roddie IC, Shepherd JT, Whelan RF: The vasomotor nerve supply to the skin and muscle of the human forearm. Clin Sci 16:67, 1957

35. Sarnoff SJ, Simeone FA: Vasodilator fibers in the human skin. J Clin Invest 26:453, 1947

36. Uvnäs B: Sympathetic vasodilator system and blood flow. Physiol Rev (Suppl 4) 40:69, 1960

37. Wetzel NC, Zotterman Y: On differences in the vascular colouration of various regions of the normal human skin. Heart 13:357, 1926

38. Wilkins RW, Eichna LW: Blood flow to the forearm and calf. I. Vasomotor reactions: Role of the sympathetic nervous system. Bull Johns Hopkins Hosp 68:425, 1941

39. Winkelmann RK, Scheen SR Jr, Pyka RA, et al: Cutaneous vascular patterns in studies with injection preparation and alkaline phosphatase reaction. In Montagna W and Ellis RA (eds): Advances in Biology of Skin, Vol II. New York, Pergamon Press, 1961

Chapter 2

Circulation to Voluntary Muscle

A knowledge of the normal vascular pattern in the voluntary muscles of the extremities and of the responses of the vessels in these sites to various types of physical, chemical, and hormonal agents is basic to the proper understanding of various pathologic states affecting such structures. This is particularly true if surgical intervention is contemplated in the control of situations resulting from local trauma.

Skeletal muscle has a rich blood supply that can readily be altered to accommodate for the marked range of metabolic needs that exists when this tissue passes from a resting state into active contraction and then back to inactivity. Circulatory adjustments are constantly being made in the extensive vascular bed in order to prevent pooling of large quantities of blood in it.

A. Anatomy of the Vascular Tree

1. Gross Morphology

The architecture and distribution of vessels to and within the voluntary muscles of the limbs vary greatly depending on specific functional needs and the degree of collateral circulation available from other sources.

Extrinsic blood supply. The types of vessel arrangements conveying blood to voluntary muscles can be divided into three groups [22]. In one, the local circulation has its origin from a number of sources (as many as five), as in the case of the deltoid, triceps, adductor magnus, vastus internus and externus, soleus, and gluteus medius and minimus. In such structures, therefore, complete block of one or two of their main arteries still leaves them with an adequate collateral circulation for the satisfaction of at least resting metabolic needs. However, even under these circumstances, the extent of vascular anastomoses cannot be anticipated until the efficiency of the patent channels is known. Moreover, there is always a possibility that despite the availability of abundant vessels, these may be so small that they are incapable of providing the muscle with enough nutrition to prevent anaerobic infection or muscle degeneration in the event of sudden occlusion of one or two main channels.

In a second group, there are only two or three arteries supplying individual muscles. Examples of such a vascular pattern are found in the gluteus maximus, the rectus femoris, the hamstrings, and the sartorius. As a result, collateral circulation to these structures is more limited than in the case of the muscles included in the first category.

In the third group, the local circulation is derived primarily from one source: Among the muscles with this vascular pattern are the crureus, the gracilis, the long head of the biceps brachii, and both heads of the gastrocnemius. It is apparent that, under such circumstances, occlusion of the single critical vessel would invariably have very serious consequences.

Since the components of the anterior tibial compartment are not infrequently affected by periods of acute ischemia from a number of different causes (see Section H, Chapter 15), specific reference to the blood supply of individual muscles located in this structure appears warranted. The circulation to the tibialis anterior is derived solely from the anterior tibial artery, whereas that to the extensor digitorum longus comes not only from this vessel but from a number of arteries which arise in the posterior compartment of the leg and penetrate the interosseous membrane. The same is true for the extensor hallucis longus except that the amount reaching this muscle from the perforating vessels is relatively small.

Intrinsic vascular patterns. When the main arterial channels penetrate the muscle mass, they form different anatomic arrangements which have been divided into five types [19]. In one, branches from a number of arteries leave the vessels at intervals throughout their length to enter the muscle, as in the case of the soleus and peroneus longus. Another pattern consists of the development of vascular arcades that originate from a single artery entering the upper end of the muscle, as is noted in the gastrocnemius. A third type involves the formation of a radiating vascular arrangement having its source from a single main artery which enters the midportion of the muscle, as in the case of the biceps brachii. In another type, there is a grouping of collateral channels arising from a number of vessels that enter the muscle throughout its length, with most of the branches usually originating from one main artery. Such an arrangement is found in the tibialis anterior, the extensor digitorum longus, and the long extensors of the leg. In the fifth category, the vascular pattern consists of an open rectangular meshwork, with occasional anastomotic connections, such an arrangement being present in the extensor hallucis longus.

2. Microscopic Morphology

As a general rule, the vascular tree penetrates the muscle mass by coursing in the intramuscular septa, branching freely to form many anastomoses that then continue as the primary arterial network. From the meshes of the latter arise smaller vessels that join with each other

to produce a secondary system of arteriolar arcades [47].

Information regarding the microscopic vascular pattern in voluntary muscle of man is fragmentary. Usually the histologic characteristics of the arterioles and capillaries are similar to those noted in other structures in the limbs. There is some question as to whether "thoroughfare channels" [23] exist, and arteriovenous shunts are rarely found, in contrast to the situation present in skin (see B-2, Chapter 1).

With regard to venous return, the venules into which the capillaries empty join with each other to form larger channels; these in general follow the course of the arterioles and then the arteries. Valves are found in the entire intramuscular venous system, including even the smallest branches, thus providing a mechanism whereby blood is effectively propelled in a proximal direction, especially during muscular contraction.

Lymphatic system. Numerous lymph channels are found in the connective tissue within the intermuscular planes, running with blood vessels [41]. Lymphatics have also been described in the intrafascicular tissue [1], which evidently play a role in conveying lymph originating in the muscles to lymph vessels. However, elements of the lymphatic system are few if any within the skeletal muscle proper.

B. Physiology of the Vascular Tree

1. Laboratory Methods for the Study of Muscle Blood Flow at Rest and during Exercise

Venous occlusion plethysmography. This is a complicated, technically difficult procedure which is used to measure the rate of total blood flow in the extremities of man [2]. When applied to the collection of data on muscle circulation, it must be modified by first administering epinephrine by ion transfer in order to suppress cutaneous circulation through the production of intense and prolonged surface vasoconstriction [13,24,25]. On the basis of the average figures for the volume of skin and muscle derived from dissections of forearms [5] and the results obtained with epinephrine by ion transfer, an equation has been arrived at which has been used to calculate resting muscle circulation [25]. However, there are several criticisms to which the procedure is open, one of which is the realization that there is no basis for assuming that at any given total forearm circulation, a fixed ratio exists between the cutaneous and the muscle blood flow [25]. At best, then, only approximate predictions can be made of muscle circulation from readings of total forearm blood flow measured by venous occlusion plethysmography.

Radioisotope disappearance rate. This method for the study of muscle circulation consists of monitoring the rate of disappearance of radioactivity following intramuscular injection of aqueous solutions of such radioisotopes as ^{24}Na, ^{85}Kr, and ^{133}Xe [36,40,42]. The last two are inert lipophilic radioactive gases that are excreted by way of the lungs, thus reducing or eliminating recirculation of resorbed radioactive matter. Although the procedure has the advantage of studying muscle circulation alone, actually it measures muscle perfusion rather than rate of blood flow and hence reflects primarily local nutritive circulation.

The technique consists of injecting the radioactive material into the muscle mass, followed by repeated external measurements of the amount of radioactivity centered over the site, using a scintillation probe. The data are registered on a ratemeter connected to a linear recorder. The rate of loss of radioactivity from the injection site is determined from the slope of the curve of disappearance.

To obtain more definitive results, it is necessary to produce local ischemia by means of a period of arterial occlusion or by a bout of exercise utilizing the muscles under study. First a 3 to 5 min count is taken at rest to determine whether the disappearance rate is linear, and then the stressing procedure is carried out. Similar counts are performed during the period of arterial occlusion or work and immediately thereafter. If, for example, isotope clearance stops while the patient is exercising, this indicates a significant reduction in muscle circulation. A postexercise disappearance rate of 4

min or more can be considered to have the same interpretation.

Delineation and quantification of distribution of radioactivity. Muscle circulation has also been studied through the intraarterial injection of macroaggregates of albumin labeled with radioactive ^{131}I. The method is based on the fact that the particles of albumin, being 10 to 100 μm in size, lodge in capillaries and arterioles and remain there until metabolized into smaller particles [38,58].

Following the injection of the radioisotope, the distribution of radioactivity in the limb is determined by scanning and by integrating the count obtained over each segment of limb. As in the case of the method utilizing the rate of disappearance of a radioisotope (see above), this procedure at best reflects nutritive rather than total blood flow.

Types of exercise. The local vascular responses to physical activity can be studied with any one of the above-mentioned methods. In the case of the upper limb, a standard exercise consists of either strong grasps on a bar, each lasting about 0.5 s and repeated over a period of 4 or 5 min, or manual compression of an ordinary sphygmomanometer bulb a specified number of times in 0.5 to 1 min, in order to raise the pressure in an air-filled bottle to a definite level (Fig. 2.1). In the case of the lower limb, the work load generally consists of the use of an ergometer connected by pulleys to a known weight which rides freely over the edge of the bed. With a downward push (extension) of the foot against a hinged vertical board, the weight is lifted upward.

2. Muscle Blood Flow during Resting and Active States

Resting blood flow readings. In normal human subjects, muscle blood flow in the forearm has been reported to be in the range of 1.8 to 9.6 ml/min per 100 ml of limb volume, using the venous occlusion plethysmographic method [25]. On the basis of ^{133}Xe clearance studies, the resting nutritive blood flow figures are 1.6 to 2.5 ml/min per 100 g of muscle mass [42].

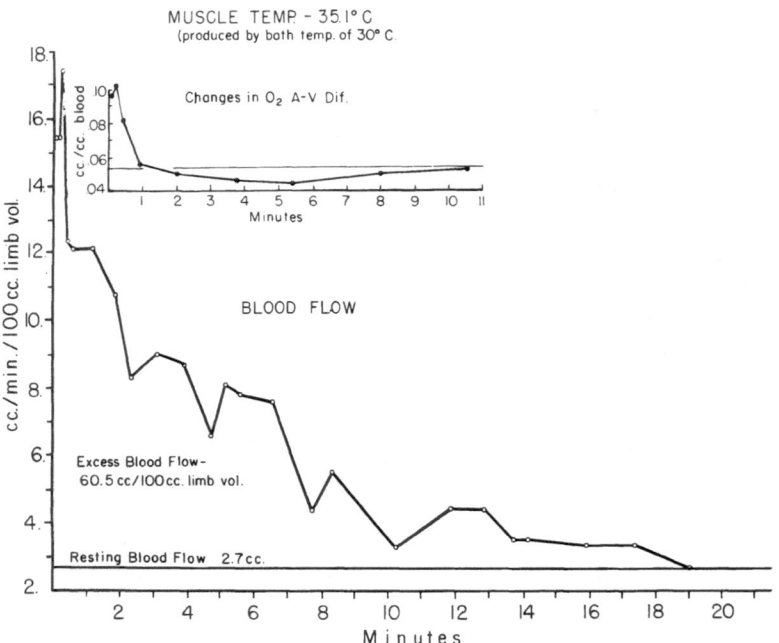

Fig. 2.1. Blood flow changes observed in the postexercise period following repeated contractions of forearm muscles, resulting from compression of a blood pressure bulb against a rising pressure. The work was done under anaerobic conditions. The curve demonstrates an initial sharp increase in forearm blood flow (measured by venous occlusion plethysmography), followed by a sharp fall and then a more gradual drop to the original resting baseline. The changes in oxygen arteriovenous differences are also shown *(upper graph)*. From Abramson DI, et al [9]. Reproduced with the permission of the Rockefeller University Press.

Vascular changes with exercise. Contraction of skeletal muscle is associated with a marked augmentation in local circulation (at times to the extent of a 20-fold or greater rise over the resting level), which occurs almost solely in the true capillary system. For example, using the radioisotope disappearance rate, moderate exercise in normal subjects has been reported to increase local blood flow to levels as high as 56 ml/min per 100 g of muscle (from a control figure of 1.6 to 2.5 ml) [42]. The magnitude of the vascular response in muscles to exercise is considered to be greater than that observed in similar types of circulatory beds anywhere else in the body [54].

During a single sustained contraction, limb volume first falls and then, after 3 to 5 min, it begins to increase at a rapid rate. In the recovery period, there is a further rise in volume, followed by a gradual fall to the resting level [33]. Blood flow begins to increase rapidly with a sustained contraction and reaches a maximal level which is maintained. During relaxation, the flow initially rises enormously and thereafter declines, at first quickly and then more slowly. Such changes have been interpreted as indicating that while a strong sustained muscular contraction compresses the vessels, the exerted force is insufficient to prevent them from dilating to a certain extent [33].

The vascular effects of rapidly repeated contractions of the muscles of the forearm have been studied under aerobic and anaerobic conditions, generally in the immediate postexercise period. Initially there is a marked increase in blood flow which subsides, at first quickly and then more slowly, to the resting level (Fig. 2.1). The magnitude of the hyperemia (blood flow repayment) and the duration of the recovery phase are directly proportional to the severity of the exercise. The marked increase in oxygen requirements of the exercising muscles is therefore taken care of, in great part, by the augmented local circulation resulting from active and passive vasodilatation. However, other mechanisms are also called upon, including a greater utilization of the oxygen in the local arterial blood, a widening of the arteriolar and capillary beds, and a rise in heart rate and arterial blood pressure (especially the systolic level), reflecting an increase in cardiac output.

There is still some controversy regarding the mechanisms responsible for the local hyperemia elicited by exercise. One which has received considerable experimental support is the release of relatively stable vasodilator substances from the active muscle fibers [31,33]. It has been suggested that these chemicals are both produced and released during the contracted state but are prevented from exhibiting an effect because of compression of the blood vessels [11]. However, the possibility that the elaboration of the substances takes place in the period of contraction but that liberation occurs only during relaxation has also been proposed [44]. Among the vasodilators which have been implicated in exercise hyperemia are histamine, acetylcholine, and adenosine triphosphate or its derivatives. Anoxia has also been considered as a possible etiologic factor.

In general terms, it can be stated that exercise hyperemia persists into the postexercise period until there is complete removal of the byproducts of increased metabolic activity and metabolic imbalance is corrected. The rate of return of blood flow to a basal level can be accelerated by physical conditioning and exercise therapy, by hyperbaric oxygenation, and by local heating [9]. (For the questionable role of inhibition of vasoconstrictor tone in exercise hyperemia and for the possible contribution of vasodilator nerves, see B-3 below.)

3. Regulation of Muscle Blood Flow

A large number of mechanisms have been implicated in the control of the circulation through muscles.

Active vasomotion. Two types of independent contraction of the minute vessels in muscle have been described in lower animals. One is a primarily slow change which is initiated by local metabolic vasodilators [45]. The other, a much faster response, probably results from neural influences since it is abolished by sympathetic denervation. Active vasomotion involves an independent unsynchronized vascular contractility producing ebb and flow of blood through the microcirculation. The alterations are related to the opening and closing of metarterioles and precapillary sphincters.

Humoral regulation. It has been proposed that circulating epinephrine formed in the adrenal medulla plays a role in the control of muscle circulation through its influence on metabolic processes. On the other hand, norepinephrine, which has little or no effect on these mechanisms and whose vascular action is primarily

vasoconstrictor, probably exerts minimal or no regulation over muscle circulation.

Central vasoconstrictor control. There is considerable controversy regarding the role of vasoconstrictor nerves in the regulation of muscle blood flow. Experimental evidence has been presented by some workers supporting the view that vasoconstrictor fibers innervate muscle blood vessels [12,13,50–53]. However, the reported data are by no means conclusive proof for this contention and, in fact, may lend themselves to other interpretations. Moreover, there are conflicting studies available which oppose such a view [5,20,49,59]. Also of importance in this regard are the findings that sympathectomy and degeneration of peripheral nerves produce no essential difference in the pattern of circulatory response of muscles to exercise [33,55]. Such results have clinical implications since lumbar sympathectomy has been advocated as therapy in arteriosclerosis obliterans (see p. 163).

Central vasodilator control. In the cat and dog, evidence has been obtained indicating that there are vasodilator nerves which innervate muscle blood vessels [21,30,56] and play an important role in the production of the marked increase in blood flow associated with muscular activity [27–29]. In man, there is experimental evidence for the view that cholinergic vasodilator nerves contribute to the vasodilatation that occurs in the muscles of the forearm during emotional stress [17,32]. Other reports are also available which are in accord with the belief that such structures do innervate the blood vessels in voluntary muscle [14,50]. However, there are no data to support the concept that, in man, vasodilator nerves normally play a part in the reflex changes in muscle blood flow during exercise or postural changes [18,53].

4. Vascular Changes Produced by Physical Agents

Since physical agents play a significant therapeutic role in the treatment of musculoskeletal disorders, it is necessary to evaluate their effects on the vascular tree in the muscles.

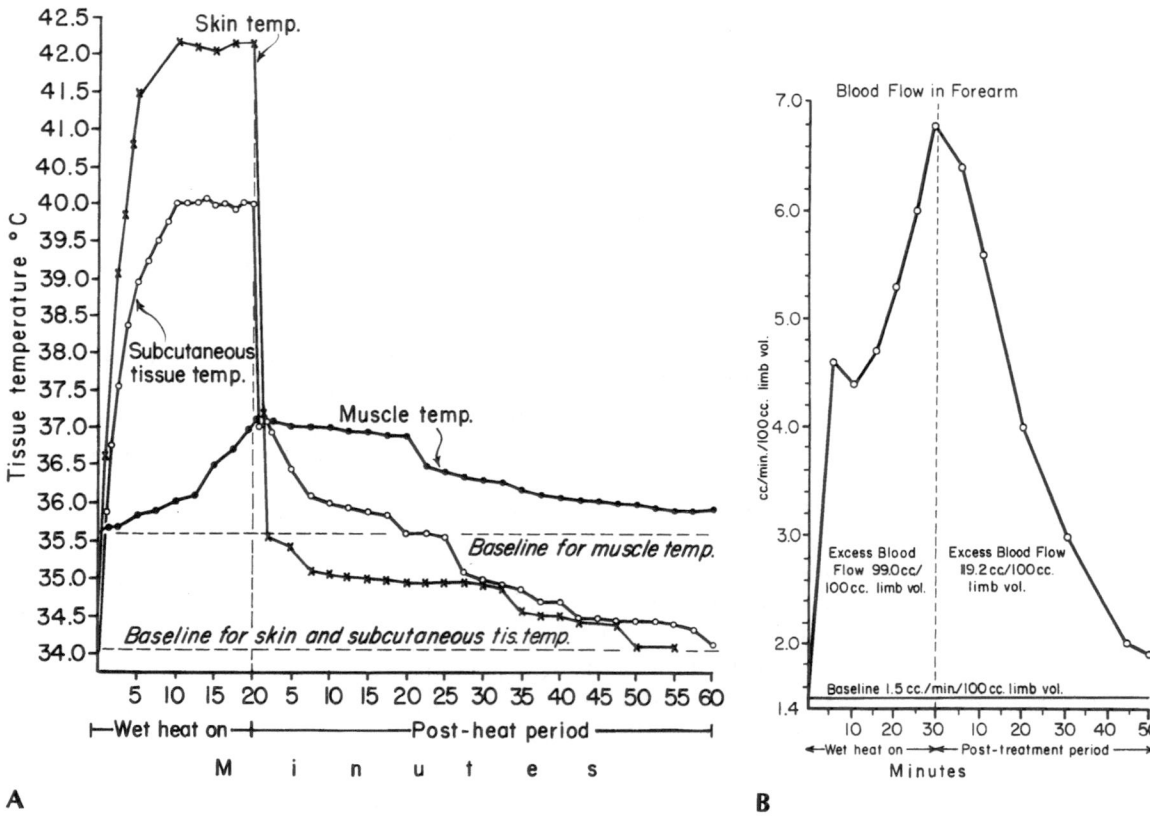

Fig. 2.2. Effect of topically applied wet heat to the forearm. **A** Tissue temperature changes produced during and after 20 min of direct heating. **B** Blood flow changes produced in the forearm by 30 min of direct heating. From Abramson DI, et al [8]. Reproduced with the permission of the Archives of Physical Medicine and Rehabilitation.

Extremes of temperature. Various types of heating procedures applied topically to the skin of the forearm have been reported to produce a definite rise in muscle temperature (Fig. 2.2A); such a response can be interpreted as being associated with a considerable increase in muscle blood flow, in view of the potent vasodilating effect that heat has on local circulation (Fig. 2.2B) [7,8,10]. Local cold when in direct contact with the skin of a limb causes a significant reduction in muscle temperature, associated with a definite fall in muscle blood flow, since it is a very powerful vasoconstricting agent (Fig. 2.3).

Short-wave diathermy. Application of this modality to the forearm elicits a significant increase in muscle temperature (Fig. 2.4A) and muscle blood flow (Fig. 2.4B), more marked than the changes observed in the skin and subcutaneous tissue [3,6].

Ultrasound. The vascular changes observed with this modality include a consistent but small increase in circulation in the forearm, with some rise in muscle temperature [4,16]. However, the available data are not clear-cut enough to state conclusively that the changes in blood flow occur in the muscles.

5. Vascular Responses to Drugs

Adrenergic agents. The reactions of the vascular bed in muscle to such substances as epinephrine and norepinephrine vary, depending upon the method of injection and the amount of the drug administered. When given intraarterially to dogs and cats, small doses of epinephrine (0.1 μg) produce vasodilatation in the limbs, whereas with larger quantities (1 to 10 μg), the initial change is vasoconstriction, followed by vasodilatation. A comparable type of vascular response is noted in the forearm and

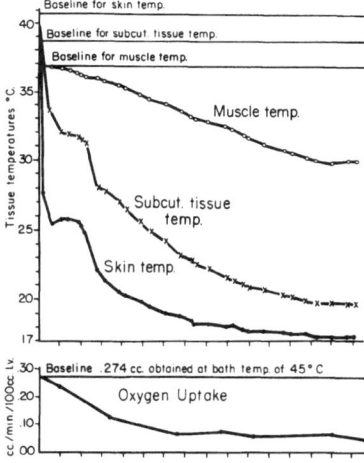

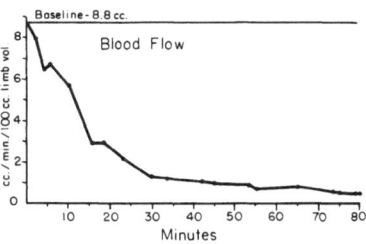

Fig. 2.3. Changes in blood flow in forearm *(lower curve)* on dropping bath temperature from 34 to 17° C. Also noted are changes in oxygen uptake *(middle curve)* and in tissue temperatures *(upper curve)*. From Abramson DI: Circulation in the Extremities. New York, Academic Press, 1967. Reproduced with permission.

calf of man, 0.002 to 0.05 μg causing an augmentation of flow and 1 to 2 μg reducing it without any change in arterial blood pressure. Norepinephrine, administered intraarterially in similar doses in dogs, cats, and man, initially produces vasoconstriction, followed by secondary vasodilatation which is less marked than that produced by epinephrine [15]. However, evidence is also available indicating that both epinephrine and norepinephrine only cause vasoconstriction of vessels in muscles [60]. Neo-Synephrine has been shown to produce vasoconstriction in the hindlimb of anesthetized dogs without secondary vasodilatation [37], whereas isoproterenol (Isuprel), another adrenergic compound, elicits marked vasodilatation under similar conditions [34].

Intravenous infusion of epinephrine (10 μg/min) in man causes a marked increase in forearm blood flow, quickly followed by a return to the control level and then a second slow dilatation. In the case of norepinephrine, first there is an augmentation in circulation in the forearm and calf and then a decrease, the vascular reactions being associated with a rise in both systolic and diastolic blood pressure and a slowing of the heart rate. Attention must be called to the fact that since these results have been obtained with the venous occlusion plethysmographic method (which measures total blood flow in the segment of limb under study), they cannot be attributed solely to alterations in muscle blood flow. There is no question that the changes in cutaneous circulation also contribute to the observed response; still it is generally accepted that the effect of epinephrine and norepinephrine on skin vessels is predominantly vasoconstrictor.

Adrenergic blocking agents. Such drugs as phenoxybenzamine (Dibenzyline), tolazoline hydrochloride (Priscoline), and phentolamine (Regitine), which block the alpha receptor end organs in the blood vessel wall, can abolish the vasoconstriction in the skeletal muscle of the hindlimb of dogs produced by stimulation of the lumbar sympathetic chain. At the same time, a dilating effect is unmasked, which can be abolished by atropine. This type of response is evidently due to stimulation of cholinergic vasodilator fibers in the dog and is ordinarily overshadowed by the predominant vasoconstricting effect of stimulation of sympathetic nerves.

Vasodilators. Acetylcholine and related compounds, which are cholinergic drugs, cause vasodilatation in skeletal muscle in the dog and in man [26]. Histamine, which is a direct myovascular relaxant, elicits the same type of response.

6. Vascular Changes Associated with Muscle Hypertrophy

Persistent use of a group of muscles over a prolonged period of time results in hypertrophy. However, when at the same time work capacity is improved, this response does not necessarily take place. For example, the athlete who is trained for endurance types of physical exertion does not possess the hypertrophied

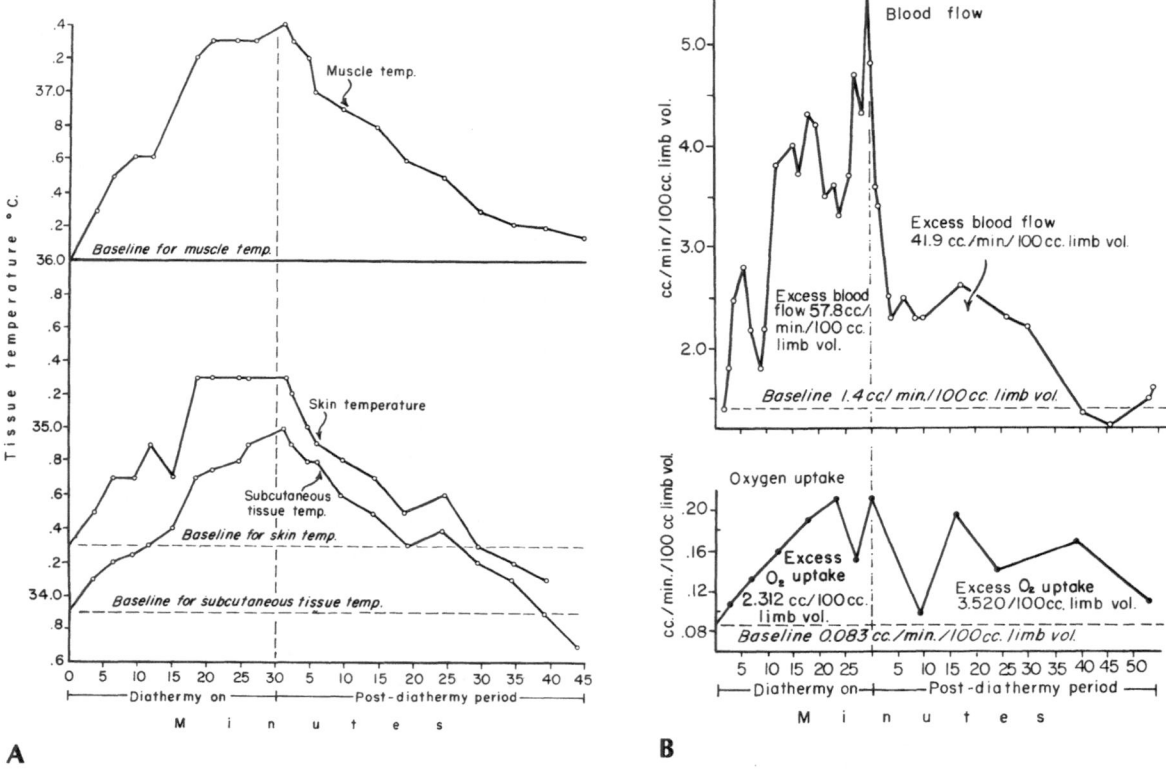

Fig. 2.4. Changes observed in the forearm during and after the application of a 30-min period of short-wave diathermy. **A** Effect on tissue temperatures. **B** Effect on forearm blood flow *(upper curve)* and oxygen uptake *(lower curve)*. From Abramson DI, et al [3]. Reproduced with the permission of Williams & Wilkins Co.

muscles of one engaged in strength activity, such as weight lifting. In this regard, it has been shown that in guinea pigs trained for running, histologic examination revealed no difference in the size of muscle cells, as compared with nonexercised animals, even though work capacity had increased. An obvious change, however, was a 40 to 45 percent growth in functional capillaries locally [48]. Other experimental work has also demonstrated that training raises the ratio of patent capillaries supplying muscle cells [57].

C. Pathology of the Vascular Tree

1. Vascular Response to Ischemia

With the onset of acute ischemia following complete occlusion of a critical artery supplying the muscle mass, the type of change will depend upon the rapidity with which the obstruction occurs, the efficiency of the existing collateral circulation, and whether the venous drainage is also occluded or patent. As pointed out in Section A, above, severity of ischemia is highly variable from one muscle to another and is related to the individual anatomic features of the vascular supply to a specific structure. If the remaining local blood circulation is inadequate to take care of the metabolic needs of resting muscle, then necrosis will result. (For the vascular changes produced in voluntary muscle demonstrating atrophy of disuse, see Section D, Chapter 23.)

2. Vascular Changes in Disease States

Atherosclerosis. Although intermittent claudication is a very common symptom in arteriosclerosis obliterans, the associated pathologic changes in the intrinsic vascular tree of the muscles of the lower limbs are generally only minor. The explanation for such an apparent discrepancy is the fact that, in most instances, the compromised circulation stems from blocks in the proximal main arteries supplying the small intramuscular branches; the latter rarely demonstrate atheromatous deposits, such lesions being uncommon in channels less than 250 μm in diameter. There may be some thickening of the walls of arteries or arterioles in an occasional muscle fiber [46].

Of interest are the findings that under resting conditions, muscle blood flow in the legs of patients suffering from intermittent claudication is approximately the same as that of normal subjects [42]. Only during exercise is a difference noted [35], the exercise hyperemia rising to 17 ml/min per 100 g of muscle, as compared with 56 ml for the normal person undergoing the same amount of physical work [42].

Hypertension. In this condition the intramuscular arteries, especially the larger and medium-sized ones, show pathologic alterations. In the arterioles thickening of the walls occurs, due chiefly to hypertrophy and hyperplasia of the muscularis coat and, to a lesser degree, of the intima and adventitia [39].

Connective tissue disorders. Abnormalities of the intramuscular vessels may be found in patients suffering from these conditions. In polyarteritis nodosa there is a pannecrosis of the medium-sized arteries, accompanied by inflammatory infiltrate and often thrombosis. Small hemorrhages may be present in the muscle, but foci of infarct necrosis are rare.

In the other connective tissue disorders, a vasculitis or perivasculitis may occasionally be seen in voluntary muscle, perhaps somewhat more often in systemic lupus erythematosus. The pathologic change consists of a loose collection of mononuclear cells, resembling lymphocytes, which surrounds the wall of a small intramuscular artery, arteriole, venule, or vein, with the wall itself apparently not involved in the process. The alteration is considered to be a nonspecific reaction which exists with great frequency, but not exclusively, in the connective tissue disorders.

3. Role of Muscle Biopsy as a Diagnostic Measure

Muscle biopsy has common usage as a means of arriving at a diagnosis in cases in which this goal cannot be reached solely by clinical study. However, there are several pitfalls associated with the procedure. For example, in certain disorders, such as arteriosclerosis obliterans (see above), pathologic changes in muscle are minimal or may be absent. Even in the case of polyarteritis nodosa, in which such abnormalities are fairly common, the chances of finding typical lesions are directly related to the size and multiplicity of the biopsies; a random specimen gives a positive result in only 30 percent of cases [43]. Of course, if correctly identified, such a report provides an indisputable diagnosis of the disease.

References

1. Aagaard OC: Über die Lymphgefässe der Zunge, des quergestreiften Muskelgewebes, und der Speicheldrüsen des Menschen. Anat Hefte 47:493, 1913
2. Abramson DI: Circulation in the Extremities. New York, Academic Press, 1967, pp 78–108
3. Abramson DI, Bell Y, Rejal H, et al: Changes in blood flow, oxygen uptake, and tissue temperatures produced by therapeutic physical agents. II. Effect of short-wave diathermy. Am J Phys Med 39:87, 1960
4. Abramson DI, Burnett C, Bell Y, et al: Changes in blood flow, oxygen uptake, and tissue temperatures produced by therapeutic physical agents. I. Effect of ultrasound. Am J Phys Med 39:51, 1960
5. Abramson DI, Ferris EB Jr: Responses of blood vessels in the resting hand and forearm to various stimuli. Am Heart J 19:541, 1940
6. Abramson DI, Harris AJ, Beaconsfield P: Changes in peripheral blood flow produced by short-wave diathermy. Arch Phys Med Rehabil 38:369, 1957
7. Abramson DI, Kahn A, Tuck S Jr, et al: Relationship between a range of tissue temperature and local oxygen uptake in the human forearm. I. Changes observed under resting conditions. J Clin Invest 37:1031, 1958
8. Abramson DI, Mitchell RE, Tuck S Jr, et al: Changes in blood flow, oxygen uptake, and tissue temperatures produced by the topical application of wet heat. Arch Phys Med Rehabil 42:305, 1961
9. Abramson DI, Tuck S Jr, Bell Y, et al: Relation-

ship between a range of tissue temperature and local oxygen uptake in the human forearm. III. Changes observed after anaerobic work, in the postexercise period. J Clin Invest 38:1126, 1959

10. Abramson DI, Tuck S Jr, Chu LSW, et al: Effect of paraffin bath and hot fomentations on local tissue temperatures. Arch Phys Med Rehabil 45:87, 1964

11. Anrep GV: Studies in Cardiovascular Regulation (Lane Medical Lectures), Vol 3. Stanford, Calif., Stanford Univ Press, 1936 p 199

12. Barcroft H, Bonnar WMcK, Edholm OG: Reflex vasodilatation in human skeletal muscle in response to heating the body. J Physiol (Lond) 106:271, 1947

13. Barcroft H, Bonnar WMcK, Edholm OG, et al: On sympathetic vasoconstrictor tone in human skeletal muscle. J Physiol (Lond) 102:21, 1943

14. Barcroft H, Edholm OG, McMichael J, et al: Posthaemorrhagic fainting: Study by cardiac output and forearm flow. Lancet 1:489, 1944

15. Barcroft H, Swan HJC: Sympathetic Control of Human Blood Vessels. London, Edward Arnold, 1953

16. Bickford RH, Duff RS: Influence of ultrasonic irradiation on temperature and blood flow in human skeletal muscle. Circ Res 1:534, 1953

17. Blair DA, Glover WE, Greenfield ADM, et al: Excitation of cholinergic vasodilator nerves to human skeletal muscles during emotional stress. J Physiol (Lond) 148:633, 1959

18. Blair DA, Glover WE, Roddie IC: Vasomotor responses in the human arm during leg exercises. Circ Res 9:264, 1961

19. Blomfield LB: Intramuscular vascular patterns in man. Proc R Soc Med 38:617, 1945

20. Brod J, Fencl V, Hejl Z, et al: Circulatory changes underlying blood pressure elevation during acute emotional stress (mental arithmetic) in normotensive and hypertensive subjects. Clin Sci 18:269, 1959

21. Bülbring E, Burn JH: The sympathetic dilator fibres in the muscles of the cat and dog. J Physiol (Lond) 83:483, 1935

22. Campbell J, Pennefather CM: The blood-supply of muscles, with special reference to war surgery. Lancet 1:294, 1919

23. Chambers R, Zweifach BW: Functional activity of the blood capillary bed, with special reference to visceral tissue. Ann NY Acad Sci 46:683, 1946

24. Cooper KE, Edholm OG, Fletcher JG, et al: Vasodilatation in the forearm during indirect heating. J Physiol (Lond) 125:56P, 1954

25. Cooper KE, Edholm OG, Mottram RF: The blood flow in skin and muscle of the human forearm. J Physiol (Lond) 128:258, 1955

26. Duff F, Greenfield ADM, Shepherd JT, et al: A quantitative study of the response to acetylcholine and histamine of the blood vessels of the human hand and forearm. J Physiol (Lond) 120:160, 1953

27. Eliasson S, Folkow B, Lindgren P, et al: Activation of sympathetic vasodilator nerves to the skeletal muscles in the cat by hypothalamic stimulation. Acta Physiol Scand 23:333, 1951

28. Eliasson S, Lindgren P, Uvnäs B: Representation in the hypothalamus and the motor cortex in the dog of the sympathetic vasodilator outflow to the skeletal muscles. Acta Physiol Scand 27:18, 1952

29. Folkow B: Nervous control of the blood vessels. Physiol Rev 35:629, 1955

30. Folkow B, Haeger K, Uvnäs B: Cholinergic vasodilator nerves in the sympathetic outflow to the muscles of the hind limbs of the cat. Acta Physiol Scand 15:401, 1948

31. Gaskell WH: The changes of the bloodstream in muscles through stimulation of their nerves. J Anat (Lond) 11:360, 1877

32. Golenhofen K, Hildebrandt G: Psychische Einflüsse auf die Muskeldurchblutung. Pflügers Arch Ges Physiol 263:637, 1957

33. Grant RT: Observations on the blood circulation in voluntary muscle in man. Clin Sci 3:157, 1938

34. Green HD, Shearin WT Jr, Jackson TW, et al: Isopropylnorepinephrine blockade of epinephrine reversal. Am J Physiol 179:287, 1954

35. Hirai M, Shionoya S: Considerations on occlusive diseases of the leg arteries and determination of muscle blood flow by ^{133}Xe clearance method. J Cardiovasc Surg 16:35, 1975

36. Holzman GB, Wagner HN Jr, Iio M, et al: Measurement of muscle blood flow in the human forearm with radioactive krypton and xenon. Circulation 30:27, 1964

37. Johnson HD, Green HD, Lanier JT: Comparison of adrenergic blocking action of Ilidar (Ro 2-3248), Regitine (C-7337), and Priscoline in innervated saphenous arterial bed (skin exclusive of muscle) and femoral arterial bed (muscle exclusive of skin) of anesthetized dog. J Pharmacol Exp Ther 108:144, 1953

38. Jones EL, Wagner HN Jr, Zuidema GD: New method for studying peripheral circulation in man. Arch Surg 91:725, 1965

39. Kernohan JW, Anderson EW, Keith NM. The arterioles in cases of hypertension. AMA Arch Intern Med 44:395, 1929

40. Kety SS: Measurement of regional circulation by the local clearance of radioactive sodium. Am Heart J 38:321, 1949

41. Kozma M, Gellert A: Mikroszkópos adatok az izom nyirokerek kérdéséhez. Kiserl Orvostud 9:147, 1957

42. Lassen NA: Muscle body flow in normal man and in patients with intermittent claudication evaluated by simultaneous ^{133}Xe and [24]Na clearances. J Clin Invest 43:1805, 1964

43. Maxeiner SR Jr, McDonald JR, Kirklin JW: Muscle biopsy in the diagnosis of periarteritis

nodosa: An evaluation. Surg Clin North Am 32:1225, 1952

44. Mertens O, Rein H, Garcia Valdecasas F: Gefässwirkungen des Adrenalins im ruhenden und arbeitenden Muskel. Arch Ges Physiol 237:454, 1936

45. Nicoll PA, Webb RL: Vascular patterns and active vasomotion as determiners of flow through minute vessels. Angiology 6:291, 1955

46. Pearson CM: Incidence and type of pathologic alterations observed in muscle in a routine autopsy survey. Neurology 9:757, 1959

47. Pearson CM: Circulation in skeletal muscle. In Abramson DI (ed): Blood Vessels and Lymphatics. New York, Academic Press, 1962, p 518

48. Petrén T, Sjöstrand T, Sylvén B: Der Einfluss des Trainings auf die Häufigkeit der Capillaren in Herz und Skeletmuskulatur. Arbeitsphysiol 9:376, 1936

49. Rapaport SI, Saul A, Hyman C, et al: Tissue clearance as a measure of nutritive blood flow and the effect of lumbar sympathetic block upon such measures in calf muscle. Circulation 5:594, 1952

50. Roddie IC, Shepherd JT: The reflex nervous control of human skeletal muscle blood vessels. Clin Sci 15:433, 1956

51. Roddie IC, Shepherd JT: Nervous control of the circulation in skeletal muscle. Br Med Bull 19:115, 1963

52. Roddie IC, Shepherd JT, Whelan RF: The vasomotor nerve supply to the skin and muscle of the human forearm. Clin Sci 16:67, 1957

53. Roddie IC, Shepherd JT, Whelan RF: Reflex changes in vasoconstrictor tone in human skeletal muscle in response to stimulation of receptors in a low-pressure area of the intrathoracic vascular bed. J Physiol (Lond) 139:369, 1957

54. Sapirstein LA: Effects of various factors on blood flow. In Abramson DI (ed): Blood Vessels and Lymphatics. New York, Academic Press, 1962, p 521

55. Shepherd JT: The blood flow through the calf after exercise in subjects with arteriosclerosis and claudication. Clin Sci 9:49, 1950

56. Uvnäs B: Sympathetic vasodilator outflow. Physiol Rev 34:608, 1954

57. Vannotti A, Magiday M: Untersuchungen zum Studium des Trainiertseins; über die Capillarisierung der trainierten Muskulatur. Arbeitsphysiol 7:615, 1934

58. Wagner HN Jr, Jones E, Tow DE, et al: A method for the study of the peripheral circulation in man. J Nucl Med 6:150, 1965

59. Wilkins RW, Eichna LW: Blood flow to the forearm and calf. I. Vasomotor reactions: Role of the sympathetic nervous system. Bull Johns Hopkins Hosp 68:425, 1941

60. Youmans PL, Green HD, Denison AB Jr: Nature of vasodilator and vasoconstrictor receptors in skeletal muscle of the dog. Circ Res 3:171, 1955

Chapter 3

Circulation to Bone

Circulation of blood through bone has a dual function: to supply nutrition to this structure and to contribute to the maintenance of homeostasis by acting as a depot for many ions and cations of body fluid. Although bone is a highly vascular tissue, experimental and clinical data regarding the architecture of its arterial and venous systems and the physiologic and pathologic responses of the local vessels are in many instances contradictory and fragmentary.

A. Anatomy of the Vascular Tree

1. Methods for the Morphologic Study of Osseous Circulation

The complex physical characteristics of mineralized bone make investigative anatomic studies of the osseous circulation difficult to carry out mainly because of the many technical barriers that must be overcome. One which gives some definitive information is a modification of the Spalteholz technique. This consists of the injection of an opaque substance into the local extraosseous arterial tree and then clearing the tissues, to produce transparency, by placing the bone in a material with a refractive index similar to that of collagen [3,79]. Stereoscopic microangiograms of the cleared preparations have also been used in order to obtain three-dimensional studies of the injected vessels [5,59]. However, all the perfusion proce-

dures supply only limited information regarding the vascular architecture in bone since they distort vessel-tissue relationships and do not allow for visualization in depth [86]. In an attempt to minimize such criticisms, electron microscopy, microscopy with ultraviolet light using fluorescent bone markers, autoradiography with tritiated thymidine, and x-ray diffraction, among others, have been proposed as adjunctive measures.

Another avenue of investigation involves the suppression of a portion of the extraosseous blood supply, followed by a study of the resulting change in bone. In this manner, gross information is obtained regarding the normal role of the suppressed source. The method has been used to determine separately the functions of the various intraosseous systems of vessels: the nutrient, the metaphyseal, the epiphyseal, and the periosteal. It provides additional information to that derived from other procedures [14,78].

2. Normal Architecture of Osseous Circulation

Because of the impervious nature of mineralized bone, a special type of blood vessel system is required to supply it with nourishment and to allow for exchange of important electrolytes between it and other body tissues.

Nutrient artery. In the case of long bones, this vessel supplies more than 50 percent of the

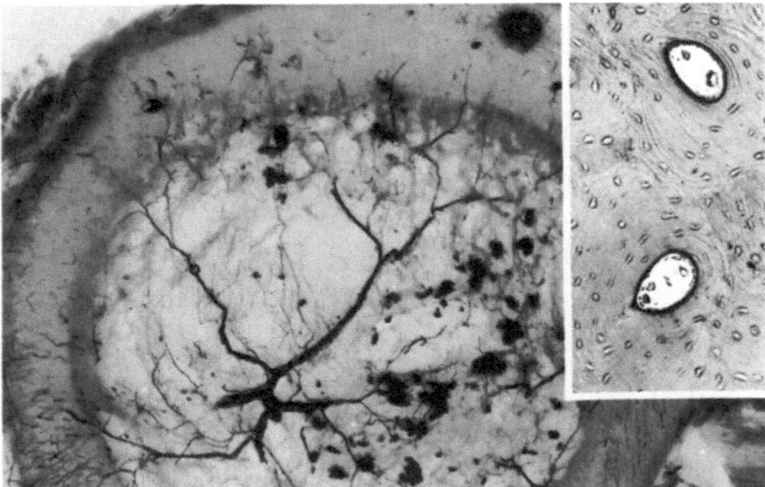

Fig. 3.1. Nutrient artery with lateral branches coursing centrifugally toward the cortex. Further subdivisions are found in the cortex which supply the vessels of the haversian canals *(inset)*. *Inset,* capillary vessels of the haversian canals supplied by lateral branches of the nutrient artery. Two capillaries are found in the superior haversian canal and three in the inferior canal. From Kelly PJ, Peterson LFA: In Abramson DI (ed): Blood Vessels and Lymphatics. New York, Academic Press, 1962. Reproduced with permission.

total blood flow. At times, as in the human femur, there are two nutrient arteries. After entering the diaphysis, the vessel divides into ascending and descending branches; these give off lateral twigs that pass radially to enter the cortex of the diaphysis (Fig. 3.1). The terminal ramifications of these vessels provide a major share of the circulation passing through the capillaries of the haversian canals. Branches of the nutrient artery are also the main source of blood for the large sinusoidal system of vessels in the bone marrow.

Epiphyseal-metaphyseal vascular system.
The ends of long bones are supplied by arteries that have their origin in vessels arising in neighboring soft tissue. During growth, the epiphyseal plate acts functionally to separate the epiphyseal circulation from the metaphyseal circulation, with unconnected systems of perforating arteries delivering blood to the two portions of bone. Those that supply the epiphysis are concerned with proliferation of the cartilage growth plate, whereas the metaphyseal system plays a role in resorption of hypertrophied and calcified cartilage cells and in laying down bone in the process of achieving longitudinal growth. After growth is completed, the blood vessels which supplied the epiphysis and metaphysis separately now develop extensive

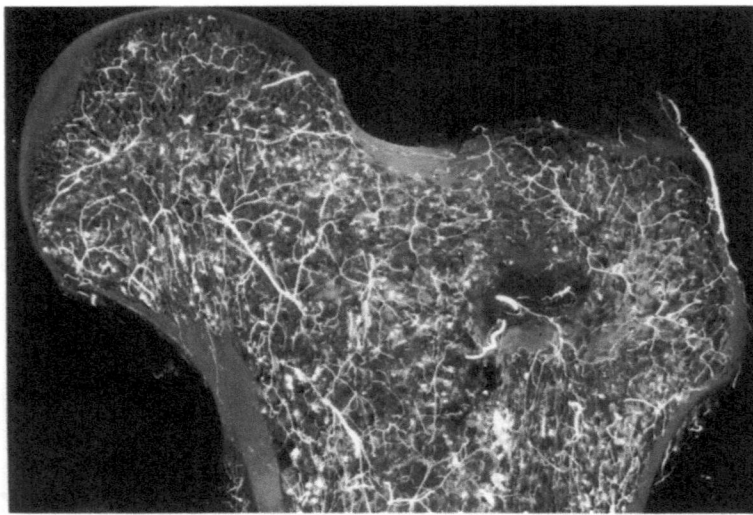

Fig. 3.2. Microangiogram of femoral head of the dog. The arterial arcades are seen in the subchondral region. The pattern of vessels is typical for cancellous bone. × 2.75. From Kelly RJ, Peterson LFA: In Abramson DI (ed): Blood Vessels and Lymphatics. New York, Academic Press, 1962. Reproduced with permission.

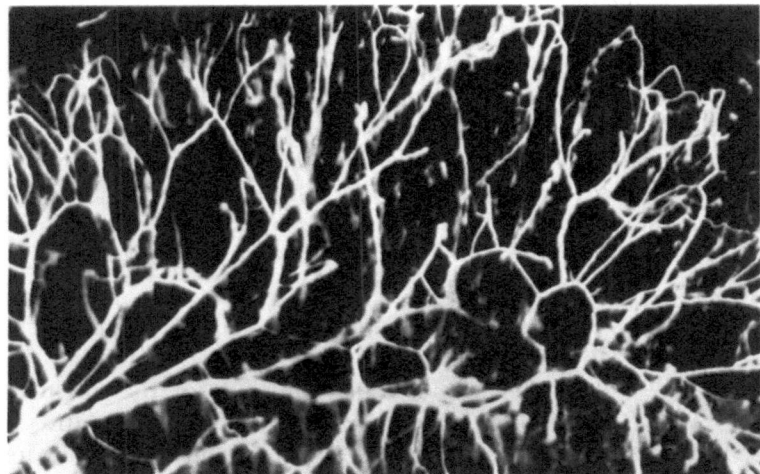

Fig. 3.3. Photomicrograph of the epiphyseal arteries within the femoral head of a patient aged 75 years. Tiers of arches are noted, running from the main lateral epiphyseal vessels below to the articular surface above. × 2.6. From Trueta and Harrison [79]. Reproduced with the permission of the Journal of Bone and Joint Surgery and Livingstone, Ltd.

anastomoses with one another and with channels arising from the nutrient artery. Together they contribute 20 to 40 percent of the total body supply to the bone [77]. In fact, these perforating vessels are able to support the diaphysis if the periosteal and nutrient circulations are suppressed [47].

The perforating epiphyseal vessels arise from all sides of the bone and enter the epiphysis through small foramina. They branch to form arterial arcades which divide and subdivide (Figs. 3.2 and 3.3). The subchondral circulation originates from the smallest of these, which then terminate in capillary loops beneath the articular cartilage.

The vessels supplying the metaphysis arise from arteries that enter from different sides of the bone and from terminal ramifications of the nutrient artery. As the channels approach the epiphyseal growth plate, they branch and subdivide further into numerous thin-walled vessels, finally ending in capillary loops.

Haversian system. In the cortex, the haversian canal in the center of the osteon contains, on the average, one to two thin-walled nonmuscular capillarylike vessels (Figs. 3.1 and 3.4A) and occasionally an arteriole and an accompanying vein (Fig. 3.4B). From the capillary, nutrition diffuses out to the osteocytes of each osteon

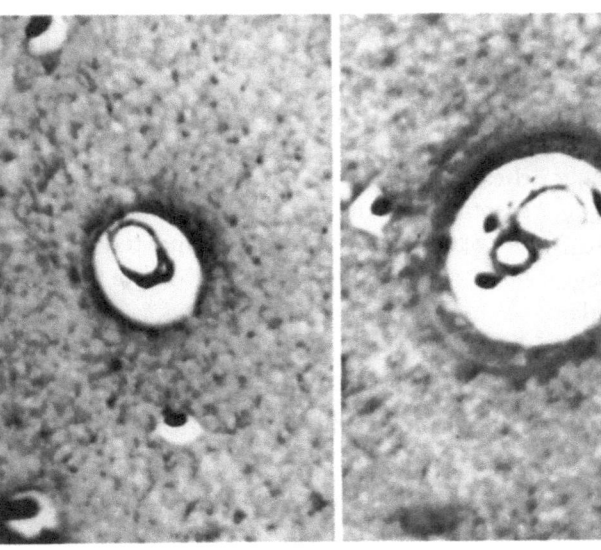

A   B

Fig. 3.4. Photomicrographs of blood vessels in haversian canals in cross section of the radius of a dog. **A** Canal in center contains a single large capillary. **B** Canal in center contains two vessels: a very small arteriole and a small venule. The stippled appearance of the intercellular substance of the bone is due to the presence of canaliculi cut in cross section and obliquely. A few bone cells may be seen in lacunae. × 800. From Ham [34]. Reproduced with the permission of the Journal of Bone and Joint Surgery.

and to the interstitial bone through canaliculi containing fine cellular processes arising from a bone cell. Such an arrangement allows for ready interchange between cells and vessels of the haversian canals [34]. The segment of cortex thus supplied is generally not greater than the width of 20 cells, and as a result structures at the periphery are prevented from suffering from lack of circulation.

Periosteal vessels. These channels are very difficult to visualize and hence to study. The system is made up primarily of fine capillaries and arterioles which require refined techniques, such as electron microscopy and ultraviolet microscopy, for productive investigation [78]. Although experimental suppression studies have revealed that the outer third of the diaphysis receives its blood supply from periosteal vessels which penetrate the cortex via haversian canals [77], this observation has not been widely accepted. In fact, significant periosteal blood supply to the upper portion of the cortex has been denied by several investigators [16,17], the alternate possibility being offered that periosteal vessels are in continuity with the cortical vascular tree. In the presence of injury or disease involving the nutrient arteries, however, there is general agreement that the periosteal vessels now assume great importance. This vascular system can, therefore, be considered in the light of a reserve source of nutrition to bone but not called upon under ordinary conditions.

Vascular bed in the medullary canal. The capillaries in the bone marrow have been found to be much larger than capillaries elsewhere (25 μm, as compared to about 10 μm). These vessels empty into extremely thin-walled wide venous sinusoids. Such anatomic findings may have significance with regard to fat embolism (see B-1, Chapter 16). It is not difficult to imagine a situation in which the fragile sinusoids, as well as the thin-walled fat cells, are ruptured either by a fracture of a long bone or by the marked jarring of the entire skeleton that occurs in a serious traumatic episode. Under such conditions, released fat particles could readily enter the local and then the systemic venous system.

Whether the sinusoidal bed is a closed or an open circulation has not been unequivocally determined. Of interest in this regard is the observation that the sinusoids do not appear to possess a supporting structure or extracellular reticulum [83,89]. It is generally accepted that these channels form the principal functioning vascular bed for the circulating blood in bone marrow. In a sense, they correspond to the capillaries in other organs [22].

Venous drainage. The veins of the bones are thin walled and much greater in number than the arteries. The sinusoids of the medullary space drain either directly into the central venous sinus (the vein accompanying the nutrient artery in the medullary space) or into other larger tributaries which then also empty into the central venous sinus. The continuation of the latter, the nutrient vein, passes through the nutrient canal with the nutrient artery and enters the extraosseous venous system. Although this vessel plays a significant role in removal of blood from bone it is by no means the major one, since a number of other drainage routes are available, such as the veins which accompany the epiphyseal arteries at the ends of long bones.

Sympathetic innervation of blood vessels. Current knowledge of the anatomic innervation of the osseous blood vessels by the sympathetic nervous system is scanty and fragmentary. Myelinated and nonmyelinated nerves are found entering the bone through the nutrient canal, accompanying the nutrient artery and vein or veins [40]. In the bone marrow, nerve bundles are frequently observed forming fine plexuses in the adventitia of vessels, even extending to the capillaries. That the sympathetic nervous system plays an important role in the regulation of osseous blood flow is supported by numerous experimental studies.

3. Anatomic Alterations of Osseous Circulation following Fractures

The circulatory changes which occur in a fracture site consist of a significant enlargement of the vascular bed (active hyperemia, hyperplasia of vascular tissue), which begins 4 to 5 days after the injury and reaches a peak at about 9 days. The response subsides gradually to control levels when union of the fracture has taken place.

The initial change is the development of a network of vessels in the region of involvement, with most of the channels arising from the surrounding soft tissues and penetrating the callus [86]. The circulatory response is generally most obvious on the dorsal and lateral aspects of the fracture site, where soft tissues are generally more plentiful [31]. The new vascular bed is made up of two types of vessels: One consists of arteries with long, irregular, and tortuous radiating branches, most numerous at the level of the fracture line, which are formed fairly early. The other is composed of slender, regular, and straight or slightly curved channels which are most commonly found in the denser and older callus at the level of the fracture, as well as in sites corresponding to callus deposition on the periosteal surface of the long bone [31].

Following experimental fracture of the forelimbs of dogs, large arteries have been found to develop from the vascular tree in the marrow cavity which then enter the fracture site. With time, they anastomose with periosteal branches, first through the uniting callus and later through vascular channels that penetrate the cortex itself [62].

As healing progresses, there is an increase in both medullary and periosteal circulations through the formation of new blood vessels. In this manner, adequate blood supply becomes available to the uniting callus and to the injured cortex at the fracture site. In most cases the necessary vascularization is chiefly derived from the medullary arterial tree, but if this circulation is destroyed the periosteal system of arteries takes over.

The growth of vessels into the cartilaginous callus is associated with the appearance of bone deposition, in the form of small halos developing around the vascular channels [86]. The halos enlarge and coalesce until the entire callus is ossified, the change occurring by the 12th day. After full development of the ossification process, the rich vascularity of the callus gradually recedes, with the result that the circulatory pattern begins to resemble that of adjacent normal bone. In the response of the body to a fracture, bone formation only takes place in vascularized areas of the callus [86].

4. Anatomic Alterations of Osseous Circulation Due to Vascular Diseases and Aging

Arteriosclerosis obliterans. Areas of necrosis found in bone of geriatric patients have been attributed to vascular insufficiency [42,66]. In the presence of a slowly developing occlusive process, however, the corresponding formation of a collateral circulation may diminish the importance of vascular obstruction as a cause for such an abnormal change [42]. The diffuse vascularization of compact and cancellous bone frequently noted in limbs amputated for gangrene secondary to arteriosclerosis obliterans has led to the suggestion that under such circumstances, cortical circulation reverses from a centrifugal to a centripetal flow, resulting in periosteal arterialization of compact bone [15].

Aging. This state, by itself, appears to produce an increase in the number of empty lacunae [29], a positive correlation existing between the alterations in these structures and ischemia. The anatomic changes suggest a causal relationship between reduced circulation and increasing numbers of dead cells [54].

B. Physiology of the Vascular Tree

1. Laboratory Methods for the Functional Study of Osseous Circulation

Direct methods for the measurement of blood flow to bone in experimental animals are performed only rarely because of numerous technical difficulties [46]. In man, all of these problems are compounded and many are insoluble, with the result that at present there is no satisfactory way to measure bone blood flow directly.

Intramedullary pressure measurements. These are made by inserting a cannula into the medullary cavity of a long bone of an experimental animal and utilizing a Statham pressure transducer, fed through carrier amplifiers, to collect the data. The method has been used primarily to study the effect of drugs on intramedullary pressure. A correlation has been reported between this measurement and bone blood flow [64].

Thermoelectric methods. One of these, the coupled thermistor probe, when inserted into the medullary cavity of an animal, gives qualitative information regarding the changes in local osseous circulation [12]. The instrument consists of two matching thermistors in a narrow bore needle balanced across a bridge. The method has certain limitations, among which is the fact that it can sample only a small amount of tissue and so reflects a purely local change in blood flow; moreover, it does not give any indication as to the direction of the circulation in bone. Also, if blood coagulates around the instrument, its sensitivity is decreased.

Vital microscopy. This procedure, which has been used to study the circulatory dynamics in bone marrow [10,52], involves examination of a living vascular bed in animals under conditions as undisturbed as possible. The method requires grinding down a small portion of the covering compact bone to tissue-paper thickness to permit investigation of the intramedullary vascular structures through the use of transilluminated light and a microscope. The fibula of the rabbit readily lends itself to such a study.

Radioisotope studies. A number of procedures currently being investigated as tools for the measurement of bone blood flow in animals all utilize radioactive tracers but in several different ways.

One method is based on the clearance of radioactive isotopes after they have been deposited in the medullary cavity of bone. Since there are no lymphatic vessels in this structure, the assumption is made that the rate of clearance of the radioisotope represents a measurement of capillary circulation in the site of deposition of the material. The main disadvantage of such an experimental approach is that it does not enable the examiner to determine easily what proportion of the isotope disap-

pearance is due to blood flow and what proportion results from tissue diffusion and metabolism.

Another technique is based on the bone-seeking characteristics of various isotopes of calcium and strontium. With such a procedure, the volume of blood or plasma "cleared" of the radioactive substance per minute is considered to be indicative of bone blood flow [4, 19,28,82]. The rationale for the method is the assumption that the process is complete and that the extraction rate for the isotope by bone is 100 percent or, in other words, that the concentration of the injected material is zero in the venous blood draining the bone. Under such circumstances, the clearance values and the bone flow values are considered to be identical, a premise questioned by other workers (see below).

The above method has been modified by simultaneously injecting ^{85}Sr and a nondiffusible dye, Evans blue (T-1824), into the nutrient artery of the tibia of experimental animals [19]. Blood is then collected from the femoral vein during the next 5 min and the percentage of the injected dose of each substance is determined. From such data, the extraction ratio for ^{85}Sr has been calculated as 76 percent [19].

Another modification consists of injecting ^{47}Ca into the jugular vein of dogs, sacrificing the animals 10 min later, and analyzing the skeleton for isotope content [82]. Again, this method is based on the assumption that the extraction ratio for the isotope by bone is 100 percent.

A method utilizing the Fick principle and involving administration of ^{45}Ca or ^{85}Sr has also been described [61]. With it the total activity in the bone is obtained and then this figure is corrected for the activity present in the marrow vascular spaces at the time of sacrifice of the experimental animals. Information on the latter point is collected through the simultaneous injection of ^{51}Cr-labeled red blood cells.

It is generally accepted that the bone blood flow readings based on the use of bone-seeking isotopes are all significantly lower than the actual perfusion values. This discrepancy results from the fact that the extraction rate of the isotope by the bone is not 100 percent [19,82], and hence the premise that clearance figures can be equated with perfusion rates is negated.

If extraction is far from complete, then it is necessary to collect samples of representative venous blood draining the bone so as to obtain a proper correction factor. However, such a step has not been successfully carried out because of technical difficulties.

Bone blood flow has also been studied using the measurement of ^{42}K or ^{86}Rb, the results being compared with the distribution of ^{24}Na-labeled microspheres. After the intravenous injection of a specific quantity of isotope the arterial dilution curve is obtained, such information being used to determine cardiac output. One minute after administration, the animal is sacrificed, followed by weighing and digesting the bone in concentrated nitric acid. Aliquots of the sample are assayed for radioactivity in a well-type scintillation counter. The fractional portion of the total injected isotope found in the sample under study is multiplied by the cardiac output to obtain the perfusion rate in the specimen of bone. The data are presented as a fraction of the injected dose of the isotope in 100 g of tissue.

The above procedure has a number of advantages but also several weaknesses. It is a useful diagnostic tool because it requires no surgery near the bone under investigation and no anesthetic; moreover, it has an extraction ratio that exceeds that of bone-seeking isotopes [49]. On the other hand, certain variables detract from the value of the method since they affect the concentration of the radioisotope in the bone. Among these are the quantity in the blood, the amount of diffusion into the interstitial fluid, the degree of exchange of interstitial isotope on the surface of bone crystals, and the quantity incorporated into bone by metabolism [9].

Methods applicable to study in man. One of the few investigative tools available for indirect measurement of osseous blood flow in human subjects is venous occlusion plethysmography. This procedure, which is ordinarily utilized to obtain total blood flow readings for the skin and muscles of the limbs [1], has been modified so as to be applicable to the indirect determination of the rate of local circulation in long bones like the humerus [26,27,39]. However, certain objections have been raised to the use of this approach [65]. In view of the vascular anatomy of bone, at best it is of value only for qualitative examination of osseous blood flow.

Another indirect method used in man consists of the intraosseous injection of a radiopaque dye and the determination of its rate of clearance [23]. The latter is converted to rate of blood flow using a theoretical exponential correlative curve.

2. Vascular Responses and Blood Flow

Bone marrow. Vascular responses in this structure have been studied in the rabbit using vital microscopy [10,52]. It has been found that blood enters arterioles and then capillaries, which in turn empty into fusiform or hexagonal sinusoids; from the latter, the blood drains into the collecting venules. Or a shorter course may be utilized: from capillaries directly into collecting venules. Contractile tissue is located at both ends of the sinusoids, the movement of blood in these vessels generally being inversely proportional to their diameter. The velocity of blood cell flow in marrow has been found to be 1.5 ml/s in arterioles, 0.5 ml/s in capillaries, 0 to 0.2 ml/s in sinusoids, and 0.1 to 0.3 ml/s in venules [10].

Haversian systems. Vital microscopy has revealed that the rate of flow in the haversian capillaries in the fibulae of rabbits is more rapid than in similar-sized vessels in the bone marrow [10]. Also of interest is the finding that if two vessels are present in a haversian system, the flow in one is in the opposite direction to that in the other, with the slower rate being present in the larger vessel [10]. The rate of blood flow in diaphyseal bone is 0.5 to 0.8 ml/s in capillaries and 0.2 to 0.5 ml/s in venules [10].

Blood flow in total bone. The readings obtained by various methods in different types of experimental animals vary considerably. In the rat, using the Fick principle and ^{45}Ca uptake by bones, the readings have been reported to be between 10 and 30 ml/min per 100 g wet weight of bone [28]. In the femur of the dog, with the same method, the data indicate blood flows of 8.5 ml/min per 100 g of fresh bone by one group of investigators [19] and 8.22 ± 0.46 ml by another group [61]. In the femur of the rabbit, the readings are 10.4 ml/min per 100 g of fresh bone [19].

Osseous blood flow in man. With the use of venous occlusion plethysmography, blood flow through the humerus of normal human subjects has been found to be in the range of 1.9 to 5.9 ml/min per 100 ml of tissue [26]. In patients with pulmonary hypertrophic osteoarthropathy the readings rise to 10.6 ml/min per 100 ml of tissue [39]. By means of a technique of clearance of radiopaque dye, data collected from the femoral head indicate that blood flow is between 3 and 7 ml/min per 100 g of tissue [55].

3. Mechanisms Involved in Control of Bone Circulation

Neural influences. Extensive experimental evidence supports the view that bone blood flow is, in part, controlled by sympathetic vasomotor neural mechanisms. For example, perfusion experiments utilizing the nutrient artery of the isolated tibia of the dog have shown that electric stimulation of nerve fibers to the bone results in a reduction in local venous blood flow [25]. Similar observations have been reported in rabbits following stimulation of a sympathetic nerve trunk [69]. Another finding in accord with the above view is a fall in intramedullary blood pressure in cats and dogs after electric stimulation of the distal cut end of peripheral nerves to a limb [36,84]. Also of importance are the reports of significant increases in osseous blood flow in the hindlimbs of dogs following lumbar sympathectomy [73] and after complete section of the sciatic nerve [68]. On the other hand, sympathetic denervation in rats does not produce hyperemia in the medullary cavity [90] and supramaximal stimulation of the peripheral cut end of either the femoral or sciatic nerve of curarized animals does not have any effect on intramedullary blood flow or pressure [65]. The whole problem of the control of the sympathetic nervous system over osseous circulation therefore requires further and more definitive investigation before significant conclusions can be reached.

Hormonal influences. The administration of epinephrine to the perfusion fluid in the dog's isolated tibia preparation has been found to decrease blood outflow from the bone [25]. A fall of intramedullary blood pressure in the intact dog has also been reported under such circumstances [7]. Similar changes have been noted with norepinephrine and Pitressin, associated with reduction or cessation of bleeding from holes drilled through the cortex into the medullary cavity [71]. Such findings may indicate that the action of sympathomimetic drugs on lowering intramedullary pressure results from vasoconstriction of the nutrient artery entering the bone and not from dilatation of marrow arterioles and capillaries [71]. Quantitative study of bone blood flow in the rabbit [20] and in the dog [85] has revealed that a microgram dose of epinephrine decreases the readings by 25 to 75 percent. In man, both epinephrine and norepinephrine produce an initial fall in intramedullary blood pressure in the sternum, followed by a rise [12].

The available experimental evidence therefore strongly supports the view that vasopressor hormones, occurring normally in the body, influence the bone blood circulation. Such a mechanism must closely interact with the neural mechanism (see above), in view of the fact that hormones like norepinephrine are produced by the sympathetic nerve endings and epinephrine and Pitressin, in part, have their origin in neural glands.

Metabolic influences. In addition, considerable information derived from experimental studies in animals and man indicates that metabolic factors, such as acid metabolites, pH, and oxygen and carbon dioxide concentrations in the blood, play a very important, if not the most important, role in regulating bone blood flow. In this regard, their actions are no different from the changes produced by them in other vascular beds.

In the rabbit or the dog, raising the carbon dioxide level in the bloodstream through rebreathing expired air [20,69] or breathing in a gas mixture low in oxygen and high in carbon dioxide definitely increases bone blood flow [20,85]. A similar response is obtained by lowering the pH of the blood by the intraarterial injection of N/15 lactic acid [85] or the intravenous or intraarterial administration of a small dose of hydrochloric acid [60]. Experimental occlusion of the femoral artery first produces a great decrease in nutrient venous outflow from the femur, followed by a two- to threefold increase over the control level on reestablishment of the circulation. The augmentation in blood flow represents a state of reactive hyperemia brought on by the period of ischemia and thus is good evidence for the metabolic control of bone blood flow [67]. Of interest in this regard are the findings that the increase in local circulation following a period of ischemia cannot be abolished by either electric stimulation of the nerves or administration of vasopressor exogenous hormones, despite the fact that both steps are known to reduce bone blood flow [69] (see above). Moreover, the reactive hyperemia response persists after the peripheral nerves are transected, thus suggesting that it is not related to a neural reflex.

Other factors influencing bone circulation. Apparently systemic blood pressure can directly or indirectly alter bone blood flow. For example, a reduction in circulating blood volume, as in shock, likewise causes a decrease in osseous circulation. Acetylcholine and stimulation of the vagus nerve reduce systemic circulation and also intramedullary blood pressure and bone blood flow. However, in some situations there is no correlation between the level of systemic blood pressure and osseous circulation, as when such vasopressor drugs as epinephrine, norepinephrine, and Pitressin are administered. The reason is that these hormones have a vasoconstrictive effect on the arterial tree in bone, causing a decrease in osseous circulation (see above), at the same time that they produce an elevation in systemic blood pressure.

A number of local factors affect bone blood flow. Among those which significantly reduce osseous circulation initially are fractures, dislocations, epiphyseal separations [35], strangulation of the articular vessels in joints, embolic obstruction of osseous vessels, and severe injury to soft tissue covering bone. An increase in bone blood flow may be noted in several orthopedic disorders, among which are pulmonary hypertrophic osteoarthropathy and Paget's disease of bone. (For changes in osseous blood flow in pulmonary hypertrophic osteoar-

thropathy, see C-2, Chapter 14; in Paget's disease of bone, see D-3, Chapter 14.)

4. Effect of Experimentally Altering Osseous Circulation on Bone Growth

Numerous experimental approaches have been utilized to influence the hemodynamics of osseous blood flow, in the hope that an increased rate of growth of long bones would ensue. The reason for the solution of such a problem is apparent—its clinical application to the management of a number of musculoskeletal disorders characterized by shortened lower limbs. That irritation and hyperemia of osseous structures produce an increase in length and thickness of bone is attested to by the finding of such alterations after infections and fractures [2,70].

Production of venous stasis. The effect of protracted interference with venous outflow has been studied through ligation of the popliteal vein of the hindlimb of dogs, increases in bone length having been reported [57,58]. However, the studies have been criticized because of the lack of control readings and of statistical analysis of the data [48]. Moreover, other investigations have subsequently indicated that no significant lengthening of femora or tibiae follows such a procedure [50]. Another important point is that only ligation of the inferior vena cava and of the ipsilateral common femoral vein results in a prolonged elevation of venous pressure, whereas lower levels of occlusion merely cause transient rises [23]. The proximal application of tourniquets to the limbs of dogs has also been reported to cause an increase in length and width of the bones, a response which has been interpreted as being due to the development of venous stasis [41].

On the basis of the available evidence, apparently no definitive conclusions can be reached regarding the effect of venous stasis on osseous growth. Perhaps with the current use of direct methods for evaluating bone formation and bone resorption and of osseous blood flow measurements, the problem will more readily be resolved.

Interference with circulation to bone. Experimental ligation of the nutrient artery to bone has been found to produce stimulation of bone growth of varying degrees [87]. A similar type of response has been observed following stripping of the periosteum of the dog's femur [21,87,88], a procedure which suppresses the blood supply to the metaphyseal side of the epiphyseal growth plate [13,53,88]. As a consequence, the epiphyseal growth plate thickens due the fact that proliferation of the cells of this structure continues while endochondral ossification ceases. The clinical finding of lengthening of a long bone in children following fractures or osteomyelitis has been attributed to blockage of the nutrient and periosteal circulations, with a resulting increased arterialization in the metaphyseal region [75]. However, evidence which does not support this concept of ischemia as a cause for an increase in length of bone includes the observation that simple suppression of the circulation in nutrient vessels to the femur of rabbits does not have any beneficial effect except that for the middle portion of growth there is acceleration of the process [14]. At present, it appears warranted to state that for growth stimulation to occur, suppression of the metaphyseal blood supply must be practically complete, with both the local periosteal and the nutrient artery circulations destroyed.

Production of an arteriovenous fistula. The clinical finding of hypertrophy and overgrowth of bone in limbs of children suffering from a congenital arteriovenous fistula (see B-2, Chapter 21) has led to the investigation of the effect of experimental formation of such a lesion. In this regard, the establishment of an arteriovenous fistula in the hindlimb of puppies has been reported to cause an acceleration of longitudinal and transverse growth of the bones distal to the abnormality and a rise in medullary cavity temperature [46]. The use of quantitative analysis by tetracycline labeling patterns and microradiography has indicated that these changes occur within the first 3 weeks after the fistula has been constructed [80]. Associated with the alterations in osseous growth, are hypervascularity on the side of the lesion (as compared with the control limb) and a marked increase in the number of filled vessels and dilatation of channels in the distal portion of the femur [51]. In addition, almost immediately following the production of the fistula, a significant increase in intramedullary pressure occurs in epiphyseal, but not diaphyseal, bone [72]. Other findings are stimulation of periosteal new bone formation, with depression of endosteal new bone production, and enlargement of the medullary cavity [80]. It has been suggested that the growth stimulating effect is caused by the elevated temperature and vascularization at the site of the epiphyseal line [37]. Another factor which may play a role is the increased collateral venous channels draining the medullary cavity [56].

Arteriovenous fistulae have also been surgically produced in children, with a reported increase in growth of a short lower limb in a significant number of cases [37,44]. However, the operation may be associated with serious systemic responses, especially congestive heart failure produced at the time the lesion is surgically corrected.

Production of internal heating. The effect of heat on bone growth has been investigated using several approaches. The application of an alternating electric current to the distal end of the femur of rats for an average period of 27.8 h has been reported to produce an average increase in length of 6.3 percent, as compared with the control limb [63]; similar results have been produced in puppies by means of shortwave diathermy [24]. However, in studies on dogs using microwave diathermy, such changes have not been reported [32]. Also, ultrasound applied over the epiphyseal area of the tibia of rabbits for relatively long periods of time has been found to cause no increase in bone length [81]. It has been suggested that the beneficial response to heating of the bone found by some investigators was due to the resulting diffuse or localized hyperemia, a situation comparable to that in arteriovenous fistula, diffuse hemangioma, osteomyelitis, and fracture of the shaft of a long bone [24].

5. Effect of Muscle Activity on Osseous Circulation

Because of the interposition of the sinusoidal system of vessels between the arterioles and the veins within the rigid compartments of the bone marrow, it would be expected that a marked drop in venous pressure would ordinarily occur, resulting in a reduction in the movement of blood out of the bone into the efferent extraosseous channels. However, several mechanical factors actively combat this state of inefficient venous return, one of which is the intermittent, repeated contractions of the muscles adjacent or attached to the bone. Such a mechanism also acts to increase osseous blood flow (see below).

Muscular contraction appears to have a twofold effect. First, by blocking or impeding venous outflow, it initially causes vascular engorgement which persists until physical activity ceases [30]. As a consequence, inactive channels and lakes in the interior of bone are filled with oxygenated blood. At the same time, during contraction, muscle circulation is diminished, the blood being squeezed out of the active tissue into the underlying bone [65]. Subsequent relaxation of the muscles exerts a sucking action upon the vascular bed in the medullary cavity, thus again augmenting refilling of the medullary sinusoids with newly oxygenated blood.

Numerous other experiments support the belief that muscle tone and muscle contractions play a role in influencing osseous circulation and in propelling venous blood from the bone in the direction of the heart. For example, during the phase of active quadriceps muscle contraction in the cat, medullary pressure and osseous blood flow in the femur are increased. Moreover, surgically suppressing the capacity of the gastrocnemius of the rabbit to contract causes marked sinusoidal and venous stasis, with rapid and severe rarefaction of the calcaneus [30].

The above view stresses the importance and value of proper muscle activity in maintaining adequate circulation to the bones, a function which is closely related to the mechanism of bone deposition. Conversely, muscle inactivity may be responsible for bone resorption observed in such conditions or states as posttraumatic vasomotor disturbances (Sudeck's atrophy; see A-2, Chapter 13), anterior poliomyelitis, flaccid paraplegia, and osteoporosis after fracture and application of a cast. Overactivity, in the form of muscle spasm, may cause bone deposition and osteosclerosis, as in spastic paraplegia and severe osteoarthritis of major joints.

6. Effect of Drugs on Osseous Circulation

Vasodilator agents. Intravenously administered histamine produces an immediate reduction in capillary blood flow in the marrow of the fibula of living rabbits, followed by a rise to a level somewhat greater than the control [11]. An increase in medullary circulation and blood pressure has been reported under similar experimental conditions [65]. On the other hand, an initial fall in medullary pressure and then a very gradual recovery to a lower baseline has also been found [7,71]. Acetylcholine and sodium nitrate likewise cause a fall in medullary pressure [7].

7. Effect of Physical Agents on Osseous Circulation

Physical agents appear to have variable effects upon blood flow in bone. For example, in high doses, ultrasound can be focally destructive to this structure [45], particularly at interfaces where there is a buildup of heat. Such a response does not occur with the therapeutic application of ultrasound [43].

The reported responses to irradiation have been contradictory. The spontaneous femoral neck fractures noted in women receiving such therapy to the pelvis have been attributed to changes in blood supply [33]. On the other hand, some convincing histopathologic and clinical evidence does not support this view [8]. A stress fracture has also been proposed as a cause for the findings [6]. Experimental work in rats has indicated a reduction in the number of filled vessels from the third to the seventh day after doses of 950 rad to the hindlimbs [38]; however, studies using similar doses of x ray and microangiographic means to determine the effect on the vascular bed have revealed no significant differences between control and irradiated extremities [18].

8. Vascular Changes Produced by Local Inflammation

The vascular response to infections of the bone is essentially the same as in other parts of the body. However, because the resulting inflammatory hyperemia produces an early rise in local tissue pressure due to the structure of bone, a reduction in local blood flow soon follows, a change which is detrimental to the process of combating the infectious agent. Interestingly, the usual locations where infection commonly occurs contain sinusoids in which blood flow is the slowest [74]. A significant finding in the case of infection in the infant is that the epiphyseal growth plate is not well established until 1 year of age, and as a result disease can invade and involve this site, causing serious damage to the epiphyseal side of the developing structure [76].

References

1. Abramson DI: Circulation in the Extremities. New York, Academic Press, 1967, pp 78–108
2. Aitken AP, Blackett CW, Cincotti JJ: Overgrowth of the femoral shaft following fracture in childhood. J Bone Joint Surg 21:334, 1939
3. Barclay AE: Micro-Arteriography and Other Radiological Techniques Employed in Biological Research. Oxford, Blackwell Scientific, 1951
4. Barnes DWH, Bishop M, Harrison GE, et al: Comparison of the plasma concentration and urinary excretion of strontium and calcium in man. Int J Radiol Biol 3:637, 1961
5. Bellman S: Microangiography. Acta Radiol (Suppl) 102:7, 1953
6. Bickel WH, Childs DS, Porretta CM: Postirradiation fractures of the femoral neck: Emphasis on the results of treatment. JAMA 175:204, 1961
7. Bloomenthal ED, Olson WH, Nicheles H: Studies on the bone marrow cavity of the dog: Fat embolism and marrow pressure. Surg Gynecol Obstet 94:215, 1952
8. Bonfiglio M: The pathology of fracture of the femoral neck following irradiation. Am J Roentgenol 70:449, 1953
9. Boyd HB, Zilversmit DB, Calandruccio RA: The use of radioactive phosphorus (P^{32}) to determine the viability of the head of the femur. J Bone Joint Surg 37A:260, 1955
10. Brånemark P-I: Vital microscopy of bone marrow in rabbit. Scand J Clin Lab Invest (Suppl) 38:1, 1959
11. Brånemark P-I: Effect of nicotinic acid and histamine on capillary circulation of bone marrow in rabbit. Acta Haematol 25:71, 1961
12. Braunsteiner H, Grabner G: Der Einfluss von Adrenalin und Noradrenalin auf die Durchblutung des Knochenmarks. Gesamte Exp Med 130:289, 1958
13. Brodin H: Longitudinal bone growth. The nutrition of the epiphyseal cartilages and the local blood supply: An experimental study in the rabbit. Acta Arthop Scand (Suppl) 20:1, 1955
14. Brookes M: Femoral growth after occlusion of the principal nutrient canal in day-old rabbits. J Bone Joint Surg 39B:563, 1957
15. Brookes M: The vascular reaction of tubular bone to ischaemia in peripheral occlusive vascular disease. J Bone Joint Surg 42B:110, 1960
16. Brookes M: The blood supply of bone. In Clark JMP (ed): Modern Trends in Orthopaedics, Vol 4. Science of Fractures. London, Butterworths, 1964, p 91
17. Brookes M, Elkin AC, Harrison RG, et al: A new concept of capillary circulation in bone cortex: Some clinical applications. Lancet 1:1078, 1961
18. Carlson HC, Williams MMD, Childs DS Jr, et al: Microangiography of bone in the study of radiation changes. Radiology 74:113,1960
19. Copp DH, Shim SS: Extraction ratio and bone clearance of Sr^{85} as a measure of effective bone blood flow. Circ Res 16:461, 1965
20. Cumming JD: A method for studying the rate of blood flow through the bone marrow of a rabbit's femur. J Physiol (Lond) 152:39P, 1960
21. de Sapio FS: Scollamento del periostio ed allungamento degli arti. Ortoped Traumatol App Motore 21:339, 1953
22. Doan CA: The circulation of the bone marrow. Contrib Embryol 14:29, 1922
23. Doumanian AV: Experimental Deep Venous Insufficiency in the Dog. Master's Thesis, Univ. of Minnesota, Minneapolis, Minn. [Quoted in Kelly PJ, Peterson LFA: Circulation in bone. In Abramson DI (ed): Blood Vessels and Lymphatics. New York, Academic Press, 1962, p 546]
24. Doyle JR, Smart BW: Stimulation of bone growth by short-wave diathermy. J Bone Joint Surg 45A:15, 1963
25. Drinker CK, Drinker KR: A method for maintaining an artificial circulation through the tibia of the dog with a demonstration of the vasomotor control of the marrow vessels. Am J Physiol 40:514, 1916
26. Edholm OG, Howarth S: Studies on the peripheral circulation in osteitis deformans. Clin Sci 12:277, 1953
27. Edholm OG, Howarth S, McMichael J: Heart failure and bone blood flow in osteitis deformans. Clin Sci 5:249, 1945
28. Frederickson JM, Hanour AJ, Copp DH: Measurement of initial bone clearance of Ca^{45} from blood in the rat. Fed Proc 14:49, 1955
29. Frost HM: In vivo osteocyte death. J Bone Joint Surg 42A:138, 1960
30. Geiser M, Trueta J: Muscle action, bone rarefaction, and bone formation. J Bone Joint Surg 40B:282, 1958
31. Göthman L: Arterial changes in experimental fractures of the rabbit's tibia treated with in-

tramedullary nailing: A microangiographic study. Acta Chir Scand 120:289, 1960-1961

32. Granberry WM, Janes JM: The lack of effect of microwave diathermy on rate of growth of bone of the growing dog. J Bone Joint Surg 45A:773, 1963

33. Gratzek FR, Holmstrom EG, Rigler LG: Post-irradiation bone changes. Am J Roentgenol 53:62, 1945

34. Ham AW: Some histophysiological problems peculiar to calcified tissues. J Bone Joint Surg 34A:701, 1952

35. Harris WR, Martin R, Tile M: Transplantation of epiphyseal plates: An experimental study. J Bone Joint Surg 47A:897, 1965

36. Herzig E, Root WS: Relation of sympathetic nervous system to blood pressure of bone marrow. Am J Physiol 196:1053, 1959

37. Hiertonn T: Arteriovenous anastomoses and acceleration of bone growth, Acta Orthop Scand 26:322, 1957

38. Hinkel CL: The effect of irradiation upon the composition and vascularity of growing rat bones. Am J Roentgenol 50:516, 1943

39. Holling HE, Brodey RS, Boland HC: Pulmonary hypertrophic osteoarthropathy. Lancet 2:1269, 1961

40. Hurrell DJ: The nerve supply of bone. J Anat (Lond) 72:54, 1937

41. Hutchison WJ, Burdeaux BD Jr: The influence of stasis on bone growth. Surg Gynecol Obstet 99:413, 1954

42. Jaffe HL, Pomeranz MM: Changes in the bones of extremities amputated because of arteriovascular disease. Arch Surg 29:566, 1934

43. Janes JM, Herrick JF, Kelly PJ, et al: Long-term effect of ultrasonic energy on femora of the dog. Proc Staff Meet Mayo Clin 35:663, 1960

44. Janes JM, Jennings WK Jr: Effect of induced arteriovenous fistula on leg length: 10-year observations. Proc Staff Meet Mayo Clin 36:1, 1961

45. Janes JM, Kelly PJ, Herrick JF, et al: The effect of high-dosage ultrasonic energy on femora of the dog: A roentgenographic, histological, and microangiographic study. J Bone Joint Surg 44A:1299, 1962

46. Janes JM, Musgrove JE: Effect of arteriovenous fistula on growth of bone: An experimental study. Surg Clin North Am 30:1191, 1950

47. Johnson RW Jr: A physiological study of the blood supply of the diaphysis. J Bone Joint Surg (NS) 9:153, 1927

48. Just-Viera JO, Yeager GH: Venous stasis. I. Effects of venous resection on bone growth. Surgery 58:694, 1965

49. Kane WJ: Fundamental concepts in bone-blood flow studies. J Bone Joint Surg 50A:801, 1968

50. Keck SW, Kelly PJ: The effect of venous stasis on intraosseous pressure and longitudinal bone growth in the dog. J Bone Joint Surg 47A:539, 1965

51. Kelly PJ, Janes JM, Peterson LFA: The effect of arteriovenous fistulae on the vascular pattern of the femora of immature dogs: A microangiographic study. J Bone Joint Surg 41A:1101, 1959

52. Kinosita R, Ohno S, Bierman HR: Observations on regenerating bone marrow tissue in situ. Proc Am Assoc Cancer Res 2:125, 1956

53. Kistler GH: Effects of circulatory disturbances on the structure and healing of bone: Injuries of the head of the femur in young rabbits. Arch Surg 33:225, 1936

54. Kornblum SS, Kelly PJ: The lacunae and haversian canals in tibial cortical bone from ischemic and nonischemic limbs: A comparative microradiographic study. J Bone Joint Surg 46A:797, 1964

55. Matumoto Y, Mizuno S: Rate of the blood flow in the femoral head: A new measuring procedure and its clinical evaluation. Med J Osaka Univ 16:431, 1966

56. McKibbin B, Ray RD: Experimental study of peripheral circulation and bone growth: The pattern of venous return in experimental arteriovenous fistulae. II. Clin Orthop 53:175, 1967

57. Pearse HE Jr, Morton JJ: The stimulation of bone growth by venous stasis. J Bone Joint Surg (NS) 12:97, 1930

58. Pearse HE Jr, Morton JJ: Venous stasis accelerates bone repair. Surgery 1:106, 1937

59. Peterson LFA, Neher M, Janes JM, et al: A stereoscopic microradiographic camera with vacuum film-holder and a stereomicroscope. Proc Staff Meet Mayo Clin 34:283, 1959

60. Post M, Shoemaker WC: Bone electrolyte response to intravenous acid loads. Surg Gynecol Obstet 115:749, 1962

61. Ray RD, Kawabata M, Galante J: Experimental study of peripheral circulation and bone growth: An experimental method for the quantitative determination of bone blood flow. III. Clin Orthop 54:175, 1967

62. Rhinelander FW, Baragry RA: Microangiography in bone healing. I. Undisplaced closed fractures. J Bone Joint Surg 44A:1273, 1962

63. Richards V, Stofer R: The stimulation of bone growth by internal heating. Surgery 46:84, 1959

64. Shaw NE: Observations on the intramedullary blood-flow and marrow-pressure in bone. Clin Sci 24:311, 1963

65. Shaw NE: Observations on the physiology of the circulation in bones. Ann R Coll Surg Engl 35:214, 1964

66. Sherman MS, Selakovich WG: Bone changes in chronic circulatory insufficiency: A histopathological study. J Bone Joint Surg 39A:892, 1957

67. Shim SS: Physiology of blood circulation of bone. J Bone Joint Surg 50A:812, 1968

68. Shim SS, Copp DH, Patterson FP: The bone blood flow in the limb following complete sci-

atic nerve section. Surg Gynecol Obstet 123:333, 1966

69. Shim SS, Patterson FP: A direct method of qualitative study of bone blood circulation. Surg Gynecol Obstet 125:261, 1967

70. Speed K: Longitudinal overgrowth of long bones. Surg Gynecol Obstet 36:787, 1923

71. Stein AH Jr, Morgan HC, Porras RF: The effect of pressor and depressor drugs on intramedullary bone-marrow pressure. J Bone Joint Surg 40A:1103, 1958

72. Stein AH Jr, Morgan HC, Porras RF: The effect of an arteriovenous fistula on intramedullary bone pressure. Surg Gynecol Obstet 109:287, 1959

73. Trotman NH, Kelly WD: The effect of sympathectomy on blood flow to bone. JAMA 183:121, 1963

74. Trueta J: Acute haematogenous osteomyelitis: Its pathology and treatment. Bull Hosp Joint Diseases 14:5, 1953

75. Trueta J: The influence of the blood supply in controlling bone growth. Bull Hosp Joint Dis 14:147, 1953

76. Trueta J: The three types of acute haematogenous osteomyelitis: A clinical and vascular study. J Bone Joint Surg 41B:671, 1959

77. Trueta J: The role of the vessels in osteogenesis. J Bone Joint Surg 45B:402, 1963

78. Trueta J, Cavadias AX: Vascular changes caused by the Küntscher type of nailing: An experimental study in the rabbit. J Bone Joint Surg 37B:492, 1955

79. Trueta J, Harrison MHM: The normal vascular anatomy of the femoral head in adult man. J Bone Joint Surg 35B:442, 1953

80. Vanderhoeft PJ, Kelly PJ, Janes JM, et al: Growth and structure of bone distal to an arteriovenous fistula: Quantitative analysis of tetracycline-induced transverse growth patterns. J Bone Joint Surg 45B:582, 1963

81. Vaughen JL, Bender LF: Effects of ultrasound on growing bone. Arch Phys Med Rehabil 40:158, 1959

82. Weinman DT, Kelly PJ, Owen CA Jr, et al: Skeletal clearance of Ca^{47} and Sr^{85} and skeletal blood flow in dogs. Proc Staff Meet Mayo Clin 38:559, 1963

83. Weiss L: An electron microscopic study of the vascular sinuses of the bone marrow of the rabbit. Bull Johns Hopkins Hosp 108:171, 1961

84. Weiss RA, Root WS: Innervation of the vessels of the marrow cavity of certain bones. Am J Physiol 197:1255, 1959

85. Woodhouse CF: Nutrient artery circulation control problems in bone. Am J Orthop 5:290, 1963

86. Wray JB: Vascular regeneration in the healing fracture: An experimental study. Angiology 14:134, 1963

87. Wu YK, Miltner LJ: A procedure for stimulation of longitudinal growth of bone: An experimental study. J Bone Joint Surg (NS) 19:909, 1937

88. Yabsley RH, Harris WR: The effect of shaft fracture and periosteal stripping on the vascular supply to epiphyseal plates. J Bone Joint Surg 47A:551, 1965

89. Zamboni L, Pease DC: The vascular bed of red bone marrow. J Ultrastruct Res 5:65, 1961

90. Zinn CJ, Griffith JQ Jr: Effect of sympathectomy upon blood supply of bone. Proc Soc Exp Biol Med 46:311, 1941

Chapter 4

Circulation to Joints and Associated Structures

This chapter deals with the anatomy of the blood supply and the normal and abnormal vascular responses of the synovial membrane and capsule of joints and with the circulation to tendons. The articular cartilage is without vessels and derives its nutrients by diffusion. (For comparable data on the bony elements of the joints, see Sections A and B, Chapter 3.)

A. Anatomy of the Vascular Tree

1. Methods of Study

The most direct method of investigating the anatomy of the blood supply to joints is gross and microscopic dissection. To visualize the small-calibered vessels, some form of injection medium, such as a mixture of India ink and human serum, has been used [10,25–27]. Serial histologic sections following injection of the vascular system have also been attempted. Arteriography and lymphangiography, utilizing a constant pressure pump, have been proposed as investigative tools, although such approaches have the disadvantage of being applicable only to the study of segments of joints. It is of importance to note that with any type of injection technique, there is always a possibility of distorting the capillary bed (incomplete filling or overdistension) and obtaining an inaccurate visualization of the microcirculation.

2. Morphology of the Blood Supply to Joints

Main arterial tree. The large arteries supplying the fibrous capsule and synovium arise from a complex anastomotic network which has its origin in the main channels to the limb. These vessels also communicate freely with those to the periosteum and epiphysis, the result being one nutritional unit for the joint cavity and the adjoining epiphysis [9]. Demonstrating occasional treelike branching, the arteries anastomose at irregular intervals to form wide-meshed, rich vascular networks of vessels. From the latter arises a second vascular plexus of smaller-calibered channels which runs alongside the synovial surface in a plane parallel to the parent network [10]. There are also small branches which pass directly to the surface of the synovial membrane and which, after a short course, turn to form an irregular quadrilateral terminal pattern lying on this structure.

Microcirculation. The terminal plexus to the synovium is composed primarily of precapillary arterioles which divide into a capillary network; the latter forms a series of finely anastomosing loops immediately under the synovial lining (Fig. 4.1) [10]. The number of capillaries vary in different and even in the same species, although areas with similar types of synovial tissue appear to demonstrate the same kind of architecture of capillary structure [28]. For ex-

41

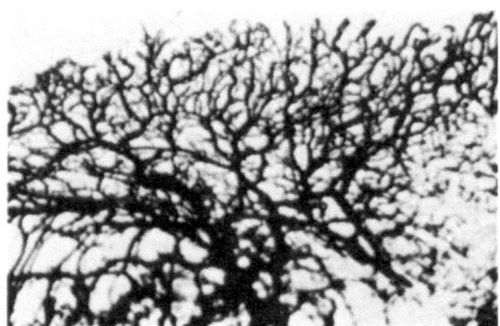

Fig. 4.1. Termination of the blood vessels of the synovial membrane covering the anterior cruciate ligament of the upper articular surface of the tibia. × 19. Visualized are precapillary arterioles dividing into a capillary network which forms a series of finely anastomosing capillary loops immediately under the synovial lining. From Davis DV, Edwards DAW [10]. Reproduced with the permission of Annals of the Royal College of Surgeons.

ample, most cellular areas possess an extensive plexus of capillaries [10,32], whereas less cellular ones, such as aponeurotic tissue, have few capillaries. Areas lining mechanically strained parts of a joint also contain a smaller concentration of vessels. Avascular structures may be surrounded by single capillary loops.

Four different vascular types have been identified in the capillary bed of the synovium [25–27]. The first consists of ordinary capillary loops, frequently with distal coiling, which are present under smooth surfaces, in villi, and in bursae and tendon sheaths. A second type, with long straight channels, forms into a wide-meshed network, resembling the vascular system of adipose tissue. A third consists of the occasional vessels seen in the portions of synovial membrane lining the joint capsule where the latter is exposed to mechanical strain. The final group is made up of channels in the periosteal synovial tissue, being similar to ordinary capillary loops with distal coil formation.

The tissues which line ligaments receive their blood supply from capillaries arising from small arteries and arterioles running longitudinally in these structures (Fig. 4.2) [10]. The minute vessels anastomose repeatedly to form numerous loops just under the synovial lining, a location which may explain the not infrequent extravasation of blood into joints (hemarthrosis) [9]. When the vessels approach the articular cavity they tend to diminish in caliber, the dimensions of the units of the innermost capillary plexus varying from 0.14 to 0.90 mm.

Arteriovenous shunts have been reported as being present on the acetabular pad of the hip

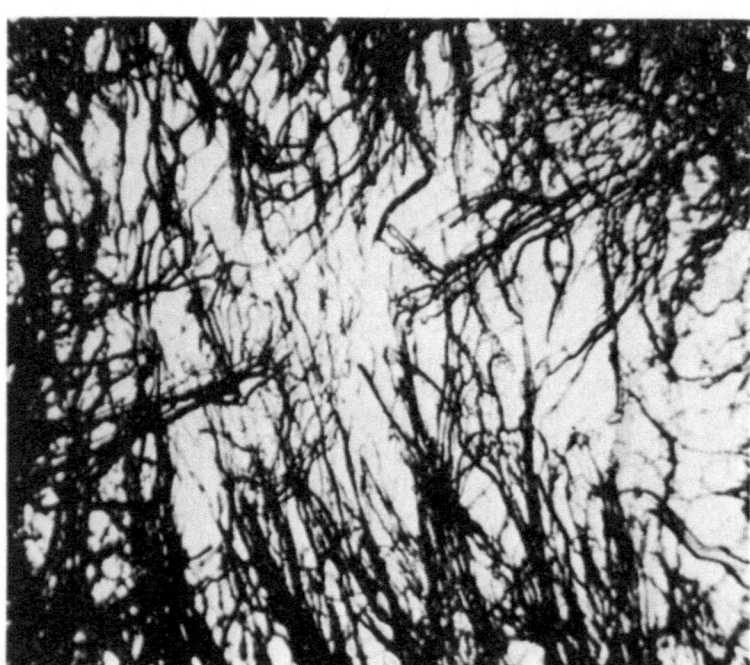

Fig. 4.2. Blood vessels of the plantar calcaneonavicular ligament in a 67-year-old man. × 24. Visualized are the numerous terminal capillary loops located around the central area which supports the head of the talus. From Davis DV, Edwards DAW [10]. Reproduced with the permission of Annals of the Royal College of Surgeons.

joint [4,30–32] and in other joints [5]. They have been divided into a group of small artery-like channels, with a definite inner longitudinal layer of smooth muscle, and into another, composed of plexiform nodules of capillaries. The latter vessels resemble the glomus tumor, located in the subcutaneous tissue of the digits (see C-1, Chapter 21), except that they possess only a few epithelioid cell components. Because of the location and arrangement of the arteriovenous shunts, the suggestion has been offered that they play an important role in the regulation of articular and, perhaps, epiphyseal blood flow [17]. Moreover, these structures have been considered to act as a shunt mechanism in the joint, reducing blood flow in one area and increasing it in another. However, the fact that the arteriovenous anastomoses are not found at birth raises some question as to their function, for it is possible that they arise in response to a specific need. Furthermore, it is necessary to point out that these structures are difficult to identify histologically and must be differentiated from arteriosclerotic intimal plaques, postmortem mural intussusception of minute vessels, and normal convoluted capillaries of the villi.

Local venous system. The size and topography of the venous channels draining synovial tissue and the fibrous capsule have been studied less extensively than the arterial tree. Large-calibered veins have been identified in the knee joint of rabbits, accompanying the arteries at their point of penetration of the capsule. These venous channels then follow the branching of the arterioles. They possess numerous valves, even in the case of the smallest-sized vessels.

Local lymphatic system. This consists of a single plexus of vessels which has a wide-meshed, irregular, and coarse polygonal pattern. From it arise numerous channels proceeding toward the articular surface and ending in lacunar enlargements. The local lymphatics are drained by vessels which pass outward to terminate in the regional deep lymph nodes [33]. Although the larger trunks are freely supplied with valves, few of these structures are seen in the lymphatics of the synovial membrane [1].

Sympathetic innervation. The sympathetic nerve supply to articular vessels is similar to that observed in other sites, with both myelinated and nonmyelinated fibers being present. The postganglionic elements run in the peripheral mixed nerves and are distributed to the articular vessels and to their epiphyseal branches. This is the only pathway available for the knee and elbow, whereas in the case of the hip and shoulder joint, some fibers also run in the adventitia of the blood vessels [15,16].

3. Morphology of the Vascular Supply to Tendons

The blood supply to tendons has been investigated in human cadavers shortly after death, using perfusion (at a constant pressure of 100 mmHg) of a silicone rubber compound, followed by the application of a dissecting microscope to obtain photographs of the specimens [34]. The blood vessels are longitudinally oriented within the tendons, with all the blood entering and exiting through the mesotenon, a thin, filmy sheet of areolar tissue attached to the undersurface of the tendon. This structure is comparable to the mesentery of the intestine, and it appears to have the same function. All the arterial branches originate in the bed deep to the tendon, pass upward into the mesotenon, branch into arcades of vessels, and then enter the tendon. Each arcade has some anastomotic connection with ones located on either side of it, but primarily it appears to be nourishing a small localized segment of tendon. For the most part, the concentration of blood vessels is located on the side of the tendon which is opposite to that on which the mesotenon is found. The relative size of blood vessels and their number in any one segment of tendon are not significantly different from those of any other. Of clinical significance is the finding that blood supply to any single segment will not support circulation in adjacent segments over more than probably 1 to 2 cm. As a result, large portions of any tendon freed at surgery must be considered to function as a free graft until a blood supply is developed by the ingrowth of vessels [34].

B.   Physiology of the Vascular Tree

Information regarding the physiology of the circulation of joints is fragmentary, due mainly to the fact that the vascular responses of the various structures are technically difficult to separate.

1.   Methods of Study

A number of physiologic means have been utilized in the measurement of joint blood flow in experimental animals. Among these are electromagnetic and bubble flowmeters inserted into vessels which contribute to the major blood supply of the joint. The femoral artery and its highest articular branch and the vein accompanying the latter have all been studied in this manner [6,7]. Isotope tracer and clearance studies, which have been useful in the determination of blood flow to bone and other organs, have not been extensively investigated with respect to the synovium. Some information has been gained, however, regarding synovial surface activity by measuring the rate of clearance of radioactive sodium injected directly into the joint [18,19,36]. Venous occlusion plethysmography has been utilized in man to measure blood flow through the normal [3] and pathologic [23] knee joint, such studies having been done under spinal anesthesia and sympathetic block and following sympathectomy. Finally, vascular responses in joints have been investigated through the changes in articular temperature [14,20–22].

2.   Vasomotor Control

The contribution of the vasomotor nerves in the regulation of blood flow to the joints has not been clearly defined. This problem has been studied in the knee joint of dogs, using an electromagnetic flowmeter, and it has been found that after cutting the local sympathetic nerve supply, the blood flow becomes approximately 50 percent greater than the resting level [6]. Stimulation of the cut end of the peripheral nerve containing the sympathetic branches produces vasoconstriction. Removal of the

sympathetic chain below the L4 level results in approximately a doubling of the local circulation; however, the change is only transient, since the readings return to or approach the control baseline within 1 h after the procedure. On the other hand, work with radiosodium clearance in dogs has revealed a marked increase in the rate of removal of the material from the knee joint, beginning the second week after lumbar sympathectomy and lasting for approximately 2 weeks afterward [37]. The changes in clearance have been interpreted as representing alterations in blood flow to the knee joint [37].

The generally accepted view is that, like other blood vessels, those to the articular structures are supplied with sympathetic vasoconstrictor fibers through which they are maintained in a state of tone [6]. In addition, the arteries appear to possess an inherent basal constrictor tone, since during the time that an increased blood flow exists due to sympathetic denervation, a further augmentation can be elicited by an intraarterial injection of a vasodilator such as acetylcholine [8].

Vasosensory fibers are found in the adventitia of joint vessels in both the capsule and the synovial tissue. They appear to play a role as a pathway for afferent pain impulses arising in the joint. There are other complex sensory endings in the vascular adventitia which may be concerned in vascular reflexes [17].

3.   Resting Blood Flow

Resting blood flow to the knee of dogs ranges between 1.5 and 7.0 ml/min [8]. However, such data have been criticized because of the possibility that in the process of cannulating a branch of the femoral artery (which was necessary in order to insert a flowmeter), the sympathetic nerves in the adventitia of the blood vessel were damaged [28]. By increasing the temperature within the knee joint of dogs and determining the rate of cooling, a normal circulation rate in articular structures has been found to be 0.75 ml/min per 100 ml of static fluid [24]. In man, the average normal resting blood flow of the knee joint at a bath temperature of 30° C has been reported as 1.3 ml/min per 100 ml of limb volume, whereas at a bath temperature of 35° C, it rises to 2.9 ml [3]. However, the results cannot be considered representative of joint blood flow, since overlying skin, subcutaneous tissue, and neighboring muscle also contributed to the vascular response.

4. Vascular Changes Produced by Exercise

Utilizing the clearance rate of sodium, it has been noted that in normal human subjects, muscular effort causes approximately an 85 percent rise in blood flow over the average figure at rest [36]. When studied by means of venous occlusion plethysmography, vigorous exercise of the knee produces an increase of 0.6 to 2.0 ml/min per 100 ml of limb volume over the resting level. Such a change, however, is in part also due to the contribution of the muscles in the segment of knee under study [3].

5. Vascular Effects of Physical Agents

Changes in ambient temperature. Although some reports indicate that there is no alteration in joint temperature on application of hot and cold packs [21], others [35] note that with the use of hot packs, the joint temperature rises simultaneously with similar changes in surrounding structures. Using the flowmeter technique, an increase in rate of flow has been found to occur only if the temperature is raised 10° C or more [7]. Rapid cooling reduces joint blood flow to about one-half the value at rest.

The effect of heat and cold on the microcirculation of the rabbit's knee joint has been investigated using vital microscopy, and it has been found that at intraarticular temperatures in the range of 36 to 37° C, the corpuscular flow in the capillary bed is discontinuous, exhibiting plasma skimming [28]. At a temperature of around 40° C, there is generalized vasodilatation, with a rapid corpuscular flow. Further temperature elevation produces stagnation of blood in the capillary bed, with a more rapid movement of corpuscles through the arteriovenous shunts. Eventually complete circulatory cessation is noted in the capillary tree. With local hypothermia, there is a reduction in the caliber of arterioles and venules, and

at an intraarticular temperature of 20 to 22 ° C, discontinuous corpuscular flow becomes more apparent, until ultimately there is no movement of blood. However, there is no corpuscular trapping, as occurs with hyperthermia. These changes in corpuscular flow on exposure to cold and heat are considered to have significance as hemodynamic phenomena, in light of the virtually complete absence of contractile elements in most parts of the capillary bed [28].

Vascular effects of indirect body heating. Application of heat to distant parts of the body has been reported to produce an increase in joint blood flow, but the changes are uniformly smaller than those which follow the direct application of heat [3]. Heating the abdomen alone to produce reflex vasodilatation causes an increase in joint segment flow of 20 percent. The clinical observation that, in the arthritic patient, relief is experienced in the involved knee joint when the upper extremities are immersed in a paraffin bath for a period of time would support the view that reflex or indirect vasodilatation produced by body heating results in an augmentation in blood flow to the joint tissues. Such a finding is also in accord with the belief that the sympathetic nervous system innervates joint blood vessels, since the increased blood flow with moderate body heating is probably effected through inhibition of sympathetic vasoconstrictor tone.

Diathermy modalities. Short-wave, long-wave, and microwave diathermy has been reported to cause a rise in temperature in joints of animals and man [29,35]. Using the radioactive sodium clearance technique, it has been found that heating the human knee joint by means of short-wave diathermy elicits a major increase in clearance, with a rise of 3 to 6° C in intraarticular temperature [19]. An augmentation in circulation which averages 100 percent has also been reported [18].

6. Vascular Effects of Chemical Agents

Using a bubble flowmeter, it has been found that the arterial inflow to the normally innervated dog's knee joint is decreased by intraarterially administered epinephrine [7], a similar response occurring in the sympathetically denervated joint [8]. At no time is a dilator response observed with epinephrine. However, in the normal human knee joint, this drug elicits an augmentation in blood flow [3]. Norepinephrine produces vasoconstriction in the innervated dog's knee joint, with a more pronounced and prolonged response being noted after sympathetic denervation [8]. An intravenous injection of Pitressin in the dog is followed by a gradual but definite reduction in intraarticular temperature [35], whereas acetylcholine injected intraarterially has a marked vasodilator effect [8]. Using the sodium clearance technique, the intraarterial injection of tolazoline hydrochloride (Priscoline) has been found to produce a definite increase in clearance and an elevation of temperature in the knee joint of patients with and without osteoarthritic changes, such data being interpreted as indicating that the drug elicits a local augmentation in circulation [11,12]. Although local anesthetics (procaine and Xylocaine) and steroids (hydrocortisone acetate and methylprednisolone) are commonly utilized intraarticularly in the treatment of joint conditions, data regarding their effect on the circulation to the synovium are not available. There is some evidence that methylprednisolone increases the viscosity and decreases the elasticity of synovial fluid. (For the effects of immobilization on the vascular responses in joints, see B-3, Chapter 23.)

7. Synovial Barrier

The exchange of fluid and other substances across the synovial membrane has important clinical implications. Nevertheless, very little work has been done on the mechanisms of transfer from the blood vessels into the joint.

There is more information, however, on the basis for the absorption of substances from the joint cavity. The lymphatics of the joint tissues, particularly of the synovial membrane, play an important role in fluid interchange, these structures being well developed in the synovial membrane [1]. The question of whether the sympathetic nervous system plays any role in fluid interchange in the joint, as reflected in

resulting changes in blood flow, is still unanswered. It has been proposed that electrolytes move freely across the synovial barrier, with the exchange of fluid being governed by the factors entering in the classical theory of Starling, perhaps modified by the existence of vasomotion in the microcirculation [2,13]. However, since the observation has been made that not all nonelectrolytes move across the barrier with equal facility, the possibility has been advanced that the role of the synovial membrane in the absorption of solutions from the joint cavity may not be purely passive and controlled by the laws of physical chemistry [1].

References

1. Barnett CH, Davies DV, MacConaill MA: Synovial Joints: Their Structure and Mechanics. Springfield, Ill., Charles C Thomas, 1961, p 89
2. Bauer W, Ropes MW, Waine H: The physiology of articular structures. Physiol Rev 20:272, 1940
3. Bonney GLW, Hughes RA, Janus O: Blood flow through the normal human knee segment. Clin Sci 11:167, 1952
4. Clara M: Die arterio-venösen Anastomosen: Anatomie, Biologie und Pathologie. Leipzig, Germany, Johann Ambrosius Barth, 1939
5. Clara M: Die arterio-venösen Anastomosen. Vienna, Springer, 1956
6. Cobbold AF, Lewis OJ: The nervous control of joint blood vessels. J Physiol (Lond) 133:467, 1956
7. Cobbold AF, Lewis OJ: Blood flow to the knee joint of the dog: Effect of heating, cooling, and adrenaline. J Physiol (Lond) 132:379, 1956
8. Cobbold AF, Lewis OJ: The action of adrenaline, noradrenaline, and acetylcholine on blood flow through joints. J Physiol (Lond) 133:472, 1956
9. Davies DV: Synovial membrane and synovial fluid of joints. Lancet 2:815, 1946
10. Davies DV, Edwards DAW: The blood supply of the synovial membrane and intra-articular structures. Ann R Coll Surg Engl 2:142, 1948
11. Davison S, Borken N, Wolf M: Elevations in temperature of joint, muscle, and skin, following injection of Priscoline intra-arterially. J Mt Sinai Hosp 21:98, 1954
12. Davison S, Wisham LH: The clearance of Na^{24} from the normal and osteoarthritic knee joint and the response to intra-arterial Priscoline. J Clin Invest 37:389, 1958
13. Edlund T: Studies on absorption of colloids

and fluid from rabbit knee joints. Acta Physiol Scand (Suppl 62) 18:1, 1949

14. Ekholm J, Skoglund S: Intra-articular knee joint temperature variations in response to cooling and heating of the skin in the cat. Acta Physiol Scand 50:175,1960

15. Gardner E: The innervation of the hip joint. Anat Rec 101:353, 1948

16. Gardner E: The innervation of the shoulder joint. Anat Rec 102:1, 1948

17. Gardner ED: Physiology of blood and nerve supply of joints. Bull Hosp Joint Dis 15:35, 1954

18. Harris R: Effect of shortwave diathermy on radiosodium clearance from the knee joint in the normal and in rheumatoid arthritis. Arch Phys Med Rehabil 42:241, 1961

19. Harris R, Millard JB: Clearance of radioactive sodium from the knee joint. Clin Sci 15:9, 1956

20. Hollander JL, Stoner EK, Brown EM Jr: The use of intra-articular temperature measurement in the evaluation of anti-arthritic agents. J Clin Invest 29:822, 1950

21. Horvath SM, Hollander JL: Intra-articular temperature as a measure of joint reaction. J Clin Invest 28:469, 1949

22. Hunter J, Whillans MG: Study of the effect of cold on joint temperature and mobility. Can J Med Sci 29:255, 1951

23. Janus O: Objective assessment of improvement in rheumatoid arthritis. Br Med J 2:1244, 1950

24. Kaplan E, Joseph NR: Determination of circulation rate in articular structures. Fed Proc 7:63, 1948

25. Lang J: Beitrag zur Gefässversorgung der Gelenkinnenhaut. Z Mikrosk Anat Forsch 60:503, 1954

26. Lang J: Bau und Funktion der Gegässe des Stratum synoviale. Anat Anz 103:13, 1956

27. Lang J: Die Gelenkinnenhaut, ihre Aufbau-und Abbauvorgänge. Morphol Jahrb 98:387, 1957–1958

28. Lindström J: Microvascular anatomy of synovial tissue. Acta Rheumatol Scand (Suppl) 7:1, 1963

29. Lonergan RC: An experimental study of diathermy. J Indust Hygiene 9:1, 1927

30. Muratori G: Anastomosi arterovenose e dispositivi vascolari di blocco nel "pulvinar acetabuli" dell'uomo. Chir Organi Mov 30:117, 1946

31. Muratori G, Bertolin A: Sulla struttura dei vasi sanguigni del "pulvinar acetabuli" dei mammiferi. Atti Soc Med Chir Padova 24:107, 1946

32. Policard A: Physiologie générale des articulations à l'état normal et pathologique. Paris, Masson, 1936

33. Sankaran B: Physiology and pathology of synovial membrane. In: Instructional Course Lectures, Miami, Fla., The American Academy of Orthopaedic Surgeons, 1963

34. Smith JW: Blood supply of tendons. Am J Surg 109:272, 1965

35. Wakim KG, Krusen FH: Influence of physical agents and of certain drugs on intra-articular temperature. Arch Phys Med 32:714, 1951

36. Wisham LH, Davison S, Gordon L: The effect of weight bearing exercise on radioactive sodium clearance from normal and osteoarthritic knee joints. Arch Phys Med Rehabil 41:587, 1960

37. Wisham LH, Dworecka FF: The effect of sympathectomy on radio-sodium clearance from the knee joints of dogs. J Cardiovasc Surg 7:66, 1966

Section 2

Study of the Circulation in the Limbs by Clinical and Laboratory Means

Chapter 5

Clinical and Laboratory Tests of Arterial Circulation

Part 1   Procedures for Study of Patency of Main Arterial Channels

---

From a clinical viewpoint, the blood supply to a limb can roughly be divided into two different types of vascular beds: [1] the distribution channels (the large arteries and their main branches) and [2] the nutritional circulation (the smaller arteries and the microcirculation), in the distal portion of which blood interacts with the tissues. In the normal individual, the terminal vascular bed is directly dependent upon the state of the larger vessels feeding it (Fig. 5.1A). When a chronic occlusive arterial disease exists, however, such a relationship no longer is present, for there may be an adequate nutritional blood flow in the face of complete occlusion of the main arteries in the limb and of the proximal vessels supplying them. This is possible because simultaneously with the progressive but slow obstruction of the main arterial channels, there is generally a compensatory growth of a collateral circulation (Figs. 5.1B and 10.1), formed in response to a state of persistent chronic ischemia of distal tissues (see C-3, Chapter 10). Hence, it is apparent that only by the combined use of procedures devised to study separately each of the two types of local circulation can a comprehensive appraisal of the actual local blood flow be reached.

The present chapter deals with a description of clinical and laboratory tests which determine the state of patency of the main arteries in the limbs, while methods for the study of the nutritional circulation are discussed in Chapter 6.

In recent years there has been a definite tendency on the part of house staff, general practitioners, internists, and surgeons to rely heavily on procedures generally only available in vascular laboratories of hospitals for confirmation of impressions that an occlusive arterial disease exists in their patients. Such an approach in many cases is costly, it frequently involves hospitalization and loss of income, and in the case of invasive methods, it may be painful and not without danger. Moreover, in most instances it is unwarranted and unnecessary, since comparable information can readily be obtained from a detailed and comprehensive vascular history and a selective physical examination utilizing palpation, auscultation, and oscillometry, all carried out in the office as outlined in Sections A, B, and C, below, and in Tables 5.1 and 5.2. With the use of such measures, techniques in physical diagnosis are also sharpened and perception of abnormal vascular manifestations in the limbs becomes more acute—characteristics that are essential to develop for the

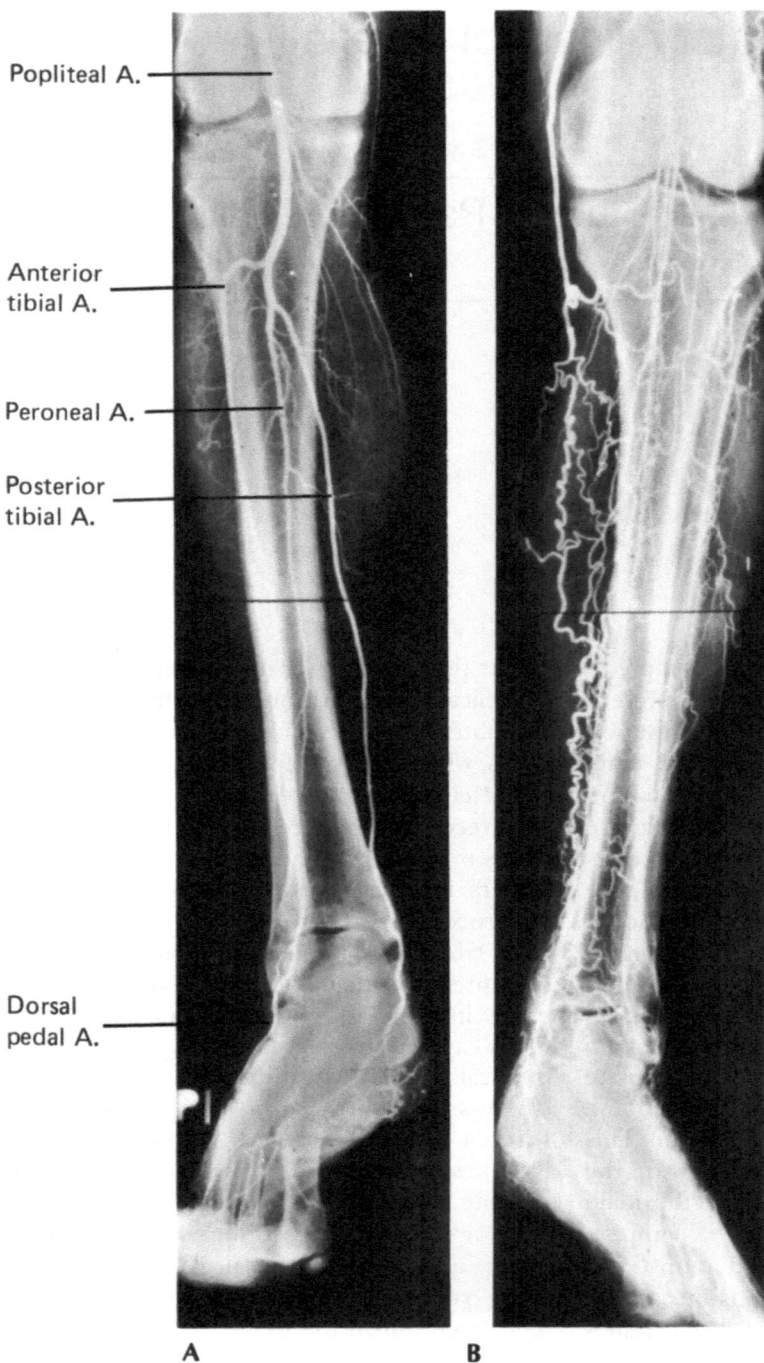

Popliteal A.

Anterior
tibial A.

Peroneal A.

Posterior
tibial A.

Dorsal
pedal A.

A   **B**

Fig. 5.1. Arteriograms of lower limbs. **A** Normal vascular tree, demonstrating visualization of the popliteal, anterior tibial, posterior tibial, peroneal, and dorsal pedal arteries. **B** Complete obliteration of the main arteries in the leg and foot, due to atherosclerosis, with replacement by an extensive collateral circulation.

neophyte in the field of circulatory disorders.

If, on the basis of a clinical study, the patient is considered to be a potential candidate for some type of reconstructive surgery, then much more definitive data regarding the vascular tree are essential, and for this purpose, it is necessary to hospitalize the patient and resort to the use of noninvasive and invasive laboratory procedures, as presented in Sections D and E, later in this chapter.

Table 5.1. Steps in History Taking.

1. Chief complaints: List
2. Relevant family history: List those conditions which are, or have a relationship to, vascular disorders (primary varicosities; congenital lymphedema; atherosclerosis in different organs and in limbs; superficial and deep thrombophlebitis)
3. Past history
   a. Excessive sweating or lack of sweating and dryness of the limbs
   b. Infrequent need to trim toenails
   c. Cold injuries (frostbite; trench foot; post-frostbite or post–trench foot syndrome)
   d. Repeated cellulitis of lower or upper limbs
   e. Attacks of superficial thrombophlebitis (types; location; outcome)
   f. Attacks of deep thrombophlebitis (types; location; outcome)
   g. Varicosities (primary; secondary)
   h. Episodes of pulmonary embolism (treatment; outcome)
   i. Swelling of lower limbs (pitting edema; lymphedema; intermittent; continuous; degree of swelling)
   j. Trauma to limbs (description of lesions; treatment; outcome)
   k. Spontaneous ulcers of legs (cause; treatment; outcome)
   l. Spontaneous gangrene of upper and lower limbs (cause; treatment; outcome)
   m. Systemic conditions associated with vascular complications in the limbs (diabetes; hypertension; sickle-cell anemia; rheumatoid arthritis; myocardial infarction)
   n. Surgical vascular procedures (sympathectomy; insertion of venous or artificial prosthesis; thromboendarterectomy; vein stripping) and outcome
   o. Nonvascular operations (herniorrhaphy; gynecologic procedures; cholecystectomy) which may be followed by deep venous thrombosis and pulmonary embolism
   p. Orthopedic or neurologic conditions affecting the limbs
4. Habits: Type, duration, and quantity, with respect to tobacco smoking; consumption of alcoholic beverages; drug addiction
5. Occupation: Possibility of injury during daily work activities; utilization of machinery or instruments capable of causing vascular disturbances (pneumatic hammers and drills; repetitive compression of palm of hand in performance of daily work duties)
6. Present history
   Vascular complaints due to arterial insufficiency
   a. Intermittent claudication: claudication distance in short city blocks; pace of walking; location of symptoms; severity of complaint; duration of symptoms after cessation of physical activity; indications of progression of the condition
   b. Ischemic neuropathy: positions initiating symptoms; location of complaints; severity of symptoms; effect on the well being of the patient; measures which cause relief of symptoms; description of complaints
   c. Ischemic pain in the presence of ulcers and gangrene: location, severity, and description of symptoms; conditions which aggravate and relieve them; effect on the well being of the patient
   Vascular complaints due to venous insufficiency
   a. Sense of tiredness, fatigue, and heaviness in the feet and lower portion of the legs associated with swelling
   b. Nocturnal cramps
   c. Local pain associated with venous stasis dermatitis or ulceration; chronic indurated cellulitis; superficial thrombophlebitis; thrombosis of collecting veins; thrombosis of venous plexuses in muscles of the calf (phlebothrombosis)
   Vascular complaints due to lymphatic obstruction, destruction, inflammation, or congenital abnormalities
   a. Sense of heaviness and fatigue in involved limb due to accumulation of lymphedema
   b. Pain and tenderness along course of lymph channels due to inflammation (lymphangitis)
   c. Pain due to breakdown of skin and formation of an ulcer

Table 5.2. Steps in the Clinical and Laboratory Study of Local Physical Findings.*

---

1. By inspection
   Arterial system in limbs
   a. Skin color in horizontal, elevated, and dependent positions (normal pink color; rubor; cyanosis; pallor)
   b. Hyperhidrosis, normal sweating pattern, or anhidrosis
   c. Signs of local inflammation (rubor and swelling)
   d. Presence of minor nutritional changes (piling up of scaly material at junction of nail plate and fleshy portion of fingertip); parchment appearance of skin; deposition of calcium (calcinosis); replacement of normal skin by scar tissue; loss of normal wrinkling over small joints of fingers; adherence of skin to subcutaneous tissue
   e. Presence of major nutritional changes (ulceration or gangrene)
   f. Nail changes (deformity; increased thickness; ridging; brittleness; deposition of pigment)
   g. Hair growth on legs, feet, and toes (normal, reduced, or absent)
   h. Presence of dermatophytosis between toes
   Venous system in limbs
   a. Varicosities; superficial thrombophlebitis; dilated veins which do not collapse on elevation of limb
   b. Swelling (location; pitting; nonpitting)
   c. Pigmentation, induration, brawniness of skin of legs; presence of stasis dermatitis or ulceration
   Lymphatic system in limbs
   a. Lymphangitis
   b. Lymphedema (location; severity; degree)
   c. Elephantiasis
2. By palpation
   Arterial system in limbs
   a. Skin temperature (differences in various toes and between the feet; presence or absence of normal gradient; abrupt changes in temperature)
   b. Determination of pulsations in subclavian, axillary, brachial, radial, and ulnar arteries in the upper limbs; abdominal aorta and its main branches; and common femoral, popliteal, posterior tibial, and dorsal pedal arteries in the lower limbs. Examination for aberrant vessels
   c. Palpation of vessels, scars, and masses for thrills
   d. Determination of texture and consistency of skin (persistence of dimpling of skin after removal of digital pressure)
   Venous system in limbs
   a. Determination of presence of superficial thrombophlebitis
   b. Determination of presence of a tender mass in calf muscles by deep palpation, as in phlebothrombosis
   c. Determination of type of swelling (pitting, nonpitting)
   Lymphatic system in limbs
   a. Determination of nonpitting quality of swelling
3. By auscultation
   Arterial system in limbs
   a. Examination for presence of bruits over the subclavian and brachial arteries in the upper limb; the abdominal aorta and its main branches; and the femoral and popliteal arteries in the lower limb (intensity, duration, and location)
   b. Examination of all local scars and masses for bruits
4. Clinical testing
   Arterial system in limbs
   a. Oscillometry performed at three levels on the upper and lower limbs
   b. Venous filling time
   c. Ulnar confirmatory test
   d. Reactive hyperemia test
   e. Subpapillary venous plexus filling time

Table 5.2. Steps in the Clinical and Laboratory Study of Local Physical Findings.* *(Continued)*

Venous system in limbs
  a. Single and multiple tourniquet tests for study of varicosities
  b. Homans' sign for study of phlebothrombosis
  c. Perthes' test for study of state of deep venous circulation
5. Laboratory testing
  Arterial system in limbs
  a. Ultrasonic echography for size and shape of abdominal aorta
  b. Skin temperature determinations
  c. Graphic representation of pulse wave
  d. Doppler ultrasonic flowmeter
  e. Contrast angiography
  f. Electromagnetic flowmeter
  Venous system in limbs
  a. Venous pressure determinations
  b. Infrared photography
  c. Doppler ultrasonic flowmeter
  d. Radioactive fibrinogen test
  e. Impedance and mercury strain-gauge plethysmography
  f. Contrast venography
  g. Radionuclide venography
  Lymphatic system in limbs
  a. Lymphangiography
6. Nonvascular adjunctive examinations
  Limited neurologic study
  a. Sensory examination of limbs
  b. Motor examination of limbs
  c. Sensory and motor nerve conduction velocity studies
  d. Elicitation of superficial and deep reflexes
  Limited orthopedic study
  a. Examination of arches of feet
  b. Range of motion of small and large joints
  c. Strength of hand grip
  d. Lasègue's sign

* A detailed description of physical findings in arterial disorders is found in Chapters 5 and 6; a discussion of those in venous disorders is presented in Chapter 7. The laboratory tests of arterial and venous efficiency are dealt with in Chapters 5 and 7, respectively.

A. Palpation of Peripheral Pulses

One of the most important steps in a vascular examination is palpation of all of the arteries of the extremities that are capable of such an examination for the purpose of determining the amplitude and force of pulsation in them. However, it is necessary to point out that information thus derived does not always give an accurate evaluation of the state of the main vessels. For example, partial obliteration of a proximal artery may still cause little or no decrease in amplitude of the pulses in the feet. Conversely, complete absence of a pulse in a vessel does not necessarily indicate that there is no flow of blood through it. In fact, the circulation may actually be adequate but nonpulsatile in character, as occurs in coarctation of the aorta in which pulsations are not felt in the femoral artery and its branches because of the long, circuitous pathway the blood must take to reach the lower limbs.

1. Alterations Produced by Systemic Disorders and Local Nonvascular Tissues

Before determining whether local vascular disorders exist on the basis of an alteration in the state of the pulsations, it is necessary first to rule out the possibility that systemic conditions or syndromes producing obstruction of great vessels proximal to the extremities are responsible for the changes. Among the constitutional diseases that produce alterations in peripheral pulsations are shock, atrial fibrillation, the terminal stage of congestive heart failure, aortic stenosis and insufficiency, constrictive pericarditis, pericardial effusion with tamponade, and myocarditis. In the lower limbs, absence of pulsations or reduction in their amplitude may be produced by such disorders of the aorta as slow thrombosis of this vessel at its bifurcation, dissecting aneurysm, and coarctation. Extrinsic pressure on the artery or its main branches by tumors or other masses will have a similar effect.

Besides the distant influences, the pulsations in peripheral arteries may be affected by local changes in nonvascular tissues. Among these are alterations in thickness and consistency of the overlying skin and subcutaneous tissue, hypertrophy of the musculature covering the vessel, and the presence of pitting and nonpitting edema. Deposition of large amounts of subcutaneous fat in the vicinity of vessels will also interfere with their palpation, as will brawniness and induration of the overlying skin.

2. Changes Produced by Local Vascular Disorders

If distant vascular influences and abnormalities of local nonvascular structures can be ruled out, then variations in the amplitude of the pulsations in the extremities can be attributed to changes in the caliber of the arteries themselves. This may take the form of temporary vasospasm or dilatation (depending on the type of modification of vasomotor control) or of permanent structural alterations in the vessel wall.

Changes in vasomotor tone. Increased vasoconstrictor tone may reduce the amplitude of pulsations in an extremity by maintaining the vessel in a greater than normal state of contraction. In fact, if vasospasm is marked enough, pulsations may be completely lost. However, removal of vasomotor control by producing a block in the pathway of the peripheral sympathetic nervous system will very rapidly result in the return of pulsations.

If inhibition of sympathetic tone exists, then the amplitude of the pulsations is increased, due to passive dilatation of the vessels. Such a change is seen when there is need for heat dissipation, as in the presence of fever or on exposure of the extremities to a high environmental temperature, and also in certain abnormal states, such as erythromelalgia, in which there is an exaggerated response to a warm environment. Vasodilatation, with bounding pulses, is likewise noted in the early stage of trench foot, frostbite, and immersion foot, and in the presence of local inflammation. Complete but not permanent removal of vasomotor influence through sympathectomy will alter pulsations in a similar manner, provided the vessels are capable of dilating.

Permanent changes in vessel wall. In the presence of a local occlusive arterial disease, the alterations in amplitude of pulsations will depend upon the degree of impingement upon the lumen of the vessel by the stenotic process. Generally, if there is less than 50 percent obstruction to blood flow, very little change in pulsations can be identified by the relatively gross means of palpating the vessel. Beyond that point, there will be significant and readily perceived reductions in amplitude and force of the pulse wave. Complete occlusion of a proximal artery supplying the one under study or a similar process in the latter will result in absence of pulsations even when blood is entering the vessel distal to the block through collateral vessels, since the pulsatile quality is lost under such circumstances. Removal of vasomotor tone through the various available clinical means will generally have little or no effect on the amplitude of pulsations in the artery in which partial or complete organic blocks exist.

3. Technique of Examination

Practical measures. In the examination of the peripheral pulses, it is necessary to compare the amplitude and force of pulsations in one artery with those in the corresponding vessel on the opposite side. Only with experience can one determine what is normal for any single vessel. At all times the examiner should be comfortable while performing the test. If he assumes a position which places a strain on his muscles, this may result in dulling of his perceptive senses and the collection of incorrect information regarding the state of the arteries. Of importance in this regard is positioning the examination table so as to allow the observer to palpate the vessels from both sides of the patient. A possibility which must always be kept in mind is that when firm pressure is utilized in palpation of an artery, the pulse in the finger of the examiner may be mistaken for that in the vessel of the patient. It is necessary to vary the pressure depending upon the depth of the artery below the skin. This precaution also applies to weak pulsations which may

not be felt if the examining fingers compress the skin with much force. How the findings are recorded depends upon individual preference. The pulsations can be described as normal, slightly, moderately, or markedly reduced, or absent; or they can be recorded as ranging from 4 to 0, with the former figure representing the maximal normal amplitude.

Neck and upper limbs. In the upper part of the body, the first vessel to be examined is the *subclavian artery,* which can readily be palpated in all but very obese or muscular individuals by cupping the fingers over the clavicle so that the tips are located behind it (Fig. 5.2A). The *axillary artery,* which is a continuation of the subclavian artery, is identified by palpating the entire axilla (Fig. 5.2B). The *brachial artery* arises from the axillary artery and can be readily palpated by partially encircling the arm in its lower third with the examining hand and compress-

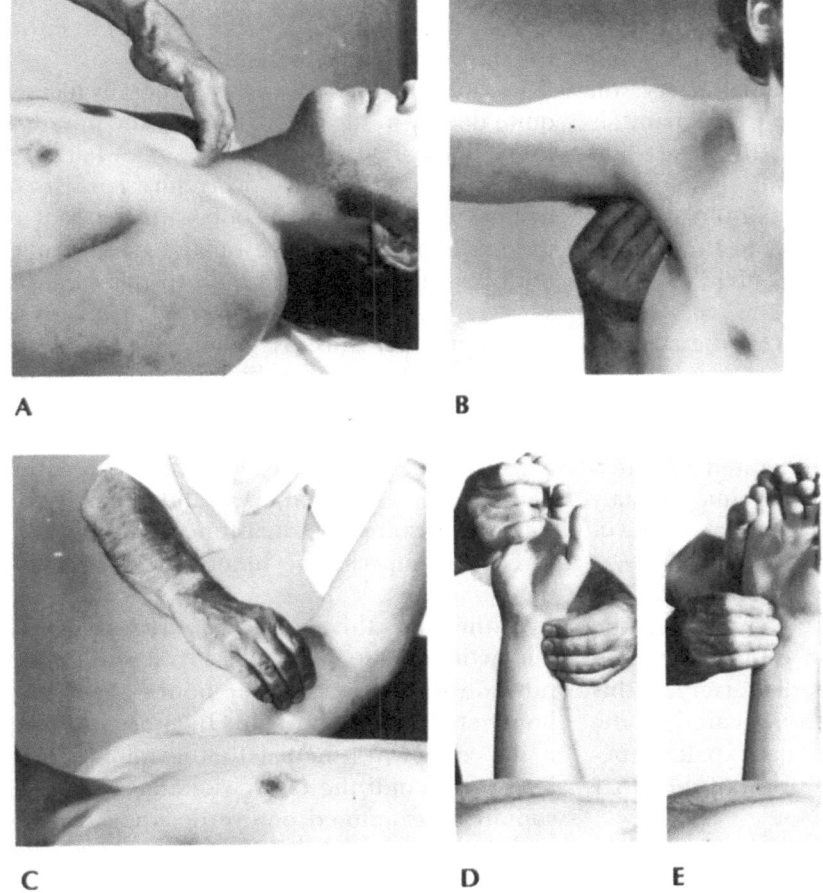

Fig. 5.2. Technique for palpation of arterial pulses in the neck and upper limbs. **A** Subclavian artery. **B** Axillary artery. **C** Brachial artery. **D** Radial artery. **E** Ulnar artery. From Abramson DI: Vascular Disorders of the Extremities. Hagerstown, Md, Harper & Row, 1974. Reproduced with permission.

ing the tissues on the medial aspect against the humerus (Fig. 5.2C). The *radial artery* is felt in the usual manner on the ventral surface of the wrist, medial to the styloid process of the radius (Fig. 5.2D). If pulsations are not palpated in this site, it is advisable to continue the examination proximally until the artery is palpated. Such a situation may arise if the vessel is occluded in its distal portion.

The *ulnar artery* can be felt at the same level at the wrist as the radial artery except that it is on the opposite side (Fig. 5.2E). Generally it is just as readily palpable as the latter. At times, however, it can only be felt with difficulty or not at all because of an aberrant location. When this is so, it is necessary to perform the ulnar confirmatory test (Allen's test) before concluding the vessel is absent. The procedure is done in the following manner: The upper extremity is elevated in order to facilitate venous drainage, and the radial artery at the wrist is obliterated by firm digital pressure. The subject then opens and closes his fist a number of times to effect further venous outflow, and with the compression of the radial artery still maintained and the fist closed, the hand is brought down to the level of the heart and the fist is now opened, no attempt being made to extend the fingers fully. If the ulnar artery is intact, there will be immediate flushing of the palm of the hand as blood enters the cutaneous microcirculation from this vessel and from the superficial volar arch. If the skin remains blanched so long as pressure is applied over the radial artery, becoming flushed when this is removed, it may then be assumed that either the ulnar artery is obliterated by a disease process or some type of anatomic anomaly exists in the connection between it and the volar arches.

By reversing the above-described procedure and digitally occluding the ulnar artery at the wrist, pertinent information can be obtained regarding the state of the radial artery at this location. The results are also evaluated on the basis of whether the palm remains pale or becomes flushed as digital occlusion of the ulnar artery is maintained.

Provided pulsations can be felt in both the radial and ulnar arteries at the wrist, slight modifications of the ulnar confirmatory test can be used to evaluate the state of the terminal vessels in the hand and fingers. For example, flushing of the palm but persistence of pallor in a finger or fingers, as digital compression of one of the two main arteries at the wrist is maintained, may indicate that the arcuate or the digital arteries, or both, are the site of an obstructive process. To confirm such an impression, on removal of digital compression of the artery at the wrist, the pallor should remain for some time and then be slowly replaced by a normal pink color. If, instead, the involved fingers immediately flush, it can be assumed that the digital arteries are patent but that the block is in a more proximally located vessel, close to its origin from the main artery.

Lower limbs. Examination of the vessels in these sites, with the possible exception of the popliteal artery, is accomplished without much difficulty. The *femoral artery* can be readily palpated in the groin below Poupart's ligament (Fig. 5.3A), its pulsations normally being greater than those of any other vessel in either the upper or lower extremities.

Because the *popliteal artery* is generally located quite deeply in the fatty tissues of the popliteal fossa, its palpation presents somewhat of a problem. A satisfactory procedure consists of having the patient lie prone with the foot of the extremity being investigated crossed over the back of the opposite limb to relax the tissues traversing the popliteal space. Considerable digital pressure is required to feel the artery, and this can be obtained by placing the fingers of the other hand over the examining fingers and pressing firmly (Fig. 5.3B). In such a manner the perceptive sense of the palpating digits is not deadened, as would occur if they were performing the dual function of exerting force to compress the tissues and of seeking the vessel.

In the foot, the *dorsal pedal artery* is usually felt in its course over the dorsal surface. Its position with respect to the bones of the foot, however, is quite variable. In most instances it lies somewhat medial to the midline (Fig. 5.4A), although the entire dorsum of the foot should be examined before deciding that the vessel is not present. The *posterior tibial artery* can be felt as it passes behind and beneath the medial malleolus. In the case of the left foot, the examiner should stand to the left of

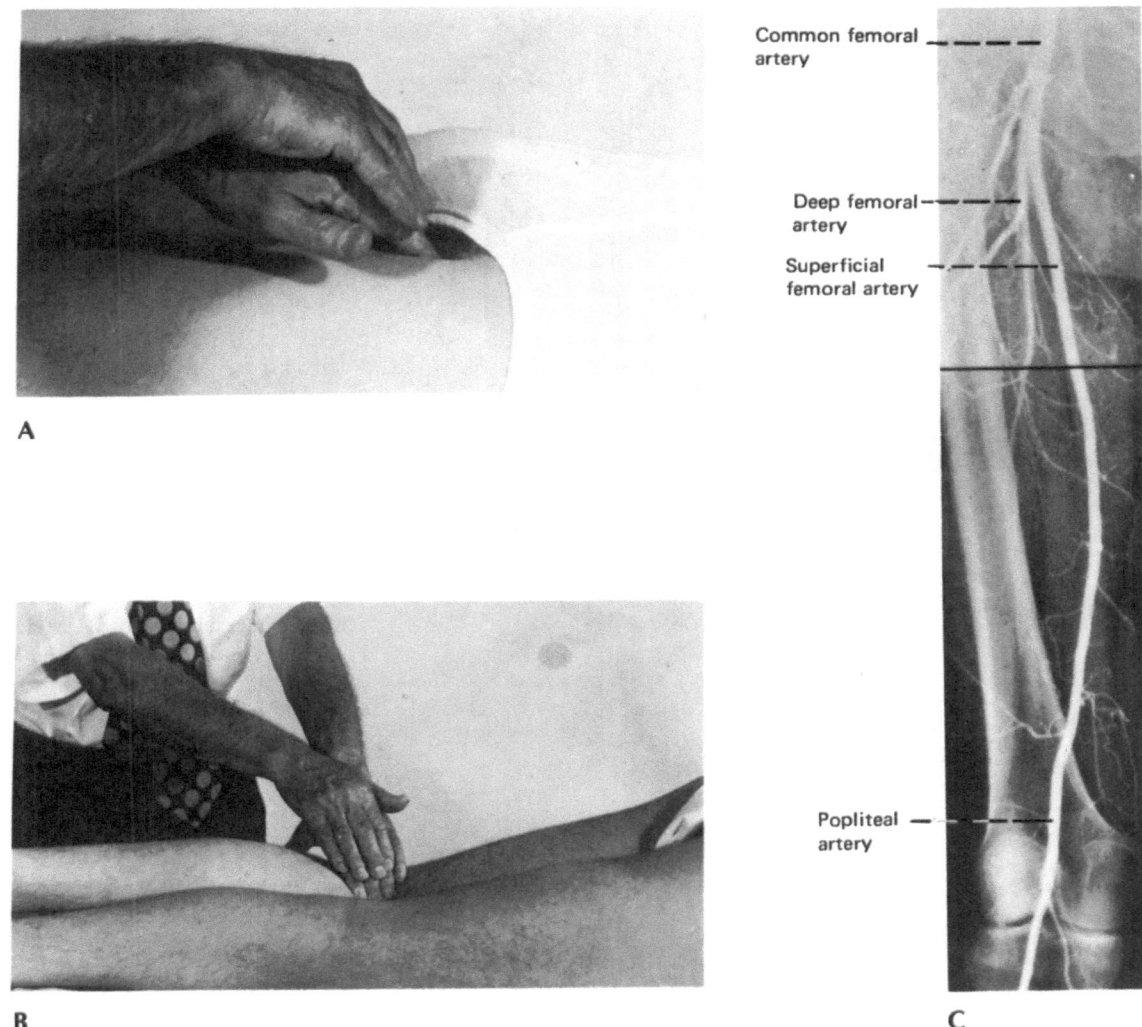

Fig. 5.3. Technique for palpation of arterial pulses in the lower limbs. **A** Femoral artery. **B** Popliteal artery. **C** Arteriographic representation of the location of the arteries. Modified from Abramson DI: Vascular Disorders of the Extremities. Hagerstown, Md, Harper & Row, 1974. Reproduced with permission.

the patient and cup the fingers of his right hand over the medial malleolus so that the fingertips slide off to enter the groove below (Fig. 5.4B). In the case of the right foot, the opposite position and the left hand of the examiner are utilized. Generally, firm pressure is necessary to feel the artery, the procedure being facilitated by simultaneously dorsiflexing and plantar flexing the foot slightly with the other hand, so as to place the vessel somewhat on a stretch.

Aberrant vessels. During the course of the examination, search for anomalous collateral arteries should always be kept in mind. With

obstruction of the popliteal artery, the lateral or medial superior genicular arteries should be looked for since under such circumstances they may become prominent in their course over the knee. In the absence of the posterior tibial artery, a large vessel may be noted along the upper border of the lateral malleolus (Fig. 5.4C) which is an enlarged perforating branch of the peroneal artery, the lateral tarsal artery.

Variations in technique. In individuals in whom absent peripheral pulsations in the lower limbs cannot be correlated with clinical manifestations, it is advisable to attempt several mea-

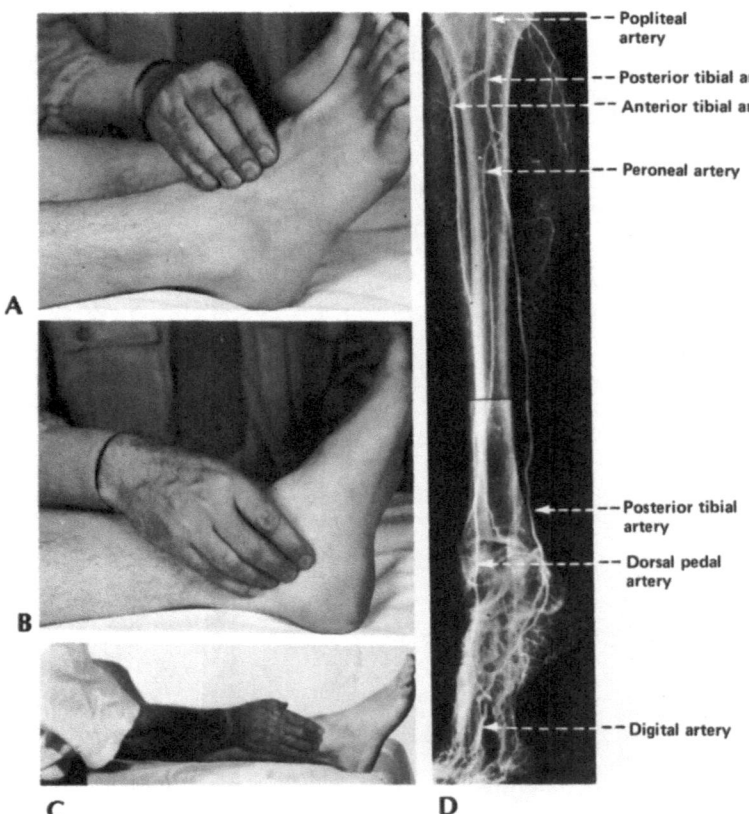

Fig. 5.4. Technique for palpation of arterial pulses in the feet. **A** Dorsal pedal artery. **B** Posterior tibial artery. **C** Penetrating branch of the peroneal artery (lateral tarsal branch). **D** Arteriographic representation of the location of the arteries in the leg and foot. **D**, from Abramson DI: Vascular Disorders of the Extremities. Hagerstown, Md, Harper & Row, 1974. Reproduced with permission.

sures in an effort to determine whether the noted changes actually represent the true degree of organic alterations in the arteries locally. One of these is to repeat the examination of the pulses with the patient sitting and his lower limbs in dependency. At times such a procedure allows for the recognition of pulsations which could not be felt otherwise. Another is to reexamine the patient immediately following a period of mild exercise. This may elicit pulsations which were not obtainable under resting conditions, probably because the increased cardiac output consequent to the physical effort now causes sufficient distension of a partially occluded artery to allow the pulse to become palpable to the examining finger. On occasion, however, a temporary loss of pulsations, previously palpated, may be noted under such circumstances. This apparent paradox may result from shunting of blood into proximally located maximally dilated vessels in the exercising muscles.

If absent pulsations are associated with signs of vasospasm, then it is advisable to effect temporary removal of vasomotor control, as by paravertebral sympathetic block or caudal block. Return of pulsations to a peripheral artery under such conditions indicates that vasospasm was responsible for the original abnormality.

Another more simple means of determining the role that vasospasm is playing in damping or obliterating pulsations in peripheral arteries is to have the patient lie down and to place a tablet of nitroglycerin, 0.4 mg (1/150 gr), under his tongue. In the presence of vasospasm, the pulses will become bounding in character within 2 to 5 min. On the other hand, if obliterative arterial disease exists, there will be little or no change in amplitude of pulsations. It is necessary to point out that after completion of the test, the patient may experience a flushed face, headache, and dizziness when he first stands.

4. Interpretation of Results

Absence of pulsations in the main arteries of the extremities does not always have the same connotation. Generally, inability to palpate the brachial, radial, ulnar, femoral, or posterior tibial arteries indicates the existence of either occlusive arterial disease or marked vasospasm. On occasion, however, the posterior tibial artery may be present but impalpable behind a prominent medial malleolus found in patients with a splayfoot. Similarly, the popliteal artery may not be felt because of anatomic alterations in the popliteal fossa. The absence of one or both dorsal pedal arteries has been reported as a normal variant in approximately 8 to 13 percent of people. When the vessel cannot be felt, it is advisable to palpate anteriorly over the ankle joint for the anterior tibial artery, of which it is a continuation.

B. Oscillometry

There is considerable difference of opinion regarding the value of oscillometry in peripheral vascular disorders. It is considered to be of little use by some workers, whereas others regard it as an important part of the vascular examination. On the basis of personal experience and observation, it would appear that the latter opinion has much in its favor.

1. Basis for Test

The oscillometer consists of a sensitive aneroid which is connected to a modified pneumatic cuff. The pulsatile change in the size of the limb with each cardiac systole produces a corresponding alteration in the air volume of the cuff. This is transmitted to the aneroid where it causes an amplified swing of the recording needle, the range of movement being noted on an arbitrary degree scale of the instrument. The increase in volume of the limb is related to the fact that more blood enters it through main arteries during the maximum ejection phase of the cardiac cycle than escapes into the proximal venous circulation; hence, the magnitude of the response as recorded by the oscillometer is an indirect index of the rate of local arterial inflow.

2. Technique

A number of satisfactory oscillometers are available commercially. All give reproducible results provided basic conditions are maintained. The environmental temperature must be constant, the readings must be collected with the subject lying down and after resting for 20 min or longer, and the cuff must be applied according to the simple directions supplied with the machine. Even under such conditions, in order to compare results obtained on a patient at different times, it is essential to use the identical instrument, since it is possible that those made by the same manufacturer at different times may vary somewhat in their sensitivity.

The pneumatic cuff is wrapped snugly around the limb, inflated to above systolic blood pressure, and then the pressure is lowered in steps of approximately 10 mmHg by means of an escape valve. Following each drop, the cuff is connected with the recording capsule and the range of movement of the needle is noted. The important reading is the one indicating the greatest excursion of the needle, the height of pressure at which this occurs appearing to have little clinical significance. Actually the pressure in the cuff acts merely as a coupling agent to transmit to the apparatus the increase in the size of the limb with each heartbeat. If the pressure is too high, this will interfere with the movement of blood into the limb. If it is too low, there will be inadequate transmission of the volume change in the extremity to the apparatus. By utilizing graded drops in pressure, the optimal change will thus be obtained, as reflected in the maximal swing of the oscillometer needle. The latter reading is considered to represent the greatest increase in the volume of the limb (at the level examined) with each heartbeat.

In every instance the cuff is applied around three sites. In the upper extremities, readings are usually obtained from the arm above the elbow, the proximal part of the forearm, and the wrist. In the lower extremities, the routine sites of application are the thigh above the knee, the calf, and the lower part of the leg above the ankle. On occasion the cuff is also applied high up on the thigh below Poupart's ligament. Placing it around the hand or foot gives information of little value, since the bony structures may support it and so interfere with the proper transmission of the pulsations to the instrument.

Normally there is a considerable variation in the results obtained from the various sites. The range is between 5 and 15 arbitrary units or higher for the arm above the elbow, the upper part of the forearm, the thigh just above the knee, and the calf; it is between 3 and 8 units or higher for the wrist and the leg immediately above the ankle. Figures which fall below the lower limit for any one of these sites should be viewed with suspicion. At times, in the obese individual the results at the thigh may be less than those at the calf, which obviously is an artifact.

When oscillometry is used to study the circulation in the lower limbs, it is always necessary to establish a reference reading obtained from an arm or forearm, provided pulsations are present in the ulnar and radial arteries at the wrist. Such a figure reflects changes produced in a normal vascular bed by any existing systemic disorders responsible for alterations in systolic discharge and hence in oscillometric data. By comparing this reading with those collected from the lower extremities, the effect on the latter of distant influences can thus be recognized and discounted.

3. Interpretation of Results

Oscillometry is an important tool in the evaluation of the arterial circulation in the limbs, provided one is fully aware of its limitations. It not only substantiates the information obtained by palpation of peripheral pulses, but it also gives a much more complete picture of the state of the main arteries than can possibly be obtained from digital examination alone. With it, a readily reproducible record is available which is expressed quantitatively, in contrast to the purely qualitative and subjective impression that results from palpation of an artery. Repeat studies at intervals using the same instrument

will give pertinent information on whether there has been any progression in the obliterative process. The procedure is also of value in determining mild degrees of impairment of arterial circulation, not reflected in sufficient reduction in amplitude of pulsations to be obvious by palpation. Similarly, it is helpful in diagnosing the presence of a block in an artery and in its location, data which are very important when embolectomy is being contemplated. Finally, the procedure is useful when local changes in nonvascular tissues make palpation of vessels difficult, as in the presence of obesity, edema, and induration and brawniness of the skin around the ankle. (For the application of the oscillometer to the problem of determining the proper level of amputation of a limb, see p. 348.)

4. Limitations of and Contraindications to Use of Method

One main limitation of oscillometry is the fact that the instruments available for clinical application are not sensitive enough to pick up oscillations in small collateral vessels, in which the pressure is lower than in the main arteries of the limb and pulsatile flow is minimal. Since in an occlusive arterial disease, this secondary system frequently carries on the principal function of supplying the tissues with nutrition, it is obvious that information derived from oscillometry alone would be of little value in determining the overall state of the local circulation. Also, there could be structural impairment of the small arteries and arterioles distal to the main channels, leading to partial anoxia of the tissues, and still with no corresponding decrease in the oscillometric measurements of the limb. Because of these inherent weaknesses of the method, oscillometry is of little value when arriving at a proper conclusion regarding prognosis.

When it is suspected that a thrombus is located in the deep venous plexuses of the calf muscles (phlebothrombosis), then oscillometry should not be performed on the lower limbs. Theoretically, at least, the application of a high pressure to the calf could conceivably be responsible for the liberation of a friable clot into the main venous circulation, with the production of a pulmonary embolism. The history of trauma to the limbs, due to lodgment of foreign bodies such as shell fragments in soft tissues in the vicinity of main arteries, is also a contraindication to oscillometry. Under such circumstances, in an attempt to obtain a reading, the application of the initially high pressure could result in injury to the vessels or the latter could go into spasm with a consequent marked ischemia of distal tissues. Finally, the presence of cellulitis or lymphangitis in the portion of limb under study prevents the use of oscillometry for obvious reasons.

C. Auscultation of Main Arteries and of Sites of Trauma

Auscultation over the main arteries in the abdominal cavity and the limbs to determine whether bruits exist gives essential information regarding the presence or absence of partial blocks in these vessels or of proximal ones which supply them with blood.

1. Pathogenesis

Bruits are acoustic vibrations, appreciated by the ear as murmurs, which are produced by turbulent nonlaminar flow of blood as it passes through a stenotic segment of artery into a normal caliber-sized vessel. The sounds are heard only when there is a pressure drop, and hence a pressure gradient, across the partially occluded portion of vessel.

Resting state. During such a period the bruit is crescendo in intensity in the early part of systole and decrescendo in the latter part. Its other characteristics will depend upon the velocity of blood flow, the degree of stenosis, and the conductance of the overlying and surrounding tissues. When metabolic needs are low (as under basal conditions), requiring only a minimal local circulation, a slight stenosis introduces no significant impedance to blood flow, and so no sound is produced. The reason is that the pressure drop across the partially occluded vessel is negligible. With more

marked narrowing of the artery the pressure drop increases and, as a consequence, the velocity of the blood flow also rises, producing vibrations even under resting conditions. The more extreme the stenosis, the louder and harsher does the sound become. At the same time, its duration is lengthened, so that with a severe degree of partial occlusion, the murmur may extend into diastole [16]. Under the latter circumstances, generally there is also an inadequate collateral circulation, a situation which contributes to the development of a very low diastolic pressure in the distal portion of the involved artery, beyond the block. Hence, a significant gradient of pressure across the point of obstruction is also present during diastole. Consequently, there is a continued rapid movement of blood through the stenotic portion, this being responsible for the production of a diastolic component to the murmur.

Physical work. During a period of increased metabolic activity, as initiated by physical exercise, even a slight stenosis may have a significant retarding effect on the resulting augmented blood flow. At the same time, the associated peripheral vasodilatation enhances the movement of blood out of the arterial tree into the microcirculation of the active tissues, thus causing an even lower pressure in the artery distal to the obstruction. As a result, the steepness of the pressure gradient across the stenotic segment increases, causing an acceleration in the velocity of the bloodstream and in the development of eddy currents and acoustic vibrations interpreted as a bruit.

With a greater degree of stenosis, physical exertion may convert a systolic bruit into one that is also heard during the initial phase of diastole [22]. Under such circumstances, there is a decrease in diastolic blood pressure in the portion of vessel distal to the partial obstruction, due to dilatation of small vessels and augmented blood flow into the active muscles. With the diastolic pressure proximal to the lesion generally being unaffected by the physical effort, the result is an increase in the pressure gradient across the stenotic segment. Such a state causes a rapid movement of blood even during diastole and hence continuation of the bruit into the early phase of this period.

It is apparent from the above that in those

cases in which there is no interference with the movement of blood through a normal artery, no murmurs can be expected to be heard by auscultation. The same holds true if there is no blood flow through a diseased vessel because of complete occlusion of its lumen by a thrombus or by extrinsic pressure.

2. Technique

Care must always be taken to place the bell of the stethoscope lightly in contact with the skin overlying the artery under study; otherwise, there will be distortion of the vessel and the production of a bruit even under normal conditions. Substitution of the diaphragm of the stethoscope tends to reduce the possibility of eliciting such an artifact because of the larger area over which the pressure is distributed.

A simple means of determining whether a murmur has significance is first to obtain an oscillometric reading at a level below the site of examination of the vessel and then at the time that a definite bruit is heard over the artery, to obtain another reading. If both are the same, it can be assumed that the murmur has its etiology in an occlusive pathologic process in the blood vessel wall. On the other hand, if the figure is now significantly less, the auscultatory finding is probably due to partial obstruction of the artery by the local extrinsic pressure exerted during the test.

Another important point to be taken into consideration is that the intensity of the bruit will, in part, depend upon the thickness of the interposed damping tissue; the less of the latter, the more likely will the murmur reach audible levels.

In the lower portion of the body, the following sites lend themselves to auscultation for bruits: on the anterior abdominal wall at the level of the aortic bifurcation and laterally overlying the external iliac artery; in the groin over the femoral artery; and in the popliteal fossa over the popliteal artery. In the upper portion of the body, bruits are sought for over the full length of the carotid arteries; over the origin of the innominate artery on the right side and the subclavian artery on the left side, at the base of the neck; over the axillary artery in the axilla; and over the bifurcation of the brachial artery somewhat above the antecubital space.

Aside from examination of the main arteries, auscultation should be routinely employed in the examination of scars located in the vicinity of large vessels, to determine whether the original trauma had produced an arterial aneurysm or an arteriovenous fistula. Injured soft tissue masses, such as a traumatized large muscle group, should also be studied for the presence of bruits, particularly if the difficulty was caused by a high-velocity missile.

3. Precautions in Interpretation of Findings

Some care must be taken in attributing proper significance to bruits heard over the peripheral arteries. Aside from the production of iatrogenic murmurs (see above), it is also necessary to keep in mind that tortuosity of a large artery, whether on a congenital basis or due to elongation and loss of elastic properties, may be responsible for the development of acoustic vibrations, despite the absence of any organic stenosis in the vessel. Other conditions in which such a situation exists are external compression of an artery, as by a tumor, an arteriovenous fistula (see F-2, Chapter 15), and an arterial aneurysm (see E-2, Chapter 15). Finally, bruits may be heard in the absence of stenosis if the flow or velocity rates are high and the vessel wall is elastic [17]. Only when all such states can be ruled out does a bruit signify a reduction in lumen size due to organic changes in the wall of the vessel.

In most instances, bruits due to stenosis of an artery are transmitted in a downstream direction from the site of origin, provided the distal portion of the channel is patent. It is for this reason that a partial occlusion of the common iliac artery at its bifurcation is associated with a murmur which may be heard either in the lower portion of the abdomen over the external iliac artery, in the groin over the femoral artery, or on occasion over the superficial femoral and popliteal arteries. A bruit originating in the common femoral artery is also audible in the groin, over the location of this vessel.

4. Information Derived from Combined Auscultation and Palpation of Arteries

Significant data can be collected if the results of auscultation are compared with those obtained by palpation. For example, a reduced femoral pulsation in the groin and a bruit heard over the lower portion of the abdomen suggest the existence of incomplete occlusion of the common or external iliac artery. Absence of a pulse in the femoral artery associated with a bruit over the external iliac artery in the lower abdomen probably indicates stenosis of the latter or of the common iliac artery and complete occlusion of the common femoral artery. When no pulse is present in the common femoral artery and no bruits are heard over the abdomen, this may mean either that the iliac arteries are also completely obstructed or that they are fully patent but that a total block exists only in the common femoral artery. Naturally, information derived from auscultation of the anterior abdominal wall has significance only if the latter does not contain a large quantity of fat.

D. Noninvasive Laboratory Procedures

1. Ultrasound Echography (Aortosonography)

Ultrasound echography is a very useful, rapid, and accurate noninvasive tool for identifying the contour, location, lumen size, and wall thickness of abdominal aortic aneurysms. It can be repeated as often as desired since the process is innocuous, and hence it is very helpful in ascertaining whether a lesion is enlarging. The technique requires the use of commercially available A-mode ultrasound equipment, with the echo pattern being displayed on an oscilloscope and photographed using self-developing film.

A standard 2.25-megacycle transducer, acoustically coupled with water-soluble gel, is applied to the anterior abdominal wall. First it is placed to the left of the midline and then moved until two strong groups of echoes, showing a slight expansile movement with an echo-free zone between them, appear on the oscillograph [4]. These images represent the near and far walls of the aorta and its lumen. From them, the overall diameter of the vessel can be determined by considering the distance between the takeoff of the first echo in the anterior wall complex and the furthest echo in the posterior aortic wall complex. By moving the transducer downward in a stepwise fashion, beginning with a site just below the xiphoid to one corresponding to the aortic bifurcation, determinations of the anteroposterior measurements of the abdominal aorta are made at various levels. Readings in lateral projections are also obtained from locations which are satisfactory for placement of the transducer.

2. Doppler Ultrasonic Flowmeter

The Doppler ultrasonic flowmeter is another noninvasive method which is of value in measuring flow velocity in major arteries in the limbs. It has the advantage of being able to obtain pertinent information at the bedside without the need to use an expensive recording apparatus.

Technique. The principle on which the method is based is the Doppler phenomenon whereby sound reflected from a moving object undergoes a shift in frequency which is proportional to the velocity of the object. The instruments available commercially all consist of a probe housing two piezometer electric crystals. One of these, driven by an oscillator, projects a 2- to 10-megacycle continuous ultrasound beam which is directed transcutaneously through the tissues overlying the artery under study. The reflected (backscattered) beam is detected by the second crystal in the probe and is converted to an electric signal. By sensing and amplifying the phase shifts that occur when the ultrasound waves are scattered by the moving cells in the bloodstream, the instrument is able to detect changes in velocity of flow, using either visual or preferably audible (loudspeaker or earphone) recordings of the flow pattern. In a patent vessel conveying blood, the frequency of the received sound differs from that of the projected one by an amount proportional to the velocity of the blood. In the absence of movement of blood through an artery, due to a complete obstruction, the frequencies of the projected and the backscattered sounds are identical.

Data are collected by placing the Doppler probe on the skin directly over a pulsating artery or in locations in which the vessels are generally palpated (see A-3, above) and noting the character of the sound. A water-soluble gel is used to conduct signals between the skin and probe. In order to tax the local vascular tree, either a period of exercise on the treadmill or 5 min of arterial occlusion are carried out and the Doppler sounds are recorded and compared with the ones obtained at rest [7].

Sounds over vessels with unimpeded flow.

Normally the sound heard over arteries is multiphasic, with a high-pitched hissing noise present during systole, followed in diastole by one or two short, medium-pitched sounds of lower intensity. An increase in blood velocity causes all of the sounds to be higher-pitched. Normal variations in rate of blood flow during the cardiac cycle can also be identified, including that associated with the dicrotic notch in the catacrotic limb of the pulse wave.

Changes produced by occlusive arterial disease.

When partial or complete block exists in the local arterial tree, characteristic changes occur in the sounds detected by the probe. A stenosing obstruction in a large artery causes damping of the systolic peak and loss of retrograde flow, giving a monophasic, low-pitched sound which extends through most of the cardiac cycle; the discrete diastolic sounds are lost. Partial obstruction of distal vessels produces a "water-hammer" effect, which consists of a short, sharp, higher-pitched sound [7]. As the probe is passed over the skin along the course of the stenosed artery under study, the intensity of the sound tends to become greater until a total occlusion is encountered, at which point and immediately beyond it all sound disappears. In the case of a stenotic lesion, the probe picks up an increase in pitch because of the greater velocity of the blood passing through the narrowed segment of vessel. Where flow is dependent solely upon movement of blood through collateral arteries, the sound heard with the instrument has a blunted and dull quality, rather than the sharp, clear-cut sound heard over a normal artery.

Evaluation of procedure in occlusive arterial disease.

The Doppler ultrasonic flowmeter is a very helpful noninvasive diagnostic tool for determining whether an occlusive arterial disorder exists, for detecting the sites of partial or complete occlusion, and for ascertaining whether progression of the obstructive process is occurring. In all these regards, the procedure appears to elicit practically the same type of information obtainable with the much less complicated and much less costly oscillometer (see Section B, above). Neither one, however, can replace contrast arteriography (see Section E, below) as a means of obtaining pertinent technical information in potential candidates for vascular reconstructive procedures, such as the extent and location of partial and complete blocks, their number, and the state of the distal runoff. Because the Doppler ultrasonic flowmeter is extremely sensitive, it is advisable to point out that an audible signal is not necessarily equivalent to a palpable arterial pulse; nor does it represent an amplified bruit.

Application of method in determining ankle blood pressure.

The Doppler ultrasonic flowmeter can be used to obtain blood pressure readings from the tibial arteries at the ankle, information of great value in the study of the arterial circulation in the foot [11]. The procedure is performed in the following manner: The probe is positioned over the posterior tibial artery just distal to the internal malleolus. A blood pressure cuff is wrapped around the middle or upper part of the leg, the pressure in it is raised to above systolic level, and then it is dropped in a stepwise fashion until there is reappearance of sound over the artery as detected by the probe. The level at which this occurs is considered to be the systolic pressure in the vessel. In a similar manner, blood pressure can be obtained in the anterior tibial and dorsal pedal arteries in the ankle and foot, respectively. If the results are equivocal, then it is necessary for the patient to perform a period of exercise on the treadmill and for the examiner to report the readings immediately after termination of the physical effort and for several minutes afterward.

In normal individuals, resting ankle blood pressure is approximately the same as that in the brachial artery. Atherosclerotic changes in the arterial tree of the lower limbs significantly reduce the level of resting ankle blood pressure, the amount of depression depending upon the degree of involvement.

Some indication of the extent and severity of the disease can also be obtained from the results elicited by exercise. In patients with either no or minor atheromatous change, physical effort generally produces an increase in ankle blood pressure. In those with a significant amount of stenosis or complete occlusion of the superficial femoral artery, but with a highly developed collateral circulation and adequate outflow, exercise is immediately followed by a moderate reduction in ankle blood pressure and a return to the control level within 5 min. In the presence of a much less efficient secondary circulation and complete occlusion of the superficial femoral artery or of involvement also of the iliofemoral artery but with good collateralization, ankle blood pressure may fall to zero after termination of exercise, to return to the control baseline in 7 to 15 min. With further progression of the occlusive disease in the local arterial tree and a poor development of the collateral circulation, exercise likewise produces an initial zero ankle blood pressure, but with the reading returning to the preexercise level only after a delay of 15 to 22 min.

3. Graphic Representation of Pulse Waves

Pertinent information regarding the local arterial circulation can be obtained from the study of the contour and amplitude of pulse wave recordings obtained from a digit or segment of limb. For this purpose, a number of instruments are available commercially, including a pneumatic cuff connected to a transducing system, a recording oscillometer, a direct writing pneumoplethysmograph (Vasograph), a simplified mercury strain-gauge plethysmograph, and an impedance plethysmograph. The last two instruments have had the widest clinical use and hence will be described below.

Mercury strain gauge. This instrument, a slender elastic tube filled with mercury, is wrapped around the extremity at the level under study. With changes in volume of the limb, there is a corresponding alteration in its circumference. The stretching or shortening of the elastic tube affects the electric resistance of the mercury column in the tube and produces an analog signal that is altered in proportion to the changes in limb volume.

Impedance plethysmograph. This apparatus utilizes paired electrodes, applied directly to the limb, which act to pass a high frequency, low-current signal through the tissues locally. Differences in the volume of blood in the extremity cause corresponding changes in the electric impedance, thus producing an analog signal which is directly related to the volume of the limb segment at the moment the tracing is recorded. Although this method, as well as the mercury strain-gauge plethysmograph, can be calibrated to give quantitative figures, such a step is unnecessary when used to detect or analyze simple waveforms at the bedside.

Interpretation of normal pulse waves. Arterial pulsations recorded from the limbs by either mercury strain-gauge or impedance plethysmography present the typical characteristics of a pulse wave. There is a rapidly rising upstroke, with a sharply rounded systolic peak occurring early in the cardiac cycle, followed by a downstroke which is concave upward and contains a dicrotic notch.

Changes in pulse waves produced by chronic occlusive arterial disease. A study of pulse waves helps in determining early involvement of the arterial tree, the site of stenosis, and progression of the obstructive process. It can also accurately predict the success or failure of bypass procedures.

In the early stage of an occlusive arterial disease, the anacrotic limb of the pulse wave tends to demonstrate a slow ascent and a reduction in amplitude. There is a rounding of the peak and the catacrotic limb manifests a slow descent, with a shallow dicrotic notch on it. As the occlusive process progresses, more rounding of the peak occurs, even to the point of becoming saw-toothed or umbrella-shaped in contour; there is also a delay in recording the curve, as compared with one obtained from an opposite normal limb. Severe stenosis manifests itself in the form of obliteration of the dicrotic notch and, in the presence of far-advanced diffuse occlusive involvement, complete absence of the pulse wave, a flat line intervening. If there are short segmental occlusions, associated with a good collateral flow and absence of small-artery disease, the pulse wave curve may be normal in all regards. However, if the secondary circulation is inadequate, then the systolic portion of the curve becomes flattened.

Placing a load upon the local vascular tree may bring out abnormalities in the pulse wave that are not noted under resting conditions. For this purpose, it is necessary to produce a period of complete anoxia of distal tissues by the application of an arterial occlusion pressure for 3 to 8 min at a proximal site. In both normal and abnormal individuals, there is an initial disappearance of the dicrotic notch in the record obtained immediately after release of pressure. Whereas rapid return of the curve to the preocclusion appearance is noted in the normal person (1 to 8 s), in the patient with chronic occlusive arterial disease there is a marked delay in the reappearance of the dicrotic notch (9 to 300 s) [2]. At the same time, the magnitude of the control peak may not be reached until 2 to 3 min after release of the arterial occlusion pressure.

The alterations in the pulse wave in chronic occlusive arterial disease reflect the changes in hemodynamics produced by an obstruction to blood flow. For example, if there is a high partial occlusion in a main artery, the end pressure in the segment of vessel proximal to the block is converted into a lateral pressure, so that blood now passes into opened collateral arteries arising in this location. Since the secondary channels are of smaller caliber, the blood encounters a greater resistance to flow. This results in a drop in systolic blood pressure distally, the magnitude of the fall being inversely related to the extent and efficiency of the functioning collateral circulation. In the presence of a patent arterial tree below the level of the block, the blood from the collateral vessels enters it, for such a pathway represents an area of decreased peripheral resistance. Hence, the fall in blood pressure due to the proximal obstruction is minimal and so the appearance of the digital pulse wave curve is little altered, if at all. On the other hand, if there is a distal obstruction also, with the result that flow to the digits must take place wholly through high-resistance, small-calibered collateral vessels, then an increased blood pressure gradient develops, the resulting reduced pressure causing significant changes in the contour and amplitude of the digital pulse wave curve.

Changes observed in vasospastic disorders. Increased vasomotor tone may be responsible for the appearance of spontaneous large, slow deflections in the pulse wave record; such findings suggest that there are rhythmic alterations in vasomotor activity. An associated change may be the existence of an active reflex following deep inspiration which is caused by vasoconstriction of small arteries and arterioles. Absence of such alterations indicates that vasomotor tone is low. In contrast with the responses in patients with chronic occlusive arterial disease, in the presence of vasospasm, a state of reactive hyperemia produced by a period of arterial occlusion pressure elicits a pulse wave curve which approaches that of the normal individual under similar circumstances (see above).

E.   Contrast Angiography

Contrast angiography is an invasive technique which is used to visualize the arterial tree in the limbs and elsewhere through the intraarterial injection of a radiopaque material, followed by radiographic study.

1.   Techniques

No attempt is made in this section to describe in detail the various angiographic procedures, since such information is readily available in monographs on the subject [5]. Instead, only a brief discussion of the different types of techniques is presented.

Radiopaque materials.   The currently available contrast media, if properly administered, are quite safe and yield excellent visualization of the arterial tree. The most commonly used preparations are the different concentrations of Hypaque-M (90%, 75%, 60%); Hypaque Sodium, 50%; Renografin-76; Renografin-60; and Angio-Conray (80%, 60%). Angio-Conray appears to be the least toxic of these substances, although actually, when utilized in peripheral angiography, there is no problem with regard to toxicity in the case of any of the commonly used contrast materials. All of them are iodine compounds which are readily excreted by the kidneys. The reason for their use in angiography is that they absorb the x-ray beam to a higher or lower degree than do the surrounding structures. Hence, when they are injected intraarterially and films are exposed to the beam, the resulting radiograph demonstrates opacification of the patent arterial tree. As a general rule, the injection is made as close to the area of interest as possible, so that the contrast medium will be delivered to the vascular bed under study in a concentrated form, this depending upon the amount of iodine present and the rate at which it reaches the site.

Despite the fact that local vasospasm may follow the intraarterial injection of the various contrast media, these substances have been found to have a vasodilating effect in dogs and in human subjects [18,23]. It is possible that the unpleasant symptoms elicited by the procedure (see below), acting as noxious impulses, are responsible for the predominant vascular constriction, while the much less powerful pharmacologic dilating effect of the contrast agents has no significant influence on the clinical manifestations.

Preliminary precautionary measures. The intraarterial injection of a large quantity of contrast medium should be preceded by intravenous administration of a very small amount as a test dose. Also, medications should always be available in the arteriographic room to combat an allergic response, including epinephrine, 1:1000; diphenhydramine hydrochloride (Benadryl); intravenous pentobarbital sodium (Nembutal); isoproterenol hydrochloride (Isuprel Hydrochloride); calcium gluconate; and caffeine sodium benzoate. Renal function tests should be performed on all patients with suspected kidney disease and those with significant renal impairment should not be subjected to angiography unless the information thus de-

rived is essential and cannot be obtained by any other means. Other prophylactic measures which have been recommended, especially for very ill patients, are avoidance of fluid restriction and intravenous mannitol infusion before and during angiography.

Abdominal aortography. The abdominal aorta and its main branches are visualized using several approaches. The one which utilizes the translumbar route gives the most definitive opacification of the vessels and accordingly is performed most often. However, reducing its value and hence its clinical application is the fact that it may be followed by several very serious complications (see E-3, below).

In contrast, intravenous aortography is well tolerated, simple, and associated with minimal complications. It involves injection of the contrast medium through a polyethylene catheter which has been inserted into the median antecubital vein and advanced to the level of the axilla. The procedure can be used in patients with a known or suspected abdominal aortic aneurysm, in whom translumbar aortography might cause very serious difficulties. In this regard, it is helpful in determining the exact location, extent, and diameter of the lesion and in ascertaining whether the process is multiple and whether the renal arteries are involved in the pathologic process. Unfortunately, intravenous aortography has several disadvantages, among which is the need to inject large quantities of the contrast medium at one time. Another point which detracts from its usefulness is that there is often poor detail in outlining the smaller ramifications of the aortic branches because of dilution of the contrast medium by the blood.

Retrograde transfemoral percutaneous aortography involves passing a catheter into the femoral artery in the groin in a cephalad direction using Seldinger's technique [20]. The instrument is then advanced to the desired level in the abdominal aorta under fluoroscopic control, and with the patient performing a Valsalva's maneuver, the contrast medium is administered with an automatic pressure injector.

Arteriography. For visualization of the arterial tree in the lower limbs, one or both femoral arteries in the groin are punctured, polyethylene catheters are passed through the needles in the direction of the aortic bifurcation, and the contrast medium is injected. Then serial films are taken. Since the proximal portion of the deep femoral artery is normally overshadowed by the common and superficial femoral arteries, it is also necessary to employ an isolated lateral view in order to determine whether this vessel is involved in the atherosclerotic process.

In the case of the upper limb, the arterial tree is visualized by percutaneous injection of the radiopaque medium into the brachial artery above the elbow, using a specially designed blunt-end 17-gauge needle with a point obturator. Through serial filming, the passage of the contrast material through various portions of the arterial tree in the limb is recorded. On occasion the axillary artery is substituted for the brachial artery, but not the subclavian artery, since this vessel has little if any sheath around it, so that bleeding is difficult to control after removal of the needle.

Pedal angiography. When it is necessary to visualize the tibial arteries at the ankle (Fig. 5.5), as in the case of a salvage operation, some modifications in technique are required, since injection of the contrast medium into the femoral artery at the groin rarely elicits the desired information. A number of different approaches are available for this purpose, one of which involves passing a small catheter (red Odman or polyethylene 205) from the common femoral into the distal segment of the popliteal artery and delivering the contrast material from this point. Another consists first of the administration of sodium thiopental (Pentothal Sodium), 0.5 to 1.0 g, intravenously, supplemented by a muscle-relaxing drug (succinylcholine, 60 to 100 mg). This is then followed by injection of the contrast medium through a Cournand needle introduced under local anesthesia upstream into the femoral artery; the use of an automatic high-pressure delivery syringe facilitates administration of the material [12]. Regulated respiration is maintained during the period of paralysis of respiratory muscles produced by

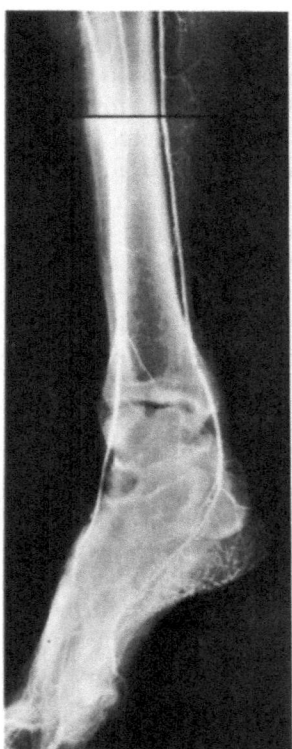 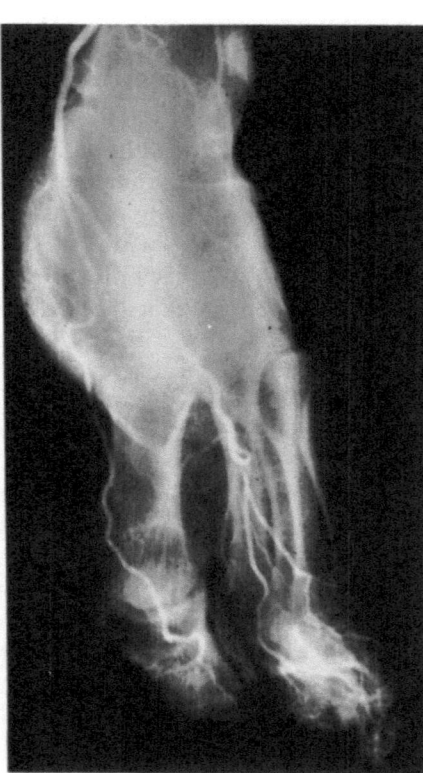

A   B

Fig. 5.5. Arteriograms demonstrating visualization of arteries in the lower portion of the leg and foot (**A**) and the digital vessels (**B**).

the muscle-relaxing drug. Other means of visualizing the vessels of the feet involve the preliminary production of reactive hyperemia [6] and the initial intraarterial injection of tolazoline hydrochloride (Priscoline).

2. Immediate Responses to Injection of Contrast Medium

As a quantity of the radiopaque material enters the local arterial tree under pressure, patients frequently experience a very unpleasant searing, burning sensation, which travels down the full length of the limb. At times it is so severe that some of them will not give permission for subsequent angiograms unless promised that general anesthesia will be employed. On the other hand, other individuals with a high threshold for pain will have very few symptoms. In those persons who voice complaints, usually peripheral vasoconstriction and contraction of voluntary muscles occur, not infrequently associated with generalized flushing of the skin and a feeling of warmth. At times there may be an erythematous eruption, nausea, vomiting, cyanosis, respiratory distress, and a fall in blood pressure. Such responses usually subside within a few minutes to an hour. However, if hypersensitivity or idiosyncrasy to the contrast medium is the cause of the reaction, the outlook may be very grave.

3. Complications of Contrast Angiography

Both local and systemic complications of angiography are prone to occur in infancy and childhood, when the vessels are particularly susceptible to spasm, and in old age, when the incidence of arteriosclerosis obliterans is high. The greatest risks are related to the mechanical aspects of the procedure, namely, the insertion of the needle or catheter and exposure of the vessel to the injection pressure.

Local responses common to all techniques. A relatively frequent complication of angiography is extravasation of radiopaque medium, with infiltration of adventitial or periarterial tissue. As a result of the accumulation of the mate-

rial, an inflammatory reaction may develop, followed by induration and fibrosis. However, since the contrast media presently being used are rapidly absorbed, such complications rarely occur, especially if moist applications and external heat are applied to encourage resorption of the material. Hematomas at the site of the injection are also usually controlled promptly.

Local destruction of the arterial wall due to catheterization is a much more serious complication of angiography since it may be followed by thrombosis of the vessel. The development of the latter requires immediate vascular reconstructive surgery if a critical artery is occluded. With the use of a needle, local dissection of the arterial wall may follow as a result of partial extrusion of the needle from the vessel. Such a lesion generally produces no serious difficulty since the blood pressure causes the intima and media to be compressed against the adventitia.

Of grave significance is the development of severe vasospasm of the local arterial tree. Such a response may be initiated by the trauma to the artery resulting from the needle puncture or from the force of the injection causing arterial distension. The noxious effect of the contrast medium may also contribute to the abnormal reaction. The clinical manifestations of intense vasospasm consist of severe pain in and blanching of the limb and, after several hours, the appearance of scattered violaceous plaques in the skin below the point of injection, these representing cutaneous and subcutaneous hemorrhages. Motor paralysis, loss of deep reflexes, and anesthesia may be present in the distal portion of the limb. In most cases there is a gradual return of sensation and movement, and in a week or 10 days, the limb becomes normal. At times, however, prolonged spasm may then be followed by arterial thrombosis and possibly the development of superficial gangrene.

Finally, infection in the form of a local abscess may arise at the site of puncture of the artery. If left untreated, it may result in thrombosis of the vessel. Hence, immediate incision and drainage must be carried out, and if occlusion of the artery has already taken place, a reconstructive procedure must be performed. However, in the presence of suppuration, the possibility of achieving a satisfactory result is slight. Because such a situation may lead to the loss of a limb, all efforts should be directed toward preventing infection by performing elective arteriography with meticulous care and sterility.

Complications of translumbar aortography. Since translumbar aortography involves a blind approach to the injection of the contrast medium into the aorta, the possibility of serious complications is greatly enhanced. For example, if the needle or catheter is inadvertently allowed to enter the lumen of a small visceral vessel leading to a single organ, injection of the concentrated radiopaque material may cause necrosis of distal tissues. Another serious consequence of translumbar aortography is paraplegia, which is likely to occur in Leriche's syndrome, in which there is delay in clearing of the contrast medium from the aorta. A number of explanations have been offered regarding the mechanism responsible for this state. Among these are the direct toxic action of the radiopaque material and damage to or thrombosis of the major radicular artery, the sole vascular supply to the upper lumbar and lower dorsal spinal cord [13]. Other complications are progressive dissection of the aortic wall producing tearing of the origins of spinal arteries and passage of the needle through the intervertebral disk into the spinal canal due to improper technique, with escape of the contrast medium into the subarachnoid space during injection. Among less serious complications are extravascular injection into soft tissues, hematoma formation, and rarely peritoneal irritation produced by intraperitoneal insertion of the needle.

Some of the above difficulties occur less frequently if an occluded tip and a side-hole needle or a catheter is substituted for the conventional end-opening aortography needle. A small test injection followed by exposure of a film is helpful in confirming that the needle is correctly positioned before making the main pressure injection, thus significantly reducing the incidence of subintimal deposition of contrast medium.

Complications of retrograde transfemoral percutaneous aortography. In the presence of severe atherosclerosis of the terminal aorta and its main branches or of aneurysms in these sites, advancement of the guide wire and catheter from the femoral artery through such vessels is very difficult and may result in serious complications. Among the latter are local arterial thrombosis, peripheral microembolism following detachment of atherosclerotic plaques, aortic perforation, formation of false aneurysms, and laceration or perforation of an aortic aneurysm. Damage to the intima may result from a "lashing" movement of the catheter tip during rapid pressure injection [14].

Systemic complications. Acute renal failure may develop if a large quantity (more than 150 ml) of the contrast medium has been injected; in fact, such a response has also been reported even with much smaller doses. It is therefore imperative to diurese the patients routinely in an attempt to remove the iodinated preparation as rapidly as possible. Careful monitoring of urinary output and of serum creatinine levels for at least 24 h after angiography has also been proposed as a precautionary measure.

4. Caution in Interpretation of Angiograms

Since the conventional use of angiography involves visualization of a two-dimensional image, the procedure may not always record a true picture of the degree of occlusion existing in a vessel. In most instances, for example, atherosclerotic lesions may appear to be less advanced than they actually are. In this regard, it is conceivable that a thin but wide layer of contrast material, filling a slitlike opening which extends across the full width of the interior of the artery, would be so oriented in profile to the roentgen beam that the lumen of the vessel appears to show no impingement by atherosclerotic plaques. Furthermore, thin, bandlike lesions which significantly obstruct an artery may be easily overlooked during angiography, although high-quality visualization performed in several projections may more readily identify them. However, even with such a measure, thin, diaphragm types of lesions may not be diagnosed if their plane does not lie tangential to the x-ray beam. Many of these are located either at the most distal or most proximal part of an atherosclerotic plaque in the aortofemoral system.

Another precaution which must be taken is to differentiate the angiographic change produced by spasm initiated by the contrast medium from an organic filling defect caused by atherosclerosis. Such a response should be suspected on finding that the shadow of the lumen of the vessel ends in a point, whereas in the case of structural disease there is a tendency for a more blunt and transverse termination, with the portion of the lumen above the obstruction showing some irregularity.

Another aspect which must be considered in evaluating information obtained by angiography is that only an anatomic picture of the vascular tree is obtained. Of importance is the fact that this may not necessarily reflect the true physiologic state of the circulation with regard to its efficiency in delivering adequate amounts of blood to the tissues. For example, when there is a slow-forming block in a proximal artery, eventually distal patent vessels are filled with blood by way of an extensive collateral circulation, a finding visualized by angiography. However, the effectiveness of such a system in conveying nutrients to the tissues is impaired because the blood passing through the circuitous, narrow, and tortuous secondary circulation bridging the block encounters high resistance. As a result, its head of pressure when it enters the distal portions of the main arterial tree is significantly reduced and so is its ability to perfuse the microcirculation. Another important criticism is that angiography does not give information on the viscoelastic properties of the vessel and on existing irregular surfaces producing turbulent flow [15], factors which play an important role during increasing rates of blood flow, as with exercise. An artifact which may influence the angiogram is the overdistension of the local arterial tree, produced by the high pressure used to inject the contrast medium. This may cause the lumen of the vessel to appear larger on the arteriogram than it actually is, thus leading to an improper interpretation of the degree of occlusive involvement of the vessels.

5. Role of Angiography and Interpretation of Abnormalities

Definitive information regarding details of the circulation which could not otherwise be determined is made available by angiography. It has application as a diagnostic aid in a large number of disorders or states. For example, it is very helpful in determining whether main vascular channels have been injured in the course of an orthopedic procedure or by trauma to a limb causing a musculoskeletal difficulty (see A-4, Chapter 15). It is also valuable, in the form of antegrade arteriography, in neurovascular compression syndromes of the shoulder girdle (see B-2, Chapter 13), and it is useful in determining the optimal level for amputation of a limb (see C-2, Chapter 24). It is helpful in making the diagnosis of congenital arteriovenous fistula and in instituting the proper surgical therapeutic approach (see B-3, Chapter 21). It may be used, although not routinely required, in the diagnosis of limb arterial aneurysm and in differentiating it from acquired arteriovenous fistula (see Sections E and F, respectively, Chapter 15). The procedure probably has its greatest clinical application in some of the conditions listed below.

Reconstructive vascular procedures. Most important is the role of angiography in the field of vascular surgery, to whose development this technique has contributed greatly. It provides information concerning the length and number of partial and complete occlusions of the local arterial tree; the adequacy of arterial inflow; and the status of the runoff circulation, i.e., the patency of the vessels distal to the lesion under study and the richness and degree of development of the collateral circulation. Such data are indispensable in the proper choice of patients with arterial insufficiency who are likely to be helped by some type of vascular reconstructive procedure. Arteriography also provides the surgeon with a guide to the institution of the most advantageous operative approach. However, even here the method should be performed only if it is intended to act immediately upon the information thus obtained (provided it is in accord with the contemplated surgical plan) and carry out the reconstructive procedure. Procrastination on the part of the patient at this point may lead to the need for another arteriographic examination should a firm commitment to have the operation be finally reached at a much later date. Another important role for angiography is that, if performed intraoperatively at the end of a reconstructive procedure, it may reveal a technical surgical error which can immediately be corrected, thus minimizing the possibility of subsequent thrombosis of the prosthesis.

Bone tumors. Angiography has also been used in the study of bone tumors and soft-tissue masses, although the current view is that with this approach it is difficult to define the exact histologic identity of many neoplasms [21].

The arteriographic appearance of a malignant tumor consists of a number of irregular, disorganized vessels and large irregular pools ("lakes") from which contrast material is rapidly shunted into the venous circulation [21]. However, some osteogenic sarcomas are highly calcified and do not display such features.

Benign neoplasms, including giant cell tumor, aneurysmal bone cyst, and osteitis fibrosa cystica of hyperparathyroidism, may be very vascular during the venous phase of the arteriogram, but the arterial phase does not show pooling and the arteries are essentially normal [19]. As a rule, benign tumors are avascular, with normal-appearing vessels being displaced around the neoplasm. However, such findings are unreliable as differential points, since malignant tumors may also be avascular. Hence, because of considerable overlap, reliance must still be placed on biopsy for a dependable means of identification of tumors.

Nevertheless, in the presence of obvious clear-cut arteriographic evidence of malignancy, generally histologic examination of the mass will confirm such a diagnosis. Also, prebiopsy arteriography is useful in demonstrating the areas of greatest vascularity. This is information of value since it has been shown that such sites are the most fruitful for obtaining a representative biopsy, especially in the presence of malignant cells [10]. The procedure likewise has application in demonstrating satellite tumors, the extent and size of the neoplasms, and evidence of recurrence—data which are helpful in surgical and radiotherapeutic management and in prognosis [21].

Inflammatory process. Such a state is characterized by a large number of normal tapering vessels which produce a uniformly dense stain [21]. In the presence of necrosis, the central portion of the lesion will appear radiolucent. The stain usually remains present longer and arteriovenous shunting is less rapid than in the normal arteriogram. Because of the variations and overlap, the differentiation of inflammatory disease from benign and malignant tumors cannot be made on the basis of arteriography alone, and hence such procedures as other types of roentgenographic studies and biopsy should also be performed.

Arteriosclerosis obliterans. This condition is easily recognized by arteriography. Atheromatous deposits within the artery produce eccentric, diffuse irregularities and narrowing which often progress to complete segmental occlusion (Fig. 5.6D). There may also be marked tortuosity of the arterial tree. Generally large numbers of collateral vessels are visualized (Fig. 5.1B), frequently bridging obstructed portions of the main artery and being responsible for opacification of patent arterial channels below the level of the block. Arteriographic abnormalities may be noted in all the arteries of the lower limb and also the proximal vessels, including the aortic bifurcation; the common and external iliac; the common, superficial, and deep femoral; and the popliteal and tibial arteries. In the upper limb, rarely are occlusions noted distal to the subclavian artery. Of diagnostic interest is the associated finding of calcification of arteries in the lower limbs, as determined by soft-tissue x-ray technique.

Arteriosclerosis obliterans with diabetes. When both of these conditions coexist at an early age, the arteriographic picture is different from that observed in the patient suffering only from atherosclerosis (see above). Although the type of change is similar, the lesions are limited to the popliteal and the tibial arteries. Rarely are they observed in the more proximal vessels. In the upper limb, the arterial tree is generally not affected.

Thromboangiitis obliterans. In this condition, also, there is patchy segmental distribution of the occlusive process, with reduction in lumen size of the involved portion of artery. After progression of the pathologic state, complete block of vessels is noted (Fig. 5.7). However, in contrast with arteriosclerosis obliterans (see

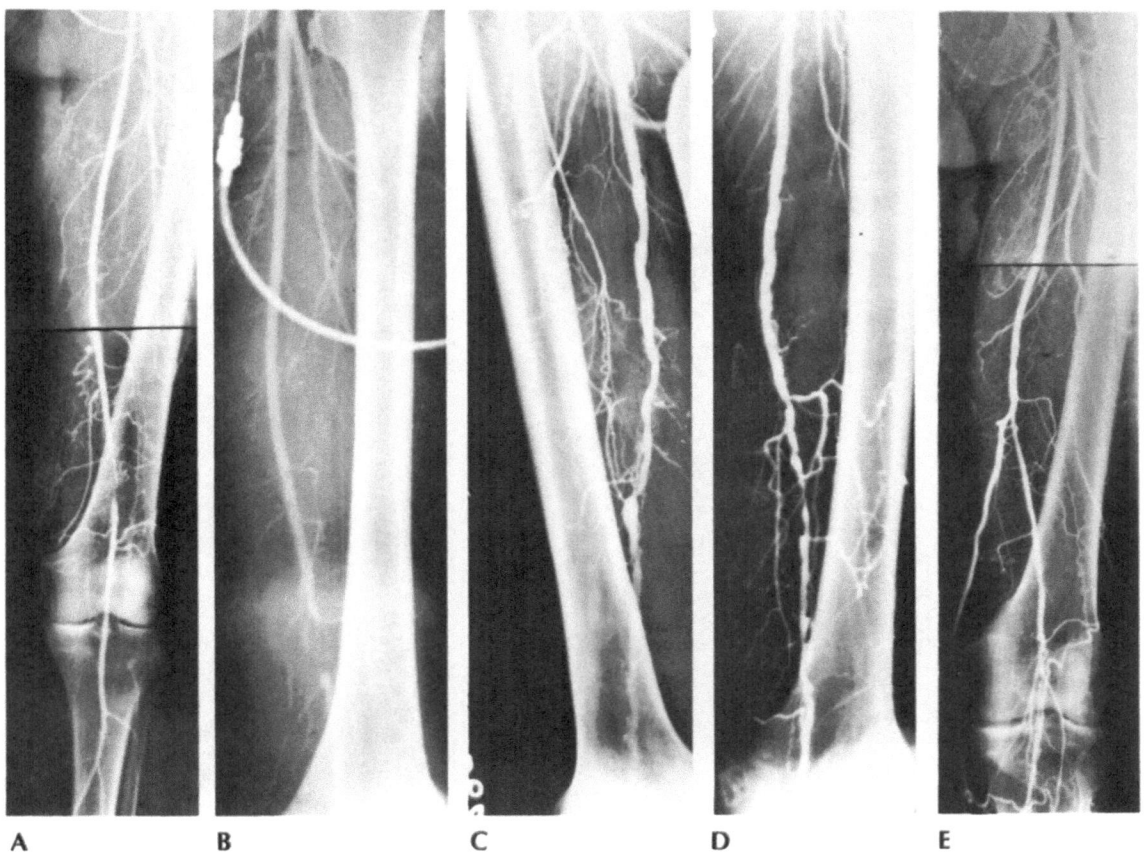

A   B   C   D   E

Fig. 5.6. Arteriographic changes found in arteriosclerosis obliterans. **A** Complete block of the superficial femoral artery in its passage through the adductor canal, a very common site for this type of lesion. **B** Similar type of obstruction to that noted in **A**. **C** Numerous partial occlusions in the full length of the superficial femoral and popliteal arteries. **D** Numerous almost complete obstructions in the superficial femoral artery. **E** Complete occlusion of the lower third of the superficial femoral artery, with enlargement of genicular vessels.

above), on either side of the obstructed segment, the arterial wall is usually smooth and without any tortuosity or filling defects. Another differential point is that, in the lower limbs, arteriography visualizes partial or complete occlusions of the popliteal and tibial arteries and their branches, while the abdominal aorta, the common and external iliac vessels, and the common, superficial, and deep femoral arteries are generally relatively free of disease (Fig. 5.7B and D). In this regard, the changes resemble those seen in young diabetics with arteriosclerosis obliterans and differ markedly from those found in arteriosclerosis obliterans alone (see above). In thromboangiitis obliterans, arteriography may also reveal stenosis and

complete occlusions of the radial and ulnar arteries and of the brachial artery at its bifurcation, whereas in arteriosclerosis obliterans, the changes in the vascular tree of the upper limb are minimal. Finally, in the uncomplicated case of thromboangiitis obliterans, there are no soft-tissue x-ray findings of calcification of arteries.

Abdominal aortic aneurysm. There is some question as to the use of angiography in the diagnosis of an abdominal aortic aneurysm. Contributing to the lack of enthusiasm for such a measure is the fact that the translumbar route cannot be utilized because of fear that the wall of the lesion might be traumatized in the course of penetrating the abdominal aorta proximally

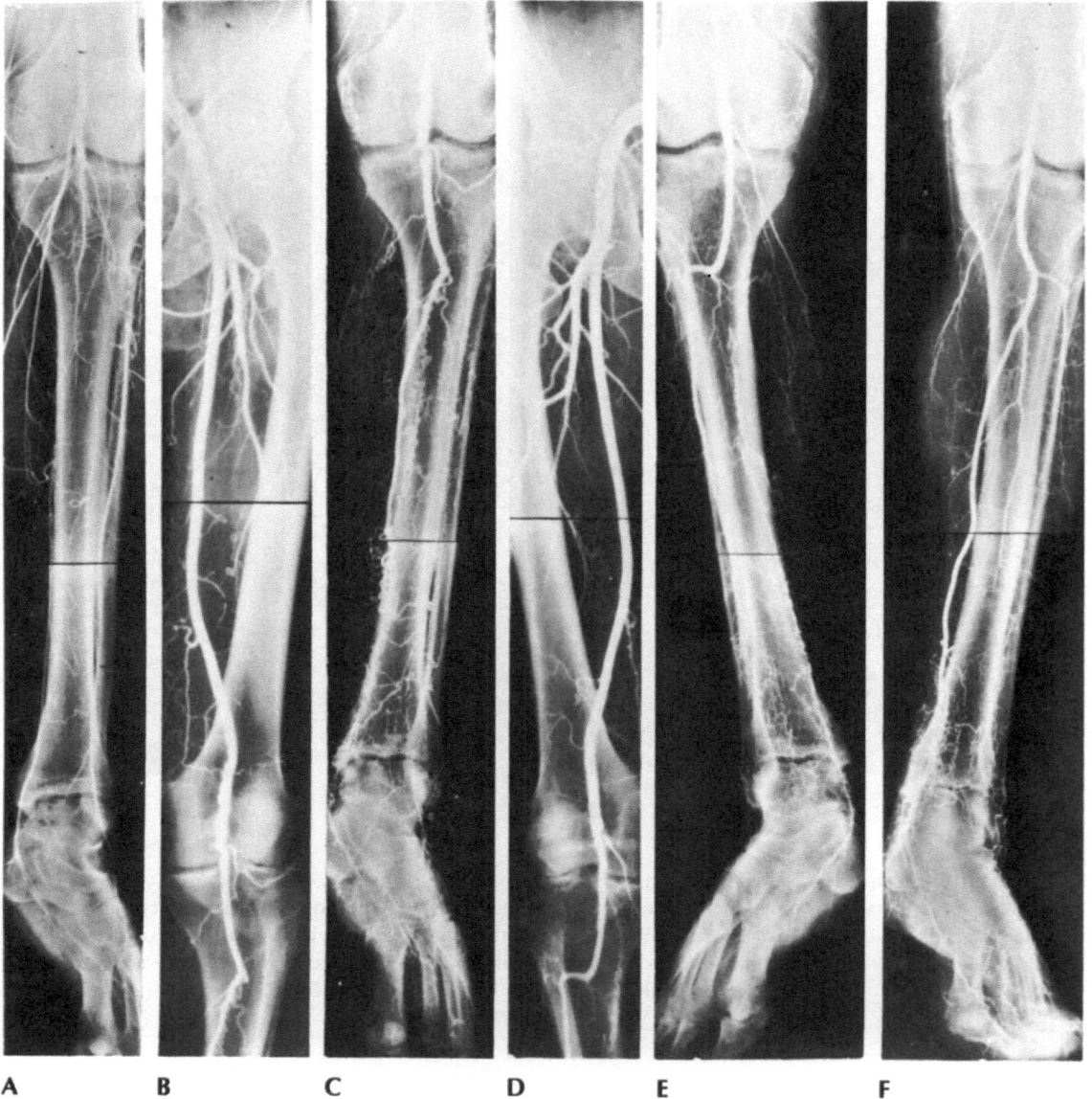

A   B   C   D   E   F

Fig. 5.7. Arteriographic changes found in thromboangiitis obliterans, with the lesions being noted at the level of the popliteal artery or distally. **A** Occlusion of the popliteal artery above its bifurcation. **B** Complete occlusion of the anterior tibial artery at its origin from the popliteal artery. **C** Same patient as in **B**, also demonstrating complete occlusion of the posterior tibial artery at about the middle portion of the leg. **D** Complete occlusion of the posterior tibial artery at its origin from the popliteal artery. **E** Same patient as in **D**, also demonstrating occlusion of the anterior tibial artery in its lower third. **F** Complete occlusion of both the anterior tibial artery (in its upper third) and the posterior tibial artery (in its lower third).

to inject the contrast medium. Hence, other approaches must be substituted, none of which is without some danger. Moreover, the information derived from angiography is limited since it only outlines that portion of the sac not filled with clot and so may even give a misleading impression of the actual size of the lesion. However, the procedure is useful in that it may visualize stenosis of renal, celiac, or superior mesenteric arteries, a situation which contraindicates ligation of the inferior mesenteric or hypogastric artery in the course of surgical treatment of the aneurysm; for under such conditions either vessel may be playing a significant role in supplying blood to the gastrointestinal tract.

6. Situations in Which Angiography Is Not Indicated

In many teaching hospitals, especially, there is a tendency to rely heavily on angiography to make or confirm a diagnosis of occlusive arterial disease, information which could readily have been obtained solely by clinical examination and oscillometry or possibly by the adjunctive use of noninvasive laboratory procedures, such as Doppler ultrasonic technique, the mercury strain-gauge plethysmograph, or the impedance plethysmograph. Such a practice should at least be discouraged or, properly, eliminated from the armamentarium of diagnostic procedures applicable to chronic occlusive arterial diseases. However, the one exception to this viewpoint is a block in the deep femoral artery causing intermittent claudication of the thigh muscles but associated with normal clinical findings in the leg and foot. Only arteriography can identify its presence.

Angiography is also unnecessary in making the diagnosis of acute arterial embolism (see A-3, Chapter 12), particularly if the viability of the limb is threatened. It provides little added information to that available from a careful physical examination, and at the same time, the delay incurred in performing it may result in progressive limb ischemia, thus interfering with salvage of the extremity by embolectomy.

In summary, angiography should not be attempted if comparable data can be obtained by physical examination and noninvasive diagnostic measures. Only if the latter have failed to yield the desired information should the procedure be carried out.

F. Electromagnetic Blood Flowmeters

Electromagnetic blood flowmeters are capable of measuring circulation in the limbs instanta-

neously, accurately, and without any difficulty. However, since the procedure requires the artery under study to be exposed, it has only limited clinical application, mainly in determining whether a newly inserted arterial prosthesis is performing properly at the time of the operation. Nevertheless, such information is indeed useful in identifying technical difficulties, thus permitting them to be remedied at once. An adjunctive measure is to study the effect on blood flow through the prosthesis of the proximal intraarterial injection of 10 mg of papaverine. The magnitude of the resulting vascular response is a reflection of the efficiency of the distal runoff and inflow capacity and of the functional state of the prosthesis.

The principle underlying the use of an electromagnetic flowmeter is based on Faraday's law [8,24], which states that when a conductor moves through a magnetic field, an electromagnetic force is generated in a direction perpendicular to both the magnetic field and the direction of movement of the conductor. The resulting voltage induced is proportional to the number of magnetic lines of force cut per unit of time. Since blood is 5 to 10 times more conductive than other tissues in the limb, its rate of movement has the greatest effect upon the recording obtained by the electromagnetic blood flowmeter. The magnitude of the reading obtained by the instrument is proportional to the strength of the magnetic field, the diameter of the vessel under study, and the mean velocity of the blood passing through it [3].

Two types of electromagnetic flowmeters are available commercially, the sine wave [9] and the square wave [1], both of which appear to have the same degree of accuracy in measuring blood flow. The technique of obtaining the readings consists of placing electrodes in contact with the outer surface of the vessel or graft under study and then establishing a magnetic field across the structure. The voltage generated by the passage of blood through the vessel is picked up by the electrodes and recorded.

There are several practical disadvantages to the electromagnetic blood flowmeter, the most important of which is that it is invasive. Moreover, the method requires expensive equipment, and the test can only be carried out when the artery is exposed during the operation.

Because of the above serious objections, attempts have been made to develop a noninvasive type which operates on the same principle as the invasive electromagnetic flowmeter, but records can be obtained from the skin surface. To accomplish this, an electromagnetic field is produced by a strong external permanent magnet and skin electrodes are used to pick up the generated voltage. The latter is considered to be proportional to the quantity of flowing blood. The resulting waveform tracing represents the instantaneous pulsatile flow through the aggregated arteries at any selected segment of limb. The available noninvasive electromagnetic flowmeters have been reported to increase patient safety and to allow for repeated measurements of blood flow and continuous monitoring. Moreover, the procedure can be performed by paramedical personnel. Whether such instruments will be able to supply the type of information obtained by the invasive electromagnetic flowmeter is questionable.

References

1. Denison ABJ, Spencer MP: Circulatory system: Methods; magnetic flowmeters. Med Phys 3:177, 1960
2. Ejrup B, Extama P, Mattila M, et al: Pulse wave registration from the big toe during reactive hyperaemia in arterial circulation disorders of the lower extremities. J Cardiovasc Surg 7:275, 1966
3. Engell HC, Lauridsen P: The use of a square-wave electromagnetic flowmeter in reconstructive vascular surgery. J Cardiovasc Surg 7:283, 1966
4. Goldberg BB, Lehman JS: Aortosonography: Ultrasound measurement of the abdominal and thoracic aorta. Arch Surg 100:652, 1970
5. Johnsrude IS, Jackson DC: A Practical Approach to Angiography. Boston, Little, Brown, 1979, p 24
6. Kahn PC, Boyer DN, Moran JM, et al: Reactive hyperemia in lower extremity arteriography: An evaluation. Radiology 90:975, 1968
7. Keitzer WF, Lichti EL, Brossart FA, et al: Use of the Doppler ultrasonic flowmeter during arterial vascular surgery. Arch Surg 105:308, 1972
8. Kolin A: An electromagnetic flowmeter: Principle of the method and its application to blood flow measurements. Proc Soc Exp Biol Med 35:53, 1936
9. Kolin A: Circulatory system: Methods; blood flow determinations by electromagnetic method. Med Phys 3:141, 1960
10. Lagergren C, Lindbom A: Angiography of peripheral tumors. Radiology 79:371, 1962
11. Lennihan R Jr, Mackereth M: Ankle blood pressure in vascular insufficiency involving the legs. J Clin Ultrasound 1:120, 1973
12. Linhart J, Dejdar R, Přerovský I, et al: Location of occlusive arterial disease of lower extremity: Possible importance of local factors in pathogenesis. Invest Radiol 3:188, 1968
13. McAfee JG: Complications of abdominal aortography and arteriography. In Abrams HL (ed): Angiography, Vol 2, 2nd ed. Boston, Little, Brown, 1971, p 717
14. Melnick GS, Gilbert GJ: Mechanical hazards in catheter aortography. Circulation 32:876, 1965
15. Moore WS, Hall AD: Unrecognized aortoiliac stenosis: A physiologic approach to the diagnosis. Arch Surg 103:633, 1971
16. Ratschow M: Importance of phonoangiography for the evaluation of arterial stenosis. Angiology 13:290, 1962
17. Rushmer RF: Cardiovascular Dynamics. Philadelphia, Saunders, 1970, p 313
18. Sako Y: Hemodynamic changes during arteriography. JAMA 183:253, 1963
19. Schobinger R, Stoll HC: The arteriographic picture of benign bone lesions containing giant cells. J Bone Joint Surg 39A:953, 1957
20. Seldinger SI: Catheter replacement of the needle in percutaneous arteriography: A new technique. Acta Radiol (Stockh) 39:368, 1953
21. Staple TW, Evens RG, Stein AH Jr: Arteriography in orthopedics. Arch Surg 97:682, 1968
22. Stead EA Jr, Greenfield JC Jr: Pressures and pulses. Physiol Physicians 2:1, 1964
23. Weatherall M: Pharmacological actions of some contrast media and comparison of their merits. Br J Radiol 15:129, 1942
24. Wetterer E: Eine neue Methode zur Registrierung der Blutströmungsgeschurndigkeit am uneröffneten Gefäss. Z Biol 98:26, 1937

Chapter 6

Clinical and Laboratory Tests of Arterial Circulation

Part 2   Procedures for the Study of Nutritional Circulation

In contrast with the examination of the main arterial tree in the limbs (see Chapter 5), information regarding the microcirculation to the tissues themselves can only be derived through indirect means. One useful approach consists of inspection and palpation, to determine skin color, skin temperature, and the nutritional state of the skin, its appendages, and subcutaneous tissue. Another involves the performance of several simple clinical tests and a few laboratory procedures. All these subjects are dealt with in this chapter.

Data derived from the use of the above listed measures are very helpful and even essential to the orthopedic or general surgeon who is contemplating the application of a cast to a limb or considering an elective operation on the toes or the foot. Besides being aware of the state of the local arteries, he or she must also be certain that there is an adequate circulation through the cutaneous arteriolar and capillary beds, as determined by the tests described below.

A. Postural Skin Color Changes

Considerable knowledge regarding the state of the cutaneous circulation can be derived from a study of skin color of the extremities in different positions. For this type of examination it is necessary to have good lighting, preferably from a natural source. The limb under examination should be exposed to a normal environmental temperature for at least 30 min before any conclusions can be drawn regarding skin color. Moreover, it is necessary to eliminate such systemic conditions as congestive heart failure, a pneumonic process interfering with oxygenation of the blood, blood dyscrasias, carbon monoxide poisoning, and shock before attributing the observed changes in skin color to alterations in local circulation.

1. Physiologic Considerations

If the relatively permanent changes produced by pigmentation are disregarded, skin color reflects the rate of blood flow through the cutaneous vessels. The two uppermost layers of venules (the subpapillary venous plexus) form a dense meshwork in the subpapillary region, and hence the color of the blood in them has a considerable influence upon skin color. As the cutaneous capillaries dilate, they too play an important role in this regard.

Under physiologic conditions, the relationship of oxyhemoglobin to reduced hemoglobin in the blood filling the superficial venules and capillaries is almost completely responsible for the tint of the skin. However, when these vessels are emptied of blood, producing cutaneous pallor, the skin becomes more transparent, thus allowing the color of the blood in deeper-lying veins to contribute to skin color. The relative amount of reduced hemoglobin compared to oxyhemoglobin in venous blood depends upon the rate of blood flow through the capillary bed. The more rapid the circulation, the greater is the quantity of oxyhemoglobin in venous blood and the redder is the skin; the slower the circulation, the greater is the quantity of reduced hemoglobin in venous blood and the more cyanotic is the skin.

2.   Skin Color in Horizontal Position

With the patient lying horizontally on an examining table and in a physiologic environment, the toes and fingers should normally demonstrate a slight pink flush. Pallor, cyanosis, and rubor generally indicate the presence of some alteration of the local vascular system, especially when the response is limited to one limb or to one or more digits.

3.   Skin Color in Elevated Position

With the lower extremities in the elevated position, the skin of the feet should continue to remain pink, although the intensity of the color may be decreased somewhat. The appearance of pallor in the distal portion of the limb is evidence that reduced arterial circulation exists. If no change occurs, it is necessary to have the patient dorsiflex his feet repeatedly at the ankle, while the examiner helps maintain the limbs in the elevated position. If moderate local arterial insufficiency exists, this added maneuver may now bring out pallor, particularly of the plantar surface of the feet and of the toes (positive plantar pallor or Samuels' test) [5].

Elevation of the upper limbs should likewise not affect the pink color of normal hands; the appearance of pallor of the fingers signifies the presence of an impaired local circulation. If no abnormal color change results from prolonged elevation and if other findings suggest

that a compromised circulation exists, it may be necessary for the patient to clench and open his fist forcibly several times while the upper limbs remain in the elevated position. The appearance of pallor in the fingers or hands indicates that there is a moderate degree of reduction in local blood flow.

4.   Skin Color in Dependent Position

After the lower or upper extremity has been elevated for some time, it is now placed in the dependent position and the changes in skin color are observed. Normally there is a return of the pink color to its previous intensity in 10 s or less (time of return of color in dependency). In a patient with arterial impairment, there is a delay in the reappearance of the skin color to as long as 45 to 60 s or more, the change being irregular and patchy rather than uniform. If varicosities are present, however, the test is of no value and may even be misleading with regard to determining the state of arterial circulation in the lower limbs. Under such circumstances, skin color will return almost immediately after the feet are placed in dependency, due to a retrograde flow of blood into the venous channels and subpapillary venous plexuses from proximal veins with incompetent valves.

Changes in skin color which appear while the lower extremity remains in dependency are also useful in the study of the cutaneous circulation. In the presence of impaired local blood flow, intense cyanotic rubor may develop slowly in the foot, a type of response generally noted in the limb manifesting a delay in return of color when first placed in dependency. The appearance of rapid cyanosis with a change to this position indicates that the tone of the superficial vessels is low or absent and that immediate pooling of blood is taking place in them.

B.   Cutaneous Temperature under Resting Conditions

Palpation of the limbs in order to determine the temperature of the skin may also give valuable information concerning changes in cutaneous circulation.

1. Physiologic Considerations

The level of cutaneous temperature is a resultant of the total amount of heat brought to the surface of the body by the blood in the cutaneous vessels and the amount lost to the environment through convection, radiation, and vaporization. If the room temperature is maintained at a constant physiologic level and drafts are eliminated, then skin temperature can be considered to be a qualitative index of cutaneous circulation.

2. Technique

As in the case of skin color, it is necessary to consider the period elapsing between the time the patient came in from outdoors and examination of the extremities. Obviously, during the winter months even the normal limb will remain cold for some time after the individual has entered the office. Therefore, one cannot draw any definite conclusions from such a finding unless a low temperature of the skin persists. Palpation should be carried out using the dorsum of the hand which appears to be very sensitive to small differences in skin temperature. The entire limb should be examined, since this maneuver may bring out sudden changes in skin temperature at different levels, as in the case of occlusion of a main artery by an embolus. If more accurate and quantitative readings are required, it is necessary to utilize a thermocouple and a recording system (see D-4, below).

3. Interpretation of Findings

Normally, in a cool environment the temperature of the toes can be expected to be lower than that of the dorsal and plantar surface of the foot; on the leg, the skin temperature progressively becomes higher as the examining hand is moved in a proximal direction. Such differences can be related to the degree of vasomotor control over the cutaneous arterioles, by far the most marked response being present in the toes.

In a physiologic environment (24° C, 74° F), the temperature of the toes of a normal person rises during the period of observation so that the limb begins to feel warm to the observer's hand; in fact, if low vasomotor tone exists, the foot may actually become hot. However, if the toes remain cold or cool after prolonged exposure to a comfortable environment, it can be assumed that there is increased vasomotor tone (vasospasm) or that organic arterial disease exists. The distinction between the two states can be made by removing vasomotor tone by any one of the available clinical methods (see D-4, below) and reexamining the feet. If vasospasm is the cause, the skin temperature will rise to a high level in the entire limb, whereas with permanent damage to the blood vessels, there will only be a slight increase due to removal of normal vasomotor tone. The persistence of a low skin temperature limited to one or several toes, with the temperature in the others rising to a high level, indicates that organic vascular disease exists in those digits displaying little or no change following sympathetic denervation.

At times, the skin temperature of a foot in which there are definite signs of occlusion of main arteries may, under resting conditions, be found to be greater than that of the opposite normal or less affected limb. Such a situation can only be explained on the basis that a very efficient collateral cutaneous circulation is present in the involved extremity, having developed in response to a state of chronic ischemia. It is therefore important to emphasize that a normal or even increased skin temperature of the feet does not necessarily rule out an organic arterial disorder affecting the large arteries in a limb.

C. Nutritional Disturbances in Skin and Its Appendages and in Subcutaneous Tissue

Valuable information regarding the cutaneous circulation can be obtained merely by inspection and palpation of the extremities.

1. Trophic Changes

The presence of healed, depressed scars on the fingers or toes, loss of portions of digits,

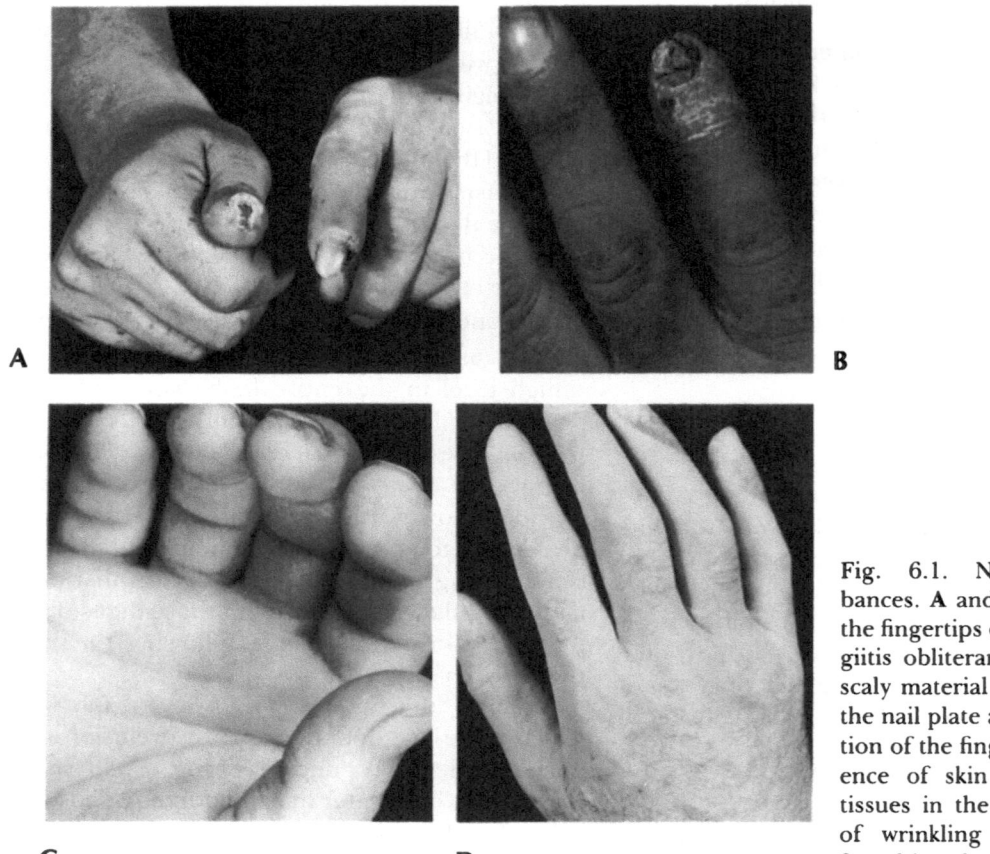

Fig. 6.1. Nutritional disturbances. **A** and **B** Ulcerations on the fingertips due to thromboangiitis obliterans. **C** Piling up of scaly material at the junction of the nail plate and the fleshy portion of the finger. **D** Firm adherence of skin to subcutaneous tissues in the fingers, with loss of wrinkling over the joints, found in scleroderma.

or the existence of large healed or open ulcers (Fig. 6.1A and B) should make one suspect that there is impairment of cutaneous blood flow. However, before reaching this conclusion, it is necessary to eliminate such etiologic factors as venous or lymphatic stasis, trauma or burns in a limb with normal blood flow, and various types of nonvascular systemic conditions associated with the production of ulcers and gangrene in the extremities.

2. State of Skin and Subcutaneous Tissue

Of significance also are the texture and consistency of the skin and subcutaneous tissue. Generally, firmness and good elasticity of these structures suggest adequate nutrition, whereas areas of softness, dimpling, or flabbiness may indicate an impaired blood supply. The absence of wrinkling of the skin over the joints

of the fingers may be due to abnormal attachment of this structure to the subcutaneous tissue, as in scleroderma (Fig. 6.1D). Other abnormal findings are thickening of the tips of the fingers and piling up of scaly material at the junction of the nail plate and the fleshy portion of the digit (Fig. 6.1C).

3. Appearance of Nails

Of interest in regard to the efficiency of the cutaneous circulation is the state of the nails of the toes and fingers. In the presence of an impaired local blood flow due to permanent organic changes in the vessels, these structures will manifest such abnormalities as deformity, brittleness and pigmentation, vertical and horizontal ridging, an increase in thickness of nail substance, and deposition of calcium. A history is generally elicited of slow growth of nails. In vasospastic conditions, such as Raynaud's disease and post–trench foot syndrome, the most frequent abnormality is thinning of the proximal nail folds with gradual merging into a widened cuticle (pterygium).

4. State of Hair

As in the case of the nails, the growth of hair on the toes is related to the state of nutrition of the cutaneous and subcutaneous tissues [2]. In the limb with a markedly impaired circulation, growth of hair may stop entirely. However, in the presence of mild or moderate ischemia, it may still be normal. The presence of hair on involved toes may at times delay amputation of the limb, on the possibility that spontaneous healing of the nutritional disturbances may still be possible. Significance can be attributed to a situation in which hair growth is absent on one foot and plentiful on the other or when it is present on some of the toes of a foot and not on others. Finally, it is also necessary to point out that in certain races, such as some Asiatic peoples and American blacks, lack of hair growth on the feet and legs is a normal finding and has no implications.

5. State of Sweat and Sebaceous Glands

Since the degree of perspiration and the state of oiliness of the feet and legs depend upon the rate of blood flow to the sweat and sebaceous glands, respectively, these manifestations can also be considered to be a reflection of the state of local circulation. Signs of normal sweating patterns and responses and absence of scaliness and dryness of the skin indicate that adequate amounts of sweat and sebum are being formed.

Increased sweating. This state may be elicited in normal people on exposure of the body to a high environmental temperature and excessive humidity if, at the same time, there is little or no loss of heat from the surface by conduction due to absence of a temperature gradient between skin and environment. It is also initiated by severe exercise, when there is need to eliminate large quantities of body heat produced by the physical exertion, and during

bouts of fever from any cause. Excessive sweating is likewise associated with periods of emotion, such as anxiety, fear, or joy. An exaggerated response is noted in the patient suffering from an anxiety state, as well as in certain congenital or familial disorders.

Excessive sweating, in the absence of emotion, a warm environmental temperature, or need for heat dissipation on any other basis, is termed hyperhidrosis. It signifies increased sympathetic activity and is generally associated with findings of vasospasm, such as coldness of the skin, cyanosis, and a subjective sense of coldness. Hyperhidrosis may also be present in some organic arterial occlusive disorders, as for example, thromboangiitis obliterans, in which the inflammatory process extends beyond the vascular components to involve the postganglionic sympathetic fibers running in the peripheral mixed nerves.

Anhidrosis. Complete absence of sweating results from a number of different mechanisms. In arteriosclerosis obliterans, the skin of the feet is dry because of the reduced circulation to the sweat glands, causing a decrease in sweat production (Fig. 6.2). Atrophy of the skin including its appendages, as in systemic sclerosis, also produces anhidrosis because of destruction of the sweat glands in the process. Elimination of sympathetic stimulation of the sweat glands, as by sympathectomy, results in a permanently dry limb. Complete destruction of peripheral nerves, including the sympathetic nervous system components, has a similar effect. Other conditions associated with anhidrosis or hyphidrosis (subnormal secretion of sweat) are heat stroke, hypothyroidism, dehydration, Fabry's disease, and Sjögren's syndrome.

D. Clinical and Laboratory Tests of Cutaneous Circulation

1. Reactive Hyperemia Test

The reactive hyperemia test is a simple, noninvasive procedure which is a useful means of collecting information regarding the state of the cutaneous circulation in the limb.

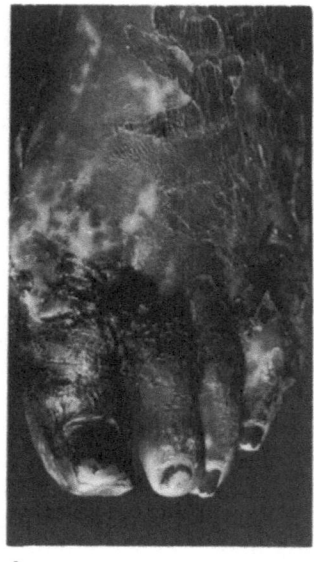

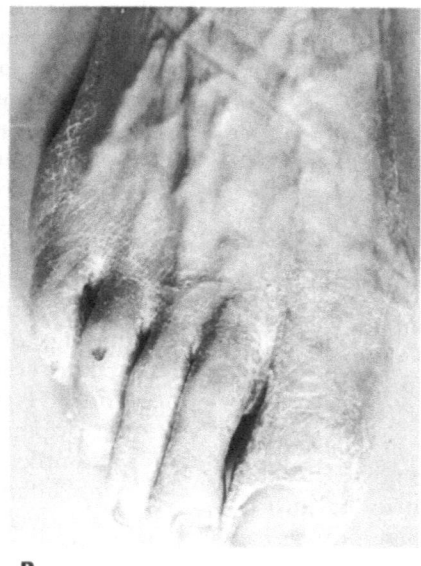

A   **B**

Fig. 6.2. Absence of sweating of the skin of the feet (**A** and **B**) producing scaliness, found in the advanced case of arteriosclerosis obliterans.

Technique. The test is performed as follows: With the patient lying on the table, an ordinary blood pressure cuff with a somewhat longer band is wrapped around the thigh or arm, the limb is elevated to drain out venous blood, and an arterial occlusion pressure is applied. The extremity is then placed in the horizontal position and the pressure maintained for a total of 3 min. At the end of this period it is suddenly released and the color changes in the skin of the limb are closely observed.

Response of the cutaneous circulation to anoxia. Normally, during a period of ischemia, a "blood flow debt" is incurred, which is then rapidly repaid, in the form of an increased supply to the tissues (state of reactive hyperemia), immediately upon reestablishment of the circulation. Clinically this manifests itself as rubor of the skin which is first noticed just below the level of the blood pressure cuff and which spreads down the limb to reach the digits in 10 to 15 s. The flush remains for 10 to 40 s and then recedes in the same order that it advanced over the skin, the entire color change being completed within 2 min.

In the presence of a reduced arterial inflow into the limb, whether due to structural disease or marked vasospasm, there is an abnormal response. The flush may be cyanotic rather than red, it is delayed in its appearance, and it slowly spreads downward in a patchy rather than uniform manner. The response may take 2 to 3 min to reach the digits, some of the latter changing color later than others, and there is usually a long delay before the alteration completely disappears. If an adequate collateral circulation exists due to a slowly forming but now total occlusion of a large artery, there may be a delayed onset of the flush, but with the development of full color (rubor). A diffuse, faint color suggests narrowing of the finer vessels [4], whereas marked mottling may indicate very severe impairment of local blood flow. If vasospasm exists, there may be a prompt appearance of the flush with good color, but this then disappears quickly. It is necessary to point out that none of the color changes, normal or abnormal, gives any information regarding the circulation in the underlying muscles, the alterations reflecting only the state of the cutaneous blood flow.

2. Venous Filling Time

A simple test for evaluation of arterial circulation in the lower limbs consists of first elevating the extremities to drain the blood out of the superficial veins, and then placing them in dependency and noting the rate of venous filling in this position. Normally the vessels on the dorsum of the feet become visible and distended within 10 s after the limb is placed in dependency (venous filling time). Delays beyond this time indicate some arterial impairment, although the test does not differentiate between functional and organic disorders unless it is repeated after removal of vasomotor tone (see D-4, below). The coexistence of varicosities eliminates the diagnostic value of this procedure since retrograde flow of blood from proximal vessels with incompetent valves causes immediate distension of superficial veins on the dorsum of the foot on placing the lower limbs in dependency.

3. Subpapillary Venous Plexus Filling Time

The subpapillary venous plexus filling time is a test for determining the state of tone or turgor in the cutaneous microcirculation. It consists of applying firm pressure for several seconds to the skin of the patient using the fingers and then studying the color changes which follow sudden removal of the force.

Normally there is first transient pallor of the area of skin previously compressed, followed by an almost immediate return (1 to 2 s) of the original pink color. If there is a reduced or absent tone in the subpapillary venous plexus or if there is venous stasis, it may take 4 or 5 s for the blood to return to the tested area, the reappearance of the pink color taking the form of an irregular, slow filling of the pale segment of skin from the periphery inward. The same type of response may be noted if the arteries feeding the skin are in a state of excessive vasomotor tone or if occlusive changes are present in the lumen of these vessels.

The above procedure is also useful in determining the state of viability of tissues. For example, if application of firm digital pressure to an apparently cyanotic area results in the temporary appearance of pallor in the compressed site, it can be assumed that the abnormal color is due to blood (with a high concentration of reduced hemoglobin) that is still present in the vascular tree; hence, the tissue is viable. However, if a similar maneuver causes no alteration in color, then irreversible changes have occurred locally, with extravasation of blood into the tissue spaces due to a marked increase in capillary permeability. Such a response indicates that superficial or deep gangrene will subsequently develop.

4. Effect of Removal of Vasomotor Tone on Skin Temperature

Since a reduction in cutaneous circulation due to vasospasm is much more amenable to treatment than that resulting from permanent structural change in the wall of an artery, it becomes of importance to ascertain to what degree this state exists in the patient with an apparent arterial disorder. Such information can be obtained by determining the elevation in cutaneous temperature produced by temporary inhibition of vasomotor tone. The assumption is made that the magnitude of the resulting change is a reflection of the increase in cutaneous blood flow which follows passive dilatation of vessels due to removal of either normal or exaggerated vasomotor tone.[1]

Technique. In order to obtain dependable readings of skin temperature, it is necessary to expose the uncovered limbs under study to a constant environmental temperature, with drafts eliminated. However, there is no need for a temperature-regulated room in order to carry out the procedure, except possibly in the summer months if the room temperature is too high to control by other means.

For the collection of accurate readings, some type of thermocouple and recording system is

---

[1] Thermography, which is also a means of studying tissue temperature, has been used in the detection of bone tumors [1,7] and of metastatic disease of bone. In fact, there is some evidence to indicate that an earlier and more accurate impression of the extent of involvement of bone by malignant disease is obtained with this method than with roentgenography [3]. The procedure also gives information as to when arterial surgery or amputation should be carried out [6]. For example, if after prolonged antibiotic treatment, hot areas are still detected, this is an indication to delay the contemplated step. It is necessary to point out that thermography requires the purchase of a relatively expensive instrument.

advisable, a number of relatively inexpensive ones being commercially available. The apparatus generally consists of a sensitive galvanometer (millivoltmeter) which records the electric currents generated when two sets of connected thermocouple junctions are exposed to different temperatures. As a reference point, one set is maintained at a constant temperature (usually that of the room), while the other is used to obtain skin temperature. Each thermocouple consists of a junction of two dissimilar metals having different coefficients of expansion. The scale on the galvanometer is calibrated in degrees centigrade or Fahrenheit, or both. The procedure is carried out as follows:

The patient is placed at bed rest for 20 min, during which time the extremities to be studied are exposed to room air to permit equilibrium to take place with the environmental temperature; then control cutaneous temperature readings are collected, with all external stimuli being reduced to a minimum. The readings are obtained from the digits, from several locations on the dorsum of the hand or foot, and from the ventral surface of the forearm or leg.

Vasomotor tone can be removed by one of several different methods, among which are procaine blocking of the stellate ganglion or the paravertebral sympathetic ganglia, reflex or indirect vasodilatation, and anesthesia of the sympathetic nerves to the lower limbs by spinal or caudal anesthesia. Partial sympathetic denervation of the toes can be obtained through anesthetization of the posterior tibial nerve in its location behind and below the medial malleolus, using a 1% procaine solution. In the upper extremity, the desired effect is produced by anesthetization of the ulnar nerve at the elbow and the median nerve at the wrist.

Interpretation of results. After removal of sympathetic control by any one of the methods already mentioned, the readings in the hands and feet of normal persons should rise to at least 30° C (86° F) and generally to between 31 and 35° C (between 88 and 95° F). In the patient with excess sympathetic activity, inhibition of vasomotor tone will cause a rise to the same levels observed in normal subjects immediately following sympathetic denervation. However, the magnitude of the increase is

much greater since the control figures are lower. In the individual with obliterative arterial disease alone, removal of vasomotor tone generally results in a rise from 23.9 or 25° C to 26.7 or 27.8° C (from 75 or 77° F to 80 or 82° F), but not higher. In other words, despite elimination of all sympathetic tone, the normal increase in arterial inflow does not occur because structural changes in the cutaneous vessels prevent adequate vasodilatation.

The various tests which temporarily remove sympathetic control over blood vessels in the extremities are therefore of value in differentiating a primarily occlusive arterial disease from one in which vasomotor tone is solely or chiefly responsible for a reduced local cutaneous blood flow. Moreover, since they also give information concerning the capacity of the vascular bed to dilate following sympathetic denervation, they are useful in arriving at a decision as to whether sympathectomy is indicated as a therapeutic measure. On the other hand, they are of no help in assessing the state of the muscle circulation.

5. Use of Radioactive Tracers

Technique. The determination of the rate of disappearance of radioisotopes from the skin involves the use of radioactive gases (^{133}Xe or ^{127}Xe) in saline which are injected locally, the radioactive material then being excreted by way of the lungs. The disappearance rate from the injection site is measured with a scintillation probe and registered on a counting device connected to a linear recorder. The rate of loss of radioactivity from the injection site is determined from the slope of the curve of disappearance.

Evaluation of procedure. This approach measures the effectiveness of the nutritive circulation in the capillary bed in the skin rather than the rate of blood flow in the arterial tree. Also important is the fact that the results cannot be expressed in volumetric units. Because of these objections, the use of radioactive tracers has a limited application as a physiologic tool for the study of cutaneous blood flow in a segment of limb.

E. Clinical Tests of Muscle Circulation

1. Claudication Time and Claudication Distance

The only available simple clinical test for determining the state of muscle circulation is the subjective response of the patient to a standard exercise. This, however, gives only a qualitative index of the severity of local arterial impairment.

In order to keep conditions as constant as possible, the examiner walks with the patient, maintaining a pace of 100 to 120 steps/min on a level surface. Using a stopwatch, the exact time of the initial development of intermittent claudication in the exercising muscles is determined (claudication time), as well as the point at which the pain is so severe that the patient must stop (absolute walking time). Another approach is to record the length of the walk in standard-sized city blocks (claudication distance). Also of value is to determine how long the pain persists following termination of the exercise, with the patient standing (pain disappearance time). The latter information appears to correlate well with the entire clinical picture: the longer the interval of recovery, the more marked is the reduction in muscle circulation.

A treadmill may be substituted for walking on the street, since with it a constant speed can be maintained. However, it has the disadvantage of placing the patient in a situation which is quite different from that which exists with normal walking. This may cause apprehension and even fear in an elderly individual and thus affect the value of the information derived from the test. Moreover, the procedure requires continuous monitoring and medical supervision.

As an adjunctive approach, in order to obtain some objectivity to the test, oscillometry (see Section B, Chapter 5) is performed before and immediately after termination of the physical effort. In the normal individual, readings are significantly increased in the postexercise period due to local dilatation in the active muscles, whereas in the patient with organic arterial disease, the response is minimal.

References

1. Farrell C, Wallace JD, Edeiken J: Thermography and osteosarcoma. Radiology 90:792, 1968
2. Naide M: Relation of growth of hair on digits to the severity of ischemia. N Engl J Med 248:179, 1953
3. Nicholson JP, Rogers RT, Tosh DC: The relative merits of thermoscanning and gamma scanning in the detection of metastatic bone disease. Br J Radiol 44:898, 1971
4. Ratschow M: Die peripheren Durchblutungsstörungen. Dresden, Theodor Steinkopff, 1949
5. Samuels SS: The early diagnosis of thromboangiitis obliterans: A new diagnostic sign. JAMA 92:1571, 1929
6. Spence VA, Kester RC, Howie G, et al: Current status of thermography in peripheral vascular disease. J Cardiovasc Surg 16:572, 1975
7. Wallace JD: Thermography in bone disease. JAMA 230:447, 1974

Chapter 7

Clinical and Laboratory Tests of Venous Circulation

Pathologic changes in the superficial and deep venous systems, particularly of the lower extremities, are relatively common complications of orthopedic difficulties (see Chapters 17–20). For this reason, it is important to be acquainted with the various clinical and laboratory tests that are useful in the study of such abnormalities.

A. Examination of the Superficial Venous System

1. Inspection and Palpation

Examination of the skin and subcutaneous tissue of the lower extremities by inspection and palpation may elicit considerable information regarding the state and ramifications of the superficial veins. In this manner, the vessels can be studied for evidence of thrombosis, inflammation, "spider" veins (Fig. 7.1), abnormal prominences, distension, pulsations, and regurgitant flow (Fig. 7.2).

Superficial thrombophlebitis. Linear red streaks in the skin, about 1 cm in width and of varying length, may indicate the presence of thrombosed subcutaneous veins with an associated phlebitis and periphlebitis. The presence of increased cutaneous temperature directly over and in the vicinity of the lesion and of a tender cordlike mass beneath the skin

helps confirm the impression. In order to differentiate a thrombosed vein from a dilated one, it is necessary to outline the entire length of the involved segment on the skin and then elevate the limb. Under these circumstances, a prominent distended vessel will collapse and become imperceptible to the examining finger, whereas an occluded one will remain unchanged.

The most likely sites for benign superficial thrombophlebitis are along the course of the two main superficial venous systems, the great saphenous and small saphenous veins. In the case of the former, the medial aspect of the thigh and leg should be inspected, whereas for the small saphenous vein, attention should be directed to the lateral and posterolateral surfaces of the leg up to the level of the popliteal space.

Dilated superficial veins. Such alterations may be a prominent finding in the early stage of acute iliofemoral thrombophlebitis. The responsible mechanism is an increase in venous pressure due to shunting of blood from the deep into the superficial venous system, in an attempt to bypass the blocked portion of vessel. Later the superficial venous network may become conspicuous as a result of the formation of a new collateral system on the lateral aspect of the thigh, the flank, and the lateral and anterior portions of the abdominal wall (Fig. 20.1A and B). Occlusion of the inferior vena cava is

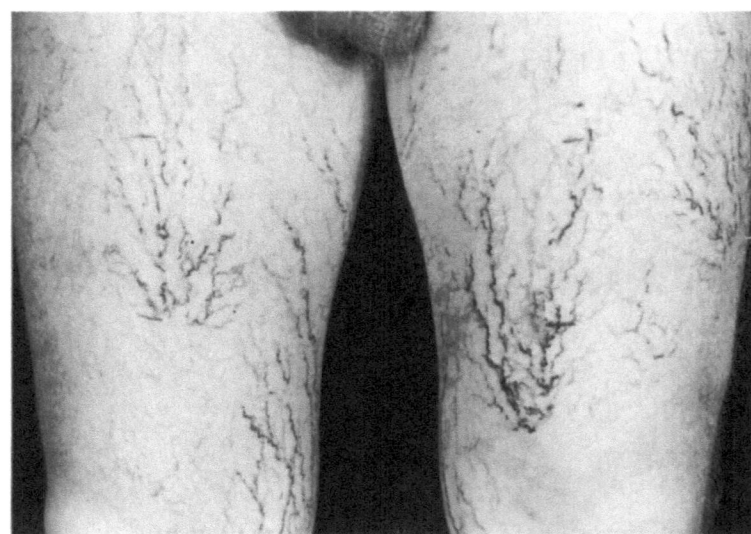

Fig. 7.1. "Spider" veins on the thighs due to enlargement of the subpapillary venous plexus.

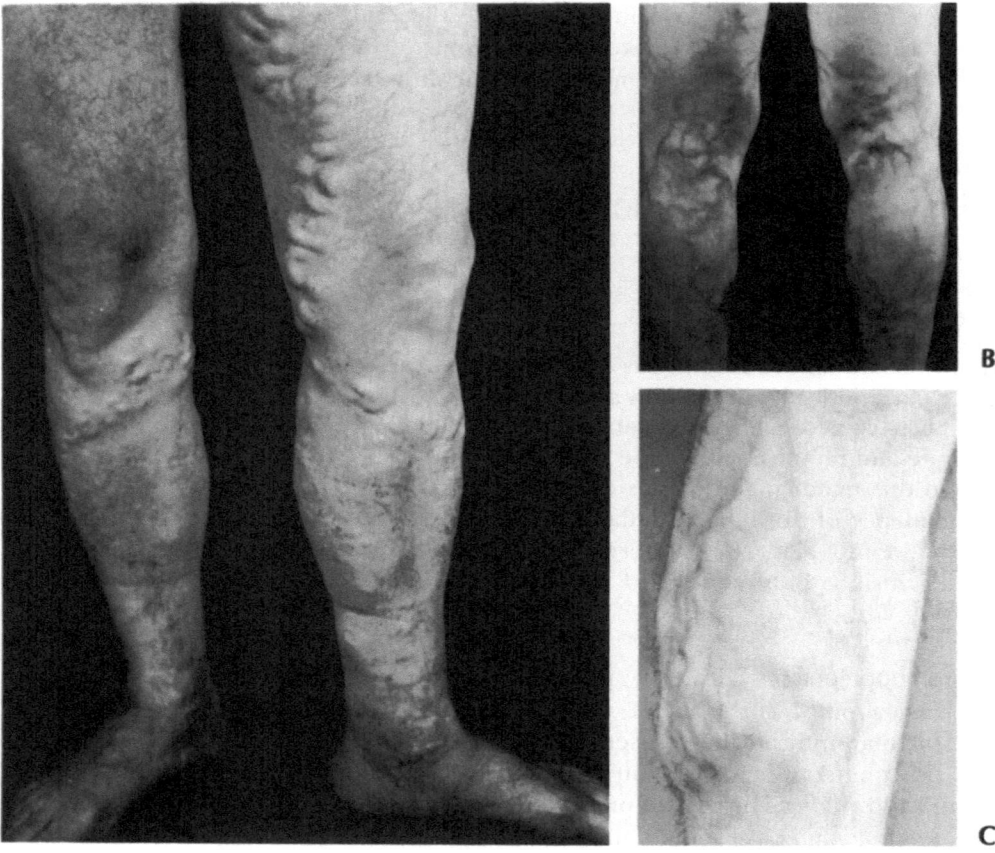

Fig. 7.2. Primary varicosities. **A** Involvement of both the great (left lower limb) and the small (right lower limb) saphenous systems. **B** Incompetency of great saphenous vein on both legs. **C** Batch of varicosities on back of leg due to incompetent communicating veins. From Abramson DI: Circulatory Diseases of the Limbs: A Primer. New York, Grune & Stratton, 1978. Reproduced with permission.

associated with the appearance of large, distended, and tortuous superficial veins on both lower limbs and on the anterior surface of the abdomen (Fig. 7.3). Following occlusion of the axillary or the subclavian vein by a thrombus (see B-2, Chapter 18), a rapidly forming collateral venous circulation is noted on the medial aspect of the involved arm and the adjoining half of the chest wall (Fig. 18.5). Slow obstruction of the superior vena cava results in the development of an extensive collateral venous network over the entire anterior chest wall which extends downward over the upper portion of the anterior abdominal wall, together with prominent large vessels in the neck and distended venules on the cheeks and nose. The sudden and apparently spontaneous appearance of dilated superficial veins on a limb may also indicate the presence of some extrinsic obstruction to venous outflow, as for example, a tumor in the chest or pelvis or a gravid uterus.

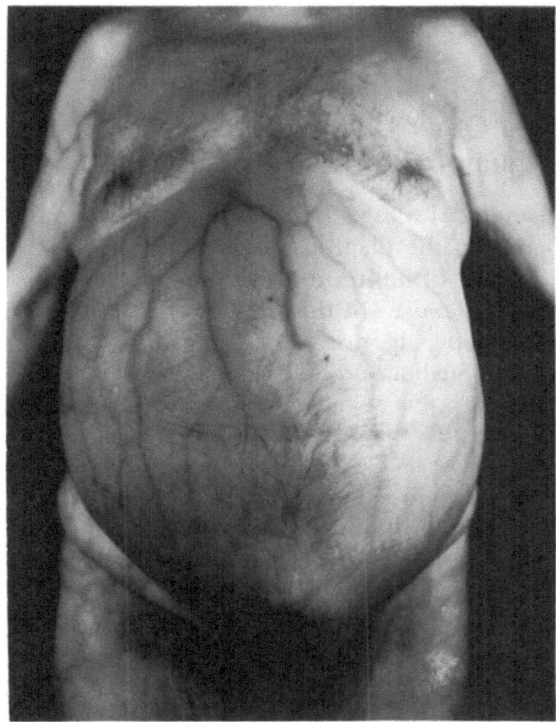

Fig. 7.3. Extensive collateral venous network on the outer aspects of the thighs and anterior abdominal wall produced by complete obstruction of blood flow in the inferior vena cava, associated with ascites. Vessels made more conspicuous by infrared photography.

2. Tests for Competency of Valves in Superficial and Communicating Veins

Since inspection and palpation alone are frequently not sufficient to differentiate between varicose and dilated veins, it is necessary to resort to several tests to make such a distinction. These procedures are also of value in accurately locating all involved vessels, information which is essential if surgical treatment of the varicose veins is contemplated.

Brodie-Trendelenburg test. This procedure, commonly known by the latter name alone, is performed as follows: After the patient lies down, the limb is elevated to empty the superficial veins, and then a rubber tourniquet is applied around the thigh just below the level of the fossa ovalis. The degree of compression utilized is much less than that which would obstruct arterial inflow or movement of blood out of the femoral vein but is sufficient to collapse the great saphenous vein. The patient now stands, with the portion of the leg displaying the varicosities facing a good light, and within 10 s the tourniquet is released. An immediate filling of the great saphenous vein and its tributaries from above downward implies that the valves in the main vessel are incompetent, probably at the level of the fossa ovalis, and that blood is leaking backward into the superficial venous system through the saphenofemoral junction. A slow filling of the vessels (30 s or more) is a normal response, being due to the upward movement of blood from the capillary system.

If, instead of removing the tourniquet almost immediately, the compression is maintained, further pertinent information can be obtained. The rapid appearance of dilated vessels in one or more areas below the level of the constricting band indicates that there has been a reflux flow into them either from an incompetent small saphenous vein or from incompetent communicating branches. If the tourniquet is now released and there is immediate greater filling of the superficial veins, this signifies that a leak is also present high in the great saphenous vein. For the sake of clarity, it is better to express the changes obtained with the procedure as indicating competency or incompetency of the valves in question, rather than as a negative or positive Trendelenburg test.

Multiple tourniquet test. This is a modification of the Trendelenburg test and is performed as follows: With the extremity elevated, four tourniquets are applied, three to the thigh so as to compress the upper, middle, and lower segments, respectively, and one to the leg just below the knee. The patient now stands and the rate of filling of the superficial veins on the leg is noted. If the response occurs rapidly with all four bands in place (in less than 30 s), it can be assumed that there are incompetent communicating vessels located below the level of the lowest tourniquet on the leg. If no change is noted, the latter band is removed. Immediate filling of the superficial veins implies that the small saphenous vein is incompetent. The same type of response resulting from removal of the tourniquet just above the knee and around the middle of the thigh indicates that the involvement is in main tributaries of the great saphenous vein. Sudden distension of veins on the leg and thigh on release of the last tourniquet localizes the difficulty to the saphenofemoral junction.

B. Clinical Examination of the Deep Venous System

1. Inspection and Palpation

Because of their location deep in the tissues (see B-2, below), normally the main venous channels in the limbs do not lend themselves to inspection or palpation. However, if they are suddenly occluded, there will result distension of the superficial veins (see A-1, above), pitting edema, and pallor and coldness of the skin (see A-3, Chapter 18).

2. Homans' Sign

Homans' sign (dorsiflexion sign) is of value in determining whether there is an acute thrombosis of the deep veins in the calf (phlebothrombosis; see A-2, Chapter 18). It consists of forcibly dorsiflexing the foot with the leg lifted off the bed, so as to place the tissues comprising the posterior portion of the calf under stress. If the venous plexuses in the muscles of the calf are thrombosed, the maneuver will cause pressure on the adjoining nerves to produce pain locally. Some degree of fullness and tension of the calf muscles as well as tenderness of the sole of the foot on pressure are frequently associated with a positive dorsiflexion sign. Symptoms in the foot may indicate that thrombi are present in the venous plexuses in the small muscles locally.

In the interpretation of the Homans' sign, the possibility of obtaining a false-positive response must be considered. For example, any type of inflammation in the vicinity of the calf may cause pain when the involved tissues are placed on stretch by dorsiflexing the foot. Therefore, before attributing symptoms produced by this maneuver to phlebothrombosis, it is necessary to rule out such conditions as superficial thrombophlebitis, chronic and acute cellulitis, dermatitis, a shortened Achilles tendon, myofibrositis, local hemorrhage, and laceration and contusion of muscles.

3. Other Diagnostic Signs of Phlebothrombosis

Among several other findings which may help confirm the diagnosis of phlebothrombosis is an area of infiltration in the region of the venous plexuses of the calf muscles, determined by deep palpation in this location (Neuhof's sign). Such a finding may exist even when Homans' sign is negative. There may also be some tenderness in the lower third of the thigh just above the level of the condyles, at the junction of the popliteal and superficial femoral veins. Another useful diagnostic point is the presence of dilated "sentinel veins" in the upper third of the leg. It has likewise been found that if a thrombus exists in the deep venous plexuses of the calf, the application of pressure as low as 100 to 120 mmHg to this site using a blood pressure cuff will elicit severe pain, whereas the opposite normal calf is generally able to withstand pressures as high as 180 to 200 mmHg without the production of symptoms [9]. It is necessary to point out, however, that, theoretically at least, such a procedure could be responsible for the dislodgment of a friable clot in the vessels, with the subsequent production of pulmonary embolism. Also of importance is the fact that the incidence of false-negative and false-positive results with this test is high.

4. Perthes' Test

Perthes' test is performed as follows: The subject stands and, after a tourniquet is placed around the thigh to compress the great saphenous vein, he either alternately flexes and extends the knee about 10 times or walks. If the deep veins are patent and competent, the exercise will cause the blood to flow into them, with the result that the superficial vessels will collapse and remain so. If the deep veins are patent but incompetent, the superficial veins will empty during the physical effort but will then refill as soon as exercise is terminated. By applying the tourniquet at different levels, information can be obtained regarding the site of incompetency. If the deep veins are not patent or if there is an increased pressure in them, the superficial vessels will become more distended during the period of exercise.

For the upper limb, the counterpart of Perthes' test consists of the following: The patient stands with both arms in the dependent position and then repeatedly opens and closes the hands with a pumping action. If there is a thrombus in the axillary or subclavian vein, such a maneuver will cause overdistension of the superficial veins on the forearm and dorsum of the hand, similar to the response to the application of a tourniquet. In the presence of a patent and competent deep venous system, the exercise will cause the superficial veins to collapse. Supporting evidence is obtained by elevating the upper limbs above the level of the head. In the case of a block in a main collecting vein, the superficial vessels will still remain distended, whereas in a normal limb they will collapse due to drainage of blood out of them.

C. Laboratory Examination of the Deep Venous System

A large number of laboratory tests are available for the study of the patency of the deep venous system, the most common of which are described below. In the case of those used primarily to determine whether thrombi exist in the deep veins of the lower limbs (Sections C-2 to C-5, below), their relative values as diagnostic aids are compared in Section C-6, below, instead of individually under each separate heading.

1. Venous Pressure Measurements

The height of the venous pressure in the limbs is a reflection of the rate of circulation through the venous system. A rise in the readings represents some interference to movement of blood through a main collecting vein proximal to the level at which the test is performed. However, no information is obtained as to whether this is the result of extrinsic compression of the vessel or of occlusion of its lumen by a thrombus. Moreover, the test does not differentiate between a rise in venous pressure caused by a systemic condition (such as congestive heart failure, constrictive pericarditis, or pericarditis with effusion) and one which follows a pathologic change in a main vein locally.

Technique. The method for obtaining venous pressure readings in the upper extremity is similar to that used in determining central venous pressure, whereas for the lower extremity, certain modifications of the standard procedure are required. These include surgically exposing a superficial vein on the dorsum of the foot under local anesthesia and cannulating it using a 14-gauge, thin-walled needle; a flexible polyethylene catheter 30 cm (12 in.) long is then treaded into the vessel through the needle. The latter is removed and the skin closed with one or two sutures previously placed. The free end of the tubing is passed through an airtight cork of a reservoir bottle so as to extend below the level of sterile heparinized saline solution half filling the container. A mercury or water manometer is connected by a three-way stopcock to a sphygmomanometer hand bulb and to a glass tube which also passes through the cork of the reservoir bottle but reaches only to above the level of the saline solution. A reading is obtained by first raising the pressure in the system to above the anticipated venous pressure and then, when the cannula is cleared of blood, lowering it very slowly. The pressure is read on the manometer scale at the instant that blood enters the translucent tubing arising from the vein [18]. Another approach involves the use of an Atlas apparatus type EM, with the pressure being transmitted by a Statham element to a Multicord 250 recorder containing an intensifier.

Venous pressure measurements under various conditions. In the horizontal position, the normal venous pressure reading in the foot is 4.8 to 8.8 mmHg (60 to 120 mm H_2O), (which range is the same as in the upper limb under similar conditions). On standing it rises to 70 to 100 mmHg, whereas during exercise it falls to around 30 to 40 mmHg, with a quick return to control levels after termination of the physical effort.

In the presence of chronic primary varicosities, the venous pressure with the patient lying down is greater than normal; on standing it is the same. However, exercise does not produce the normal lowering of the readings because of the retrograde flow of blood from the deep venous system into the great saphenous vein at the level of the fossa ovalis. If this backward movement is prevented by first applying a tourniquet around the upper part of the thigh, exercise will reduce the venous pressure so that the readings now fall in the range of normal.

In the patient suffering from postphlebitic syndrome (see Chapter 20), venous pressure readings in recumbency are normal, whereas on standing they exceed the normal range. Exercise does not cause them to fall even with a tourniquet around the thigh to prevent regurgitant flow into the superficial veins. This is so because the deep venous system is either impatent or incompetent, both states interfering with movement of blood out of the limb in the direction of the inferior vena cava.

It can therefore be emphasized that venous pressure measurements supply definitive information regarding the condition of the deep venous system and that such an approach is helpful in differentiating secondary from primary varicosities if this cannot be done by other less complicated clinical means.

2. Contrast Venography

The technique of roentgenographic visualization of the deep venous tree in the extremities through the use of radiopaque material is generally similar in principle to that utilized in angiography (see E-1, Chapter 5), except that the contrast medium is introduced into a peripheral vein. When the method was first proposed, it claimed many advocates. Then there was a swing away from its routine application. However, this technique undoubtedly still plays a very important role in the diagnosis of some of the pathologic processes affecting the deep venous system, particularly of the lower limbs.

Adverse reactions. As in the case of arteriography (see E-2 and E-3, Chapter 5), a number of precautions must be taken with venography. The first is the determination of sensitivity to the contrast medium. Certain types of patients respond poorly to the material and in them the procedure should not be used or, if necessary, performed only with great caution. If signs of an allergic reaction occur, the injection is immediately terminated and 30 mg of diphenhydramine hydrochloride (Benadryl) are given intravenously. Other adverse responses to the parenteral administration of the contrast medium are fainting, infection of cutdown sites, and extravasation of the radiopaque material into the tissues. Postinjection thrombosis and embolism, which occur in about 3 percent of cases, can generally be prevented if 5000 units of heparin are given intravenously before venography is carried out [12].

Techniques. A number of different methods have been suggested for visualizing the deep veins of the lower extremities. One consists of cannulating a tributary of the short saphenous vein after it has been exposed by a small incision under local anesthesia. The vessel used is a constant small vein present behind the external malleolus which communicates with the deep venous system. About 20 ml of the contrast material are injected through a 19-gauge transfusion cannula over a period of 60 s. Then an x-ray film, which has been placed under the leg, is exposed. The cannula is removed, the vein is tied, and the skin is closed with silk after any residual contrast material is removed with normal saline. If a 19-gauge needle is used instead of a cannula, it is generally not necessary to tie off the vein.

It has been suggested that combining fluoroscopy with the radiographic technique has many advantages over the latter alone. Through fluoroscopy the dynamic picture existing in the venous tree can be studied; at the same time, such a procedure helps to localize the involved site, so that the subsequent radiograph can be appropriately centered, thus obtaining more complete and accurate information regarding the state of the affected veins. The method consists of placing the patient on the fluoroscopic table with the foot everted and the limb slightly abducted. The small vein behind the external malleolus is exposed, as previously mentioned, and 30 ml of contrast material are injected. During the first part of this step, the response is observed fluoroscopically. By the time 10 to 15 ml have entered the vessel over a period of from 10 to 30 s, a clear outline of the deep venous system has been obtained. Then fluoroscopy is terminated, the remaining 15 to 20 ml of contrast material are injected, and an x-ray film is exposed.

Another procedure which has had clinical application obviates the need for exposing the vein surgically. With the legs dependent, a 20-gauge needle is inserted into a subcutaneous vein on the dorsum of the foot or lateral side of the ankle. The needle is connected to an infusion set containing normal saline, which is permitted to enter the vein rather rapidly so as to prevent clotting. After the needle is strapped in place with adhesive tape, the patient is placed on the x-ray table with the cassette containing the film behind the calf and thigh. Then a rubber tourniquet is applied around the leg, at the junction of the middle and lower third, with sufficient pressure to prevent the contrast medium from entering the superficial veins of the upper part of the leg and thigh. Twenty milliliters of contrast medium are slowly injected into the tubing of the infusion set just above the needle, while the tubing is pinched off at a higher level to prevent retrograde flow. An x-ray film is exposed 5 s after the full amount has been injected, and then the saline is again allowed to enter the

vein, in order to wash the radiopaque material out. It is possible to obtain a number of different views by rotating the leg after the first film is exposed and immediately taking another. If with the first radiograph the foot is rotated inward, the space between the fibula and tibia will be increased, thus making it possible to obtain a more complete picture of the deep venous system, less obscured by the shadow of the bones.

Information regarding the state of the valves in the main veins can be collected in the following manner: A venogram is obtained using either of the above methods, and then with 10 ml of the contrast medium still in the syringe, the patient performs a Valsalva maneuver. While this is being carried out, the remainder of the radiopaque material is injected into the vein. The resulting increase in intraabdominal pressure reverses the direction of the contrast medium in the veins of the pelvis and lower limbs and normally causes closure of the valve cusps and bulging of the paravalvular sinuses. As a result, there is concentration of the radiopaque material just proximal to the valves and reduction of opacity below this level. If incompetent valves are present, such changes are not noted.

Retrograde venography may be helpful in obtaining further information regarding the state of the large collecting veins [15]. This first involves slow injection of the contrast medium into the femoral vein just below the inguinal ligament. Then after two x-ray exposures have been made, the patient exercises by raising himself from the table 10 times, with another film being taken 1 min after termination of the physical effort. Clearing of the veins of contrast material following exercise can be interpreted as supporting the view that the valves locally are competent.

Finally, venography can be performed using the intraosseous route [1], since the circulation of the hematopoietic bone marrow is in direct communication only with the extraosseous deep venous system. As a result, there is no need to utilize a tourniquet around the lower portion of the limb. However, a great disadvantage to the method is that the injection of the contrast medium is always associated with severe local bursting pain.

The technique of intraosseous venography consists of anesthetizing the skin over the designated site (the tibia just above the base of the medial malleolus, the medial or lateral malleolus, or the lateral portion of the os calcis) and then, after penetrating the bone using a short-beveled bone marrow aspiration needle, injecting the contrast medium into the bone marrow cavity. In order to evaluate the function of the venous pump, one exposure is made immediately after the injection and another is taken following three vigorous contractions of the leg muscles. In normal limbs the contrast medium is no longer present in the veins of the leg in the second radiograph, but it may still be apparent in one suffering from chronic venous insufficiency.

In the case of the upper extremity, no problems are generally encountered in visualizing pathologic changes in the deep venous system, since if a block does occur, it is found in the proximal segment of the main vein. Hence, if 10 ml of the radiopaque material are injected into the median basilic vein at the elbow, this will invariably outline the large venous channels of the arm and also the axillary and subclavian veins.

Evaluation of the different techniques. With all of the described modifications, the aim is to fill the deep veins of the upper and lower limbs with the contrast material, so that they will then be visualized on the x-ray film. In the case of the procedure in which the tributary of the short saphenous vein in the foot is exposed surgically, this goal is achieved without difficulty, since the vessel communicates with the deep venous system. The same holds true for intraosseous phlebography. However, in the case of the procedure in which a superficial vein on the dorsum of the foot is entered percutaneously (the most common approach), the necessity of applying a tourniquet around the leg in order to direct the radiopaque material into the deep venous circulation may introduce a number of difficulties. For example, use of insufficient tension on the band may result in visualization primarily of the superficial rather than the deep venous system. Too much pressure may obstruct deep veins as well as superficial vessels and lead to inadequate or no filling of the deep venous system. Such a response

may incorrectly be interpreted as indicating a block in the vessels; or if there is incomplete filling of all the venous plexuses, a thrombus in one or several of them may go unrecognized.

Normal architecture of deep venous system. The pattern of the deep veins in the upper and lower extremities varies considerably in different individuals. In general, the deep tributaries of the foot and leg fuse to make up the paired anterior and posterior tibial veins (venae comitantes of anterior and posterior tibial arteries), which then join to form the popliteal vein (Fig. 7.4B and C). The latter, which may also be paired, extends upward onto the thigh as the superficial femoral vein (Fig. 7.4A) to join with the deep femoral vein to become the common femoral vein. The common femoral vein then continues as the iliofemoral and finally as the common iliac vein in the abdomen. All of the main vessels and their tributaries (except for the deep femoral vein) are visualized by the contrast medium when injected into a vessel in the foot, the popliteal and superficial femoral veins in the thigh appearing as a straight tubular filling. The valves are also brought out in the course of the vessels. In the case of the upper extremity, the contrast material normally outlines the basilic, the axillary, the subclavian, and at times even the innominate veins (Fig. 7.5).

Venographic signs of obstruction. Thrombi in the venous plexuses of the calf muscles are identified as constant, elongated filling defects which persist in shape and location in well-opacified vessels in at least two films (Fig. 18.1A). A thrombus still floating in the lumen and partly occluding it appears as a well-defined translucent area surrounded by a rim or narrow border of contrast medium (Fig. 18.1B). The latter may be so delicate that at times it seems as though it has been traced with a pencil [12]. The ends of the thrombus have rounded tips. Early in the inception of the condition, bridging collateral vessels may be sparse or almost invisible, probably because venous backflow is still effective due to the fact that the thrombus is not as yet adherent to the wall of the vessel. Partial obstruction of a collecting vein may also manifest itself in the form of a reduction in size and irregularities

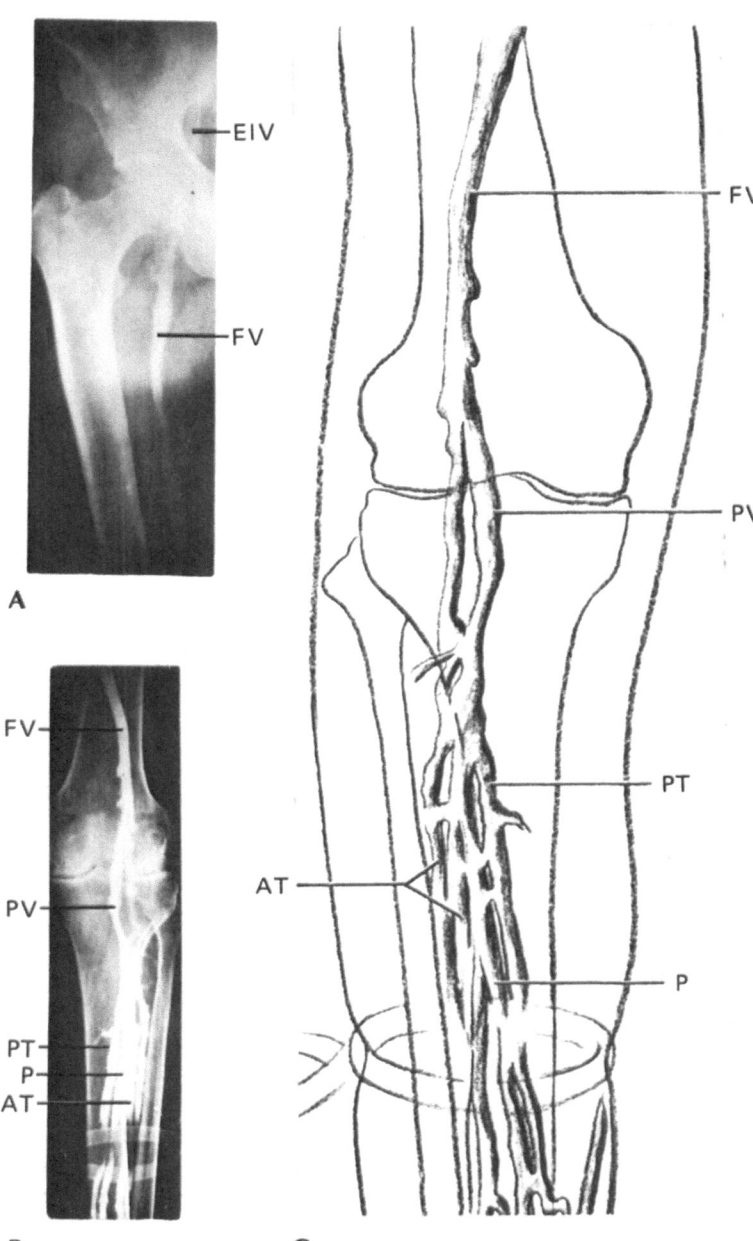

Fig. 7.4. Normal venous tree visualized by venography. **A** *EIV,* external iliac vein; *FV,* superficial femoral vein. **B** *FV,* superficial femoral vein; *PV,* popliteal vein; *PT,* venae comitantes of posterior tibial artery; *P,* venae comitantes of peroneal artery; *AT,* venae comitantes of anterior tibial artery. **C** Diagrammatic representation of the venous tree visualized in **B. A** and **B,** from Abramson DI: Vascular Disorders of the Extremities. Hagerstown, Md, Harper & Row, 1974. Reproduced with permission.

in contour of segments of the vessel. When complete occlusion occurs, the involved portion of vein shows no opacification at all, with the rim of contrast medium having disappeared. Under such circumstances, backflow cannot occur except through collateral veins which now become prominent.

Artifacts in venography. Signs of organic abnormalities in the venogram (see above) must be differentiated from changes produced by the injection of the contrast medium and from hemodynamic factors in the blood. Venospasm, which may be initiated by the radiopaque material, generally manifests itself as an almost complete obliteration of a segment of vein, with tapering distally and normal-appearing vessel on either side of the block. Perhaps with the previous use of fluoroscopy, this state will more readily be identified.

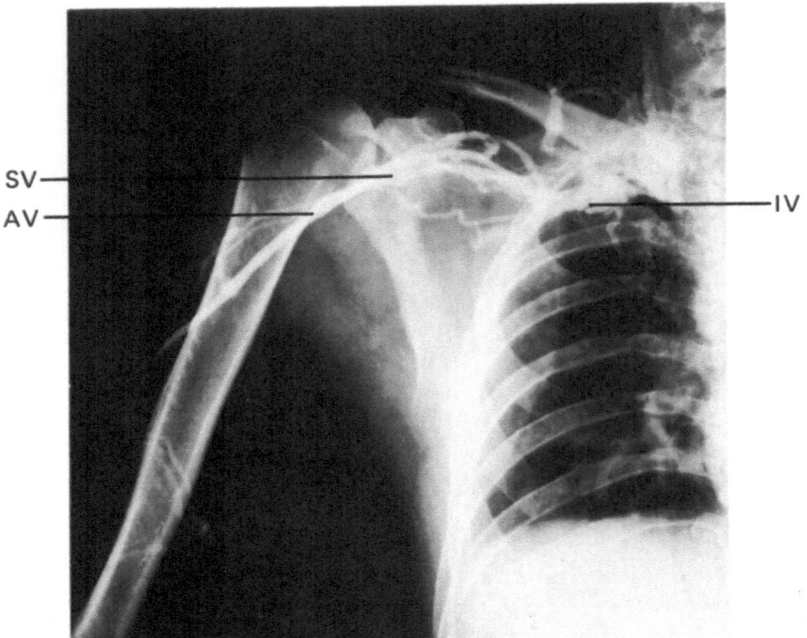

Fig. 7.5. Normal venous tree in upper limb visualized by venography. *AV*, axillary vein; *SV*, subclavian vein; *IV*, innominate vein.

Another source of error is a greater blood flow velocity in the center of the vessel, causing translucency in this area. Such an artifact can usually be excluded by an additional film of the same segment. Interpretation of the changes in the venogram may also be made difficult by the inflow phenomenon produced when a vein without contrast medium drains into one containing it. This causes a translucency to develop in the dense shadow of the main trunk, at the junction points, which appears like a finger in the central portion of the vessel [12]. Such a change is generally noticed in the large collecting vessels (the popliteal and femoral veins) and it can be differentiated from that produced by a thrombus, since the contours of the inflow phenomenon are hazy whereas those of a clot are clear-cut. Again, an additional film will help clarify the situation.

Finally, contractions of voluntary muscles toward the end of the examination may produce changes in the venogram which mimic thrombosis. As a result of expression of blood from the deep venous plexuses by the active muscles, filling defects of differing lengths appear in these vessels. With easing of muscular tension, opacification again occurs. Another situation which may cause artifacts is when muscular contractions press large quantities of unmixed blood into the deep veins. Since this complement of blood mixes only poorly with that containing contrast medium, filling defects in the deep veins are simulated. In both of the above instances, a second film can readily identify the nature of the apparent abnormality.

Indications for use of procedure. Contrast venography has application to a number of different situations. Primary among these is acute thrombosis of the deep veins of the lower limbs, particularly involvement of the venous plexuses in the muscles of the calf. In certain instances, the procedure is also useful in determining why surgical procedures for primary varicosities have not produced a therapeutic effect, as for example, by visualizing an incompetent communicating vein which is continually feeding the superficial varicosities. The procedure is likewise helpful in the treatment of varicose ulcers since it may call attention to the presence, location, and extent of incompetent perforating vessels which are producing venous stasis in the vicinity of the lesion. Similarly, contrast venography is of value in the study of chronic ulcers of the leg without any apparent etiology, since it may demonstrate an old block in the deep venous system, thus clarifying the nature of the condition.

In the case of patients who have an indefinite history of iliofemoral thrombophlebitis and in whom it is necessary to determine whether this has any basis, venography is of considerable value. It will bring out the filling defect and the presence of extensive collateral vessels bridging the gap, thus helping to confirm the diagnosis. Or it may not visualize the main vessels, but instead a number of smaller tortuous channels replacing them. The procedure is also important if varicosities are to be treated surgically and there is some question whether they are primary and hence operable or secondary to an old iliofemoral thrombophlebitis (part of the postphlebitic syndrome) and almost always left untouched. Finally, the procedure is helpful in determining valvular incompetency in the main collecting veins in the thigh and pelvis. (For further discussion of the value of contrast venography, see pp. 191 and 223.)

3. Radionuclide Venography

Radionuclide phlebography has been proposed as a substitute for contrast venography (see C-2, above) since it is a less painful and more rapid technique for visualizing thrombi in the deep veins of the lower limbs, unassociated with significant morbidity.

Technique. Scanning is performed using as a tracer human serum albumin microspheres incorporating ^{99m}Tc sulfur colloid [14]. An advantage to the injection of such a material is that pulmonary scanning can be carried out at the same time that peripheral venography is performed [21]. A refinement of the method consists of isotope labeling of 15- to 30-μm microspheres of uniform spherical shape [21], which have less tendency to adhere to venous valves than do those that are irregular.

The radionuclide is injected into a dorsal vein of the foot through a small-calibered plastic needle after double ankle tourniquets have been applied, the procedure being carried out with the patient carefully positioned under an Anger-type scintillation camera. Rapid-sequence scintiphotography of blood flow through the veins of the calf, thigh, groin, and abdomen is performed with a Gamma camera, the image being recorded simultaneously by Polaroid camera photography.

4. Radioactive Fibrinogen Test

The fibrinogen uptake test is based on the fact that the short half-life isotope of iodine, ^{125}I, can be incorporated into the molecule of fibrinogen without altering the process of conversion to fibrin. The radioactive fibrinogen is therefore capable of accumulating in areas of endothelial damage by becoming adherent to the clot as it flows past the site of involvement. As a consequence, there is a buildup of radioactivity in the vicinity of the lesion as determined by surface counting. The radiation dosage from the labeled fibrinogen is small, being less than that used in lung scans.

Technique. The procedure is performed as follows: First an oral dose of Lugol's solution or sodium iodide (100 mg) is given 24 h before the test or 150 mg of sodium iodide are injected intravenously on the same day, to protect the thyroid gland; then 100 μCi of ^{125}I-human fibrinogen (Sensor; Ibrin) are also given intravenously. After allowing 10 to 60 min for mixing, the patient's legs are elevated 10° and surface counting is carried out over selected areas of each limb, using a shielded external probe and a single-channel analyzer spectrometer. The test causes no discomfort to the patient and requires no physical effort on his part; hence it can be used in seriously ill subjects. Moreover, with the administration of a single dose it is possible to make serial measurements, since the radioactivity can be followed sequentially over a period of approximately 7 days. One drawback of this procedure is its cost.

Since the possibility of transmission of hepatitis through the labeled fibrinogen exists, all donors must be screened very carefully. They must be Australia antigen–negative and must be observed for at least several years so as to make certain that they cannot transmit hepatitis.

5. Doppler Ultrasonic Flowmeter

The principle involved in the Doppler ultrasonic flowmeter technique and the apparatus used are described in Section D-2, Chapter 5.

Basis for use of method in venous disease. The test depends on the fact that normal nonoccluded veins demonstrate spontaneous cyclic respiratory flow. Associated with a deep breath and depression of the diaphragm, a transient obstruction of the inferior vena cava in the abdomen is produced, followed by release as the breath is expired. During the latter phase, there is an increase in venous flow. Using a Doppler instrument, the changes in venous circulation can be heard at the femoral and popliteal levels as a cyclic blowing sound. By squeezing the tissues distal to the probe, an additional quantity of blood flows into the venous system, momentarily increasing the velocity of venous circulation and thus altering the quality of the sound.

In the presence of a thrombus completely occluding a collecting vein in the lower limb, the cyclic respiratory flow is significantly altered or diminished and so is the resulting sound; at the same time, no change in sound follows an attempt to facilitate venous outflow mechanically. For an obvious abnormality to be identified by the Doppler instrument, however, more than one of the collecting veins of the leg (anterior tibial, posterior tibial, or peroneal) must be occluded. Otherwise the sound due to cyclic respiratory flow is still heard, although diminished in intensity.

Technique. The probe head, held at an angle of 45°, is lightly placed in contact with the skin overlying the main veins of the lower limb (the common femoral, superficial femoral, popliteal, and posterior tibial veins), and the venous velocity signal is identified by a change in frequency related to the respiratory cycle. To facilitate collection of the data, examination of the popliteal vein is performed by placing the patient in the prone position with the knee slightly flexed and the foot resting on a pillow; for study of the other vessels, he is left on his back.[1]

---

[1] There are a number of other much less commonly used laboratory procedures available for the identification of deep venous thrombosis. However, since they are rarely utilized by the orthopedic or general surgeon, they have not been described. Among these are impedance plethysmography [7,19,22], mercury strain-gauge plethysmography, phleborheography [4,5], and thermography [3]. The relative value of most of these as diagnostic aids is discussed in Section 6.

6. Relative Value of Laboratory Tests of Acute Deep Venous Thrombosis

At this point, a comparison of the relative worth of the common laboratory procedures utilized in the diagnosis of acute deep venous thrombosis of the lower limbs appears to be in order, since perusal of individual papers randomly selected from the voluminous literature on the subject generally leaves the reader confused and uncertain as to the choice of an appropriate test for a specific situation. What gives urgency to the elucidation of the problem is that in most instances reliance solely on clinical means of making a diagnosis, as for example, in the case of phlebothrombosis (see A-2, Chapter 18), frequently results in inaccurate evaluation of the situation.

Contrast venography. This procedure is still regarded as the single most useful technique for establishing the presence of thrombi in the deep venous system of the lower limbs. It also reveals in detail the anatomy of the occluded veins and accurately differentiates between a clot obstructing a vessel and extrinsic pressure caused by a tumor interfering with movement of blood through the venous system.

However, the absence of contrast material in a deep vein is not unequivocal evidence for the existence of thrombosis. For example, such a finding may also be due to technical difficulties preventing the radiopaque medium from entering the deep channels, or it may follow spasm of veins which produces filling defects that are difficult to differentiate from changes due to structural alterations. False-negative results may also occur, as when thrombi are present in the soleal sinuses, all of which are not always opacified. Moreover, the same situation may exist in the case of the sural veins as they enter the popliteal space, since these are often only partially filled.

Because of the possibility of misinterpretation of the findings, venography should be utilized only by the expert who has had considerable experience in the recognition of artifacts. Also important in the full evaluation of the procedure is the fact that it is cumbersome, time consuming, invasive, costly, and associated with adverse and, at times, serious reactions. For these reasons, it cannot be used as a screening procedure or carried out repeatedly to supply information necessary for the proper treatment of a patient with deep venous thrombosis. (For discussion of artifacts in venography, see p. 97.)

Radionuclide venography. This method also visualizes the main veins in the limbs, but the anatomic detail is poorer than that obtained with contrast media studies. Nevertheless, it has the advantage of more clearly reflecting flow characteristics and of giving better physiologic data than does contrast venography. Also, it is helpful in detecting nonocclusive thrombi through the development of localized increases of radioactivity. It has been found useful in determining the existence of deep venous thrombosis in bedridden patients before the appearance of clinical manifestations. Moreover, the procedure has been used in followup studies on persons undergoing various forms of therapy, since it can be repeated many times without causing any ill effects. However, a serious objection to the test is that it is cumbersome and requires costly specialized equipment and trained personnel.

Radioactive fibrinogen test. This procedure has proved to be a sensitive tool for screening special populations with high risk of venous thrombosis, for studying the natural history of deep venous thrombosis, and for evaluating results of prophylactic and therapeutic regimens [8,10,13]. In contrast to radionuclide venography, it has its greatest value in identifying clots in the sinusoids of the muscles of the calf, particularly the soleus muscle [6,11]. The test also demonstrates a local increase in radioactivity in nonocclusive thrombi which lie free in the bloodstream and which may readily be liberated to form pulmonary emboli. The accuracy of the results is much poorer, however, when thrombi are located in the collecting veins of the thigh or in the iliac veins. In fact, a clot which completely occludes one of these vessels will not be identified, since under these conditions all flow ceases in the involved vein and hence the thrombus does not have the possibility of contact with the circulating radioactive material.

Several disadvantages and limitations characterize the radioactive fibrinogen test, the most serious of which is that radioactive fibrinogen will attach itself to other concentrations of fibrin besides thrombi in blood vessels, such as hematomas, local trauma, and healing wounds. False-positive results may also be noted in acute arthritis, varicose ulcers, cellulitis, and superficial thrombophlebitis. Another response which reduces the value of the procedure is the finding that false-negative results may occur in patients in whom the thrombi are over 11 days old because fibrinogen is preferentially deposited only around newly forming clots and may not accumulate once the thrombus is established. Because of this type of reaction, it has been proposed to use radioactive technetium-labeled streptokinase and technetium-labeled urokinase in place of radioactive fibrinogen, since both of these drugs continue to cause lysis of the surface of clot even in the complete thrombus, thus enhancing the possibility of late identification of the intravascular process. Finally, the test does not become positive in the presence of a developing thrombus in a vein until approximately 96 h have elapsed.

Doppler ultrasonic flowmeter. Since this procedure identifies movement of blood through main collecting veins, it is of diagnostic value solely when a large clot completely obstructs such channels, a situation which is generally readily recognized by physical examination (see Section A-3, Chapter 18). In general, the procedure is useful as a diagnostic test for relatively recent rather than for older thrombotic episodes in the veins. This is probably so because as the collateral circulation becomes more efficient, the functional impedance to venous return is relieved and any abnormal response previously reported by the apparatus then reverts to normal. Detracting from the value of the method is the fact that it does not detect clots in the small deep venous plexuses in the calf [17], the site of origin of the majority of pulmonary emboli. Nor does it identify thrombi which have propagated into the popliteal or the superficial femoral vein without obstructing the vessel [17], a situation which is also conducive to liberation of clots into the main venous system. Consequently, the Doppler ultrasound technique cannot be used as a screening method to detect early disease in the deep veins of the lower limbs. It must also be noted that with this test, false-negative results occur in almost 24 percent of the cases [16]. The fact that flow in large collaterals or large superficial veins may produce a sound which is indistinguishable from that heard over a normal major deep channel may, in part, be responsible for such a situation. One advantage of the method is that it is noninvasive and can be repeated as often as necessary without any discomfort to the patient.

Measures dependent on changes in limb size. Impedance plethysmography, mercury strain-gauge plethysmography, and phleborheography record variations in the volume of a limb or in resulting tissue resistance during respiration or after mechanical compression of a distal segment. As a group, they give information regarding the presence of clots which occlude main collecting veins. However, thrombosis of venous plexuses in the muscles of the calf is not identified because the involved vessels do not contribute significantly to removal of blood from the limb, and hence clots in them do not materially affect the normal respiratory changes in venous flow. Also, it must be pointed out that venous volume changes can be influenced by a number of different factors unrelated to venous thrombosis, such as significant local vasoconstriction, low cardiac output, shock, and occlusive arterial disease, among others. Finally, the procedures require active cooperation on the part of the patient, which may be difficult to obtain if he is acutely ill. There is also the theoretical and probably remote possibility that frequent inflation of a blood pressure cuff or mechanical compression of the foot and leg may initiate liberation of thrombi into the bloodstream.

Conclusions. The above evaluation of the various diagnostic tests for deep venous thrombosis in the lower limbs clearly points out the fact that generally it is not possible to obtain maximal information concerning the existing state using only a single approach. In order to elucidate the problem, numerous studies have been performed for the purpose of determining which combination of procedures is most effective. For example, the results of one investigation [20] indicate that whereas the diagnostic accuracy of Doppler ultrasound and impedance outflow testing was 82.9 and 70.9 percent, respectively, when each was used independently, combination of the techniques increased the accuracy to 95 percent.[2]

References

1. Arnoldi CC, Bauer G: Intraosseous phlebography. Angiology 11:44, 1960
2. Comp PC, Jacocks RM, Taylor FB Jr: The dilute whole blood clot lysis assay: A screening method for identifying postoperative patients with a high incidence of deep venous thrombosis. J Lab Clin Med 93:120, 1979
3. Cooke ED, Pilcher MF: Thermography in diagnosis of deep venous thrombosis. Br Med J 2:523, 1973
4. Cranley JJ, Canos AJ, Sull WJ, et al: Phleborheographic technique for diagnosing deep venous thrombosis of the lower extremities. Surg Gynecol Obstet 141:331, 1975
5. Cranley JJ, Gay AY, Grass AM, et al: A plethysmographic technique for the diagnosis of deep venous thrombosis of the lower extremities. Surg Gynecol Obstet 136:385, 1973
6. Flanc C, Kakkar VV, Clarke MB: The detection of venous thrombosis of the legs using ^{125}I-labelled fibrinogen. Br J Surg 55:742, 1968
7. Gazzaniga AB, Will DI, Shobe JB, et al: ^{125}I-fibrinogen uptake and bilateral impedance rheography: Diagnosis of postoperative venous thrombosis. Arch Surg 108:66, 1974
8. Hirsh J, Gallus AS: ^{125}I-labeled fibrinogen scanning: Use in the diagnosis of venous thrombosis. JAMA 233:970, 1975
9. Lowenberg RI: Early diagnosis of phlebothrombosis with aid of a new clinical test. JAMA 155:1566, 1954
10. Negus D: The diagnosis of deep-vein thrombosis. Br J Surg 59:830, 1972
11. Negus D, Pinto DJ, Le Quesne LE, et al: ^{125}I-labelled fibrinogen in the diagnosis of deep-vein thrombosis and its correlation with phlebography. Br J Surg 55:835, 1968
12. Nissl R: Acute thrombosis. In May R (ed): Sur-

[2] A recently described dilute whole blood lysis assay test has been proposed for use as a screening method for identifying postoperative patients who have a high incidence of thrombophlebitis, thus reducing the need for more costly diagnostic procedures [2]. The value of this approach must await further study.

gery of the Veins of the Leg and Pelvis, Philadelphia, Saunders, 1979, Chap 5

13. Pollak EW, Webber MM, Barker WF, et al: Autologous ^{125}I-fibrinogen uptake test in the detection and management of venous thrombosis: A prospective study. Arch Surg 109:48, 1974

14. Rhodes BA, Stern HS, Buchanan JA, et al: Lung scanning with ^{99m}Tc-microspheres. Radiology 99:613, 1971

15. Shumacker HB Jr, Moore TC, Campbell JA: Functional venography of the lower extremities. Surg Gynecol Obstet 98:257, 1954

16. Sigel B, Felix WR Jr, Popky GL, et al: Diagnosis of lower limb venous thrombosis by Doppler ultrasound technique. Arch Surg 104:174, 1972

17. Sigel B, Popky GL, Wagner DK, et al: A Doppler ultrasound method for diagnosing lower extremity venous disease. Surg Gynecol Obstet 127:337, 1968

18. Walker AJ, Longland CJ: Venous pressure measurement in the foot in exercise as an aid to investigation of venous disease in the leg. Clin Sci 9:101, 1950

19. Wheeler HB, Pearson D, O'Connell D, et al: Impedance phlebography: Technique, interpretation, and results. Arch Surg 104:164, 1972

20. Yao JST, Henkin RE, Bergan JJ: Venous thromboembolic disease: Evaluation of new methodology in treatment. Arch Surg 109:664, 1974

21. Yao JST, Henkin RE, Conn J Jr, et al: Combined isotope venography and lung scanning: A new diagnostic approach to thromboembolism. Arch Surg 107:146, 1973

22. Young AE, Henderson BA, Phillips DA, et al: Impedance plethysmography: Its limitations as a substitute for phlebography. Cardiovasc Radiol 1:233, 1978

Section 3

Clinical Disorders

Chapter 8

Differential Diagnosis of Physical Findings and States

Part 1   Pitting Edema; Lymphedema; Ulceration; Gangrene

There are a number of abnormal states which are found in both vascular conditions and in musculoskeletal disorders, the most common of which are pitting edema, lymphedema, ulceration, and gangrene. The present chapter is devoted to a discussion of the pathogenesis and differential diagnosis of these entities.

A.   Pitting Edema

Pitting edema is a state in which there is an abnormal accumulation of water in the tissue spaces (expanded interstitial fluid volume) due to the fact that drainage of the fluid is not keeping pace with its formation. The swelling is soft, is usually located in the distal portion of a limb, and is easily reduced by recumbency and elevation of the involved extremity. However, if left unchecked, pitting edema may develop characteristics of lymphedema (see Section B, below).

1.   Factors Normally Preventing Edema Formation

Before presenting the mechanisms responsible for pitting edema, it is necessary first to review

the factors which operate to maintain the lower limbs free of swelling during the course of daily physical activity, including relatively long periods of sitting and standing.

Osmotic resistance of blood proteins. The osmotic pull of the proteins in circulating blood exists because capillaries (except in the liver and perhaps in a few other sites) do not permit substances composed of large molecules, such as albumin, globulin, and the various formed elements of the blood, to pass through their walls. As a result, a mechanism is at hand whereby some of the fluid which would ordinarily move out of the lumen of the vessel is prevented from doing so by the osmotic pull of the impermeable materials. Such a force is relatively uniform throughout the arterial tree and is normally equivalent to 26 mmHg.

In the arteriolar end of the capillary, the blood pressure or filtration pressure is approximately 32 mmHg, as compared with the osmotic resistance of 26 mmHg, leaving an effective filtration pressure of 6 mmHg. Hence, the direction of flow of fluids is from the lumen of the capillary toward the tissue spaces. This results in a concentration of blood proteins in the venous end of the capillary, with a consequent increase in blood osmotic resistance in this site. Simultaneously, a reduction in filtration or blood pressure is taking place as the blood passes through the capillary bed. With conditions thus reversed at the venular end of the capillary, there is now a movement of fluid from the tissue spaces into the bloodstream.

Contribution of physical activity. Another important factor in the control of edema formation is the pumping action exerted by contracting voluntary muscles in the lower limbs on the neighboring thin-walled veins. Because the numerous valves in the latter prevent retrograde flow, the result during walking, for example, is propulsion of the stream of blood in an upward direction toward the heart. As a consequence, the venous pressure in the superficial veins falls, so that its transmission back into the venular end of the capillary is minimal. The very thin lymphatic channels, also possessing valves, are similarly influenced, thus reducing lymph stasis and facilitating the removal of fluid and large protein molecules from the tissue spaces.

Adjunctive mechanisms. Several other factors are involved in maintaining the lower extremities edema-free. One is the contribution of respiration to the movement of venous blood out of the lower limbs, due to an increase in negative pressure in the chest during inspiration associated with a simultaneous increase in positive pressure in the abdomen, both responses resulting from depression of the diaphragm. Such a mechanism empties the large veins in the abdomen which then permits the movement of blood from the lower limbs into them. Hence, venous pressure in the superficial veins in the lower extremities is reduced. The distension and recoil of the large arteries with each heartbeat also play a role in the removal of fluid from the lower limbs since this mechanism has a pumping effect on the neighboring thin-walled collecting lymphatic channels, thus facilitating removal of lymph from the tissue spaces. Elevation of an extremity reduces the filtration pressure in the capillaries to a level below that exerted by the osmotic resistance of the blood proteins and, at the same time, this position facilitates blood and lymph movement out of the limb. Finally, the blood continuously entering the venous system from the

arterial tree propels that already present in a proximal direction, with the valves in the veins preventing retrograde flow.

2. Physiologic and Pharmacologic Edema

Dependency edema. Despite the existence of the various mechanisms available for movement of blood out of the lower limbs, the body is still constantly on the verge of edema formation, particularly in the case of the feet and ankles. Such a tendency is exaggerated when an extremity is maintained in dependency for a protracted period of time, and as a result its distal portion may manifest physiologic edema. This type of response is frequently noted in normal people after long trips on trains, jet planes, or automobiles (traveler's edema, deck ankles). The alteration is caused by the prolonged additive effects of hydrostatic pressure existing in dependency on capillary filtration pressure and of the loss of the normal pumping mechanism exerted on the thin-walled veins and lymphatics by exercising voluntary muscles in the lower limbs. In the case of very long periods of dependency, there is the added factor of disuse which contributes to edema formation by initiating a state of vasospasm. (For the mechanism responsible for edema formation under these circumstances, see A-3, below.)

There are certain limiting factors to the accumulation of fluid in dependency edema. One of these is tissue pressure which eventually rises to a level that is higher than the augmented capillary filtration pressure in dependency, at which point no further swelling develops. Normal or heightened muscle tone also acts as a deterrent to edema formation by preventing further accommodation of tissues to external forces and thus raising the pressure in the intercellular spaces.

Dependency edema is generally more marked in the summer months, probably due to the vasodilating effect of heat on the cutaneous arterial, arteriolar, and venous trees. This change leads to an increase in local arterial blood flow and a decrease in resistance of the veins to stretching. Because of such responses, the venous system becomes more distended, with a resulting increase in venous pressure, transmitted back as an elevated capillary filtration pressure. At the same time, less blood pressure is dissipated in moving the blood through the now-dilated arteriolar bed, so that the filtration pressure at the arteriolar end of the capillary is higher. Moreover, in a warm environment, there is a disinclination to perform physical exercise, and consequently the pumping effect of contracting muscles on the thin-walled veins is diminished and venous pressure rises on this account. All of these factors contribute to an increase in effective capillary filtration pressure and hence edema formation.

Dependency edema is also part of the clinical picture of a number of unrelated abnormal states. For example, it is observed in the hemiplegic patient in the upper and lower paralyzed limbs and in both lower extremities of the paraplegic and the quadriplegic. The schizophrenic patient who maintains his arms immobile against the sides of his body for hours or even days likewise demonstrates swelling of the hands and even of the forearms.

Although ordinarily a patient with arteriosclerosis obliterans or thromboangiitis obliterans does not manifest edema of the lower extremities, he may if he is suffering from ischemic neuropathy or impending or existing gangrene and has learned that sleeping in a chair with the lower limbs maintained in dependency brings relief from the very severe pain experienced while lying horizontally in bed. Besides the persistent effect of dependency on increasing filtration pressure in the capillary lumen and the immobility of the lower limbs for protracted periods of time, there is also the contributing factor of greater capillary permeability related to the existing marked impairment of local circulation. As a result of all these mechanisms, increased movement of fluid from the bloodstream into the tissue spaces occurs, to produce edema.

Drug edema. Ingestion of certain medications, such as corticosteroids and adrenocorticotropins, estrogen, progesterone (including birth control agents), testosterone, and aldosterone-like substances, may also result in edema formation. Antihypertensive drugs, including guanethidine sulfate (Ismelin), hydralazine hydrochloride (Apresoline), the *Rauwolfia* prepa-

rations, methyldopa (Aldomet), and diazides, may have a similar effect. Antiinflammatory medications, such as phenylbutazone (Butazolidin), can cause swelling of the feet and lower portion of the legs.

3. Edema Associated with Arterial Vasospasm

Under certain conditions, edema of the distal portion of a limb is found in association with arterial vasospasm, as for example, in the acute phase of trench foot and frostbite (see Section D, Chapter 13), as a chronic manifestation of the post–trench foot and postfrostbite syndromes, and in major causalgia and posttraumatic vasomotor disorders (see A-1 and A-2, respectively, Chapter 13).

There are several mechanisms involved in the production of the swelling found in vasospasm. One of these is the reduced pumping action exerted by the large arteries in the limb on the neighboring thin-walled lymphatic channels, due to a damping or even loss of the normal distension and recoil of the vascular tree with each heartbeat. Another is anoxia of the capillary wall because of the decreased arterial inflow, resulting in greater permeability of this structure and more rapid movement of fluid into the tissue spaces from the bloodstream. Disuse makes a contribution since it initiates a reflex arc involving the peripheral sympathetic nerves as the efferent arm, thus further exaggerating the already-existing state of vasospasm. Finally, since the clinical entities mentioned above are generally associated with severe pain, the patient, in order to minimize the symptoms, holds the involved limb in dependency and immobile, making no attempt to contract his voluntary muscles. As a consequence of these factors, also, edema formation is accelerated.

4. Edema of Venous Origin

Edema is a common finding in several venous disorders of the extremities, the mechanism responsible for the change being somewhat different in each.

Edema due to occlusion of or extrinsic pressure on main collecting veins. In the initial stage of popliteal, iliofemoral, subclavian, or axillary thrombophlebitis, pitting edema is a prominent sign (Fig. 18.3). However, in severe cases the skin is so tightly stretched by the fluid in the tissue spaces that pitting is produced only with difficulty. Compression of a main collecting vein by external pressure, such as by a rapidly enlarging pelvic tumor, may produce similar local changes in an extremity.

The chief mechanism for the production of swelling following sudden, complete obstruction of a main vein is interference with the movement of blood out of the limb. As a result, there is stasis in the large and small channels distally, producing a rise in pressure within their lumen, sometimes to a level four or five times as great as normal. The elevation in venous pressure is reflected back into the full length of the capillaries as an augmented capillary filtration pressure, thus facilitating the movement of fluid from the bloodstream into the extravascular spaces. At the same time, such a change prevents the normal movement of tissue fluid into the venular portion of the capillary.

Another factor accelerating the rate of edema formation is associated venospasm, which tends to raise venous pressure even more. The response is due to the initiation of a reflex arc as a consequence of the occlusion of a main venous channel, the efferent limb of the pathway being the peripheral sympathetic nervous system innervating medium- and small-sized veins. The resulting high venous pressure is reflected back into the microcirculation and contributes to the production of anoxia of capillary endothelium, followed by greater permeability of this structure. The latter change facilitates the movement of fluid out of the capillary lumen into the tissue space. Contributing to the altered capillary permeability is the ischemia of vascular structures resulting from the reduction in arterial inflow produced by vasospasm.

Interference with lymphatic drainage from the limb also plays a role in the edema formation which follows thrombosis of a collecting vein. The responsible mechanism is inflammation and occlusion of the neighboring large lymphatic vessels located in the popliteal space, the groin, or the axilla by extension from the periphlebitic reaction which always is present

under such circumstances. The resulting lymphatic stasis is further exaggerated by the greater burden placed on the lymphatic system through loss of the normal means of removal of fluid by way of venous channels. Another factor augmenting lymph stasis is the arterial spasm which accompanies the venous spasm and is due to the same etiology (see above). As a consequence, there is a reduction or even a complete loss of pulsations in the main arterial trunks in the limbs, thus eliminating the normal pumping action on the neighboring thin-walled lymphatics supplied by the rhythmic distension and recoil of the arteries with each cardiac cycle. Hence, stagnation of tissue fluid and accumulation of protein occur in the perivascular spaces, a situation conducive to edema formation because of the osmotic pressure exerted by substances of high molecular weight, preventing resorption of tissue fluid into the vascular tree.

Postphlebitic edema. The swelling of the postphlebitic syndrome (Fig. 20.2A), which occurs as a sequela in patients generally improperly treated during the acute stage of iliofemoral thrombophlebitis, is due to an inefficient venous system, incapable of moving the blood from the lower extremities into the large collecting veins in the abdomen on assumption of the upright position. The main cause is the absence of an adequate collateral venous circulation in the face of an impatent or incompetent deep venous system.

Edema associated with primary varicosities. In the presence of primary varicosities of the lower limbs, venous stasis eventually develops. Because of the marked distension of the superficial veins and the poor support they normally possess, these vessels enlarge and become tortuous, in the process of which the valves locally also become incompetent. The elevated venous pressure is reflected back into the capillary tree as an increased capillary filtration pressure. As a result, there is swelling of the ankle, which forms during the day and disappears after a night's rest. At times the edema may extend upward onto the lower portion of the leg. The degree of swelling in primary varicosities is generally related to the period of time that the patient has remained in the upright position, particularly standing, during the previous day. Walking, with the associated pumping action exerted on the superficial veins by the contracting muscles, produces much less edema. (For a discussion of edema produced by application of a cast, see Section A, Chapter 22.)

B. Lymphedema

Lymphedema, the second clinical type of edema, is a firm swelling of a limb which is not particularly affected by elevation, in contradistinction to pitting edema (see Section A, above).

1. Pathogenesis

Plasma circulates continuously from blood to interstitial spaces, with most of the capillary filtrate being returned to the venous end of the capillary. The remaining small percentage is removed by way of the network of lymph vessels, the lymph eventually entering the subclavian veins by way of the thoracic duct and the right lymphatic duct. Such a mechanism offsets the loss of plasma from the blood capillaries.

When clinical lymphedema develops, this signifies a situation in which absorption of lymph into the lymphatic system and its removal from the limb are faulty, although the rate of formation of this constituent is normal (low output failure). As the large molecules in the tissue spaces accumulate, they begin to exert a significant and progressive increase in osmotic pressure or pull which results in water retention and edema formation in the extracellular compartments.

2. Etiologic Factors

Lymphedema is found in two types of conditions. In one, an anomaly of the lymphatic system exists, consisting of either an absence of formed lymph channels (aplasia), unconnected lymph spaces, a reduced number or size of lymph channels (hypoplasia), or widening, enlargement, and tortuosity of lymph vessels (hyperplasia) producing incompetency of their valves. In the second group of conditions responsible for lymphedema, this state develops as a result of either an inflammatory process affecting the collecting lymphatic channels, destruction of critical lymph vessels by trauma, or obstruction to the flow of lymph by malignant metastasis to critical lymph nodes in the axilla, popliteal space, or groin (Fig. 8.1D). Total occlusion of main collecting veins, producing marked interference with venous outflow, may compromise a latent inadequacy of the lymphatics to the point of producing lymphedema because of the greater load now placed on the latter system.

3. Clinical Entities

Primary lymphedema. This state, resulting from anomalous development of the lymphatic system, is found in several clinical disorders. Congenital lymphedema is probably the most common type. Typically, in this entity there is diffuse swelling of a lower limb first noted at birth or shortly thereafter (Fig. 8.1A). The edema is firm and initially subsides with prolonged elevation of the limb. Later, however, this does not occur, and at the same time there is a gradual enlargement of the circumferences of the limb. Associated with the condition, delineated pink areas of capillary angioma may be found on the buttock or other portions of the lower extremity. If more than one member of a family develops congenital lymphedema of a lower limb, the condition is termed congenital familial lymphedema (Milroy's disease). Except for this difference, clinically both conditions are similar in all respects.

Lymphedema praecox is seen most often in girls or young women, appearing during or after puberty. The swelling is first noted around the ankles and then extends upward onto the legs, eventually to affect the entire length of the limbs. The edema is enhanced by prolonged standing, by warm weather, and during the menstrual period. As the swelling progressively becomes more marked, the weight of the leg increases. As a result, the patient begins to complain of a sense of heaviness and discomfort in it and notes a reduced ability to perform strenuous physical exercise. Also of great importance is the fact that the large un-

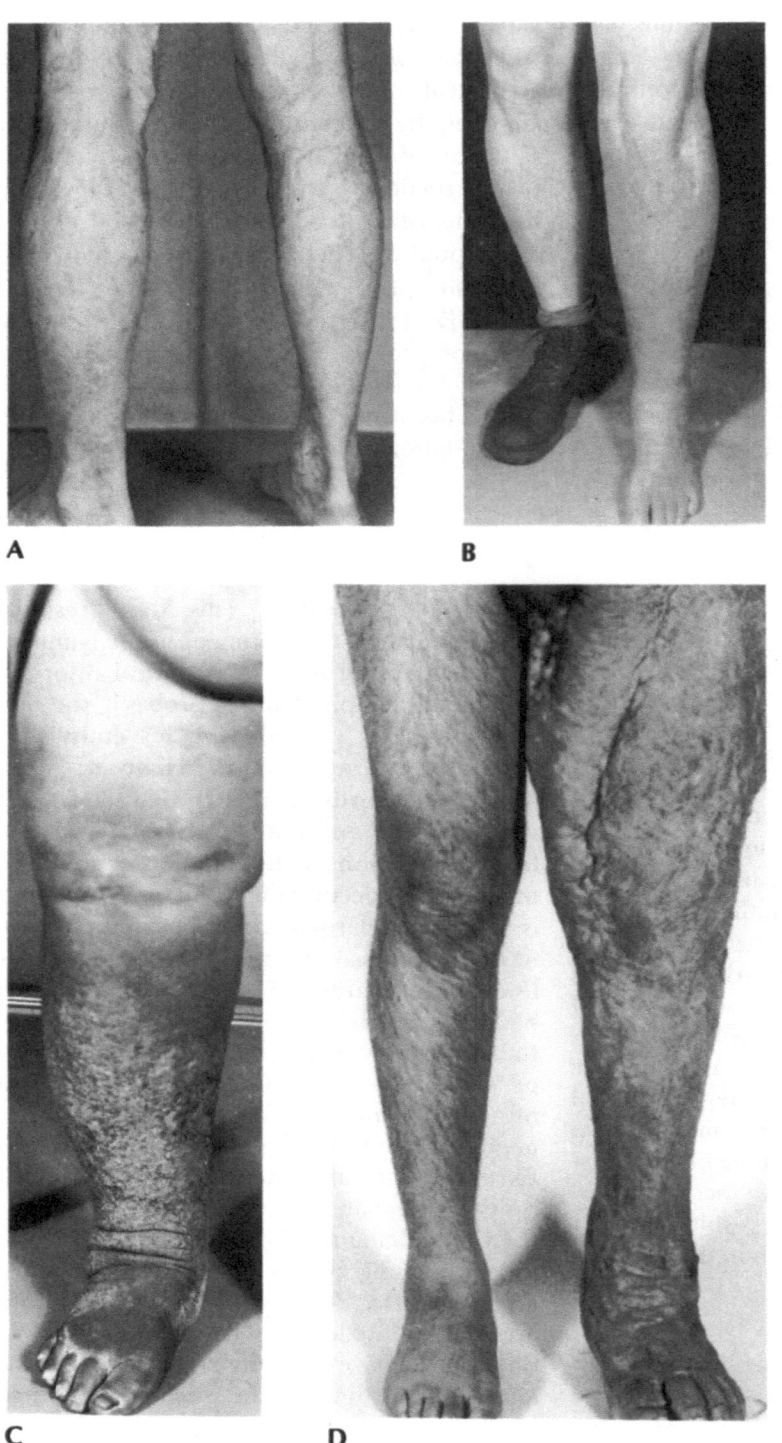

Fig. 8.1. Lymphedema of various types. **A** Primary lymphedema (congenital lymphedema). **B** Secondary lymphedema following destruction of main lymph channels in the leg (at the level of the knee) by shell fragment wounds. **C** Secondary lymphedema due to repeated attacks of cellulitis, followed by lymphangitis and lymphadenitis. **D** Secondary lymphedema and fibroedema following metastasis of carcinoma to inguinal lymph nodes. **B,** from Abramson DI: Circulatory Diseases of the Limbs: A Primer. New York, Grune & Stratton, 1978. Reproduced with permission.

sightly lower limb, which is difficult to hide from view, has a devastating psychologic effect upon the young female patient.

Secondary lymphedema. Destruction or obstruction of regional lymph nodes by metastasis of malignant tumors is a fairly common cause of secondary lymphedema. Typically, the onset of swelling is painless and slowly progressive, the edema first being noted in the portion of limb located just below the site of the involved lymph nodes. Later there is extension of the process distally. With involvement of the skin locally, this structure assumes a hard and indurated consistency and then becomes firmly adherent to underlying tissues.

Because of the scarcity of lymph channels in the limbs and the inability of these structures to regenerate, local injury, even if limited, may result in the development of lymphedema, particularly if the trauma occurs where vessels converge to enter superficial and deep lymph nodes (Fig. 8.1B). Extirpation of regional lymph nodes with destruction of lymph channels, as in the course of a radical mastectomy, may have the same effect. Of course, in the case of the latter procedure, there are other possible factors which may contribute to the development of edema of the upper limb, such as simultaneous thrombosis of the axillary vein due to local trauma, infection, and postirradiation fibrosis, among others.

Inflammatory lymphedema, following cellulitis, erysipelas, or filariasis, results from repeated episodes of lymphangitis and lymphadenitis, associated with systemic responses (high fever, chills, malaise) (Fig. 8.1C). Ultimately fibrosis and thrombosis of the lymph channels ensue. If the attacks of cellulitis and lymphangitis continue uncontrolled, fibroedema will replace the lymphedema and the acute episodes of inflammation then generally subside. A common etiologic agent in inflammatory lymphedema is a streptococcal invasion of the lymph channels.

4. Treatment

Most important in the management of both primary and secondary lymphedema is an attempt to prevent or eliminate those factors conducive to lymph retention in the limbs. If such an approach is not successful, then measures should be instituted to control or reduce the accumulation of the fluid in the tissue spaces.

Need for control of lymphedema. Maintenance of the affected limb in as an edema-free state as possible is the goal of the therapeutic program, for otherwise varying degrees of disability and serious consequences may result. For example, the swollen limb is more susceptible to recurrent lymphangitis, lymphadenitis, and thrombophlebitis than is one in which the edema has been controlled. Furthermore, persistent, chronic swelling of a considerable degree may be followed by fibroedema (Fig. 8.1D) and elephantiasis which are irreversible processes. Also, on occasion, long-standing brawny edema of a limb may become the site of a lymphangiosarcoma, a highly malignant lesion. Even in the absence of serious complications, a swollen limb results in limited usefulness and discomfort and may have considerable psychologic impact on the patient because of the cosmetic deformity.

Therapy for existing cellulitis and lymphangitis. The management of an acute inflammatory process, whether it is the initial attack or a recurrence, involves the immediate institution of an antibiotic program, preferably penicillin or a derivative, for control of the infection. Generally such an approach is very effective in this regard. However, it is necessary to point out that the patient may already be sensitized to a mold, since frequently dermatophytosis of the web of the toes is present, which acts as the portal of entry for streptococci responsible for the lymphangitis. Therefore, the physician should be aware of such a possibility when he administers a mold extract, in order to be prepared to control any allergic responses that might develop. Besides systemic medication, local therapy, in the form of wet heat, should be utilized to localize the inflammatory process and reduce the lymphangitis and lymphadenitis. Also, the patient should be at complete bed rest, and existing dermatophytosis should be actively treated (see D-1, Chapter 11).

Prophylactic measures. Since patients with both primary and secondary lymphedema appear to be very vulnerable to repeated episodes of streptococcal lymphangitis and lymphadenitis, each subsequent attack aggravating the existing lymphedema, it is essential to control such a situation. For this purpose, such individuals should be placed on continuous prophylactic use of penicillin G, utilizing the regimen found effective in rheumatic heart disease. In most individuals, as little as 400,000 units taken orally twice a day is adequate for maintenance therapy. The limb previously involved should be carefully examined for areas of increased cutaneous temperature. If these are found, then the dosage of penicillin G should be increased to three or four times the usual amount for several days. Such a step generally causes the local areas of heat to disappear within 24 to 72 h, at which point the maintenance dose of penicillin is resumed.

Besides the above procedures, the patient should be instructed in the local care of the involved limb, a continuing problem for the remainder of his or her life. Following a radical mastectomy, for example, the homolateral upper limb must be carefully protected from any type of injury. In the performance of such household duties as washing dishes, the patient should wear loose-fitting rubber gloves and avoid strong detergents. At no time should the cuticles of the nails be cut, either by a manicurist or by the patient, because of the fear of developing an infection followed by lymphangitis. A wristwatch should be worn on the unaffected side for the same reason. The patient should not use the involved limb in the performance of strenuous work or to carry a heavy purse or a valise. Nor should the extremity be utilized for injections, venipuncture, or blood pressure recordings. If the patient smokes, the cigarette should be held by the opposite hand so as to minimize the possibility of inadvertently developing a burn in an area vulnerable to infection. The skin of the hand should be kept soft with lanolin. Finally, the patient should be instructed to see a physician at the first sign of swelling, redness, or unnatural warmth of the extremity.

In the case of an edematous lower limb, all types of local skin infections should be avoided. The patient should always use socks and shoes when ambulatory. If dermatophytosis is present, this should be vigorously attacked. In or-

der to eradicate it, an autogenous vaccine may be necessary.

Physical methods for control of swelling. If considerable swelling is present in a lower limb, it may be necessary initially to place the patient at complete bed rest, without bathroom privileges, and elevate the involved extremity by placing it at a 45° angle using a specially designed sling and overhead pulleys on a Balkan fracture frame. When no further reduction in size of the limb is noted, the patient is permitted to become ambulatory again. To prevent reaccumulation of fluid, a strong elastic support, such as a pure 100 percent pararubber bandage, 7.5 cm (3 in.) wide, is wrapped around the limb (in the same manner as an Ace bandage) over a cotton stocking. The support should be removed in the afternoon and reapplied with the patient lying down, but not exactly superimposed so as to minimize ridging. At night the patient should sleep with the foot of the bed elevated about 15 cm (6 in.). As adjunctive measures, a salt-poor diet and occasional diuretics are helpful.

Mechanical methods have also been utilized to reduce the swelling. One produces directional compression of the lower limb from toes to thigh, using 14 rubber cuffs. The compression (50 to 80 mmHg) is applied 20 times/min, the pressure wave (produced by means of a distributor valve) moving the fluid in the limb proximally. Another method consists of intermittent application of compression pressures (30 to 40 mmHg) to the limb by means of a boot or sleeve. A treatment period can last for 5 to 6 h during which time fluid is expressed from the limb. Both procedures, with some modifications, can be used for the control of lymphedema of both the upper and lower limbs.

Surgical therapy. This approach to the control of lymphedema should be considered only as a last resort, when conservative methods have not been effective and the progressive enlargement of the involved lower limb has become a disabling affliction, significantly interfering with daily physical activities. A number of operative procedures have been described for this purpose, all requiring the anatomic information derived from a preliminary lymphangiogram [10,11]. The surgical techniques can be divided into two groups. In one the chief object is to improve function by the development of new lymph pathways; in the other, the purpose is to excise or reduce the amount of diseased structures in the limb.

The early efforts dealt with methods to facilitate lymphatic drainage by embedding various types of material into the subcutaneous tissue (lymphangioplasty), including silk, nylon strands, strips of fascia or cellophane, and wires. The rationale for such an approach was the hope that growth of lymph channels would occur along the course of the foreign bodies. Unfortunately, none of these procedures has proved to be of any value in the removal of lymph. Another more recent approach consists of lengthening the intact omentum, which possesses a rich lymphatic and vascular supply, and attaching it to the tissues of the involved lower limb after passing it through a formed tunnel [9]. The purpose with this approach is also to facilitate lymph drainage from the affected limb. However, there is some question as to whether bridging lymphatic channels develop in such a preparation and that clinical improvement results from its use [3]. Finally, an operation has been proposed in which anastomoses are constructed between three to nine lymphatic vessels and the great saphenous vein. The technique has been utilized in cases of lymphatic channels blocked at a definite level and with lymphangiographic visualization of normal valves and permeability of the vessels elsewhere. A recent study has reported an average reduction of 76 percent in the degree of edema using the procedure, the success of the operation being proportionate to the number of anastomoses achieved [5].

Among the purely excisional types of procedures is the Charles' operation in which all skin and spongy subcutaneous tissues are removed down to the muscle and then the latter is covered by split skin grafts obtained from a healthy area of the body. It is applicable only for cases in which there are severe and advanced skin changes in the involved limb.

Another procedure, the Thompson buried dermis flap operation, combines attempts to encourage lymph drainage with removal of involved tissues. The excess loose, spongy, edematous subcutaneous tissue is excised and a flap of skin is buried in the muscles of the limb near the deep neurovascular bundle. The edge of the flap is shaved, as in the Thiersch method, so as to avoid the complications which may arise from burying epidermis. Whether the burial of the flap leads to definite anastomoses or linkage between superficial and deep lymph channels is questionable. Nevertheless, it is believed by some investigators that the Thompson procedure gives the best results of all the operations available [3]. A modification of it is the Homans' operation in which simple flaps are used, without any overlap or intermuscular burial. Another involves overlap of the shaved flap and no intermuscular burial, with the buried dermis flap lying under the other skin flap and not between the muscles.

C. Ulceration

Although ulcers of the lower limbs are usually the result of either an inadequate arterial circulation (see B-3, Chapter 11) or interference with venous outflow (see B-11, Chapter 20), such lesions may also be present in a number of unrelated nonvascular conditions. Among these are congestive heart failure, local trauma associated with fractures, peripheral neuropathy and other neurologic states, chronic systemic infections such as syphilis and tuberculosis, and blood dyscrasias. In most instances the initiating factor is an injury, but some of the lesions may occur spontaneously. The discussion below will be limited primarily to those types of ulcers not described in other chapters.

1. Ulcers of Functional Arterial Disorders

In long-standing functional vasospastic states, the repeated short periods of impaired circulation, due to temporary spasm of small arteries or arterioles, may eventually lead to sufficient alteration in the cutaneous blood flow to make the skin vulnerable to ulceration.

Ulcers of Raynaud's disease. These lesions are typical of the type of trophic disturbance observed in vasospastic states. The ulcer is usually located in the distal portion of the fingers

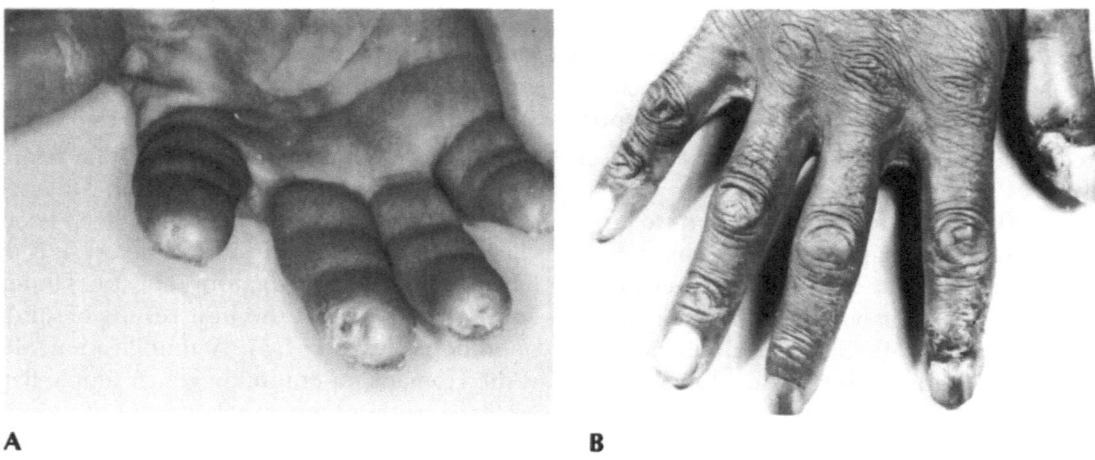

A   **B**

Fig. 8.2. Ulcerations of Raynaud's disease, found at tips of fingers (**A**) and around edges of nails (**B**).

(Fig. 8.2) and is almost always associated with severe excruciating pain locally. The history of typical color changes in the involved digits, elicited by exposure to cold or emotional excitation, and the absence of organic blocks in the main vessels to the limb are of value in differentiating the ulceration of Raynaud's disease from that of an occlusive arterial disorder. (For a discussion of the pathogenesis and clinical manifestations of Raynaud's disease, see Chapter 10, p. 143.)

Ulcers of livedo reticularis. Infrequently ulcers are noted in livedo reticularis, a vasospastic disorder characterized by a mottled, blotchy appearance of the skin, particularly of the lower extremities. The persistent reticular cyanotic discoloration produces a meshwork effect which outlines normal skin. The abnormal manifestations reflect a state of marked spasm of the arterioles in the deep cutis and upper layer of subcutaneous tissue and atonic dilatation of the capillaries and venules, due to the existing ischemia of the skin. As a consequence of these changes, there is stasis of the local circulation. In the chronic state, the clinical picture is associated with certain pathologic alterations in the cutaneous microcirculation [1], consisting of proliferation of the intima of the arterioles and perivascular infiltration, producing thickening of the vessel walls; in some instances the lumina of the vessels may be occluded [7].

The ulcerations due to livedo reticularis are found in the legs [8], generally on the posterior surface. They first appear either as tender nodules in the skin or as purplish areas on which blisters may develop. The latter then break down, producing superficial ulcers which may enlarge to 2 to 4 cm (1 to 2 in.) in diameter in the course of several weeks or months. During the period of formation of the lesions, there is considerable local pain present. The ulcers generally become indolent and persistent, responding poorly to therapy utilized for venous stasis lesions.

The ulcers of livedo reticularis are clinically not specific and may resemble those of several conditions, such as chronic chilblain, nonspecific vasculitis (Fig. 8.3), erythema induratum [8], hemolytic anemia, and hypertensive ischemic ulcer. However, in none of these disorders is the typical reticular mottled skin discoloration of livedo reticularis noted.

2. Ulcers of Hematologic Origin

Ulcers of sickle-cell anemia. Ulcerations of the lower extremity are not infrequently found in this condition [4], particularly in adults. The site of predilection is around the ankle or the anterior surface of the lower half of the leg. The lesion may be single or multiple, affecting one or both lower limbs. Typically it manifests a punched-out appearance and may show pigmentation and cicatrization. The presence of a chronic ulcer on the leg of a black individual,

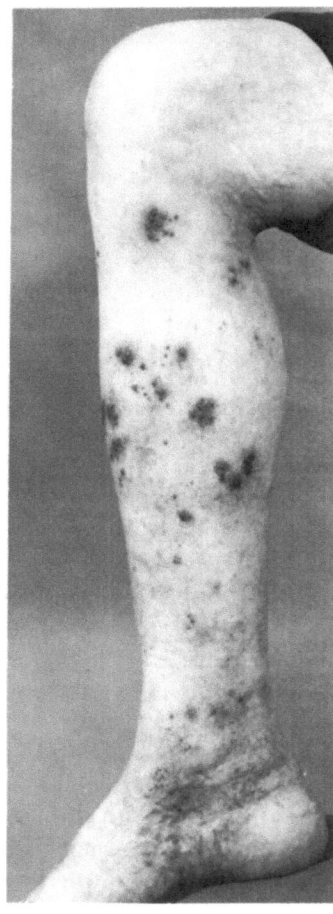 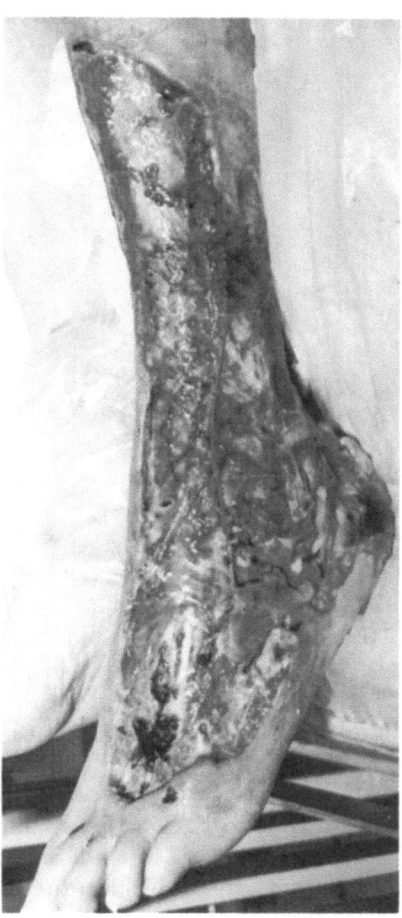

A   **B**

Fig. 8.3. Types of ulcers produced by nonspecific vasculitis of the cutaneous circulation. **A** Localized lesions. **B** Extensive involvement, with destruction of skin of foot and leg.

associated with sickling of red blood cells in the peripheral blood, slightly jaundiced sclerae, hepatomegaly, splenomegaly, and arthralgias, supports the diagnosis of sickle-cell anemia as the cause of the lesion. Signs of arterial, venous, and lymphatic involvement are absent.

The mechanism responsible for the production of the recurrent lesions is not known, although occlusion of the cutaneous microcirculation by plugs of sickled cells has been suggested. The relatively low oxygen content of blood in the veins of the lower portion of the legs, together with stasis in these vessels, increases the tendency of the red blood cells to sickle. As a consequence, the viscosity of the blood locally increases, which causes further impairment of circulation around the ankle.

Response of the ulcer to various therapeutic regimens is generally poor. Bed rest and eleva-

tion of the leg, pressure dressings, histamine by ion transfer, repeated small transfusions of packed or sedimented red blood cells, and the use of various stimulating ointments are indicated. At times sympathectomy or excision and grafting may be necessary. Even if healing of the ulcer occurs, there is always a good possibility of a recurrence in the same or a neighboring site.

3. Ulcers Associated with Metabolic Disorders

Neurotrophic ulcers. An unusual type of ulceration is that associated with a number of unrelated neurologic conditions, such as peripheral neuropathy from various causes (particularly diabetes), cord lesions, tabes dorsalis, myelodysplasia, and syringomyelia. The common de-

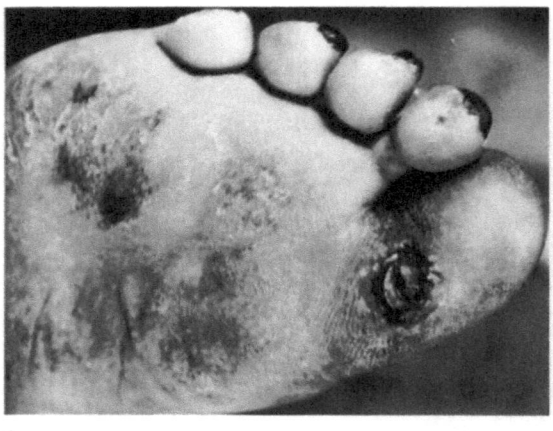

A

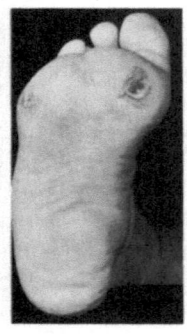

B

Fig. 8.4. Neurotrophic, painless ulcers of diabetes mellitus, in the presence of an adequate local arterial circulation (**A** and **B**).

nominator in this state, regardless of the etiologic factor, is damage to sensation, either central or peripheral in origin. (For a discussion of peripheral neuropathy, see Section B, Chapter 9.)

The lesion is generally found under a callus, either at the base of the great toe on the plantar surface of the foot (Fig. 8.4), in the region of other metatarsal heads, at the base of the fifth toe, or on the heel. It is most often present in the limb suffering from hypalgesia and loss of sensation and rarely in one with hyperesthesia. Commonly, as a result of thinning out of the fat pads over the metatarsal arch in the foot, callosities are formed as space replacements, followed by the production of the ulcer. The lesion results from continuous pressure of the thickened keratin material on a devitalized dermal area, and in this sense it can be considered to be a traumatic ulcer. The altered dynamics of the foot leading to overloading of the forefoot, the dryness of the skin which follows autosympathectomy due to the associated peripheral neuropathy, and the decrease in pain sensation from the same cause all contribute to a situation conducive to the formation of the neurotrophic ulcer.

The lesion usually starts with the appearance of erythema, and then the site becomes swollen and fluctuant, followed by the production of a true abscess. The latter generally opens outward, with drainage of seropurulent secretion which is thin and malodorous. Although the ulcer may look small, it frequently is found to undermine extensively below the skin, possess-

ing a deep funnellike base which may reach as far as the underlying bone. In fact, in the advanced case, there is often loss of the metatarsal heads, with multiple areas of low-grade cortical osteomyelitis of the metatarsal or phalangeal bones.

The diagnosis of a neurotrophic ulcer is made on the basis of marked destruction of soft tissues and even of the bones of the foot, associated with little or no pain, a normal circulation in the limb, and neuropathy in the form of impaired or absent vibration sense perception and other sensory losses and a decrease or absence of ankle jerks. A careful neurologic examination is necessary in order to establish the diagnosis and also to map out the zones of abnormal sensation. Sensory alterations which follow dermatome patterns are found in patients suffering from radicular lesions, myelodysplasia, and old injuries of the cord. In diabetic neuropathy, such neurologic changes are not noted.

The presence of roentgenographic abnormalities may be helpful in making the diagnosis of a neurotrophic ulcer. The alterations are generally of a degenerative character, consisting of bony atrophy, periosteal thickening, and sclerotic changes in the joints. There may also be joint destruction with displacement.

The conservative treatment of neurotrophic ulcers is frequently not successful; also, recurrences are not uncommon. Of greatest importance is removal of pressure from the involved area. Infection should be aggressively attacked and necrotic tissue must repeatedly be removed by debridement. If extensive local bony destruction exists, surgical intervention with excision of the necrotic tissue is indicated. In view of the excellent local blood supply generally present, healing can be expected to occur in most instances. At times, more heroic procedures are required, such as disarticulation of the involved digit, tenotomy of the flexors of the toe, and resection of the metatarsal heads with or without disarticulation.

D. Gangrene

As in the case of ulceration of ischemic origin, the presence of gangrene in a limb indicates that the cutaneous circulation to the involved area is compromised to the point that even the low metabolic needs of resting skin cannot be satisfied. Such a situation may indicate either a reduction in circulation to all the tissues of the limb or only a decreased blood flow limited to a small portion of the skin and subcutaneous tissue—the site of the lesion. In general, the impairment in blood flow is of a greater degree than is the case for ischemic ulceration, thus producing more extensive irreversible changes.

In most instances the initiation of the gangrenous process is heralded by the onset of severe constant pain in the involved region (see A-5, Chapter 10) and by the appearance of a cyanotic hue to the skin which is not altered by digital pressure, as well as by a marked reduction in local skin temperature. Subsequently the affected tissues may become distended with fluid and almost fluctuant, particularly if the process is located in the distal portion of a digit. If there is no superimposed infection, absorption of the fluid occurs, producing mummification of the tissues ("dry gangrene"); little or no odor is present. Gradually the superficial layers become dry and brittle, the same process taking place in the deeper structures, such as the bone. A clear-cut line of demarcation may appear between viable and nonviable tissues.

If the lesion becomes secondarily infected, then the course of events is somewhat different. Inflammation is generally noted at the border of the necrotic and normal tissues, and this may penetrate some distance into surrounding structures. Lymphangitis may also be associated with the spread of the inflammatory process. The dry appearance of the lesion is lost, to be replaced by a stage of breakdown of necrotic tissue by bacterial action and the production of purulent material ("wet gangrene").

1. Factors Producing Gangrene of Arterial Occlusive Disorders

Irreversible and progressive structural alteration in the walls of main arteries or in their subdivisions, leading to severe ischemia and eventually gangrene, may exist in thromboangiitis obliterans, arteriosclerosis obliterans, polyarteritis nodosa, and other generalized vascular conditions. Occlusion of a main artery by an embolus or ligation of a traumatized vessel may also produce gangrene of a distal portion of the involved limb, since under such circumstances the local circulation is greatly compromised. (For a discussion of venous gangrene, see p. 267.)

Aside from a gradually increasing state of anoxia due to the natural advancement of an obliterative process, there are several other factors which may initiate gangrene in an extremity with mild to moderate impairment in blood supply. Most potent among these are the local application of heat and the prolonged exposure of a limb to moderate cold. If a limb suffering from an occlusive arterial disease is placed in forced extension, as in the treatment of an orthopedic condition, this may also precipitate death of tissue. (See C-2, Chapter 22, for further discussion of this subject.)

2. Drug-induced Gangrene

Following intraarterial injection. A number of medications, generally administered intravenously without adverse reactions, may produce gangrene of the hand or foot when inadvertently injected intraarterially. Increasing the incidence of this type of response is the tendency of the drug addict to utilize an artery when he no longer has veins available for the injection of narcotics or other substances.

Among the drugs which have been administered intraarterially with disastrous results are amphetamine sulfate (Benzedrine), amobarbital (Amytal), secobarbital, pentobarbital (Nembutal), meperidine hydrochloride (Demerol), sodium sulfobromophthalein (Bromsulphalein), chlorpromazine hydrochloride (Thorazine), promazine hydrochloride (Sparine), ether, hydroxyzine hydrochloride (Atarax), thiopental sodium (Pentothal) [6], and propoxyphene hydrochloride (Darvon).

With all of the above medications, tissue response occurs within a few minutes after the intraarterial injection is completed. The patient begins to experience severe pain in the hand or foot, associated with blanching and coldness and paralysis of muscles, followed by the appearance of frank gangrene of the digits. Examination reveals absent pulses in distal structures and corresponding changes in oscillometric readings. Later the tissues become edematous, this response resolving in 4 to 5 days.

The basis for the rapid production of necrosis is not clear. It has been suggested that the high concentration of the drug causes chemical endarteritis in the capillaries, arterioles, and small arteries, followed by thrombosis, acute ischemia, and death of tissues. With intravenous administration, such a situation does not exist because of thorough mixing and dilution of the drug by the venous blood before the material reaches the microcirculation.

Following intravenous injection.
Several medications, even when administered intravenously, may produce necrosis of tissues. An example is the continuous infusion of norepinephrine (Levophed) [14]. This measure may result in gangrene of fingers or toes, as a result of the intense and prolonged vasoconstriction of the smaller cutaneous arteries and arterioles. The same type of necrosis may occur locally following extravasation of the solution into the subcutaneous tissues.

Following oral administration.
Such vasoconstricting drugs as ergotamine tartrate, when given by mouth for a prolonged period of time, may cause marked spasm of the arterial tree, resulting in gangrene of the fingers and toes.[1] The patients are usually women, younger than 40 years of age, who are on the routine use

[1] A similar response may follow the repeated rectal administration of suppositories of ergotamine tartrate and caffeine (Cafergot).

of ergotamine tartrate, generally for the treatment of migraine headaches.

The clinical picture of ergot-induced arterial insufficiency is fairly typical. First the pulses in the main arteries in the limbs disappear, followed by the onset of intermittent claudication and the appearance of cyanotic mottling, associated with reduced cutaneous temperature. If the medication is continued, the color changes become irreversible and necrosis of the skin develops.

Many cases of ergot poisoning are recognized merely by a high level of suspicion when signs of acute arterial insufficiency appear in a young patient known to be taking ergot alkaloids. If there is any question about the diagnosis, arteriography is helpful in elucidating the problem. The changes consist of generalized narrowing of the arteries with little irregularity in the contour of the lumen. At times the spasm of the vessel is so severe that the lumen becomes about 1 mm in width and yet the contour remains regular. The visualization of a collateral circulation, as is observed in most cases of chronic occlusive arterial disorders, is absent.

Pharmacologically the ergot compounds produce direct vasoconstriction. There is also an effect on the endothelium of the arteries which causes permanent damage. As a consequence of such changes, widespread stasis in and thrombosis of distributing arteries and the microcirculation occur, with subsequent necrosis of skin and subcutaneous tissue if the ischemia is severe. The vascular spasm is unaffected by sympathetic denervation.

It is important to point out that several conditions are known to aggravate the vasoconstrictor effect of ergotamine. Among these are fever, thyrotoxicosis, pregnancy, hepatic disease, malnutrition, renal disease, hypertension, and an existing chronic occlusive arterial disease in the limbs. The pharmacologic effect of ergotamine is potentiated by smoking, oral contraceptives, and drugs which depress the function of the liver (phenothiazine derivatives, troleandomycin).

Treatment of ergot poisoning consists of immediate discontinuation of the drug and management of the local difficulty. Generally there is a complete regression of the process if this approach is initiated before gangrene ensues.

Sodium nitroprusside has been reported to have beneficial effects in patients manifesting signs of impending gangrene [2]. The medication is given intravenously by infusion pump at the rate of 50 μg/min until signs of improvement persist.

3. Gangrene Produced by Mechanical Obstruction or Compression of Arteries

Spasm and thrombosis of arteries. Gangrene may develop in a limb due to persistent mild mechanical compression of a critical artery. This factor either directly interferes with blood flowing through the vessel or it initiates spasm of the vascular circular muscle fibers which has the same effect. For example, forced extension of a limb, as in the treatment of an orthopedic condition, may cause sufficient reduction in local circulation to produce a nutritional disturbance even in the presence of a previously normal blood supply (see B-3, Chapter 22) (Fig. 8.5). On occasion, the repeated irritation of the subclavian artery by one of the neurovascular compression syndromes of the shoulder girdle may result in spasm and thrombosis of this vessel, followed by gangrene of the fingers (see B-4, Chapter 13).

Hemorrhage into tissues. Gangrene of tips of digits may be produced by extravasation of blood into the cutaneous and subcutaneous tissues locally, as in the case of certain blood dyscrasias like hemophilia. Occlusion of a peripheral artery may also result from extensive bleeding into a confined space causing compression of the vessel, followed by loss of viability of the affected tissues. In the case of blood dyscrasias, a contributing factor to the development of gangrene may be associated thrombosis of the small arteries due to changes in blood constituents. (For discussion of gangrene following severe injury of tissues, including vascular elements, see Chapter 15.)

Annular bands. Congenital constricting bands are rare developmental anomalies which may cause complete or partial amputation of the involved structures (Fig. 8.6B), particularly digits (Fig. 8.6A). Not infrequently they are associated with other congenital anomalies, such as

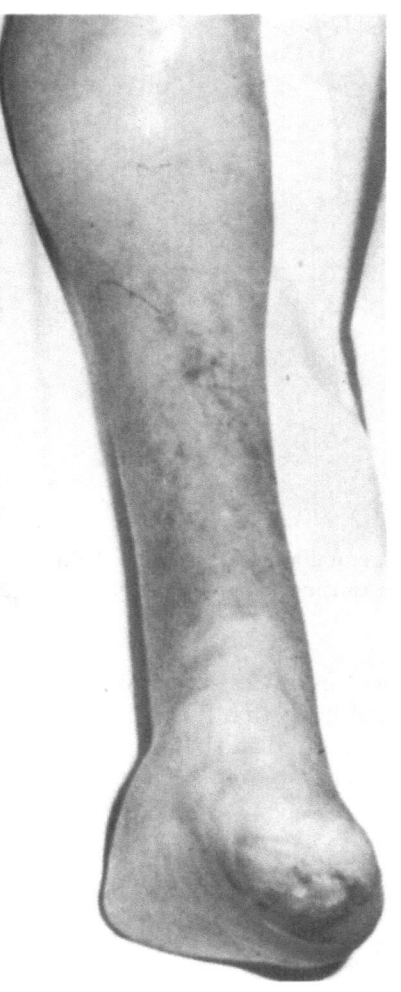

Fig. 8.5. Effect of sudden, strong extension of the left knee of a patient suffering from rheumatoid arthritis, resulting in arterial spasm, gangrene of the foot, and the need for a local amputation. Adequate arterial circulation to the limb was present before the maneuver.

syndactyly, clubfoot, cleft palate, harelip, aplasia cutis, and placental malformations. Histologic study of congenital bands favors the concept of abnormal histogenesis, a form of congenital collagen dysplasia, rather than a scar [12].

In ainhum (dactylolysis spontanea) [13], a disease which is found primarily in dark-skinned races, there is a formation of a linear, fibrous band at the digitoplantar fold of the fifth toe, which eventually produces encirclement of the digit (Fig. 8.6A). As this structure

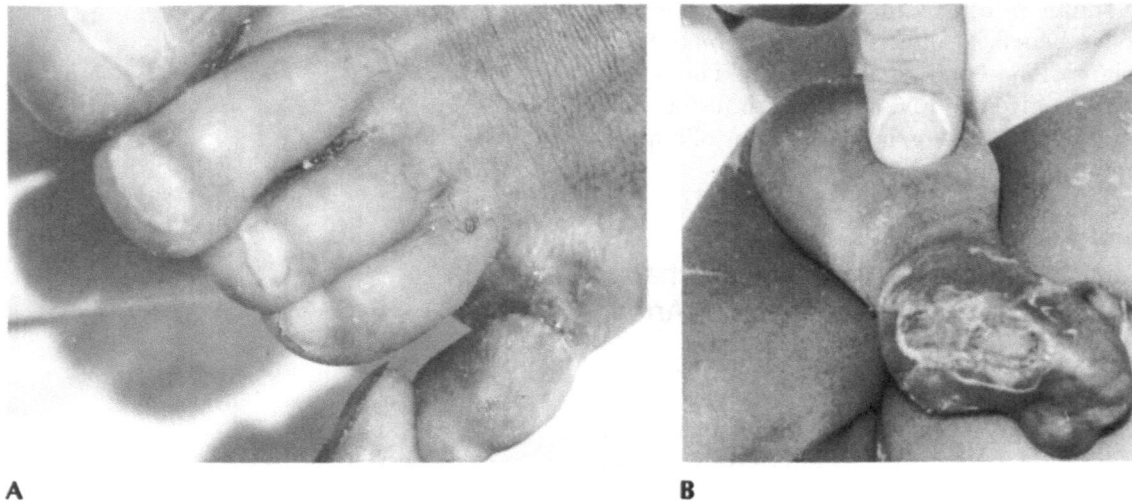

A   **B**

Fig. 8.6. Congenital annular bands. **A** Ainhum, with typical ringlike constriction of fifth toe. **B** Congenital band at ankle causing gangrene of foot.

grows deeper, it causes strangulation of the tissues beyond it, so that the distal end of the toe becomes enlarged and bulbous, followed by spontaneous amputation of the devitalized part.

References

1. Barker NW, Hines EA Jr, Craig WMcK: Livedo reticularis: A peripheral arteriolar disease. Am Heart J 21:592, 1941
2. Carliner NH, Denue DP, Finch CS Jr, et al: Sodium nitroprusside treatment of ergotamine-induced peripheral ischemia. JAMA 227:308, 1974
3. Chilvers AS, Kinmonth JB: Operations for lymphoedema of the lower limbs: A study of the results in 108 operations utilizing vascularized dermal flaps. J Cardiovasc Surg 16:115, 1975
4. Cummer CL, LaRocco CG: Ulcers of the legs in sickle-cell anemia. Arch Dermatol Syph 42:1015, 1940
5. Degni M: New technique of lymphatic-venous anastomosis for the treatment of lymphedema. J Cardiovasc Surg 19:577, 1978
6. Engler HS, Purvis JG, Kanavage CB, et al: Gangrenous extremities resulting from intraarterial injections. Arch Surg 94:644, 1967
7. Farber EM, Barnes VR: Livedo reticularis. Stanford Med Bull 13:183, 1955
8. Feldaker M, Hines EA Jr, Kierland RR: Livedo reticularis with ulceration. Circulation 13:196, 1956
9. Goldsmith HS: The treatment of postsurgical lymphedema. Surg Clin North Am 49:407, 1969
10. Kinmonth JB: Lymphangiography in man: Method of outlining the lymphatic trunks at operation. Clin Sci 11:13, 1952
11. Kinmonth JB: Lymphangiography in clinical surgery and particularly in the treatment of lymphoedema. Ann R Coll Surg Engl 15:300, 1954
12. Raque CJ, Stein KM, Lane JM, et al: Pseudoainhum constricting bands of the extremities. Arch Dermatol 105:434, 1972
13. Riley LH Jr, Cantrell JR: Clinical and pathological observations in three cases of ainhum. Arch Surg 79:1013, 1959
14. Weeks PM: Ischemia of the hand secondary to levarterenol bitartrate extravasation: Method of management. JAMA 196:288, 1966

Chapter 9

Differential Diagnosis of Physical Findings and States

Part 2 Soft-tissue Calcification; Peripheral Neuropathy; Neurotrophic Arthropathy; Petechiae and Ecchymosis; Cutaneous and Subcutaneous Masses

---

This chapter, like Chapter 8, deals with the pathogenesis and differential diagnosis of abnormal states found both in vascular and musculoskeletal disorders.

A. Soft-tissue Calcification

Soft-tissue calcification is an abnormal accumulation of lime salts in a tissue in amounts which are demonstrable on microscopic, roentgenographic, and even naked-eye examination [13].

1. Pathogenesis

The exact mechanism responsible for the development of aggregates of calcium carbonate and phosphate, derived from the components present in blood and tissue fluid, is not known. Ordinarily, there is a dynamic equilibrium between the amount of calcium and phosphorus in the bloodstream, which in turn is dependent upon the absorption of these ions from the gastrointestinal tract, their resorption from or deposition in the bony storehouse, and their excretion by the kidneys and bowel [13]. At a normal carbon dioxide tension, the blood serum and interstitial fluid are essentially saturated with calcium and phosphorus ions. In the presence of an increase of calcium without a compensatory decrease of phosphorus, or with the reverse situation, precipitation of insoluble calcium phosphate occurs. Injured tissue is receptive to deposition of calcium salts because of the associated presence of a lowered carbon dioxide tension, a situation which allows fewer calcium and phosphate ions to be held in solution.

2. Types

Abnormal calcium deposits in soft tissues have been classified in the following manner [5].

Metastatic calcification. In this category, the abnormal response is due to an altered calcium and/or phosphorus regulation remote from the site of deposit of the salt. Generally, the calcium and phosphorus concentrations in the serum are elevated, and precipitation of calcium phosphate, usually in an alkaline medium, develops in normal tissues. These changes may be associated with hyperparathyroidism, vitamin D intoxication, pseudohypoparathyroidism, destructive bone diseases (leukemia, multiple myeloma, osteomyelitis, Paget's disease, metastatic carcinoma), and renal insufficiency.

Vascular calcification. Calcium deposits may take place on ulcerated atherosclerotic plaques in the intima of arteries or in the media of such vessels, as in Mönckeberg's sclerosis (see C-2, Chapter 11). The vascular changes are intensified in conditions in which there are elevated serum calcium levels, such as hyperparathyroidism and vitamin D intoxication.

Dystrophic calcification. In this group calcification occurs usually with localized injury due to a known etiologic agent. This process takes place in devitalized tissues, such as infarcts and areas of necrosis or fatty degeneration. Associated conditions are infection, granulomas, parasitic infestation, foreign bodies, and congenital defects. The deposition of the calcium is facilitated by a local increase in alkalinity or by an elevation of serum calcium or serum phosphorus values.

In the case of indolent, nonhealing ulcers of the legs due to protracted venous stasis, there may be actual deposition of bony plaques in the base of the lesions and in the surrounding tissues [6,7]. Such a change may be responsible for failure to achieve healing of the condition regardless of the therapeutic program attempted.

Calcinosis. This type is divided into two categories: calcinosis universalis, a rare disease, chiefly of childhood; and calcinosis circumscripta, found in association with Raynaud's disease, progressive systemic sclerosis, dermatomyositis, systemic lupus erythematosus, and rheumatoid arthritis. In calcinosis universalis, calcification starts in the subcutaneous tissue and then spreads to the deeper connective tissue septa, muscles, tendons, and fasciae. The process tends to be symmetric, beaded, and arranged in long bands. Calcinosis circumscripta is generally found in older female patients, and it is usually confined to the terminal phalanges of the fingers and the extensor surfaces of the elbows and knees. At times there may be large conglomerations of calcium deposits in other parts of the body. In calcinosis, the avidity of calcium for degenerated tissue is clearly demonstrated.

Heterotopic bone formation. In this type, serum calcium, phosphorus, and pH values are generally normal. The process is found in many sites, including insertions of tendons, postoperative abdominal scars, and soft tissues of paraplegics. Typical of the condition is myositis ossificans progressiva, which usually appears before the age of 6 years and is characterized by progressive ossification of connective tissues of muscles. A local type of heterotopic bone formation is traumatic myositis ossificans secondary to hematoma formation. After injury to deep muscle tissue, edema and cellular proliferation are superseded by masses of collagen which accept the deposition of calcium salts, followed by the appearance of osteoid, cartilage, and bone [1]. Most frequently involved is the quadriceps of the thigh, followed by the brachialis above the elbow.

B. Peripheral Neuropathy

Peripheral neuropathy is an acute or chronic degenerative condition of either the peripheral nerves, the autonomic nervous system, or the central nervous system.

1. Etiologic Agents

Diabetes mellitus is by far the most common cause of peripheral neuropathy. Among other etiologic agents are toxic substances (alcohol, lead, mercury, arsenic, methyl-n-butyl ketone, thallium, acrylamide, and n-hexane, an organic compound found in glues); drugs (nitrofurantoin, chloroquine, isoniazid, hydralazine hydrochloride, thalidomide, and phenytoin sodium); and systemic disorders (spontaneous myxedema, pernicious anemia, vitamin deficiency, and constitutional responses to tetanus antitoxin administration, among others).

2. Pathology and Pathogenesis

The lesions in the nerves in peripheral neuropathy are degenerative in nature, and hence the commonly used term, peripheral neuritis, which implies an inflammatory process, is an improper designation. The predominant change in diabetic peripheral neuropathy is a demyelination, with relative preservation of axons in the peripheral nerves and dorsal nerve roots and secondary alterations in the spinal cord. In the peripheral nerves, the sensory components are much more affected than the motor fibers. Fibrosis is not an obvious abnormality. A common finding is neurogenic atrophy of small bundles of voluntary muscle in the leg and foot. The cause of the pathologic changes is still uncertain. One view considers the abnormalities to be a primary degeneration of nervous structures due to metabolic factors. Another attributes the changes to microangiopathy.

3. Clinical Manifestations

Since most peripheral nerves contain sensory and motor fibers which are involved to varying degrees in peripheral neuropathy, the patient generally demonstrates both sensory and motor abnormalities. These follow the course and anatomic distribution of the peripheral nerves involved.

Symptoms. The complaints are usually located in the distal portions of the limbs, particularly the digits. They range from paresthesias, such as numbness, tingling, and prickling, to burning, aching, or sharp, intense pain. Frequently, tenderness is present along the course of the nerves.

Signs of sensory involvement. The objective findings consist of impairment of touch, vibration, position, and temperature sense. However, hyperesthesia may also be present. Of course, if the condition has progressed to the point of complete functional severance of the nerve, pain is absent and loss of sensation is complete.

Signs of motor involvement. In some patients, the prominent abnormalities consist mainly of

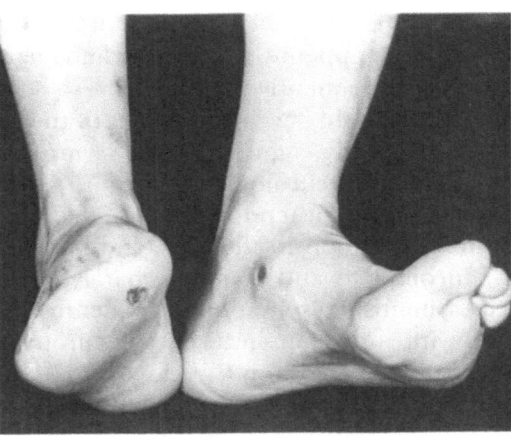

Fig. 9.1. Paralysis and atrophy of small muscles of the feet in a patient with peripheral neuropathy due to diabetes mellitus.

those due to motor impairment. They may range from mild weakness to complete paralysis, in the form of a foot drop or a wrist drop. If paralysis exists, it is always of the flaccid type and is ultimately associated with atrophy of the muscles (Fig. 9.1) and loss of deep-tendon reflexes. No abnormal reflexes are elicited.

Vascular manifestations. Since the sympathetic fibers in the peripheral mixed nerves are also affected in peripheral neuropathy, signs of increased and then decreased or even absent vasomotor tone are present. With early irritation of the sympathetic nerves, the skin becomes cold, blue, hyperhidrotic, and even edematous (see A-3, Chapter 8). As the process advances and the sympathetic nerves degenerate, autosympathectomy is produced; the limb is now warm, well-colored, and dry. The peripheral pulses are bounding and the oscillometric readings obtained from various levels on the extremity fall into the high normal range.

4. Types of Peripheral Neuropathy

Diabetic neuropathy. In diabetes mellitus there is primarily involvement of the nerves of the lower limbs, although neurologic changes may also be present in the upper extremities, the trunk, and other parts of the body. The chief complaint is severe pain, usually worse at night, which may result in sleeplessness, poor appetite, weight loss, and mental depression. Frequently the limbs are so sensitive to pressue that even the weight of the bed clothes markedly aggravates the symptoms. The associated neurologic signs consist of diminished or absent tendon reflexes, decreased vibratory sensation in the toes, and paresthesias. Incomplete and complete paralysis may occur. Diminished sensation is frequently associated with such complications as neuropathic arthropathy (see Section C, below) and neurotrophic ulcers (see C-3, Chapter 8). Prolonged nerve conduction velocity is a common laboratory finding, as well as an elevation of total protein content in the spinal fluid. The latter change may be related to the fact that spinal cord changes are present in association with the degenerative peripheral neuropathy.

The cause of the neurologic derangement in diabetes is unknown. It may represent either a toxic metabolic state, degenerative vascular changes in the peripheral nervous system, or a combination of these factors. The possibility of microangiopathy affecting the vasa nervorum has been advanced, but evidence has also been presented supporting the view that there is no correlation between the nervous and the arteriolar and capillary alterations and hence that the basis of the demyelination is not vascular [2]. Histologic examination of autopsy material [9] is in accord with the possibility that multiple small infarcts in the peripheral nerve trunks are the cause for the clinical picture. Although much of the available data indicate that diabetic peripheral neuropathy develops most frequently in long-standing, poorly controlled cases, this state has also occurred during good chemical control and may, in fact, be precipitated following institution of proper diet, insulin, or tolbutamide (Orinase) [3,4,11]. Various stress factors have also been proposed as a cause of neuropathy [4,11].

Nutritional neuropathy.

In this state paresthesias and pain in the feet, impaired sense of position to the point of ataxia, exquisite tenderness of the legs, and diminished to absent deep-tendon reflexes are prominent findings. However, motor weakness and foot drop and wrist drop may also be present.

In chronic alcoholism the inadequate diet is probably responsible for a deficiency of the B complex vitamins and for the appearance of peripheral neuropathy. The latter may on occasion be acute and progressive, with an unfavorable outcome.

Other systemic disorders.

A number of other generalized conditions can produce localized neuropathies. Leprosy may involve any peripheral nerve, although the most common lesions are found in the median, ulnar, and sciatic nerves. In polyarteritis nodosa (see C-2, Chapter 13), rheumatoid arthritis (see C-5, Chapter 13), Sjögren's syndrome, Wegener's granulomatosis, and Degos-Kohlmeier's syndrome, the existing ischemia due to a vasculitis may affect several or many peripheral nerves. Serum sickness may be associated with trigeminal neuropathy, as well as with involvement of the brachial plexus. The exotoxin of diphtheria affects both the cranial nerves and the peripheral nerves to the limbs. Porphyria is typified by peripheral neuropathy in addition to its gastrointestinal symptoms. Viral brachial nerve neuropathy has also been noted.

Guillain-Barré syndrome (acute idiopathic polyneuritis; Landry's paralysis) may follow an upper respiratory infection and is usually ushered in by paresthesia and weakness of the legs progressing to paralysis, associated with a significant rise in spinal fluid protein. The neuropathy ascends to the upper limbs, the trunk muscles, and the cranial nerves (with accompanying bulbar symptoms). Sensory changes may be minimal. The condition is a true peripheral neuritis since an inflammatory process is present. The nerve roots and the sensory ganglia, as well as the peripheral nerves, may be involved.

Toxic neuropathy.

Chronic poisoning by heavy metals, such as lead, mercury, and arsenic, may cause a toxic neuropathy which involves multiple peripheral nerves. The changes with lead or mercury poisoning are generally noted in motor nerves, resulting in wrist drop and less commonly foot drop. Practically no sensory abnormalities are observed. Encephalopathy may also be part of the clinical picture of lead intoxication, with findings of diffuse brain disease. In arsenical neuropathy, both sensory and motor changes are present.

Trauma to or compression of peripheral nerves. Direct injury to a peripheral nerve may produce neuropathy, the same response occurring if there is compression of this structure by a tumor. Prolonged pressure over a superficial segment of nerve, producing mechanical and ischemic effects, may lead to temporary or persistent sensory or motor disturbances. Such a situation may exist during protracted surgical anesthesia and in an alcoholic bout during which the back of the arm is kept against a table edge, causing pressure on the radial nerve and a resulting peripheral neuropathy (Saturday night palsy). Sitting for an extended period of time with the knees crossed may compress the peroneal nerve against the fibula so as to produce peroneal nerve palsy with foot drop. Ulnar nerve neuropathy and palsy may follow persistent positional compression of the ulnar nerve.

Another example of pressure neuropathy is the neurologic findings in the neurovascular compression syndromes of the shoulder girdle (see Section B, Chapter 13). In these conditions, either a cervical rib, a hypertrophied scalenus anticus muscle, or some other mass presses upon the components of the brachial plexus when the precipitating position is assumed.

Meralgia paresthetica is an example of neuropathy of a purely sensory peripheral nerve, the lateral femoral cutaneous nerve arising from the second lumbar root. The symptoms consist of paresthesias and pain over the anterolateral aspect of the thigh. It is believed that the lateral femoral cutaneous nerve is in some way compressed as it passes through the fascia lata.

5. Differential Diagnosis

Ischemic neuropathy. Peripheral neuropathy must be differentiated from ischemic neuropathy which is due to a very severe degree of ischemia of peripheral tissues (including the mixed nerves) produced by a chronic occlusive arterial disease, generally arteriosclerosis obliterans of the lower extremities. Although the symptoms of the two conditions are frequently similar (sense of coldness, numbness, or burning in the feet, paresthesias of the toes, and shooting, lancinating pain), the precipitating

factors are different. In ischemic neuropathy the complaints appear soon after the patient lies down in bed in preparation for sleep and are immediately alleviated by placing the lower limbs over the edge of the bed, sitting up, or standing. None of these positions has an effect on eliciting or controlling the symptoms of peripheral neuropathy, since the latter may appear spontaneously. With regard to physical findings, ischemic neuropathy is always associated with signs of a markedly reduced local arterial circulation, such as absent pulsations in the feet, oscillometric readings of zero above the ankles and frequently at higher levels, changes in the skin indicating the existence of a precarious nutritional circulation, and absence or reduction of vibration sense perception in the toes. In the uncomplicated case of peripheral neuropathy, the circulation in the feet is normal, while neurologic findings are much more extensive, including absence or reduction of pin prick and cotton wool sensation and of deep-tendon and vibration sense perception. Ankle jerks and knee jerks may be absent or decreased and signs of atrophy of small muscles of the foot are present. Less marked but similar changes may be noted in the hands. When a patient with diabetes and peripheral neuropathy also suffers from arteriosclerosis obliterans and ischemic neuropathy, both etiologies are probably responsible for the abnormal neurologic symptoms and signs.

Radiculitis. Displacement of an intervertebral disk in the cervical or lumbar region causes a radiculitis rather than a peripheral neuropathy because it is the spinal roots which are compressed. The neurologic changes are segmental rather than coinciding with an area subserved by a peripheral nerve, as occurs in peripheral neuropathy.

Upper motor neuron paralysis. In this state, the paralysis is spastic, with hyperreflexia and pathologic reflexes present. Moreover, sensory disturbances are not noted unless sensory pathways are involved in the same lesion.

6. Treatment

Therapy in peripheral neuropathy depends on the cause. Exogenous toxins must be eliminated and nutritional and vitamin deficiencies corrected. If the neuropathy is due to compression of a peripheral nerve, the etiologic agent should be removed by surgical means.

Medications. For arsenic and mercury poisoning, dimercaprol (BAL) should be given by deep intramuscular injection to bind the metals for excretion and thus remove them from their toxic combination with the body sulfhydryls. This drug has also received clinical trials in acute idiopathic polyneuritis, diabetic polyneuropathy, and polyneuropathies of obscure origin. However, its value in such conditions has not as yet been determined. It is important to point out that BAL is contraindicated in most instances of hepatic insufficiency. The drug also produces a rise in blood pressure accompanied by tachycardia.

Since vitamin B_{12} is specifically effective in pernicious anemia, where elements of peripheral neuropathy are also present, it has been used with varying reports of effectiveness in nutritional and diabetic polyneuropathy, as well as in acute porphyria. Vitamin B_1 (thiamine chloride) in large doses (800 mg daily), when given over a prolonged period of time, appears to reduce the symptoms of diabetic peripheral neuropathy. Among other medications which have been used in this state are phenytoin sodium (Dilantin), promethazine hydrochloride (Phenergan), phenylbutazone (Butazolidin), prednisone, and clofibrate (Atromid-S).

Since very severe pain may be present in peripheral neuropathy, it is necessary to attempt to control this with medication. However, the use of narcotics in large doses must be avoided in order to prevent addiction. If at all possible, aspirin and codeine should be substituted. Because the symptoms are worse at night, sedatives such as chloral hydrate and barbiturates should be given to the patient before retiring.

Adjunctive procedures. Aside from drug therapy, general supportive measures should be instituted. These include bed rest and physical therapeutic modalities to prevent muscle contractures. In the presence of foot drop, the ankle joint and foot should be properly protected with a foot-drop brace until spontaneous improvement appears. In the interval, range-of-motion exercises of the ankle joint should re-

peatedly be carried out during the course of the day, in order to prevent ankylosis and fibrosis of the joint tissues.

C. Neuropathic Arthropathy

Neuropathic joint disease (Charcot's joint) is a chronic progressive degenerative arthropathy affecting one or more joints in the limbs and the vertebral joints, associated with various neurologic disorders. Common to all of the latter conditions is a disturbance in sensation to the affected structures.

1. Etiology and Incidence

In the past, tabes dorsalis of syphilitic origin was the usual cause of painless deformities of the joints of the limbs, particularly, the knees and, less often, the hips and ankles. The spine, in the lower dorsal and lumbar region, was also involved. In most instances there was more than one joint affected. However, with the decline in the incidence of tertiary syphilis, the greatest number of cases of Charcot's joint disease are now seen in the tarsus and other articulations of the diabetic foot [8]. This type of abnormality also occurs in approximately 20 to 25 percent of patients with syringomyelia. In children the sensory disturbance resulting from myelomeningocele is the most frequent basis of neuropathic arthropathy affecting the joints of the lower limbs. Charcot's joints have also been found in congenital indifference to pain, nutritional deficiency, myelopathy of pernicious anemia, spinal cord compression, hereditary sensory neuropathy, peripheral nerve section, peripheral nerve disorders, leprosy, chronic alcoholism, poliomyelitis, birth defects (idiopathic myelodysplasia), and trauma.

2. Pathogenesis

Although the exact causative agent is not precisely understood, it is believed that loss of the normal response to pain and derangement of proprioceptive mechanisms lead to relaxation of supporting structures and chronic instability of the joint. At the same time, the joint is deprived of protective reactions to minor injuries of daily activity or more important stresses to which it is liable, because of the underlying neurologic disease. Also, the sensory defects lead to a type of premature degenerative joint disease [10].

3. Pathology

The Charcot's joint demonstrates signs of destructive and hypertrophic changes which resemble those of other types of degenerative joint disease. There is erosion of the lining cartilage, together with necrosis of menisci and formation of loose bodies. Later in the disease, marked and extensive marginal osteophytic growth develops, perhaps in response to the hypermobility of the neuropathic joint.

Beneath the articular surface of the joint, in the zone of provisional calcification, are found proliferation of cartilage (which demonstrates signs of undergoing calcification) and, in some areas, even dense bone formation. Associated changes are subluxations, dislocations, and fractures of articular facets, osteophytes, epicondyles, and condyles. All of these alterations produce marked disorganization of the osseous components, bizarre overgrowth of marginal bone and callus, capsular contraction, and stretching of supporting ligaments [10]. There are also atrophic types of Charcot's joints with bone disorganization.

4. Clinical Manifestations

In the diabetic the lesion usually develops insidiously, generally being associated with prominent signs and symptoms of peripheral neuropathy (see Section B, above), but with no indications of an impaired circulatory status of the involved limbs. Not infrequently an associated finding is the presence of neurotrophic ulcers (see C-3, Chapter 8) on the plantar surface of the foot. Early in the condition the limb is excessively perspired, but later anhidrosis appears as autosympathectomy occurs (see B-3, above). At first there are thickening and swelling of the foot, accompanied by little if any pain, redness, or warmth. As the process continues, the enlargement of the foot becomes more marked, the change being associated with deformity and a tendency to

flattening, eversion, and external rotation (diabetic foot). Eventually there is extensive disruption of the ankle, the astragalotibial joint, the tarsometatarsal or metatarsophalangeal joint, or any combination of these structures (foreshortened foot) [8].

In the case of Charcot's joints due to etiologies other than diabetes, the distribution of affected joints is determined by the underlying neurologic lesion. With involvement of knees or shoulders, large effusions are common. At times tap of the synovial fluid reveals it to be sanguineous, although generally no abnormalities are found. Consistently there is abnormal hypermobility (torsion) of the joint. When the spine is the site of neuropathic arthropathy, abnormalities of form and function may be much less obvious.

5. Roentgenographic Findings

X-ray examination is a very important means of determining the degree of joint damage in the well-developed case of Charcot's joint. However, in the early stage of this disorder, the findings may be minimal except for the commonly present effusion. In the advanced stage, there is evidence of destructive and hypertrophic changes in the involved joint, including erosion of the articular cartilage, fragmentation of subchondral bone, and proliferation of new bone at the margins of the joint. Frequently chip and compression fractures exist and free bodies are present in the joint cavity. The soft tissues are thickened and contain scattered calcifications. With further progression, there may be complete disintegration of the osseous structures.

Roentgenographic examination of the affected foot in the well-developed case of Charcot's joint due to diabetes reveals extensive fragmentation and lysis of the bones, especially the tarsals and proximal ends of the metatarsals. The shafts of the latter often become tapered and may fracture. Bony fragments may be scattered around in a loose and irregular fashion.

6. Treatment

Local therapy. The basic approach to the neuropathic foot is immobilization of the affected joint and restriction of weight bearing [10]. Immobilization of the spine is accomplished by a corset or brace, whereas the knee joint can be placed in a caliper brace. In the case of the hip joint, non-weight bearing by resorting to crutches is helpful. Early in the condition, immobilization provided by plaster casts may produce significant improvement.

Operative measures are limited to amputation or arthrodesis of weight-bearing joints. In the foot, a Syme's amputation (see C-5, Chapter 24) may, at times, be justified. Thigh amputation in the case of genicular involvement is less successful and rarely recommended. Arthrodesis of Charcot's joints frequently results in failure because of infection, nonunion, or both. However, in the relatively young adult the possibility of a successful fusion makes the attempt worthwhile. Antibiotics are prescribed if infection is present, as well as incision and drainage.

Subsequently physical therapeutic procedures and orthopedic appliances are helpful. Among these are soapsuds soaks, special shoes devised to relieve pressure on involved structures, prostheses, braces, crutches, and canes. Elevation of the affected limb at frequent intervals may give some relief.

Supportive therapy. If diabetes is the causative agent, medical control of the condition is imperative. Large doses of thiamine chloride, 200 mg four times a day, may be helpful in the treatment of the underlying peripheral neuropathy (see B-6, above). If the condition is caused by a neurologic disorder, this should be managed medically, if possible.

D. Petechiae and Ecchymosis

Petechiae and ecchymosis are found in both arterial and venous disorders of the limbs, as well as being part of the clinical picture of a relatively large number of nonvascular disorders. They represent escape of blood from capillaries into the skin or mucous membranes.

1. Petechiae in Vascular Conditions

Pathogenesis. Petechiae in vascular disorders are generally due to a change in the permeability of the capillary wall, allowing formed elements of the blood to enter the tissue spaces. Other underlying mechanisms are an increase in vascular fragility and obstruction of small blood vessels by microemboli (bacterial or nonbacterial), followed by damage to their walls and extravasation of blood. A most common cause in chronic occlusive arterial disease is a local state of anoxia of all tissues including the minute vessels, with the change in the latter producing a greater permeability of the capillary wall. The petechiae are found on the distal portions of the lower limbs. Although the material deposited in the skin is hemoglobin, the range of color changes usually associated with a hematoma or a hemorrhage into the tissues is not noted in the case of these lesions. They are not altered by the application of digital pressure to them or by elevation of the limb, the results being distinguishing points from reversible cyanosis.

Prognosis. The appearance of spontaneous petechiae in vascular disorders has different prognostic implications depending upon the underlying mechanism. In the presence of an occlusive arterial disease, whether acute or chronic, an extremely guarded outlook is warranted with regard to viability of the limb, for generally such a response is followed by actual gangrene of the affected structures. In the case of venous involvement, such as severe primary varicosities, the appearance of petechiae on the medial aspect of the lower portion of the leg has no special significance except that later pigmentation may develop in the site, due to the deposition of hemosiderin derived from the breakdown of hemoglobin. This type of change is conducive to ulcer formation.

2. Petechiae in Nonvascular Disorders or States

Hematologic and nonhematologic conditions. Petechiae are associated with various types of thrombocytopenic purpura (idiopathic or symptomatic) and with nonthrombocytopenic purpura. Among the conditions in which the latter is found are Henoch-Schönlein purpura (Fig. 9.2), chronic nephritis, cardiac or hepatic disorders, food allergy, metabolic conditions,

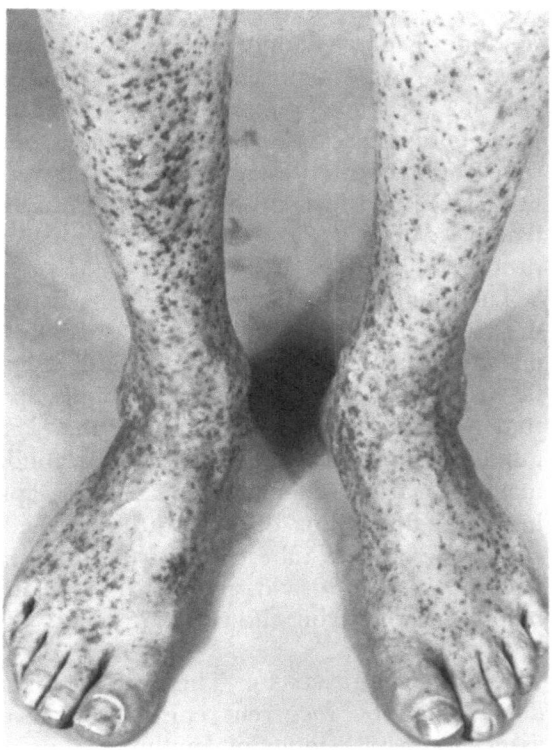

Fig. 9.2. Henoch-Schönlein purpura.

vitamin C or P deficiency, and infectious diseases. The etiologic agent in these abnormalities may be failure to maintain normal repair of the capillary wall, due to low levels of prothrombin and fibrinogen and a reduced platelet count.

Protracted periods of bed rest. Patients who have been at prolonged bed rest for whatever cause and are then placed on an ambulation program may initially demonstrate crops of petechiae on the lower portion of the legs. Possibly the long period of inactivity is responsible for alterations in capillary permeability, the assumption of the upright position resulting in an increase in hydrostatic pressure sufficient to produce movement of blood through the capillary wall and into the tissue spaces. No special significance is attached to this type of response, and with continued ambulation the petechiae disappear.

Drug purpura. A number of medications are responsible for the production of petechiae.

Among these are the steroids, stilbestrol, quinine and quinidine, antibacterial agents, reserpine, meprobamate, and thiazide diuretics. The response is probably due either to a perivascular lymphocytic vasculitis, capillary damage from a direct toxic effect of the medication, or an allergic reaction. Large doses of heparin and of oral anticoagulants may also be associated with the appearance of fine petechiae on the lower part of the legs and on the dorsum of the feet.

Local injury. Trauma to normal tissues may be responsible for subcutaneous ecchymosis. This is particularly true for obese women who have considerable deposition of subcutaneous fat, a very poor support for the capillaries found under the skin. Hence, these vessels are readily traumatized by even minor injury, resulting in local areas of subcutaneous hemorrhage, especially on the thighs and legs.

Larger vessels, such as veins, may also rupture following injury or mild or marked contraction of voluntary muscles locally. A frequent location for such a response is deep in the calf muscles, the resulting clinical picture resembling phlebothrombosis (see A-2, Chapter 18). The color changes in the skin due to the breakdown products of hemoglobin are generally noted several days after the acute episode, being located some distance below the actual point at which the hemorrhage took place (not infrequently just above the malleoli). If the patient is bedridden at the time of the hemorrhage and remains so, the ecchymosis may be observed in the skin over the calf muscles.

E. Cutaneous and Subcutaneous Masses

1. Classification of Entities

A number of vascular and nonvascular disorders are associated with the presence of palpable masses in the limbs. Among the vascular disorders typified by pulsating lesions are arterial aneurysms (spontaneous and traumatic), arteriovenous fistulae (congenital and acquired), and the small aneurysmal masses found in polyarteritis nodosa. Nonpulsating but soft vascular or lymphatic masses consist of clusters of varicose veins, lymphatic tumors, glomus tumor, and hemangioma. Examples of nonpulsating hard vascular masses are the various types of superficial thrombophlebitis and chronic indurated cellulitis. Others have a varying degree of acute or chronic panniculitis in the subcutaneous tissue, as typified by Weber-Christian disease, erythema induratum, erythema nodosum, erythrocyanosis, and chronic chilblain.

Among the nonvascular disorders characterized by the presence of nodules in the limbs are xanthomas, fatty tumors, fibromas, neurofibromas, fibrosarcomas, Hodgkin's disease, and sarcoidosis. In the case of most of these conditions, it is necessary to resort to histopathologic study of biopsy material to arrive at the proper diagnosis, since this cannot be made purely on clinical grounds; however, even such a procedure does not always establish the true basis for the lesion.

This section deals with a discussion of the vascular entities in the above list not presented elsewhere. Descriptions of the other clinical conditions can be found by reference to the Index.

2. Clinical Entities

Erythema induratum. This is a chronic disorder which is characterized by nodules and ulcerations in the lower extremities. It is generally considered to be due to tuberculosis (Bazin's disease), although a nontuberculous type has also been described (nodular vasculitis). The disease occurs most often in girls during adolescence and less frequently in men. Histologically typical tubercles are found in the lesion with caseation in the center. There may also be marked necrosis of fat and extensive fibrosis.

The first clinical manifestation of the condition is the appearance of bluish-red, deep-seated nodules in the skin and subcutaneous tissue of the legs, particularly the calves. When ulceration occurs, the nodule first becomes tender and painful and assumes an irregular shape, with a ragged, undermined edge and a granulating base secreting a watery discharge.

As healing slowly occurs in the original lesions, new ones generally appear, these subsequently developing superimposed ulcerations. Eventually the areas are epithelialized, leaving atrophic depressed scars surrounded by pigmentation. With repeated attacks, edema may form in the legs and feet, probably as the result of lymphatic obstruction due to the inflammatory process.

The diagnosis of Bazin's disease is dependent upon the existence of signs of tuberculosis elsewhere in the body. In this regard, it may be necessary to obtain chest radiographs, sputum examinations, tuberculin testing, and guinea pig inoculations of material from abnormally appearing regional lymph nodes. Rapid healing of the lesions following the use of medications of value in tuberculosis (streptomycin, para-aminosalicylic acid, and isoniazid) is also helpful in identifying the etiologic agent.

Weber-Christian disease. This is a rare disorder typified by recurrent episodes of fever associated with single or multiple crops of subcutaneous nodules, located in the limbs, particularly the legs. Also designated as relapsing febrile, nodular nonsuppurative panniculitis, the condition has an unknown etiology. However, a number of possible causative agents have been proposed, among which are the halogen compounds (iodides, chlorides, and bromides), exposure to trauma and cold, faulty fat metabolism, antigen-antibody reactions, infections, and antitrypsin deficiency. The disease is found most often in obese women between the ages of 30 and 50 years.

The pathologic changes consist of nonsuppurative necrosis of fat cells in the subcutaneous panniculus and elsewhere, associated with infiltration of the tissues with lymphocytes, monocytes, and polymorphonuclear leukocytes. The interlobar areas and the walls of vessels may demonstrate fibrinoid degeneration, similar to that observed in connective tissue disorders (see Section C, Chapter 13).

The clinical manifestations of Weber-Christian disease are not typical. In some patients the prominent findings are local pain and tenderness, whereas in others there are also systemic responses. The condition is characterized by repeated attacks, some lasting as long as several months, followed by spontaneous remissions. Despite the frequent bouts of fever, the white blood cell count is generally normal, or there might even be a leukopenia.

The subcutaneous nodules may vary in size from 0.5 to 5 cm in diameter and may or may not be tender. At first the skin over the lesions is red, but then the color changes to a brownish discoloration. There is a tendency for neighboring nodules to coalesce, forming indurated plaques under the skin; at times necrosis of the lesion may develop. With progression of the disease, the affected subcutaneous fat becomes atrophied, producing depression and deformation of the skin. Swelling of the limb is a prominent associated finding.

Weber-Christian disease must be differentiated from cellulitis, superficial thrombophlebitis, asymptomatic lipomatosis, and Dercum's disease. A distinguishing point between Weber-Christian disease and erythema nodosum (see below) and erythema induratum (see above) is that in the latter two conditions the nodules do not show signs of atrophy, although in the case of erythema induratum they may ulcerate.

A large number of therapeutic approaches have been suggested for Weber-Christian disease. Among these are antibiotics, steroids, x-ray therapy, and local excision of the nodules. Continuous intravenous infusion of heparin has been reported to prevent the appearance of nodules in some of the patients [12]. Rarely is Weber-Christian disease a cause of death. When this occurs, there is widespread involvement of adipose tissue throughout the body. (For a discussion of nodules in rheumatoid arthritis, see C-5, Chapter 13.)

Erythema nodosum. This condition is a non-specific syndrome typified by the transient appearance of cutaneous and subcutaneous nodules resembling bruises, associated with fever, malaise, and migratory arthritis. It has numerous etiologies, among which are acute rheumatic fever, syphilis, tuberculosis, upper respiratory infections, diphtheria, measles, brucellosis, sarcoidosis, malaria, ulcerative colitis, and infectious mononucleosis. Various drugs, such as sulfonamide compounds, iodides, certain oral contraceptive drugs, and bromides, may also be responsible for the appearance of the syndrome in sensitive individuals. It is seen primarily in women between 20 and 30 years of age, generally in the spring and autumn.

The pathologic changes found in a biopsied nodule consist of infiltration of lymphocytes and polymorphonuclear leukocytes about the vascular network in the middle and lower portions of the corium and adjacent subcutaneous fat. The vessel walls are edematous and the capillaries are dilated.

Typically the nodule of erythema nodosum is superficial, firm, red, hot, and tender and about 1 to 2 cm in diameter. It is found in the subcutaneous tissue, with the overlying skin becoming shiny and raised. Eventually the lesion assumes a bruised appearance following the onset of swelling and erythema. Each nodule lasts for a few days to 6 weeks or longer. As involution occurs, the color of the lesion may change from the original bright red hue to purple, yellow, green, and then brown. At no time do the nodules ulcerate although at times they seem to fluctuate. They are usually found on the anterior surface of the legs in the pretibial region and less frequently on the soles of the feet, the calves, knees, and thighs; occasionally they are present on the upper part of the arms.

Associated with the presence of the nodules are systemic reactions in the form of arthritis of the ankles, knees, wrists, fingers, and elbows. There may be malaise and a fever of 37.2 to 38.3° C (99 to 101° F). Roentgenographic examination of the chest may reveal bilateral hilar lymphadenopathy and occasionally diffuse pulmonary mottling.

Since erythema nodosum is a self-limiting condition, no specific therapy is indicated. Symptomatic control of the pain associated with the arthralgias may be necessary.

References

1. Aegerter EE, Kirpatrick JA Jr: Orthopedic Diseases: Physiology, Pathology, and Radiology. Philadelphia, Saunders, 1963, p 344
2. Dolman CL: Morbid anatomy of diabetic neuropathy. Neurology (Minneap) 13:135, 1963
3. Ellenberg M: Diabetic neuropathy precipitated by diabetic control with tolbutamide. JAMA 169:1755, 1959
4. Ellenberg M: Diabetic neuropathy: Considera-

tions of factors in onset. Ann Intern Med 52:1067, 1960

5. Hilbish TF, Bartter FC: Roentgen findings in abnormal deposition of calcium in tissues. Am J Roentgenol 87:1128, 1962

6. Lippmann HI: Subcutaneous ossification in chronic venous insufficiency: Presentation of 23 cases: A preliminary report. Angiology 8:378, 1957

7. Lippmann HI, Goldin RR: Subcutaneous ossification of the legs in chronic venous insufficiency. Radiology 74:279, 1960

8. Miller DS, Lichtman WF: Diabetic neuropathic arthropathy of feet. Arch Surg 70:513, 1955

9. Raff MC, Asbury AK: Ischemic mononeuropathy and mononeuropathy multiplex in diabetes mellitus. N Engl J Med 279:17, 1968

10. Rodnan GP, Maclachlan MJ, Brower TD: Neuropathic joint disease (Charcot joints). Bull Rheum Dis 9:183, 1959

11. Rundles RW: Diabetic neuropathy. Medicine 24:111, 1945

12. Tsaltas TT, Wise RI: Etiology and treatment of Weber-Christian's disease. Clin Res 18:465, 1970

13. Wheeler CE, Curtis AC, Cawley EP, et al: Soft tissue calcification with special reference to its occurrence in the "collagen diseases." Ann Intern Med 36:1050, 1952

Chapter 10

Description and Pathogenesis of Symptoms and Signs of Arterial Insufficiency

This chapter deals primarily with a description of, and the abnormal mechanisms responsible for, the more common symptoms and, to a lesser extent, the typical signs found in chronic and acute arterial disorders of the limbs. Also included is the differentiation of the complaints from those of musculoskeletal or related origin which mimic them.

In the collection of data on vascular symptoms and signs is it essential to follow a consistent plan, as outlined in Tables 5.1 and 5.2, for otherwise there is always the possibility that important information will inadvertently be omitted.

A. Clinical Manifestations of Chronic Ischemia

1. Intermittent Claudication

Description of symptom complex. The most common and most classic complaint of patients suffering from any type of chronic occlusive arterial disorder affecting the lower limbs is pain in exercising muscles (intermittent claudication; exercise pain). This symptom may take the form of a sensation of tightness or compression, a cramp, a feeling as though the leg is enclosed in a vise, an inability to make further volitional contractions of the active muscles, a sharp pain, or a dull ache. Not infrequently,

it is described as a sense of local tiredness or fatigue provoked by the physical effort. At times, the discomfort assumes the form of numbness occurring most commonly in the toes, either alone or in association with pain in the exercising muscles. Invariably intermittent claudication is noted after the patient has walked a certain distance at a specific pace (claudication distance, measured in short city blocks) and is not present while he is sitting, lying down, or standing. In fact, in most instances, relief is experienced soon after he stops and stands still, shifting the weight of his body to the uninvolved limb. Usually if the individual continues to walk after experiencing pain, the symptoms will build up in intensity until he is compelled to stop. Occasionally, however, the symptoms level off, and the patient is able to ambulate for long distances with only a moderate amount of discomfort. The explanation may be that he slows his pace or adopts a shuffling gait.

Pathogenesis. Intermittent claudication has its origin in contracting muscles that are receiving an insufficient flow of oxygenated arterial blood to satisfy their markedly increased metabolic requirements (15 to 20 times greater than those of the resting state). As a consequence, there is a local production of stable abnormal substances, the exact chemical or physiochemical nature of which has not been identified.

135

The increase in concentration of such materials with each subsequent muscular contraction ultimately causes stimulation or irritation of sensory nerve endings in the tissue spaces in the active muscle mass, with the production of pain. Since the onset and severity of the symptoms are directly related to the magnitude and rate of development of an oxygen debt in the exercising muscles, it follows that if the patient walks at a fast pace or uphill or carries a heavy valise or groceries, the nonsymptomatic latent period will be reduced, with the result that he will develop pain sooner than when he is walking more slowly on a level surface, unencumbered by any packages.

On termination of the exercise, metabolic requirements rapidly return to a resting level, so that now the blood flow is again adequate for basic tissue needs. At this point there is no further buildup of pain-producing substances, while the amount which has accumulated during the physical effort either diffuses into the bloodstream or is destroyed locally. With a lowering of the concentration of these substances and then their disappearance, the symptoms begin to fade away. The duration of the period of recovery is related to the size of the oxygen debt incurred during the physical exertion and the efficiency of the systemic and local compensatory cardiovascular mechanisms to cope with it subsequently. Such information is of value, since it is related to the degree and severity of the existing impairment of local circulation.

However, at least two nonvascular factors affect the severity of intermittent claudication and its duration after termination of exercise. One of these is the patient's threshold for pain, this increasing or decreasing claudication distance depending upon his reaction to the symptoms. Another is the concurrent metabolic activity of the tissues of the extremity. The fact that neither type of response can be accurately considered or evaluated makes the distance a patient can walk only a crude reflection of the severity of the impairment in local arterial circulation.

Conditions or states in which intermittent claudication is found. Exercise pain may be present in a variety of different states and disorders and even at times in normal individuals. In the case of the latter group, the symptom may be experienced if the work load is so great that the resulting rise in metabolic requirements of the active tissues cannot be adequately met, even by maximally dilated normal arteries in the limbs and a highly efficient cardiovascular system.

Certain systemic conditions may be associated with exercise pain despite the presence of a normal arterial tree in the lower limbs. Such a situation exists in anemia of a severe degree, the basis for the symptom being a lack of adequate carriers of oxygen to the exercising muscles. In congenital heart disease in which there is unsaturation of the blood, the oxygen supply to the muscles may also be deficient during bouts of physical activity. Patients with severe congestive heart failure may complain of intermittent claudication because of a reduced cardiac output, local capillary changes, and perhaps altered tissue fluid content, all factors which interfere with the movement of adequate amounts of oxygen out of the capillary bloodstream into the tissue spaces. Individuals with a severe degree of hyperthyroidism may have comparable symptoms due to the heightened metabolic requirements of all their tissues, including voluntary muscle, this situation being exaggerated during periods of physical activity. Myxedema has also been cited as a cause of intermittent claudication, with relief following thyroid therapy.

The most common etiologic agent for the production of exercise pain is, of course, a chronic occlusive arterial disorder, such as arteriosclerosis obliterans or, much less frequently, thromboangiitis obliterans, in which there is partial or complete obstruction of blood flow either in the large proximal arteries supplying the local arterial system, in the vascular channels in the muscles, or in both groups. Intermittent claudication may also exist in patients in whom critical arteries have been ligated following trauma; an embolus has occluded a vessel; and an acquired or congenital arteriovenous fistula is present which is diverting blood from the active muscles.

In the rare case of popliteal artery entrapment syndrome, intermittent claudication may be experienced in the calf. The cause of this condition may be one of several anomalous positions for the popliteal artery. In one, the vessel runs medially to the medial head of a normal gastrocnemius muscle instead of between the two heads of this structure. In another, it is in its normal location, but the gastrocnemius or the plantaris muscle has an aberrant origin or an accessory head; or the medial head of the gastrocnemius has a lower and more lateral insertion than normal, separating the artery from the vein or both vessels from the nerve.

Regardless of the type of anatomic variation, in every instance the trapped artery suffers injury as the patient walks, either because it is squeezed by the contraction of the gastrocnemius muscle or because it is compressed between the muscle and the bone. As a result, insufficient blood supply reaches the exercising muscles and intermittent claudication is produced. If the condition remains untreated, the repeated trauma to the artery may produce degeneration of its wall, followed either by aneurysmal dilatation or plaque formation and possibly thrombosis [8]. Occlusion of the artery occurs gradually, allowing for the development of a rich collateral circulation around the knee. Such a compensatory change is responsible for the important diagnostic finding of a significant increase in local skin temperature ("hot knee") [2,5]. Palpation of the knee generally reveals the presence of large collateral arteries, especially on the posterior and lateral aspects of the joint. Pulsations in the arteries of the foot and oscillometric readings on the leg are either significantly reduced or absent. Arteriography will confirm the presence of a partial or complete block in the popliteal artery and an aberrant location of the vessel if it is still patent. Before thrombosis occurs, simply flexing the knee acutely by gastrocnemius action may produce paresthesias in the toes, while forced plantar hyperextension or dorsiflexion of the foot will result in loss of distal pulses [16].

2. Symptoms That Mimic Intermittent Claudication

Orthopedic involvement of foot and ankle. Pain in the foot, due either to severe *pes planus, callosities, verrucae,* or *arthritis* of the ankle joint, may superficially resemble intermittent claudication of the intrinsic muscles of the foot. However, the important distinguishing point is that such

a symptom is related to weight bearing and not necessarily to walking. Another difference is the fact that the pain persists for some time after the exercise is terminated, in contrast with the rapid subsidence of the symptom of intermittent claudication under such circumstances. Furthermore, it usually does not stop the patient after a set distance, nor is it as severe as typical intermittent claudication. Finally, the circulation in the foot is always normal in the above conditions.

Another orthopedic condition of the foot which may produce symptoms that mimic intermittent claudication is *inflammation* of the *conjoined tendon* as it arises from the tuberosity of the os calcis, a condition frequently associated with bony spur formation. A prominent complaint in this disorder is localized tenderness in the heel which appears when the patient stands and continues for a while after he lies down. At the same time, no abnormalities of local circulation are noted.

Metatarsalgia (Morton's toe) must also be considered in the differential diagnosis of intermittent claudication limited to the small muscles of the foot. In this disorder, walking with shoes on produces a sudden, sharp, crippling, burning sensation in the toes, usually originating between the third and fourth metatarsophalangeal joints; at times the pain radiates up the calf as far as the knee. Of diagnostic importance are the findings of a crepitant mass between the third and fourth toes, near the ball of the foot, and the production of typical pain when this tumor is pinched between metatarsal heads. Relief occurs when the shoe is removed and the foot is massaged. Also of value in recognizing the condition is the temporary alleviation of pain following injection of 0.5 ml of 1% procaine through the web space into the neuroma. Local arterial circulation is normal in metatarsalgia.

Trauma to a group of muscles may result in the formation of a hematoma, which if untreated may lead to the development of *myositis ossificans*. In the case of involvement of the lower limbs, walking will produce pain in the affected muscles, which disappears soon after the patient stops and stands still or more rapidly when he sits down. Differentiation from intermittent claudication is based on the history of trauma to the limb and the rapid appearance of a mass, followed by bone formation in the injured muscles (usually the quadriceps, less frequently the hamstrings), as determined by radiography. No local signs of arterial insufficiency are noted in myositis ossificans.

The symptoms associated with *tennis leg* have on occasion also been mistaken for intermittent claudication. However, the condition develops acutely shortly after some type of injury to calf muscles, such as partial tearing of the medial gastrocnemius muscle belly at or near the musculotendinous junction. Initially there is severe pain in the posteromedial part of the calf, midway between the knee and the ankle, on taking a step. Shortly after the injury, a defect can be felt in the medial muscle belly of the gastrocnemius. After a few days, ecchymosis is observed over the medial portion of the calf, extending distally along the Achilles tendon to the ankle, associated with slight edema. No signs of local arterial insufficiency are noted.

Intermittent limping may be mistaken for intermittent claudication affecting the calf [13]. The term refers to a sequence of events in which the patient finds that after walking several blocks, he must come to a complete halt because of a cramplike pain or sense of exhaustion in one or both legs.

Among orthopedic conditions which may cause intermittent limping is a shortened Achilles tendon or triceps surae muscles, producing an inability to dorsiflex the foot, and an imbalance of the metatarsal heads. Intermittent limping may be acquired, as in women by the use of high heels, or it may be congenital. Another mechanism which may be responsible for it is disuse of the foot because of fear of eliciting pain in an arthritic ankle joint on movement. Under such circumstances, extreme contraction of the gastrocnemius and its tendon will result, producing symptoms on walking. The same type of response may exist if a painful plantar wart is present, causing the patient to assume a protective habitus over a long period of time. There should be no difficulty differentiating any of the above conditions from arteriosclerosis obliterans, since they do not present findings of involvement of the arterial circulation in the lower limbs. At the same time, there are positive signs, as well as therapeutic results with various nonvascular measures, to suggest that other etiologic factors exist.

It is necessary to point out that in the elderly individual, orthopedic disorders may be associated with arteriosclerosis obliterans. Under such circumstances, a history can be elicited of pain in the lower limb or lower back on standing and a definite increase in severity of symptoms on walking. At the same time, there will be physical findings suggesting the presence of both types of conditions.

Involvement of nerve roots.

Irritation of large nerve trunks innervating the structures in a lower limb, as in the case of *herniated lumbar disk*, may cause symptoms which mimic intermittent claudication located in the buttock. Of diagnostic importance is the fact that the orthopedic complaint becomes worse on change of posture, as from the horizontal to the upright position, but not particularly on walking. Furthermore, although originating in the buttock, this pain radiates down the lower extremity along the course of the sciatic nerve. Associated findings are signs of pressure and irritation of nervous elements, such as reduced vibratory sense perception and decreased sensation to cotton wool and pin prick (most obvious in the toes); absent or diminished ankle and knee jerks; weakness in extension of the great toe; spasm of the muscles of the back; atrophy of the leg and thigh muscles; tilting of the pelvis; and positive Lasègue's and crossed Lasègue's signs. On the other hand, findings of impairment of arterial circulation are absent. For these reasons, no difficulty should be encountered differentiating the pain due to compression of large nerve trunks from intermittent claudication limited to the muscles of the buttock, thigh, or leg.

Joint abnormalities.

The pain associated with *arthritic disorders* may at times be mistaken for intermittent claudication. However, it is articular or periarticular in location rather than limited to the site of the exercising muscles. It may be experienced at rest, especially during inclement weather, or it may follow immediately after motion of the joints is initiated. In the case of osteoarthritis, the symptom may disappear with sustained activity. Signs of sympathetic hypertonus, such as coldness, cyanosis, and hyperhidrosis, may be present in certain cases of rheumatoid arthritis (see C-5, Chapter 13), but these can be readily distinguished from the findings of obliterative vascular disease through the use of tests for removal of vasomotor tonus (see D-4, Chapter 6). The fact that in arthritic conditions the main peripheral arteries are intact and demonstrate normal pulsations is of prime importance in the differential diagnosis. At times, tomograms and bone scans may be necessary to verify the presence of an arthritic joint.

Neurogenic intermittent claudication. This state, which is also called intermittent ischemia of the cauda equina and pseudoclaudication syndrome, results from some type of abnormality of the lumbar spine, generally a herniated nucleus pulposus [1,17] or a vertebral spine bony alteration [7]. As a cause for the symptoms, it has been suggested that ischemic neuropathy develops during exercise due to compression of nerve roots in the cauda equina by either protrusion of the involved lumbar disk [1], pressure induced by marked hypertrophic ridging in the intervertebral canal [3], or congenital narrowing (stenosis) of this structure [18,19]. Another explanation is that there is a relative neural ischemia during physical exercise [7].

In the case of neurogenic intermittent claudication, the pain in the lower limb is initiated by walking and relieved by rest, in which regard it resembles true intermittent claudication. However, the distance the patient covers before experiencing it may become smaller and smaller with subsequent attempts. Moreover, the pain is neuritic in type, being described as a sensation of numbness, tingling, weakness, or incoordination, and it may not be localized to a muscle mass, as consistently occurs in true intermittent claudication. Also of significant diagnostic importance is the finding that in neurogenic intermittent claudication, identical symptoms to those experienced on walking may likewise develop in the hip or thigh on straightening the back while in bed or on prolonged standing [9]. Furthermore, if the symptoms are initiated by walking, relief is generally obtained only on sitting down or lying down,

and not on standing, and this will not occur until 20 or 30 min have elapsed. Such responses are different from those observed with true intermittent claudication (see A-1, above).

In neurogenic intermittent claudication, signs of the usual type of herniated lumbar disk, such as a positive coughing or sneezing effect or a positive straight leg–raising maneuver, are not present. However, ankle jerks may be absent or reduced, or they may disappear temporarily during exercise. Also, elevated cerebrospinal fluid protein may be observed. Because of the lack of clear-cut findings of a herniated disk, at times it may be necessary to perform a myelogram in order to demonstrate a partial or complete block in the lumbar region. Most important as a differential point is the fact that in the presence of neurogenic intermittent claudication, the arterial circulation in the involved limb is normal.

Muscle enzyme deficiency disorders. In several muscle disorders due to a lack or reduction in enzymes, pain is experienced in exercising muscles. Among these are muscle phosphorylase deficiency (McArdle's syndrome) [12], muscle phosphofructokinase deficiency, and muscle glucosidase deficiency. Besides painful cramps produced by physical effort, definite weakness, easy fatigability, and stiffness are experienced in the active muscles. The diagnosis of McArdle's syndrome can be made by determining the absence of a rise in venous blood lactate levels after ischemic exercise of the arm [12]. Signs of local arterial insufficiency are not noted in the muscle enzyme deficiency disorders.

Avitaminosis. Difficulty in walking may be present in patients suffering from severe *vitamin B$_1$ deficiency*. At the beginning, weakness is experienced only when walking many blocks, but as the condition becomes more marked, even covering a distance as short as 100 feet may have a profound effect. Associated findings are burning of the soles of the feet, numbness of the dorsum of the feet, and, at times, foot drop. Signs of impairment of local arterial circulation are absent. The significant therapeutic response to hyperalimentation may help in making the diagnosis.

3. Ischemic Neuropathy

In a small number of patients suffering from a severe, long-standing chronic occlusive arterial disorder, ischemic neuropathy, a symptom complex present at rest, may begin to be experienced. It is generally so intense as to overshadow any other ischemic difficulties and it is an ominous indication of advanced or end-stage local arterial insufficiency.

Description of complaints. The symptoms of ischemic neuropathy are typical for stimulation or irritation of nervous elements. They consist of paresthesias, formication, prickling, tingling, or a sense of numbness or coldness in the toes. On occasion a severe lancinating sensation which travels down the limb may be felt. Usually the complaints are severe enough to interfere with sleep and proper rest.

Pathogenesis. The symptoms generally appear when the patient lies down in bed, in preparation for sleep. Their onset may occur because in such circumstances, the hydrostatic mechanism, which is present on standing or sitting and helps drive blood into the diseased and partially obliterated vessels of the lower limbs, no longer operates. At the same time, there is a drop in systemic blood pressure. Due to both these alterations, the peripheral nerves, already in a chronic state of anoxia from the existing impairment of local circulation, become even further anoxemic and therefore more irritated; as a result, neuritic symptoms develop. Sitting up and placing the lower limbs in dependency, attempting to sleep in a chair, or walking around the room will all produce almost immediate temporary cessation of complaints; these, unfortunately, return to their previous state of severity within 15 min after the reclining position is again assumed.

Conditions or states in which symptoms are found. Ischemic neuropathy may be part of the clinical picture of the far advanced case of arteriosclerosis obliterans and much less often thromboangiitis obliterans. It may also be experienced by patients who are suffering from a severe degree of arterial insufficiency due to other pathologic states, such as ligation of a main artery following trauma, sudden thrombosis of a vessel, or arterial embolism. In the case of chronic occlusive arterial disorders, the neuritic symptoms generally appear after intermittent claudication has been present for many years.

4. Symptoms That Mimic Ischemic Neuropathy

Orthopedic disorders. The rest pain of ischemic neuropathy must be differentiated from complaints present in several orthopedic conditions. Among these are myositis, fibrositis, and disorders of the bone, including Paget's disease, gout, osteoid osteoma, periostitis, decalcification following hyperparathyroidism, chronic osteomyelitis, multiple myeloma, and other tumors in bone. X-ray studies and blood chemistry examination should prove of value in the differential diagnosis of most of these disorders. Another important diagnostic point is that signs of impairment of arterial circulation are absent. In contrast, rest pain in an occlusive arterial disease indicates the existence of a marked state of anoxia, and in all instances it is associated with obvious signs of a severe degree of involvement of the circulation.

Pressure on or injury to peripheral nerves. Among possible etiologic agents which may produce pressure on nerve trunks proximal to the extremity are arthritis of the spine, bursitis, neoplasms within the spinal cord, tumors of the cauda equina, and herniated nucleus pulposus in the lumbar region. All of these conditions elicit neuritic pains in the limbs at rest and hence must be differentiated from ischemic neuropathy. Again, the abnormalities exist in the presence of a normal local arterial circulation. (For a differentiation of ischemic neuropathy from peripheral neuropathy which may mimic it, see B-5, Chapter 9.)

Restless leg syndrome. This symptom complex is a generally common occurrence in young women, although it is also found in other individuals. It consists of unpleasant, distressing paresthesias and formication in the calves and lower portion of the legs and occasionally in the thighs. There may also be a sensation of coldness in the feet, muscular weakness, and fatigue. The complaints are experienced when the person is lying in bed and less often when sitting. Because of their intensity, they may interfere with proper rest. In order to obtain relief, the patient generally makes voluntary twitching movements with the lower limbs, gets out of bed and walks around, or waves the legs several times while sitting on the edge of the bed.

Despite the severity of the clinical picture, frequently there are no objective signs of a vascular, neurologic, or orthopedic dysfunction being present, with the result that a functional basis must be entertained. In support of such a possibility is the finding that many patients suffering from the restless leg syndrome also manifest nervous fatigue, emotional tension, and agitated depression. However, it is necessary to point out that the condition has also been found in persons in whom microemboli consisting of cholesterol crystals have occluded portions of the microcirculation in the lower limbs. Among other organic conditions associated with the restless leg syndrome are diabetes, iron-deficiency anemia, prostatism, vitamin deficiency, acute poliomyelitis, peptic ulcer, malignancy, and acute porphyria.

5. Pain of Gangrene or of Ischemic Ulceration

Description of symptoms. Impending or existing nutritional changes in the limbs almost invariably produce severe pain in the site of involvement. The symptom is frequently continuous, although at times it may be lancinating and intermittent. It is present at rest but may become worse on walking. This is due to stretching of the involved structures and to shunting of blood from the affected site into dilated muscle vessels, thus exaggerating the existing ischemia of nerve endings.

Generally the pain also becomes more marked when the patient lies down in bed in preparation for sleep. Under these circumstances there is a reduction in blood pressure (and hence in head of pressure in the affected arteries in the limb) and a loss of the beneficial effects of hydrostatic pressure moving blood into the foot in the standing or sitting position.

As a consequence, arterial inflow is further impaired and the degree of ischemia of nerve elements in the vicinity of the lesion is increased. Moreover, when the patient is in bed, the number of impulses from his body and of stimuli from his environment bombarding his sensorium are significantly reduced, permitting him to concentrate his attention fully on the pain originating in the lesion which, as a result, becomes exaggerated in his mind.

The severity of the pain associated with an ischemic ulcer or gangrene may vary depending upon the underlying pathology. Generally such a lesion located on a toe of a patient with thromboangiitis obliterans produces much greater and more intense pain than does one of the same extent in an individual suffering from arteriosclerosis obliterans. If the atherosclerosis is associated with peripheral neuropathy due to diabetes mellitus, pain may be even less or possibly absent. In fact, under such circumstances, if the ulcer or gangrene is located on the plantar surface of the foot, the patient may not even be aware of its existence until his attention is called to it by the appearance of secretion or blood on his sock. On the other hand, on occasion the whole clinical picture is exaggerated by the peripheral neuropathy if functional sensory pathways still exist.

Another factor which influences the severity of the complaints is the patient's response and tolerance to pain. Some individuals appear to experience only minor symptoms from trophic lesions, whereas in others, they become excruciating.

As a general rule, the greater the extent and depth of the gangrenous or ulcerative area, the more marked is the pain. However, in some patients, a superficial lesion may be associated with more severe symptoms than one which penetrates into deeper tissues. An explanation for such a response is presented in the section on pathogenesis, below.

If an ischemic ulcer or gangrene is present in the involved lower extremity of a hemiplegic patient, the amount of pain associated with such a lesion may be increased. Evidently the trophic disturbance acts as a trigger mechanism to initiate a severe degree of thalamic pain, a not uncommon phenomenon in a paralyzed limb. There may be an accompanying involuntary flexion of the leg at the knee (probably due to a spinal reflex), which further exaggerates the severity of the symptom.

Because the marked reduction in cutaneous circulation responsible for the presence of a serious nutritional disturbance is almost invariably associated with a similar change in muscle circulation, the patient suffering from an ulcer or gangrene generally also complains of long-standing intermittent claudication in the legs or feet.

Pathogenesis. The ischemic lesion usually produces severe pain locally, in part because the surrounding inflammatory reaction causes irritation or partial destruction of small sensory fibers located in the transitional zone between viable and necrotic structures. Also of importance is the underlying marked anoxia of tissues, including nervous elements. The more extensive the involvement, the larger is the transitional zone; hence the greater are the number of peripheral nerve endings affected by the ischemia and the more marked are the symptoms. The explanation for the severe pain occasionally associated with a superficial ulcer may be that in such circumstances the numerous cutaneous nerve endings are irritated and still capable of conducting pain impulses, whereas in the case of a lesion which also involves underlying structures, these structures are no longer viable.

6. Pain of Chronic Vasospasm or of Vasodilatation

Description of symptoms. Severe, excruciating, burning pain in the distal parts of limbs may be present in conditions in which persistent abnormalities of vasomotor tone are the etiologic agent. The most marked symptoms exist when increased sympathetic tone is present. The complaints are associated with other signs of this state, such as coldness, cyanosis, hyperhidrosis, increased reactivity of the vascular tree to cold, and at times edema (see A-3, Chapter 8).

Reduced sympathetic tone may also result in a severe degree of burning, but this is associated with a feeling of warmth. Under such circumstances, the limb is red, hot, and at times

tender, and signs of augmented local blood flow are prominent.

Pathogenesis. The symptoms associated with a chronic state of vasospasm stem from ischemia of cutaneous nerves as a result of a reduced local blood supply produced by the increased vasomotor tone. Support for this view is the finding that on removal of sympathetic control, as by peripheral nerve block or paravertebral sympathetic block, frequently the complaints are minimized or even abolished. However, it is necessary to point out that pain may also be present when no obvious signs of local anoxia exist. A possible explanation for such a situation is that sympathetic afferent, as well as efferent, fibers are present in the peripheral mixed nerves and that these are responsible for the spread of impulses from the involved site to the spinal cord and brain. It would appear, therefore, that the relief of pain in vasospastic states produced clinically by sympathetic denervation may be due to the blocking of afferent impulses from the involved structures, as well as to elimination of vasospasm.

The mechanism responsible for abnormal vasodilatation is not known, although the possibility has been offered that such a response is the result of some disturbance in the vasomotor center in the medulla, this hypothesis being based on the fact that the alterations in the limbs are usually bilateral. The commonly present burning sensation is probably the result of vascular tension produced by the increased blood flow; this, in turn, causes pressure on and irritation of neighboring nerve endings. There is also a possibility that greater peripheral serotonin activity exists [4].

Conditions or states in which symptoms are found. Pain associated with vasospasm is part of the clinical picture of such vasospastic conditions as major causalgia, posttraumatic vasomotor disorders, trench foot, frostbite, post–trench foot syndrome, and postfrostbite syndrome.

Vasodilatation, due to a decrease in vasomotor tone, is found as the chief manifestation of primary erythromelalgia. Such a response may also be noted in the initial stage of trench foot, immersion foot, and posttraumatic vasomotor disorders.

B. Clinical Manifestations of Acute Ischemia

1. General Characteristics

Following sudden cessation of blood flow through a critical artery in a limb, there is a variable period of time at the beginning during which little or no local circulation is present in the arterial tree primarily supplied by the involved vessel. As a consequence, the distal tissues suffer from a state of acute anoxia. Regardless of whether the causative agent is functional (vasospastic) or organic (permanently occlusive), the early clinical picture is approximately the same. Such a situation persists during the period in which the abnormal mechanism operates without the appearance of compensatory vascular mechanisms. (For the conditions which influence the degree and intensity of the acute ischemia and hence the severity of the symptoms, see C-1, below.)

Clinical disorders manifesting acute anoxia. Among these are functional or vasospastic diseases, such as spasm of a critical artery due to trauma or a similar change in a digital artery precipitated by exposure to cold or emotional excitation, as in Raynaud's disease or Raynaud's syndrome. Organic disorders capable of producing a comparable clinical picture are arterial embolism, rapid spontaneous arterial thrombosis, traumatic arterial thrombosis, and laceration and severance of main arteries.

2. Acute Anoxia on a Vasospastic Basis

Involvement of main channels. Transient spasm of a critical artery produces marked ischemia of the distal tissues supplied by the vessel, in many instances the response being of a completely reversible nature. The findings observed in acute vascular spasm (traumatic vasospasm) are typical for the clinical picture present in this state. The arteriospasm may be either neurogenic or myogenic in type. (For the pathogenesis of the two types of acute vascular spasm, see C-2, Chapter 15.)

Involvement of small channels. Typical of the clinical picture of sudden spasm of small noncritical arteries are the findings noted in Raynaud's disease or Raynaud's syndrome. The resulting changes are due to temporary, episodic, and completely reversible total obliteration of the lumen of digital and interosseous arteries on exposure of the body or limbs to cold or following emotional excitation [15]. Since other portions of the local vascular tree are not affected by the stimuli, the abnormal alterations are limited to the digits, particularly the fingers and, much less frequently, the toes. As in the case of functional occlusion of large, critical arteries (see above), the symptoms and physical findings result from the state of severe ischemia of the distal portions of the digits, due to cessation of local arterial inflow.

Generally, during the period in which spasm of the digital and interosseous arteries exists, the patient experiences a sense of coldness, numbness, or tightness in the involved digits. At times, the complaints may be associated with actual diminution of sensory acuity due to local anoxia of nerve endings. In some instances there may be unpleasant sensations in the fingers which are difficult to describe.

With reestablishment of the circulation (on release of the spasm of the digital arteries), the patient becomes aware of burning, paresthesias, tingling, or throbbing in the tips of the fingers. Such symptoms are probably related to the return of function in the peripheral nerves previously made temporarily nonfunctioning by the acute state of ischemia.

The local alterations observed during an episode of digital artery spasm are characteristic, consisting of color changes limited to the digits, which are first present in the tips and later in the proximal portions. Initially, the involved finger or fingers become cadaveric white due to cessation of arterial blood flow and emptying of the cutaneous capillaries and subpapillary venous plexuses of blood. At the same time, the state of local anoxia may produce active spasm of the cutaneous microcirculation which further accentuates the existing waxy pallor.

Cyanosis may replace the pallor in the affected digits or it may be the initial and sole sign. This type of color change has been attributed to a number of different mechanisms, none of which has been unequivocally accepted. One of these involves the possibility that the spasm of the digital artery is intermittently released during the attack, permitting blood to enter the capillary bed and the subpapillary venous plexuses at a slow rate. The resulting stasis in the cutaneous microcirculation affords the opportunity for more effective removal of oxygen from each unit of blood passing through the skin; as a consequence of the accumulation of a greater than normal concentration of reduced hemoglobin in the capillary and venous blood, cyanosis develops. Another theory proposes that during an attack, blood is trapped in the subpapillary venous plexuses, the removal of oxygen from it resulting in the cyanotic hue to the skin. Spasm of digital veins, preventing local venous outflow from the finger, has also been considered as an etiologic agent in the production of the color. In fact, it has been postulated that in the patient in whom cyanosis is the only change, without the previous appearance of pallor, the alteration could result solely from venospasm, without the contribution of digital artery spasm. Another possibility is opening up of arteriovenous shunts with secondary ischemia of cutaneous capillary beds [14].

On removal of the agent responsible for the attack (exposure to cold or emotional excitation), pallor or cyanosis disappears slowly, to be replaced either by rubor followed by a normal color, or only by the latter change. The exaggerated redness of the skin reflects a state of reactive hyperemia, resulting from a marked dilatation of the local arterioles, capillaries, and venules and a more rapid movement of highly oxygenated blood through the cutaneous and subcutaneous microcirculation. In this period there is a repayment of the oxygen debt incurred during the preceding episode of digital arterial spasm.

No unanimity exists regarding the mechanism responsible for the spasm of the digital arteries. It is highly questionable that the sympathetic nerves innervating these vessels are implicated, since color changes can be elicited even after sympathetic denervation. A better possibility is that there is an inherent fault in the arteries themselves which causes them to be excessively reactive to various types of noxious stimuli. It has also been proposed that norepinephrine in abnormal amounts is produced locally at the alpha-receptor endings in the blood vessel wall and that this substance, in turn, causes intense spasm of the digital arteries [15].

3. Acute Anoxia on an Organic Basis

Pathogenesis. Initially, the complaints associated with sudden, complete, and permanent interference with blood flow through a critical artery in the limbs are due primarily to the resulting marked ischemia of nervous structures, just as in the case of spasm of main arteries (see above).

Clinical manifestations. The symptoms are particularly marked in the most distal portions of the limb, the fingers and toes. They consist of paresthesias, a sense of numbness or burning, and/or pain which is generally severe (acute ischemic neuropathy). The underlying mechanism is irritation of the sensory fibers in the peripheral mixed nerves by the existing anoxia. A "dead" feeling may also be experienced in the entire hand or foot. The complaints are present at rest, particularly when the patient lies down in bed, whereas standing or sitting may produce some reduction in their severity. This is so because hydrostatic pressure in the lower limbs operating under the latter conditions causes an increase in blood flow in patent collateral arteries, thus helping to nourish the involved nervous structures. On the other hand, walking exaggerates the symptoms, due to shunting of the small quantity of available blood from the skin and subcutaneous tissues, including the peripheral mixed nerves, into the now dilated arterioles in the exercising muscles of the foot and leg.

Associated with the acute ischemic neuropathy present in the distal tissues, there may be pain at the level of the arterial occlusion. Although generally of short duration, this symptom probably results from spasm of the affected vessel and from the production of a periarterial inflammatory reaction locally initiated by the pathologic change occurring within the artery.

In contrast with acute spasm of an artery in the limb, total obstruction of the vessel by an organic occlusive process is not reversible. Hence the associated changes are much more severe and may be followed by nutritional disturbances, such as ulceration or gangrene, if the available collateral circulation is not efficient enough to provide adequate circulation to distal tissues (see Section C, below).

In general, there is a good correlation between the severity of the complaints and the extent and degree of the abnormal physical findings. This is in contrast with vasospasm in which the symptoms are not as great as would be anticipated on the basis of the intensity and depth of pallor of the skin in the affected limb.

C. Anatomic Responses of the Arterial Tree to Ischemia on an Organic Basis

1. General Factors Influencing Efficiency of Collateral Circulation

After sudden or slow organic occlusion of a critical artery in the limb, maintenance of viability of distal structures will initially depend solely on the ability of the remaining patent vessels to take over the function of supplying the tissues with adequate circulation. The effectiveness of this vascular bed is dependent on a number of different factors: the previous role of the affected vessel; the rate at which the occlusion occurred; the anatomic state of the remaining arteries; the efficiency with which the vascular readjustments take place; the degree of existing spasm produced by the vascular episode; the number and size of branches above and below the site of occlusion; the pressure gradient present proximal and distal to the obstruction; and the amount of time which has elapsed since the occlusion [20].

2. Anatomic Vascular Responses to Acute Anoxia

Available mechanisms. If a critical artery is suddenly occluded by an embolus or a rapidly developing thrombus or if its continuity is destroyed by trauma, there is relatively no time for an adequate new collateral circulation to develop. As a result, the only means of supplying the limb with blood is through preexisting pathways, i.e., main distributing branches of both large and medium-sized arteries that arise from the involved vessel proximal to the site of pathologic change and those that reenter the main vessel distal to it [11].

Character of occlusion. The site of involvement of the obstruction plays a significant role since its location may affect the number and size of the available branches arising proximally. Also of importance is the length of the occlusion. If this is short, the arterial blood is returned to the main artery distal to the occlusion by a variable course in alternate channels, but with little loss of blood pressure and volume flow in overcoming internal resistance. On the other hand, if the length of obliteration is considerable, the arterial blood may never enter the main artery again, such a situation resulting in a great loss of blood pressure and of volume flow because of the high peripheral resistance encountered by the blood as it reaches the tissues via small arterial and arteriolar vascular beds [6]. In general, proximal propagation of secondary thrombosis stops at the origin of the first large collateral branch, whereas distal spread may be extensive, even to the point of occluding the mouths of all the reentry vessels [11].

Influence of superimposed spasm. Sudden obstruction of a critical artery by an embolus or by acute trauma to a vessel is frequently associated with reflex spasm arising from stimulation of the sensory fibers in the arterial wall, a response which tends to reduce even further the blood flow into the distal part of a limb. Although this type of vascular change usually disappears within a few hours, still it may be sufficient during the early critical period to contribute significantly to loss of viability of tissues. In addition, if the spasm persists, it may be followed by secondary thrombosis of the vessel. In the case of trauma to an artery, frequently inflammatory changes occur in the arterial wall to produce a mild panarteritis, but the alterations are generally not severe enough in themselves to cause occlusion of the channel.

Hemodynamic changes initiated by obliteration of a critical artery. The efficiency of the secondary circulation depends on several mechanical factors. First is the transformation of the high end pressure in the obstructed artery into a lateral pressure in the branches arising proximal to the obstruction. Circulation through these vessels is further facilitated by the pressure gradient that exists across the collateral vessels and the distant capillary beds. However, other mechanisms interfere with blood flow through the collateral arteries, such as the smaller diameter of the branches, as compared to that of the obstructed artery from which they arise. Moreover, the blood must traverse a much longer and more circuitous pathway than previously in order to nourish distant tissues. Also, more vessels are involved in accomplishing this purpose, thus increasing the total area of vessel wall in contact with the blood. All these factors contribute to increased peripheral resistance to the flow of blood in a distal direction.

Despite the various obstacles to the mainte-nance of adequate peripheral circulation after sudden cessation of flow through a critical artery, in some instances vascular readjustments rapidly take place, permitting the development of some blood supply to distant tissues. However, in general the sequence of events leads to necrosis of the limb unless circulation through the main vessel is rapidly reestablished, as by embolectomy in the case of arterial embolism or by reconstructive surgery following loss of continuity of the artery through trauma.

Hemodynamic changes initiated by obliteration of a noncritical artery. If the vessel involved is not the sole means of supplying the distal tissues with blood, the compensatory mechanisms are usually adequate to prevent necrosis of tissues. However, the patient may subsequently suffer from intermittent claudication due to insufficient blood supply to the muscles of the lower extremities during periods of physical activity involving them. With passage of time, this complaint may become less severe

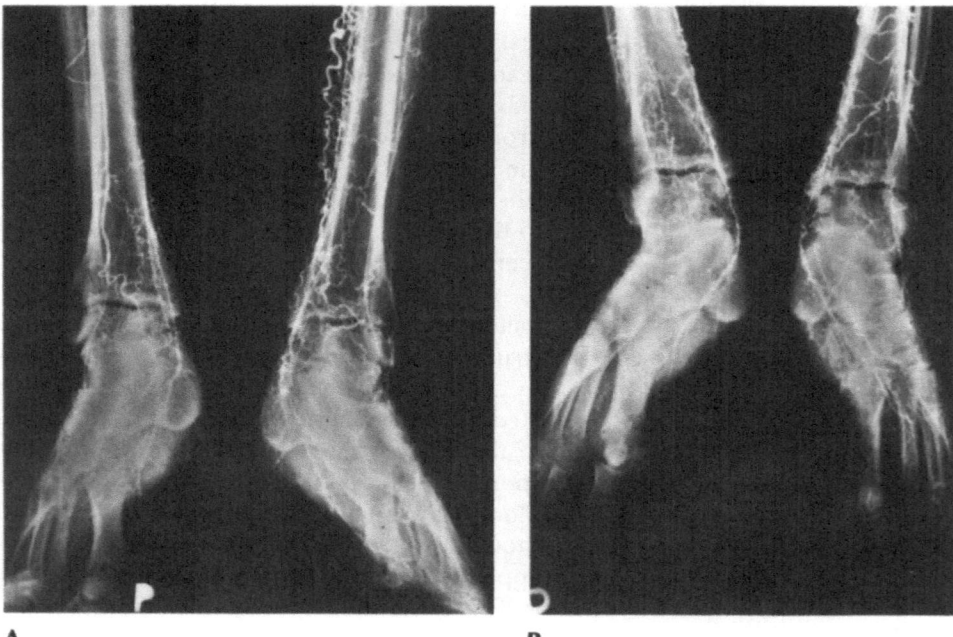

A   B

Fig. 10.1. Development of an extensive collateral arterial circulation to the lower portions of the legs and feet in patients with arteriosclerosis obliterans in whom occlusion of the local main arterial channels occurred very slowly (**A** and **B**). Adequate circulation is brought to the feet by this secondary vascular tree.

or even disappear as a result of the ingrowth of a new collateral system in the muscles.

3. Anatomic Vascular Responses to Chronic Anoxia

Situations in which a slowly forming collateral circulation develops. When there is a slow progression of an obliterative process in a main artery, as frequently occurs in chronic occlusive arterial disorders (arteriosclerosis obliterans; thromboangiitis obliterans), very often the concomitantly developing secondary local circulation (Figs. 5.1 and 10.1) will be adequate to take care of the metabolic needs of the tissues under resting conditions, with possibly intermittent claudication being experienced on physical exertion. A similar type of situation exists in the presence of an acquired arteriovenous fistula (see Section F, Chapter 15), in which most of the blood reaching a limb is shunted through the abnormal communication into the main venous circulation.

Basis for growth of collateral circulation. Several views have been proposed with regard to the stimulus responsible for the development of collateral vessels. One postulates that the most potent factor is a state of chronic anoxia in tissues deprived partly of blood supply. Another explanation is the production of a local chemical stimulant. In a third view, the mechanistic theory, it is assumed that the growth of collaterals, with a resulting increase in local blood flow, is dependent on gradients in blood pressure in the arterial tree set up by occlusion of the main vessel. According to this concept, a fall in pressure occurs in the capillary beds distally, with the result that blood is attracted to these areas from arteriolar beds of branches arising from the involved main artery above the level of the obstruction. In response to the greater blood flow, the branches dilate, thus contributing to the formation of a secondary circulation. Other factors playing a role in the development of collateral vessels are the age of the patient, the condition of his heart, the systemic blood pressure, and the viscosity of the blood.

Derivation of secondary network. Collateral arteries arise from several sources. One is the existing secondary branches in the area of involvement which are already functioning and which, as a result of the added stimulus, now dilate and anastomose with each other (main collateral branches). Another set consists of multiple muscular branches that anastomose with one another, to serve as the midzone arteries in the collateral circulation (accessory collateral branches) [10]. This arterial system probably undergoes proliferation following occlusion of the major artery, although the possibility also exists that it was always present but not functioning. Most of the midzone collateral vessels arise in muscles possessing extensive vascular attachments to extrinsic arterial channels. Those with limited vascular communications, obtaining their blood supply from single or a small group of arteries, are a poor source of midzone collateral vessels.

There are several other sources from which a collateral system can be derived. Supplemental branches, which originate from either main or accessory collateral channels, develop and run parallel to the obliterated artery. Twigs from the main collateral branches may form bridging pathways around the site of occlusion (Fig. 5.6). Obstruction of the terminal portion of an artery may be followed by the development of small collaterals which arise proximally to the involved site and pass distally in an approximately parallel course to the obstructed artery. Finally, a main artery may enlarge so that its branches will now supply an area previously provided for by the subdivisions of the obliterated vessel.

Characteristics of collateral vessels. This system of arteries differs from normal vessels in several respects. The channels are irregular in their course, they have a "corkscrewlike" appearance, and they vary significantly in size, most having small lumens (Fig. 10.1). They cross and recross (without purpose) and anastomose quite freely with one another. Such anatomic architecture is conducive to the development of a significant resistance to flow, thus supporting the impression that the collateral arterial bed is a poorly efficient means of supplying the distal tissues with blood. Nevertheless, it is frequently the only available mechanism to accomplish this need and often is very successful in achieving such a goal.

References

1. Blau JN, Logue V: Intermittent claudication of the cauda equina: An unusual syndrome resulting from central protrusion of a lumbar intervertebral disc. Lancet 1:1081, 1961
2. Bouhoutsos I, Goulios A: Popliteal artery entrapment: Report of a case. J Cardiovasc Surg 18:481, 1977
3. Brish A, Lerner MA, Braham J: Intermittent claudication from compression of cauda equina by a narrowed spinal canal. J Neurosurg 21:207, 1964
4. Catchpole BN: Erythromelalgia. Lancet 1:909, 1964
5. Chavatzas D, Barabas A, Martin P: Popliteal artery entrapment. Lancet 2:181, 1973
6. Conley JE, Kennedy WF: Collateral arterial circulation in the legs. AMA Arch Surg 81:348, 1960
7. Evans JG: Neurogenic intermittent claudication. Br Med J 2:985, 1964
8. Insua JA, Young JR, Humphries AW: Popliteal artery entrapment syndrome. Arch Surg 101:771, 1970
9. Kavanaugh GJ, Svien HJ, Holman CB, et al: "Pseudoclaudication" syndrome produced by compression of the cauda equina. JAMA 206:2477, 1968
10. Krahl E, Pratt GH, Rousselot LM, et al: The collateral circulation in the arterial occlusive disease of the lower extremity. Surg Gynecol Obstet 98:324, 1954
11. Levin PM, Rich NM, Hutton JE Jr: Collateral circulation in arterial injuries. Arch Surg 102:392, 1971
12. McArdle B: Myopathy due to a defect in muscular glycogen breakdown. Clin Sci 10:13, 1951
13. Mufson I: Intermittent limping–intermittent claudication: Their differential diagnosis. Ann Intern Med 14:2240, 1941
14. Nielubowicz J, Zajac S, Szamowska R, et al: The origin of Raynaud's phenomenon. J Cardiovasc Surg 19:607, 1978
15. Peacock JH: Peripheral venous blood concentration of epinephrine and norepinephrine in primary Raynaud's disease. Circ Res 7:821, 1959
16. Servello M: Clinical syndrome of anomalous position of the popliteal artery: Differentiation from juvenile arteriopathy. Circulation 26:885, 1962
17. Silver RA, Schuele HL, Stack JK, et al: Intermittent claudication of neurospinal origin. Arch Surg 98:523, 1969
18. Verbiest H: A radicular syndrome from developmental narrowing of the lumbar vertebral canal. J Bone Joint Surg 36B:230, 1954
19. Verbiest H: Further experiences on the pathological influence of a developmental narrowness of the bony lumbar vertebral canal. J Bone Joint Surg 37B:576, 1955
20. Winblad JN, Reemtsma K, Vernhet JL, et al: Etiologic mechanisms in the development of collateral circulation. Surgery 45:105, 1959

Chapter 11

Spontaneous Organic Occlusive Arterial Diseases

Part 1 Arteriosclerosis Obliterans and Aortoiliac Arterial Occlusive Disease

---

This chapter deals with spontaneously developing chronic occlusive arterial disorders, primarily atherosclerosis of the arteries of the lower limbs (arteriosclerosis obliterans) and of the abdominal aorta and its main branches (aortoiliac arterial occlusive disease; Leriche's syndrome). The discussion of thromboangiitis obliterans, which once was prevalent in the United States and is now rarely observed by the orthopedic or general surgeon, will be limited to its differentiation from arteriosclerosis obliterans. Further information regarding this interesting clinical entity can be obtained from other sources [2]. Only the fundamentals of medical and surgical treatment will be considered since a more detailed presentation would be inappropriate considering the scope of the volume. The main purpose of this chapter, therefore, is to make readily available background information upon which can be formulated a safe therapeutic program for an orthopedic problem affecting the lower limbs of elderly persons, particularly in the light of the high incidence of local arterial insufficiency that exists in such individuals.

A. General Considerations

1. Incidence

Arteriosclerosis obliterans is by far the most important of the chronic occlusive arterial diseases. It is predominantly present in patients between the ages of 50 and 70 years; however, it may also be seen in the third and fourth decades of life. When the atherosclerotic change is located in the aortic bifurcation or both common iliac arteries, the disease process is found one decade earlier than would be expected if the same type of lesion were present elsewhere, i.e., in the vessels of the lower extremities.

With regard to atherosclerosis of the arteries of the lower limbs, there is no evidence to indicate that any one group of individuals is affected to a much greater extent than others. Nor is there any striking sex predisposition, although the condition appears somewhat more frequently in males than in females. In the case of Leriche's syndrome, the incidence of the disorder is much greater among men than among women (ratio of 10:1); rarely is the American black so afflicted.

Arteriosclerosis is a generalized multifaceted process which affects the brain and heart much more often than the extremities. However, at times the changes may be limited to the lower limbs alone, and therefore the absence of the pathologic process elsewhere should not eliminate this entity from the differential diagnosis of an obliterative vascular disorder of the lower extremities.

2. Etiologic Factors

A number of views have been advanced regarding the cause of atherosclerosis but none has received general acceptance. It is the belief of some workers that the pathologic changes are associated with, or caused by, an error in metabolism of fat and other lipids. Abnormal vascularization of the arterial wall has also been implicated as an etiologic factor. The possibility has been offered that the production of arteriosclerosis is the result of prolonged stress or strain to which the arteries are subjected during the life of the individual and hence that it is part of the natural aging process. Other factors which have been proposed but not fully evaluated are the hereditary quality or family predisposition, the habitus or constitution, sex and the role of sex hormones, smoking, low levels of high-density lipoprotein–bound cholesterol, endothelial injury, and alterations of endothelial permeability related to the presence of hypertension or to the breakdown of platelets.

There is little question that endothelial cells are significantly involved in the production of atherosclerosis. For example, they are known to bind and metabolize lipoproteins. They also appear to be the site of localization of lipoprotein lipase, an enzyme that may be very important in the binding of lipoproteins to the vessel wall and in the transport of cholesterol and triglycerides into this site [36]. Moreover, increased endothelial permeability, probably due to injury, may result in the unrestricted influx of macromolecules, such as low-density lipoprotein, into the subendothelium and media. The subsequent complex interactions among platelets, platelet constituents, and low-density lipoprotein may be responsible for the development of the plaque, followed by intimal thickening.

3. Pathology

The typical pathologic changes in arteriosclerosis obliterans are degenerative in nature. Associated alterations are a marked increase of connective tissue components (collagen, elastic fibers, proteoglycans) and large deposits of both intracellular and extracellular lipids [29,34,43,47]. Three different types of lesions may develop: the fatty streak, the fibrous atherosclerotic plaque (see below), and the complicated lesion [42].

Atheroma formation. The most common and most significant alteration is the atheromatous plaque located in the subintimal tissue. It is found chiefly in large and medium-sized arteries and may extend into vessels of smaller caliber, particularly in patients also suffering from both diabetes and hypertension.

The atheroma has the appearance of a raised yellowish mass extending beyond the endothelial surface into the lumen of the vessel. Histologically the lesion is initially composed of proliferating endothelial cells, fibroblasts, foam cells, and large quantities of lipid material. Later, calcium deposition may occur. The distortion of the intima which follows the process favors thrombus formation. When the latter occurs, the clot goes through the various stages of organization, eventually producing complete occlusion of the lumen. More rapid arterial thrombosis may follow sudden hemorrhage, a predisposition which exists in atherosclerosis. Recanalization of the proliferating mass may subsequently take place. (For a discussion of arterial thrombosis, see Section B, Chapter 12.)

Associated with the alterations in the intima are changes in the media and adventitia. Those in the media consist of atrophy and necrosis of muscle fibers, followed by thinning of the coat and replacement by collagenous fibers and then by calcium deposits. In only a small percentage of cases do the latter produce the ring-like arrangement of Mönckeberg's sclerosis. The adventitial alterations include fibrosis, an increased vascularity, and frequently a mononuclear infiltrate which is predominantly lymphocytic.

In the case of Leriche's syndrome, the histologic alterations consist of atheromatous intimal proliferation, medial sclerosis, and periarterial fibrosis, with various degrees of chronic inflammation. The latter type of change causes the vessel to become adherent to the prevertebral fascia and the neighboring veins (including the inferior vena cava) and lymph nodes, as well as the sympathetic chain. One anatomic difference from the abnormalities noted in arteriosclerosis obliterans is that the occlusive process is segmental, with little or no sclerotic changes present on either side of the involved portion of artery. In most instances the pathologic change originates in the common iliac arteries and progressively involves the aortic bifurcation and terminal aorta. Much less often it is first found in the aorta, below the point of origin of the inferior mesenteric artery, and then it spreads downward into the iliac arteries.

B. Clinical Manifestations

It is difficult to place individuals with arteriosclerosis obliterans or aortoiliac arterial occlusive disease into categories on the basis of severity of symptoms or of extent of the occlusive process. This is probably because only rarely does a patient in an early stage of the disease seek medical advice for complaints referable to the limbs. The reason is that the initial rate of occlusion of the main arteries is generally so slow that, as a reduction in the size of the lumen occurs, this is balanced by a corresponding increase in growth, ramification, and efficiency of new collateral channels (see C-3, Chapter 10).

1. Symptoms

Arteriosclerosis obliterans. If the pathologic process is accelerated while the collateral circulation fails to keep pace, then the patient will begin to experience pain in the lower extremities on walking (intermittent claudication) (see A-1, Chapter 10). Infrequently, as a late symptom, there may be rest pain (particularly in bed), characterized by hyperesthesia, burning, coldness, tingling, or lancinating sensations in the toes; such complaints are typical of ischemic neuropathy (see A-3, Chapter 10). If the occlusive disorder progresses further, symptoms due to nutritional disturbances may appear. These are in the form of severe continuous pain

locally, caused by actual destruction of tissues (see A-5, Chapter 10).

Aortoiliac arterial occlusive disease. Because the obliterative process in this disorder is so insidious, the clinical picture develops and progresses very slowly, even though complete obstruction of the aortic bifurcation ultimately results. This is due to the fact that there is always growth of an abundant collateral circulation which bridges the occluded segment; of importance, also, is the fact that the distal vascular tree generally remains open and available for transporting nutrition to the tissues of the feet. However, the compensatory secondary blood supply is rarely adequate to take care of the markedly increased metabolic needs of exercising muscles, and hence a prominent symptom of the condition is intermittent claudication (see A-1, Chapter 10), usually experienced in both buttocks. Not infrequently, the initial pain on walking is located in the calves, then in the thigh muscles, and finally in the buttocks if the patient continues to exercise. At times, intermittent claudication may be present only in the calves, with no extension to proximal muscle groups. In the younger age group, a very significant early abnormality is an inability to maintain erection of the penis, probably due to failure of adequate blood flow to the corpus cavernosum, supplied by the internal pudendal artery. When this symptom first appears in patients who are in the fifth and sixth decades of life, it is not as diagnostic of aortoiliac occlusive arterial disease, since it may also be due to physiologic changes related to the aging process. Because of associated ischemia of the sacral cord, there may be paresthesias present, in the form of sacral formication and perineal pain.

2. Signs

Arteriosclerosis obliterans. The physical findings are generally clear-cut in the patient with this disorder who has obvious symptoms referable to the local circulatory system. Reduced or absent pulsations are present in the main arteries of one or both lower extremities, associated with low or absent oscillometric readings at various levels (see Sections A and B, Chapter 5). Signs of impaired cutaneous blood flow are particularly marked in the feet (see Chapter 6). These consist of a positive plantar pallor test, a delay in the venous filling time and in the return of color in the feet, and the appearance of intense cyanosis when the limbs are maintained in dependency; the involved foot or feet may be dry and cooler than normal. Attacks of Raynaud's phenomenon may appear in the digits on exposure to cold. With progression of the pathologic process, eventually the impairment of local circulation may become so great that the metabolic needs of the tissues are not satisfied even at rest, and under such circumstances slight trauma to the skin may be sufficient to initiate an ulcerative lesion or gangrene.

Aortoiliac arterial occlusive disease. In this condition, physical examination generally reveals typical findings. Arterial pulsations are absent in the femoral, popliteal, dorsal pedal, and posterior tibial arteries bilaterally, and there may be a loud systolic bruit heard over the aorta above the level of the umbilicus and over one or both common iliac arteries. It may also be present over the spinous processes of the lumbar vertebrae. If occlusion of the aortic bifurcation or of the iliac arteries is incomplete, murmurs may be heard over the femoral arteries in the groin, and reduced pulsations may be felt in this region. Oscillometry generally demonstrates zero readings at various levels on the thighs and legs. However, if the occlusive process has been very slow, allowing for the formation of large collateral arteries, low readings may be obtainable from the thighs.

3. Impending or Existing Nutritional Disturbances

Before actual destruction of tissue becomes apparent in arteriosclerosis obliterans, there may be some difficulty in identifying the basis for ischemic symptoms experienced in the foot. Of help is the fact that usually some type of color change, either cyanosis or pallor, is noted in the site from which pain impulses arise. A definite reduction in cutaneous temperature is generally also present, as compared with the surrounding tissue.

When an ischemic ulcer or gangrene (Fig.

11.1) develops in a patient with arteriosclerosis obliterans, invariably this is associated with definite signs of a marked reduction in local circulation. The changes consist of absence of pulsations in the feet, reduced or absent oscillometric readings at distal levels of the involved limb, and signs of impairment of blood flow to the skin (abnormal nail growth, sparse or absent hair growth, loss of subcutaneous tissue, abnormal color changes, and low cutaneous temperature).

In most patients with Leriche's syndrome, the nutritional circulation in the feet usually appears adequate, with normal hair and nail growth, cutaneous temperature, and skin color. If the development of the collateral circulation has not kept pace with the rate of occlusion of the vessel, then ischemic changes may be present. These include a lowered skin temperature, dependent rubor, pallor of the plantar surface of the feet on prolonged elevation, and signs of reduced blood flow to nails, hair, and sweat and sebaceous glands. Only rarely are such nutritional disturbances as spontaneous ulceration or gangrene of the feet noted. There may be some signs of muscle wasting.

4. Contribution of Diabetes Mellitus

The coexistence of diabetes with arteriosclerosis obliterans significantly alters the clinical picture of the latter and its prognosis.

Rate of progression of disorder. A most important result of the presence of diabetes is that there is an acceleration of the occlusive process in the vascular tree of the lower limbs, so that signs of arteriosclerosis obliterans may be found even in very young diabetics [8]; in contrast, the onset of uncomplicated atherosclerosis usually occurs in the fifth and sixth decades of life. Moreover, the incidence of ulceration of the feet (Fig. 11.2) with superimposed infection is markedly increased in patients who are suffering from both conditions, as compared with those with atherosclerosis alone. In fact, of all the complications of diabetes requiring hospitalization, ischemic lesions of the lower limbs are the most common.

Location and types of pathologic changes. Diabetes likewise contributes to a lower level of

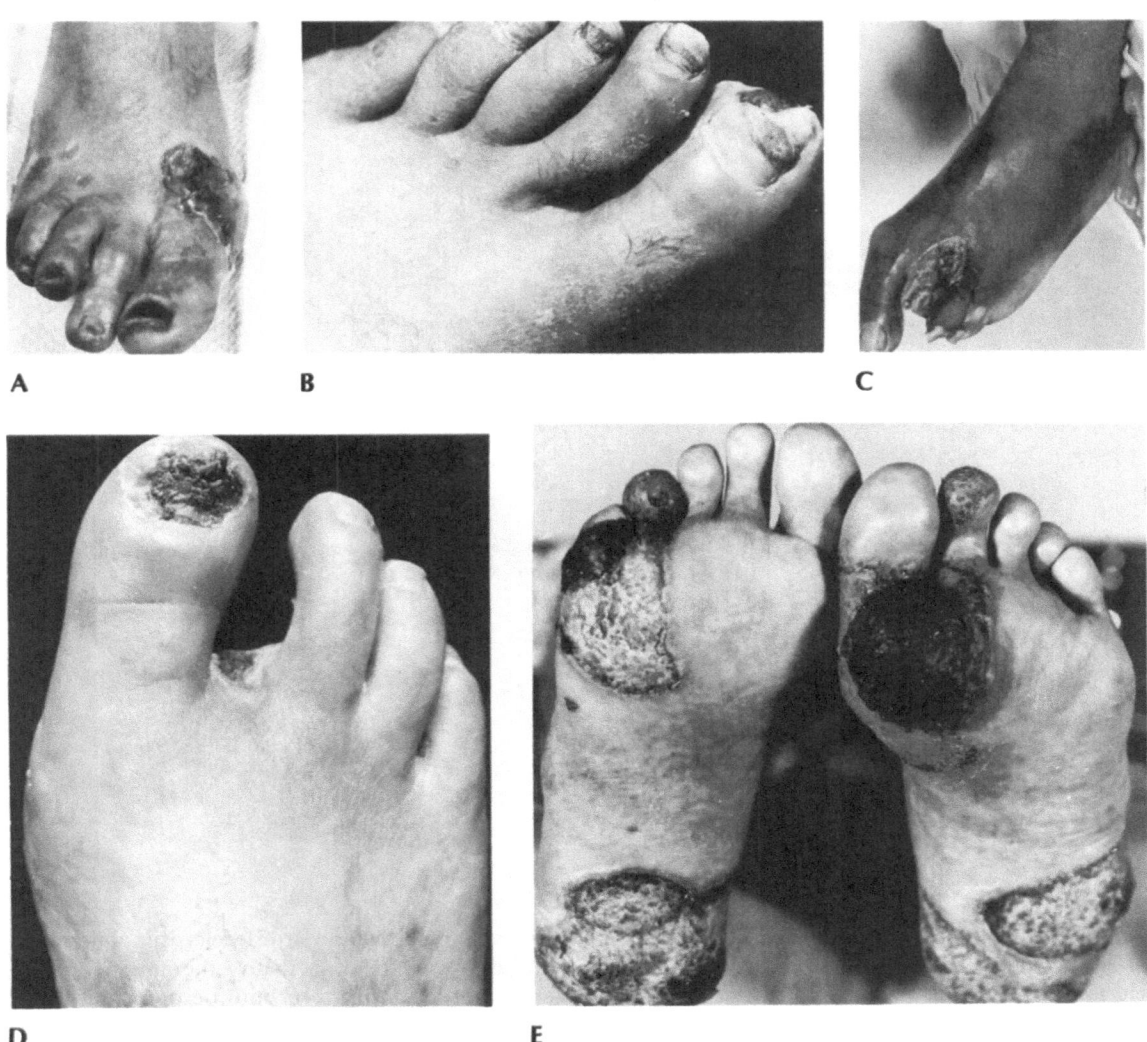

Fig. 11.1. Nutritional changes of varying degrees of severity in patients with a markedly compromised arterial circulation to the feet due to arteriosclerosis obliterans. **A** Necrotic plaque at the base of the great toe, showing signs of demarcation from surrounding viable tissue. **B** Necrosis limited to tip of great toe and involving the terminal phalanx. **C** Gangrene affecting the second and third toes and extending onto the foot proper. **D** Gangrene of nail-bed of great toe. Site of previously amputated second toe shows signs of nonhealing. **E** Extensive gangrene of toes, plantar surface, and heels of both feet, with superimposed infection.

occlusion in the vascular tree. Whereas in arteriosclerosis obliterans alone atherosclerotic plaques may be found in the abdominal aorta, the iliac arteries, the common femoral arteries and their main branches, and the terminal vessels, when arteriosclerosis obliterans occurs in the young diabetic, involvement is rarely noted proximal to the popliteal arteries [42]. Associated with changes in the latter vessels and their main branches are extensive obstructions in the

terminal arterial bed and also in the microcirculation in the form of thickening of the basement membrane (microangiopathy) [25,39,46]. Whether microangiopathy is specific for diabetes, as proposed by some workers [25], or whether the capillary basement membrane thickening is a nonspecific reaction of the vessel to some form of injury operating through a multifactorial process, as suggested by others [46], has still to be elucidated, although the

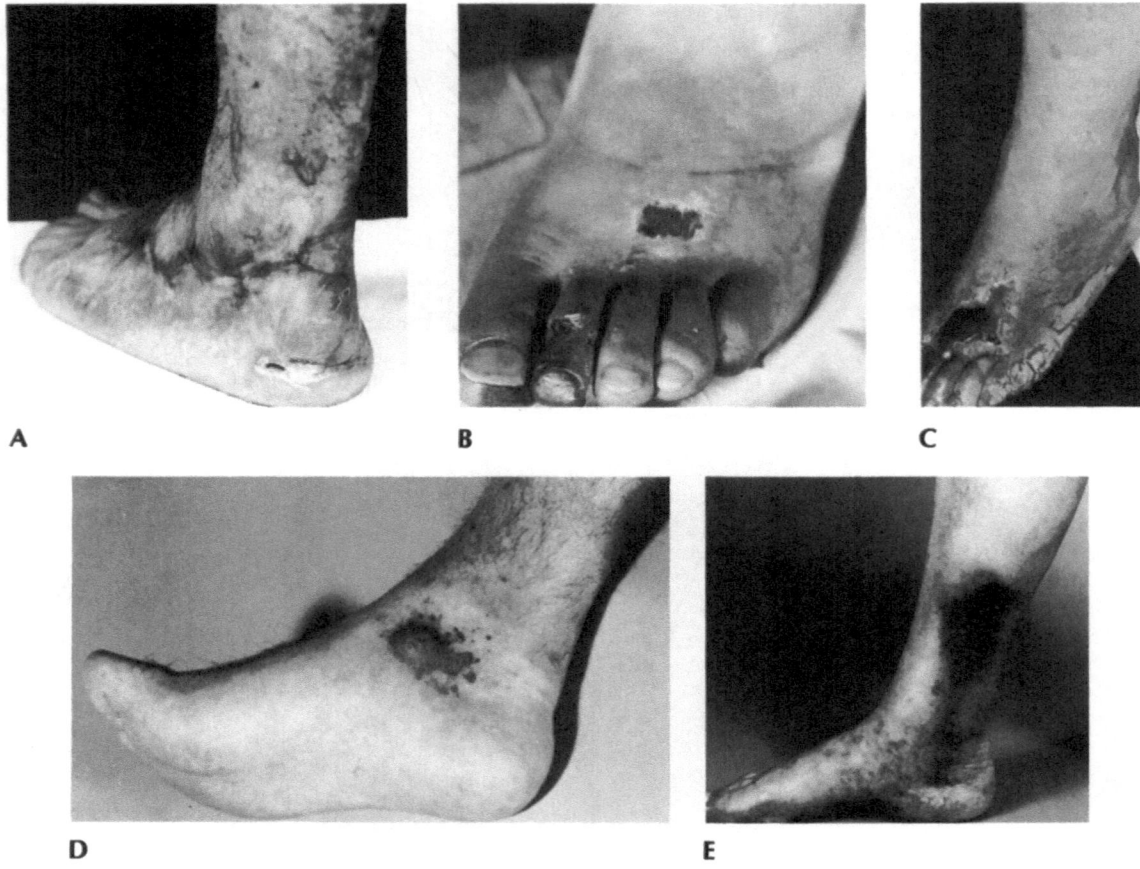

Fig. 11.2. Nutritional changes in patients with both diabetes mellitus and arteriosclerosis obliterans. **A** Healing infection and ulceration, with lesion on heel unresponsive to conservative therapy. **B** Localized lesions on second toe and on dorsum of foot. **C** Extension of lesion from second toe onto foot proper. **D** and **E** Nonhealing ulcerations over the internal malleolus and surrounding tissues.

available evidence appears to support the latter view. What is important is that only rarely is there any morphologic evidence indicating that capillary basement membrane thickening is associated with a reduction of capillary lumen diameter [46]. If this can be substantiated, then it can be assumed that so-called small-vessel disease of diabetes does not interfere with blood flow and hence is not responsible for the existing state of ischemia present in this disorder. Of course, a possibility to be considered is that the pathologic change in the capillary bed influences tissue nutrition by interfering with diffusion through the wall of the vessel [14]. It has been suggested that basement membrane thickening is due to the deposition of fibrin within the wall of the capillary [21].

Hematologic changes. Abnormalities of the blood may, in part, be responsible for the circulatory insufficiency found in diabetes. Although whole-blood viscosity (packed cell volume) in diabetics under stable well-controlled conditions has been found to be no different from that of normal subjects, during ketoacidosis the associated dehydration may lead to a greater increase in blood viscosity, a result which has been noted by several workers [10,30]. Although the subject of alterations in the physical properties of red blood cells in diabetes has only superficially been studied, there is some evidence that these structures may be abnormally rigid, thus failing to negotiate the capillary bed [14]. Increased platelet aggregation has been demonstrated in diabetics, particularly those with neuropathy [31], and also increased platelet adhesiveness [28], changes which favor thrombus formation.

Alterations in the response to infection. The patient with both diabetes and arteriosclerosis obliterans reacts poorly to infection, probably because there is an undermining of the natural defenses of the body and of the resistance of the tissues to noxious agents. The existence of diabetes appears to encourage cutaneous inflammation, perhaps through a number of mechanisms: dehydration, an altered immunologic capacity of blood and fixed tissue cells, and an abnormal state of cellular nutrition. There is also a delayed leukocytic migration to the site of injury [24], which may result in subnormal handling of infection at the cellular level. However, since the introduction of insulin and antibiotics, the difference in response to infection between the diabetic and the nondiabetic individual has been abolished to a great degree. There is now evidence that a well-controlled diabetic is no more susceptible to infection than the nondiabetic [27].

Influence of diabetes upon the clinical picture. The patient suffering from both diabetes and arteriosclerosis obliterans may experience the same vascular symptoms as the one with arterial insufficiency alone, mainly, intermittent claudication, ischemic neuropathy, and pain associated with trophic changes. However, the complaints experienced in exercising muscles are generally present in the feet and less often in the calf because of the more distal location of the atherosclerotic process; rarely are they noted in the thighs. Since peripheral neuropathy may frequently also exist (due to diabetes), at times it is difficult to differentiate this state from ischemic neuropathy due to impaired arterial circulation; in fact, in some patients both conditions may be present. Finally, the pain resulting from ulcers or gangrene may be much less than in the case of a similar-sized lesion in the individual with arteriosclerosis obliterans alone. This is probably due to the coexistence of peripheral neuropathy interfering with the transmission of afferent impulses over peripheral mixed nerves. At times, when the latter structures are entirely destroyed or made nonconductive by the pathologic process, pain may be absent.

Because of the greater tendency for secondary infection to develop in the site of an ischemic ulcer or gangrene, the lesion in the diabetic with arteriosclerosis obliterans generally becomes moist and soft ("wet gangrene"). In contrast, such a complication in arteriosclerosis obliterans alone rapidly loses fluid by absorption and becomes mummified ("dry gangrene"). In the diabetic with arteriosclerosis obliterans, there may also be a rapid spread of the inflammatory process to surrounding tissues, into regional lymph channels, and along the anatomic planes of the foot. (For discussion of the neurotrophic ulcer associated with diabetes, see p. 118; for discussion of neuropathic arthropathy, see p. 128.)

C. Differential Diagnosis

1. Thromboangiitis Obliterans (Buerger's Disease)

At times there may be considerable difficulty differentiating arteriosclerosis obliterans from thromboangiitis obliterans. However, in most instances, certain clear-cut differences exist between the two disorders. Among these is the fact that the onset of thromboangiitis obliterans occurs primarily in male patients between the ages of 16 and 40 years (average 29.3 years), whereas arteriosclerosis obliterans (without diabetes) has its inception in persons who are 45 to 70 years old (average 58.9 years) [3]. However, if diabetes coexists, then arteriosclerosis obliterans may appear at a much younger age (see B-4, above). Thromboangiitis obliterans is rarely present in women and blacks, a distinction not noted in the case of arteriosclerosis obliterans. Moreover, in about 40 percent of cases, there is a history or the presence of repeated episodes of superficial migratory thrombophlebitis generally involving the lower limbs, a finding never reported in arteriosclerosis obliterans [3]. A history of tobacco smoking is always obtained in thromboangiitis obliterans but not necessarily in arteriosclerosis obliterans. In about 20 percent of patients with thromboangiitis obliterans, ulcerations or gangrene may occur on the fingers, frequently requiring digital amputation (Fig. 11.3), a finding not seen in arteriosclerosis

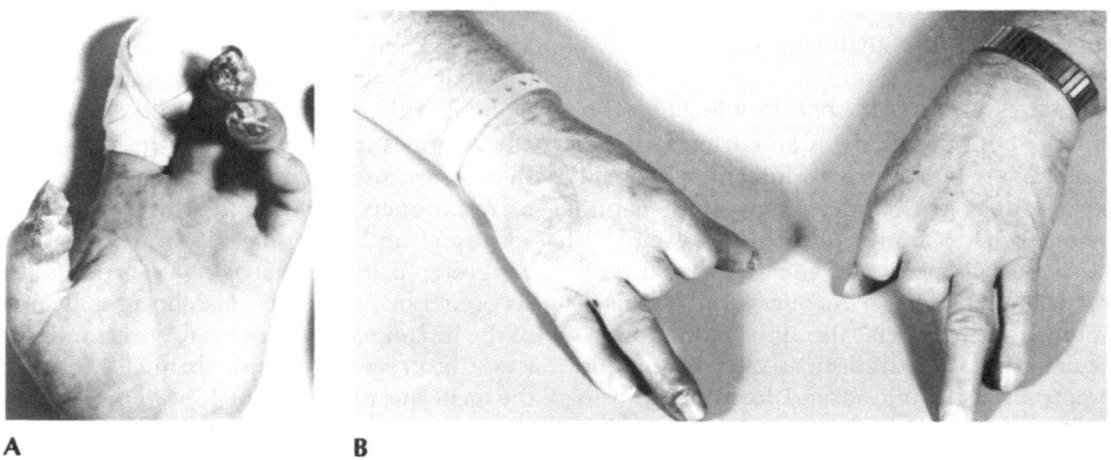

A   **B**

Fig. 11.3. Thromboangiitis obliterans. **A** Gangrene of fingers. **B** Amputation of fingers of both hands because of gangrene and nonhealing ulceration.

obliterans. Finally, of importance in differentiation are the angiographic changes of partial or complete occlusion noted in the brachial, radial, and ulnar arteries in thromboangiitis obliterans and the absence of such changes in arteriosclerosis obliterans. In the lower limbs, the blocks in thromboangiitis obliterans are found in the popliteal arteries and distally (Fig. 5.7), whereas in arteriosclerosis obliterans, they are located in the aortic bifurcation, the iliacs, and the common, superficial, and deep femoral arteries, as well as in the arteries of the leg and foot (see E-5, Chapter 5) (Fig. 5.6).

2. Mönckeberg's Sclerosis

Mönckeberg's sclerosis is a clinical entity in which there is deposition of calcium in the media of muscular arteries in the lower limbs of young and middle-aged persons, as determined by roentgenography (Fig. 11.4). Because there is no impingement upon the lumen of the involved vessels, no interference with arterial inflow results [22], and hence no symptoms or signs of impaired blood supply to the lower limbs are present. However, the possibility has been raised that the condition constitutes the earliest phase of plaque formation [32]. The diagnosis of Mönckeberg's sclerosis is frequently made following the use of soft-tissue x-ray technique for some other purpose.

The findings consist of straight lines of cal-cium about 1 cm apart, deposited along the internal elastic lamella, with a fine granular haze between them. There are gaps in the lines, producing a segmental appearance. The uniform deposition of the dense calcium forms a chain of rings similar to a goose neck [38], the process outlining the arteries and their main branches (Fig. 11.4). In the small vessels the deposition of calcium is more granular and the segmentation is more readily apparent. The changes resemble the dense calcification seen in the smaller arteries of diabetic patients with arteriosclerosis obliterans. However, they differ from those observed following deposition of calcium in sites of ulceration of atherosclerotic plaques in the intima. In the latter, the roentgenographic changes appear to run in the long axis of the blood vessel in the form of patchy calcification.

D. Treatment

1. Conservative Therapy

Because of the extensive collateral circulation that generally develops in the course of years in the majority of patients with arteriosclerosis obliterans and aortoiliac arterial occlusive disease, the first and frequently only approach to therapy consists of conservative measures. This applies particularly to persons suffering from

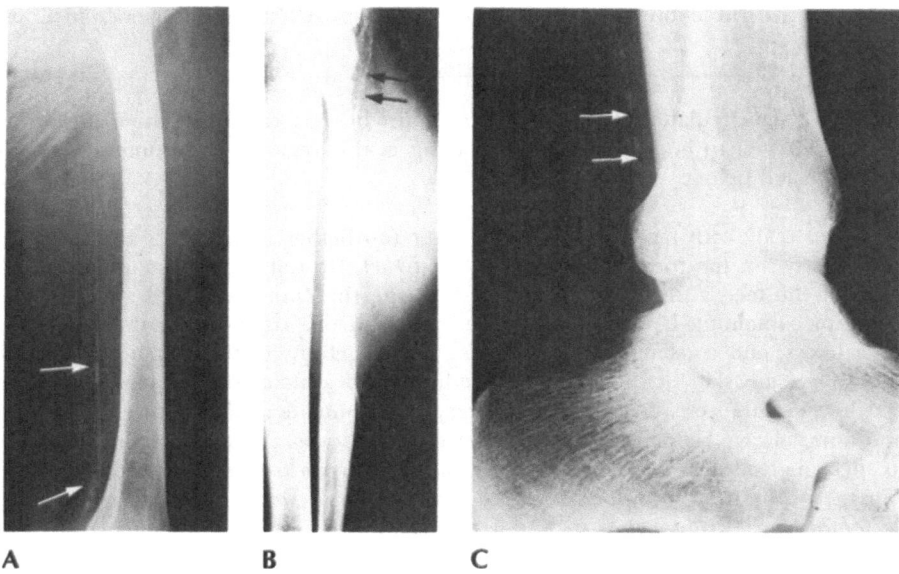

Fig. 11.4. Mönckeberg's sclerosis visualized with soft-tissue x-ray technique, noted in sites indicated by arrows. **A** Calcification of superficial femoral artery. **B** Calcification of upper segment of posterior tibial artery. **C** Calcification of posterior tibial artery above the ankle.

mild nondisabling intermittent claudication and demonstrating no signs of beginning nutritional disturbances in the feet. The same regimen is also applicable to individuals who are poor operative risks because of the coexistence of advanced cerebral, cardiac, or malignant disease.

General medical measures. There appears to be considerable difference of opinion regarding the value of reducing serum lipids by whatever means for the purpose of preventing or slowing the development of arteriosclerosis obliterans. The evidence is more convincing for the view that in patients with hyperlipoproteinemia, trials of hypolipemic therapy are indicated. At the same time, attempts should be made to reduce weight if obesity exists. Aside from the possible beneficial effect upon the metabolic processes of the body, such a step by itself may increase claudication distance.

General measures for local care of limbs. Detailed instruction in meticulous foot hygiene is essential in the prevention of ulceration and gangrene. Since the actual steps must be carried out by the patient himself, he should be supplied with a list of directions, as outlined in Table 11.1, and clearly made aware of his role in the problem. However, it is also the duty of the physician to explain in detail the reasons for the various steps presented in the table and the possible serious consequences of neglecting them (Fig. 11.5). A significant part of the first office visit should be devoted to this task. Of special importance is emphasis on the deleterious effects of concentrated heat or protracted exposure to low environmental temperatures and on efforts to prevent injury to the lower limbs, especially the feet. It should be stressed that even slight abrasions must receive special and careful attention.

When diabetes coexists with arteriosclerosis obliterans, local care of the feet is even more important than in the case of arterial insufficiency alone, because of the increased susceptibility of the patient with both conditions to infection. If peripheral neuropathy has also developed, the situation is even more precarious, since pain is not experienced after continuity of the skin has been destroyed by a noxious agent. As a result, the presence of a trophic lesion may initially not be recognized by the patient, especially when it is located in a site not readily accessible to his inspection, such as the plantar surface of the foot. For this

Table 11.1. General Home Care Directions for Patients Suffering from Arterial Insufficiency in Lower Limbs (with or without Diabetes).

Since you are suffering from poor circulation in your feet, you must be very careful of them. If you are also diabetic, it is necessary for you to be even more painstaking in this regard. At all times, you must follow exactly the directions listed below.

1. Carefully wash your feet daily with face soap in tepid water (no higher than 90° F) and dry them completely, especially between the toes, using a clean soft towel. Do not use hot soapy water and do not rub the skin of the feet. After washing, gently massage the entire foot and apply a small quantity of hand cream containing lanolin to replace the natural oils removed by the bath. This prevents dryness, scaliness, and cracking of the skin. Try not to get any of the cream between the toes since this will soften the skin of the web and predispose to athlete's foot. Small strands of lamb's wool placed between the toes daily may help prevent accumulation of moisture in the web.

2. When you are outdoors, always keep your feet warm. Use wool socks or wool-lined shoes in the winter and cotton socks or stockings in warm weather. Change your socks or stockings daily. Before retiring, cover your feet with loose-fitting bed socks or oversize, heavy wool socks.

3. When the outside temperature drops below 0° F, don't leave your house. If it is not as cold, dress very warmly, wearing heavy underwear, wool socks, fur-lined boots, and warm mittens. Never find yourself in a situation during the winter months when you have to wait longer than 15 min for public transportation or for help for your disabled automobile. Try to seek shelter in a warm, enclosed environment. In the summer, do not expose your lower limbs to the direct rays of the hot sun, since you are more susceptible to blister formation and second-degree burns than are people with normal circulation.

4. Always wear square-toed or round-toed shoes made of soft leather, with plenty of room (but not overlarge) and no pressure whatsoever on toes or bunions. Undue pressure can be determined if you stand while wearing your shoes and have a relative examine them in this position. If the shoes appear too tight, holes should be cut in the leather over the sites of pressure to relieve the compression. Don't break in new shoes all at once. On the first day, wear them for a half-hour and then a half-hour longer every day thereafter.

5. Before you put your shoes on, examine them. Look for such things as nailheads or nailpoints extending through the insole, a wrinkled lining, or a pebble under the insole.

6. Your toenails should be cut by a competent person after they have been softened by immersion of the feet in lukewarm soapy water. The trimming should be done in a very good light using clippers. The nails should be cut straight across; the corners should not be cut down. If your feet are taken care of by a podiatrist, be sure to tell him that you have reduced circulation to the lower limbs.

7. Never apply any type of concentrated heat to your lower limbs, such as hot water bottles, electric heating pad, immersion of feet in hot water, hot bath, short-wave diathermy, infrared lamp, ultraviolet light, or heat cradle.

8. Don't cut your corns or calluses. Never use corn plasters or other corn remedies on your feet. Instead, take pressure of shoes off corns, bunions, or calluses, using pads or larger shoes. Your podiatrist may be able to help you in this regard. However, he should only attempt minimal surgical treatment of corns or calluses, only steps which are absolutely essential to make you more comfortable. He should not perform operative procedures on your feet.

9. Besides corn remedies, never use strong antiseptic drugs or caustics on your feet, such as tincture of iodine, Lysol, or carbolic acid. Never apply any type of adhesive tape or adhesive paper directly to the skin of the feet. If a bandage is required, it is kept in place by means of adhesive tape applied to the cloth.

10. Don't wear circular garters or allow any type of elastic band to be placed around the leg, foot, or toes.

11. Avoid getting athlete's foot. Of help in this regard is never to go without shoes, not even at home or on the beach. This will also prevent you from stubbing your toes or stepping on tacks in the bedroom or bathroom at night or stepping on lighted cigarettes, broken glass, shells, or stones on the beach. Sustaining even a minor bruise on the sole of your feet may be very serious, since it may produce a nonhealing ulcer which will incapacitate you.

Table 11.1. General Home Care Directions for Patients Suffering from Arterial Insufficiency in Lower Limbs (with or without Diabetes). (*Continued*)

12. See your doctor as soon as you discover a blister, infection of the toes, athlete's foot, ingrowing toenails, or trouble with bunions, corns, or calluses. Don't self-treat the difficulty.
13. Examine your feet when you take your shoes off at night. Look for chafed spots, pressure points, blisters, cracks between the toes, and excessive dryness and scaliness of the skin of the legs and feet. If your eyesight is poor or if you have difficulty inspecting the sole of your feet, have some member of your family do this routinely.
14. Do not smoke cigarettes, cigars, or a pipe or use tobacco in any other form.

reason, it is essential to have both lower limbs carefully and routinely examined by a member of the family who is fully aware of the seriousness of even minor abrasions of the skin in a diabetic with impaired arterial circulation to the extremities. Besides this precaution, all the items listed in Table 11.1 should be discussed in detail.

Approach to control of fungal infections. Prophylactic measures should be followed in regard to dermatophytosis and, if already present, the condition should be treated aggressively but still cautiously. The reason for such precautions is that a fungal infection in the web between the toes may act as a portal of entry for bacteria, which is frequently followed by the formation of a penetrating ulcer that involves the foot proper and that may ultimately require an amputation of a portion of the limb.

An important step in the prevention of dermatophytosis is keeping the web between the toes dry, especially after a bath or shower; sprinkling a mild fungicidal powder in between the toes is helpful in this regard. The patient should be warned never to walk on the floor without shoes and stockings; when he uses a public shower he should wear wooden shower clogs, and after drying carefully between the toes he should also sprinkle a fungicidal powder into the web spaces.

If dermatophytosis exists, the approach depends on the severity of the infection. If it is of a mild degree, unassociated with any regional or systemic responses, only local therapy is necessary. First a 3% Vioform cream should be applied to facilitate removal of crusting. Then fungicides should be used to control the scaling. Among these are a combination of 20% zinc undecylenate, 2% undecylenic acid, and talcum (Desenex) and propionates and caprylate compound (Sopronol). The ointment form should be applied at night and powder in the

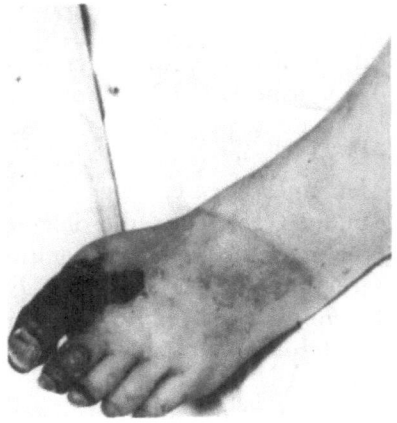 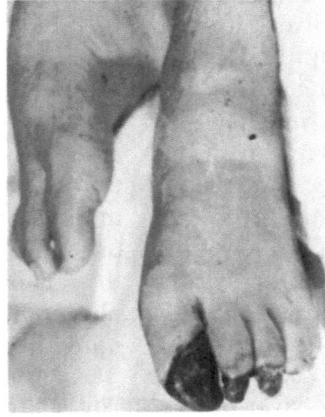

A B

Fig. 11.5. Thermal burns causing gangrene. **A** Result of application of a hot-water bottle to the foot of an 82-year-old woman suffering from arteriosclerosis obliterans. **B** Result of the application of a heating pad to a 15-year-old boy suffering from a neuromuscular dystrophy with a sensory deficit in the foot.

morning. In order to prevent reinfection, socks previously used should be boiled and new shoes should be worn. The daily application of the fungicidal powder should be continued indefinitely.

If the fungal infection has resulted in an acute inflammation associated with a lymphangitis, the patient should be placed at complete bed rest and the involved toes separated using halves of small corks. The feet should be immersed in pans of fungicidal soaks, including solutions of potassium permanganate (first 1:8000 and later 1:4000 concentration); silver nitrate, 0.125 to 0.25%; and boric acid, 3%. Initially the treatment is given twice daily for 30 min and later once a day before retiring. If fever and malaise are also present, penicillin is administered, although the physician must be alert to the possibility that a local sensitivity response or a generalized allergic reaction may follow. To control the fungal infection by systemic means, griseofulvin is administered orally in daily doses of 0.75 to 1.0 g for about 4 to 8 weeks, followed by a reduced amount for several weeks.

Treatment of local nonvascular lesions. Blisters produced by wearing improper shoes or by other types of compression should be treated very carefully (Fig. 11.6). If the lesion is intact and not enlarging or under tension, all local pressure should be removed from it and the area covered with dry sterile gauze. These steps are carried out in the hope that the fluid ultimately will be spontaneously absorbed and epithelialization will occur under the raised nonviable skin. As a consequence, no ulcer will develop in the involved site.

If the blister has already ruptured either spontaneously or following trauma, then it is best to remove the wrinkled overlying skin which may otherwise harbor bacteria and cover the denuded area with sterile gauze after cleansing it with a mild antiseptic (hydrogen peroxide, alcohol, Betadine solution). Or if the lesion appears to be enlarging and undermining surrounding skin or demonstrates increasing tension, then under aseptic conditions it should be punctured to relieve the pressure, and the superimposed nonviable layer of skin should also be debrided. The site is then cleansed with a mild antiseptic and covered

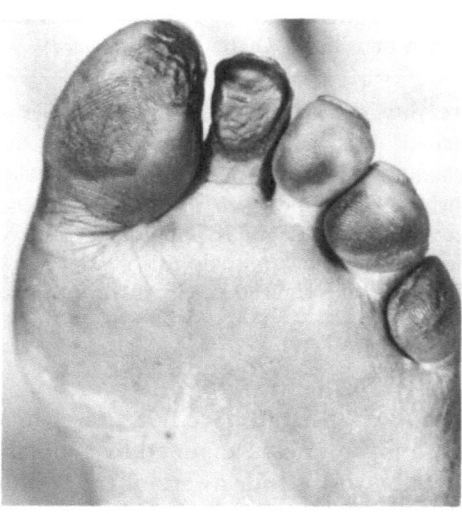

Fig. 11.6. Hemorrhagic blisters on the foot of a diabetic, a response frequently noted in this type of person. The lesions have been protected from pressure, in the hope that the fluid would be absorbed spontaneously.

with sterile gauze. Unfortunately, in both types of cases, in the presence of impaired local circulation, an ulcer will almost invariably develop. Such a possibility clearly emphasizes the need to exert great care in protecting the foot from even mild trauma.

Abstinence from smoking. As a general rule, if at all feasible, tobacco smoking should be stopped by the patient suffering from arteriosclerosis obliterans. In this manner, the vasoconstricting effect of the habit on the cutaneous blood supply, especially to the toes, is eliminated and local circulation is thus increased. Such a response is especially important when an ulcer or gangrene is present on the foot or elsewhere. Also, not infrequently claudication distance becomes greater after several months of abstinence. However, the deleterious effect of tobacco smoking on accelerating the rate of progression of the occlusive process observed in thromboangiitis obliterans is not noted in arteriosclerosis obliterans.

Physical activity. Patients should be encouraged to walk and exercise as much as possible, since such measures are excellent stimulants to the growth of a collateral circulation in the muscles of the lower limbs. If, instead, they assume a life of physical inactivity, this is generally followed by muscle atrophy due to disuse (see Section D, Chapter 23) and further impairment in walking. At the same time, such an attitude leads to mental deterioration and the adoption of the role of an incurable invalid.

As a rule, the patient should first walk to the point of experiencing pain in the exercising muscles; then, if at all feasible, he should continue walking for a short distance in order to build up an oxygen debt, even though such a step ordinarily causes a sharp rise in intensity of the symptom. At this point he stops the exercise and rests until all discomfort has disappeared, following which he repeats the same sequence. In many instances, after several weeks of such a program, the patient finds that he is able to cover the greater distance without any longer experiencing pain. By continuing the regimen of graded exercises, he frequently is able to obtain a significant increase in claudication distance. At no time, however, should he walk far enough to cause symptoms that are unbearable; if he does, resting may not produce rapid disappearance of the pain.

Certain physical accommodations can be made to intermittent claudication. If the patient finds that he is unable to perform daily activities without great inconvenience because of having to stop frequently, he should reduce his pace and thus be able to walk further, although taking a longer time to do so. Using a cane to reduce the weight of the body on the involved limb will also increase claudication distance. Walking stiff-legged, without bending the knees and contracting the calf muscles to any extent, will delay the onset of the pain provided it is located in the muscles of the leg. The use of lifts placed on the heel of the shoes may be of value, since this modifies the gait and causes the patient to use the thigh muscles instead of the gastrocnemius muscle to throw his foot forward. Finally, the use of external short-leg braces that restrict or eliminate ankle motion may increase walking ability.

Drug therapy. Over the course of years a number of medications have been utilized in the treatment of intermittent claudication, but it is questionable as to whether any of them produce a significant increase in walking ability. Among those which have received extensive clinical trial are the beta-receptor–stimulating agents, such as nylidrin hydrochloride (Arlidin) and isoxsuprine hydrochloride (Vasodilan) administered orally. Experiments have shown that both drugs dilate the arterioles in skeletal muscle. However, since the reported increases rarely are greater than doubling of the resting blood flow, it is apparent that a response of such magnitude would have very little effect on enhancing local circulation to the level necessary to satisfy the fifteen- or twentyfold rise in metabolic needs of muscles when exercised.

Conservative therapy for ulceration or gangrene. If, despite special efforts to maintain the continuity of the skin of the feet intact, an ulcer or localized gangrene develops, the conservative therapeutic program already described must be modified. First, physical activity must be curtailed since walking may stretch inflamed tissues, causing pain, and may facilitate movement of bacteria into the local lymphatics and veins. At the same time, the resulting dilatation of blood vessels in the exercising muscles of the feet and elsewhere will act to divert blood away from the skin in the vicinity of the lesion, thus retarding the local healing process and demarcation of normal from nonviable tissue. To achieve the desired goals, the patient is advised to sit in a chair with the lower extremities in dependency and to ambulate only when absolutely necessary, using crutches and no weight bearing on the involved limb. He should also carry out a series of exercises with the other three extremities and the body several times a day. In this manner, the systemic blood pressure and hence the head of pressure in the affected blood vessels will not fall. Prolonged periods of bed rest during the day should be discouraged so as to prevent the deleterious effects of deconditioning on the local vascular tree and on other portions of the body (see Section B, Chapter 23).

Of great importance in the maintenance of the patient's morale is control of the pain originating in the ischemic lesion, which not infrequently is excruciating (see A-5, Chapter 10). For this purpose, it may be necessary to resort to the use of narcotics, although such an approach should be avoided as much as possible.

At times a slow-drip intravenous injection of 500 to 1000 ml of 0.1 or 0.2% procaine or of 5% ethyl alcohol may control the symptoms. If the patient has a low threshold to pain, the problem is made much more difficult, with the result that the possibility of an amputation has to be considered at a time when such a step is not warranted on the basis of the extent and seriousness of the nutritional disturbance.

With regard to the treatment of the lesion itself, the first step is control of local infection, a problem which generally is not very great in the case of the patient with arteriosclerosis obliterans without diabetes. To utilize appropriate antibacterial agents for this purpose, a culture of the secretion is made from the ulcer or area of gangrene so as to carry out sensitivity studies. In order to obtain meaningful data, it is necessary to do the following: The site of involvement is debrided of superficial necrotic tissue, cleansed with a mild antiseptic, and covered with sterile gauze for 24 h. At the end of this period, care is taken in removing the dressing without affecting the accumulated secretion under the gauze. The latter is then utilized in the procedure of determining the appropriate antibacterial agent. Unfortunately, because of the poor blood supply in the vicinity of the lesion, it is generally difficult to achieve a high enough local concentration of the medication to be very effective against the infection. Nevertheless, such a possibility should not deter one from instituting oral or parenteral administration of the proper medication. Local application of an antibiotic in an ointment form is generally of little value especially if the base and sides of the ulcer are covered by necrotic tissue or coagulated secretion. At the same time, prolonged contact with an oily base may produce maceration of surrounding poorly viable tissue and thus encourage extension of the lesion. This objection does not hold if the antibiotic is applied by aerosol spray. If no improvement is noted in the control of the infection after a week's trial with the appropriate antibiotics, it may be necessary to perform another culture and sensitivity study on the basis that the bacterial flora may have changed in the interval.

With regard to other local therapy, the lesion should be cleansed daily with a mild antiseptic and, if a whirlpool bath, filled with an antiseptic solution, is available, the limb should be immersed in it for about 20 min. At home, a pan large enough to hold the foot comfortably is substituted. This is first filled with tap water and then boiled for 5 min. After the water becomes lukewarm, 4 ml (1 teaspoonful) of tincture of green soap or pHisoHex soap are added and the foot is immersed in the container for 20 min. With either procedure, after the soaking, the foot is removed and dried very thoroughly especially between the toes and a cream containing lanolin is applied to the skin except on the toes, in the webs between the toes, and in the vicinity of the lesion. The ulcer is cleansed with a mild antiseptic and, while the tissues are still soft from soaking, attempts are made to remove as much necrotic tissue as possible using a pair of small, fine clippers (tissue nippers) utilized by podiatrists for other purposes. When the debridement is performed properly, it should elicit little or no pain, and no bleeding should ensue. At all times, the step is limited to the removal of necrotic tissue or coagulated secretion; no viable structures are ever included in the procedure.

The described sequence should be repeated daily until a granulating base becomes visible and the sides of the ulcer are free of necrotic tissue. Until such a situation is achieved, signs of healing will not occur. Evidently the presence of devitalized tissue and of secretion from the wound encourages the growth of bacteria locally, thus preventing the formation of granulation tissue and subsequent epithelialization. If difficulty is encountered in removing eschars because of firm adherence to the base and sides of the ulcer, it may be necessary to utilize local application of a proteolytic enzyme (Elase ointment) for 24 h before attempting debridement. However, it is necessary to point out that medications of this type which are in an ointment base may also cause maceration of surrounding structures.

The next step consists of attempts to facilitate epithelialization of the lesion once the crater of the ulcer is filled with granulation tissue almost to the level of the surrounding skin. Sympathetic blocking agents like phenoxybenzamine hydrochloride (Dibenzyline) should be given a clinical trial since they cause transient dilatation of the cutaneous arteries and arterioles, especially in the digits, provided, of course, that these vessels are not partly or completely occluded by atherosclerotic plaques. The direct application of a myovascular relaxant, 2% nitroglycerin ointment (Nitrol ointment), to the base of an involved toe may be effective in increasing blood flow into the digit by its vasodilating action upon the digital arteries. That the drug passes through intact skin is attested to by the frequent nitrite headache the patient experiences with such therapy. The medication is applied three times a day for an hour each time. At the same time, the lesion is dressed less frequently so as to minimize injury to delicate granulation tissue and epithelial cells.

The use of stimulating ointments is generally of little value. However, in some patients the local application of a 5% crude coal tar ointment may accelerate the rate of epithelialization. The medication is left on the ulcer for periods of 24 h after it is determined that there is no sensitivity to it in the form of local itching, burning, or other types of pain soon after application.

Percutaneous vascular recanalization. This approach to therapy for atherosclerotic stenosis of main vessels of the lower limbs was originally described by Dotter and Judkins in 1964 [16]. However, up to recently it has had only fragmentary trials in the vascular clinics in the United States, with most of the definitive work having been carried out in Europe, particularly Switzerland and Germany [49]. Currently more attention is being paid to the method by the vascular surgeons in the United States.

The procedure consists of the nonsurgical dilatation of stenosed arteries or of the creation of a new lumen in occluded vessels (recanalization) by means of balloon-tipped or double-lumen catheters inserted intraluminally under local anesthesia. In response to the resulting central expanding force exerted against the clot and debris partially or completely filling the vessel, the foreign material is compressed and flattened against the intact arterial wall and redistributed longitudinally.[1] As a consequence, the lumen of the artery is enlarged or reformed, thus permitting reestablishment of

---

[1] Recently this theory has been questioned and other possibilities proposed, all of which require further evaluation.

local circulation. Before the procedure is performed, the patient, is systemically heparinized.

The final evaluation of percutaneous vascular recanalization must await many more clinical trials, especially in the vascular clinics in the United States.

2. Surgical Therapy

Lumbar sympathectomy. On the basis of the available experimental and clinical studies on human subjects, certain conclusions can be drawn concerning the therapeutic effectiveness of this procedure. With regard to intermittent claudication, it appears to have little or no effect on increasing walking distance. This would be in accord with the physiologic data indicating that alterations in sympathetic tone do not play a role in the changes in muscle blood flow elicited by physical exercise [37]. Nor does the operation prevent the appearance of ulcers or gangrene when performed as a prophylactic measure. In this regard, it has been shown that the loss of vascular tone after sympathectomy is only temporary, the initial marked increase in cutaneous blood flow, particularly in the digits, lasting only for a short period of time [6, 17,26]. Thereafter a small augmentation (less than double the control readings) persists [20]. There is no evidence available to support the view that sympathectomy enhances the extent and efficiency of the collateral circulation [19]. Finally, with respect to the treatment of existing ulceration or gangrene, the operation, by removing vasomotor tone from cutaneous vessels and increasing local blood flow, may be of some value in demarcating or healing the lesion. This is so provided first that the trophic disturbance is limited to a toe or toes and has not as yet involved the foot proper and second that the vessels locally are not filled with clot and are still capable of dilating when sympathetic nervous system control is eliminated.

Lumbar sympathectomy is rarely of value in the patient who is suffering from both diabetes and arteriosclerosis obliterans. One reason for this is that in the diabetic who also has peripheral neuropathy, autosympathectomy may already exist as a result of destruction of the peripheral mixed nerves containing the sympathetic fibers, and hence sympathectomy would contribute nothing further toward increasing the blood supply. Moreover, since diabetes frequently affects the terminal blood vessels (microangiopathy), removal of sympathetic control over this type of vascular bed will not result in any significant increase in local blood flow. However, when peripheral neuropathy is not present, sympathectomy may relieve rest pain [18] and help small ulcerations of the toes or feet to heal. It may also facilitate healing of the operative site after amputation of toes, provided that it is performed at the same time or shortly thereafter.

Thromboendarterectomy. This procedure has been utilized for many years, although since the advent of vascular grafts (see below) it has assumed less importance as a means of reestablishing circulation in large vessels in which segmental thrombosis exists. When a small block occurs in the artery and calcification is not demonstrated, it is to be preferred to a graft, whereas utilization of the procedure for a long stretch of thrombosed vessel is not indicated in most instances. When used in femoropopliteal occlusions, the method is much less successful than in the case of wide-calibered channels, and thrombosis is liable to occur.

Thromboendarterectomy, in the presence of arteriosclerosis obliterans, has its greatest applicability to blocks in the deep femoral artery and the adjoining proximal portion of the common femoral artery. The reason for this is that generally only the first centimeter of the deep femoral artery is involved in the atherosclerotic process, while its branches remain patent. As a result, the procedure is frequently effective in reestablishing circulation in the terminal vessels, which in turn communicate with the popliteal artery and its branches. Also, proximal blood flow develops through connections with subdivisions of the common iliac artery.

Thromboendarterectomy has also been utilized for aortoiliac arterial occlusive disease since the obstructions are usually segmental, short, and localized. The advantage of the procedure is that it is not necessary to introduce foreign material into the body, a measure which has attendant risk. Moreover, the operation takes less time than does the insertion of a graft and the damage to the existing circulation is not as great. However, there may be more post-

operative complications, including recurrence of the stenosis.

Thromboendarterectomy is used infrequently in the young patient with diabetes and arteriosclerosis obliterans, since for the most part the occlusive disease is distal to the popliteal artery. Arterial blocks so situated do not readily lend themselves to such a surgical measure. Even in those individuals in whom arterial insufficiency preceded the appearance of diabetes for many years and in whom there are occlusions at higher levels in the arterial tree (the common and superficial femoral arteries), attempts to remove such blocks surgically are generally ineffective. The reason is that in these individuals, diabetes has also produced obliterative changes in the runoff distally and in the terminal circulation, with the result that treatment of the proximal obstruction has very little if any effect on increasing the nutritional circulation to the tissues of the foot. Nevertheless, some clinical studies are available which emphasize the beneficial effects of such procedures. In fact, it has been stated that the results of vascular surgery for large artery disease in diabetics are as good as those obtained in nondiabetics.

Among the complications of thromboendarterectomy is aneurysmal dilatation of the weakened arterial wall. Such a response may also occur if medial calcification is prominent. Inadequate closure of the incision in the vessel, because of the poor state of the remaining coats of the wall, may lead to serious hemorrhage which is difficult to control. A frequent sequela of the technique is subsequent thrombosis of the thromboendarterectomized segment of vessel, due to platelet aggregation and fibrin deposition or to fragments of material left by the instrument. Such complications can be recognized and corrected at the time of surgery by utilizing intraoperative angiography [23]. Postoperative fibrosis, producing constriction of the lumen, may also result in thrombosis of the vessel.

Restoration of arterial continuity with a graft. At present this procedure is generally accepted as the most effective surgical approach to the problem of increasing circulation to an ischemic lower extremity suffering from arteriosclerosis obliterans, provided all of the criteria for a successful result (see below) are satisfied.

Potentially good candidates for a graft procedure fall into several general groups. One consists of relatively young people, who, although demonstrating a stationary process as determined by clinical means, are unable to conduct their daily business activities because of marked limitation in walking. Another category is composed of individuals, regardless of their age, who are manifesting rapid deterioration in walking ability, indicating marked progression of the arteriosclerotic process. However, if such a change occurs early in the disease, it should be observed carefully before considering any surgical therapy, because it may then be followed by a stationary period. The presence of rest pain (ischemic neuropathy) indicates the existence of a marked impairment of circulation, and hence an individual with such a symptom should be considered as a possible candidate for a graft procedure. Finally, if there are signs of impending trophic changes or if ulcers or gangrene already exist, with the lesions being limited to a toe or toes, a graft procedure appears indicated. If there has been extension of the necrotic process onto the foot proper, such as operation is also useful since it may permit removal of the involved tissues with subsequent healing of the operative site, thus acting as a preferred substitute for a major amputation. If such a goal cannot be achieved, the increased blood flow, even if only temporary, may be sufficient for healing of the stump at a lower than anticipated level of amputation.

In the case of the patient suffering from aortoiliac arterial occlusive disease, the appearance of nutritional disturbances or a rapid deterioration in walking ability is sufficient indication for reevaluation of the local circulation, with the possibility of reconstructive surgery being seriously considered. The patient with this condition who suffers from disabling intermittent claudication and is unable to be gainfully employed or take care of the activities of daily living should also be considered a candidate for a surgical procedure, provided there are no general contraindications for such a measure.

After the general criteria are satisfied, it is now necessary to determine whether the pathologic vascular changes are such that the insertion of a graft has a good possibility of

significantly increasing blood flow to the foot. It is therefore necessary to subject the potential candidate for the operation to further studies, including aortography or arteriography (see Section E, Chapter 5). The results may prove valuable in the final determination of operability and in the selection of the site and method of operation. It is important to ascertain the following: (1) the size of the vessel involved; (2) the site of the primary occlusion; (3) the existence of other obstructions in the arteries that supply the limb; (4) the condition of the vessel above and, particularly, below the site of the primary occlusion; and (5) the extent of the available collateral circulation and the adequacy of the runoff into the vessels of the leg and foot.

In the case of occlusion of the superficial femoral artery, a femoropopliteal graft carries with it a good possibility of a successful result, provided, of course, that a segmental thrombosis and a patent terminal distributional system exist. The patient with extensive disease of the arteries proximally and distally is a poor candidate for a graft procedure.

For blocks below the groin, an autogenous reversed great saphenous venous graft appears to be the only type which has the potential of retaining patency for a relatively long period of time (Fig. 11.7). The use of a Dacron prosthesis as a substitute has a very great possibility of thrombosis of the graft shortly after its insertion. Recently human umbilical cord vessels [11,12] and expanded polytetrafluoroethylene prostheses [9,45] have been proposed for patients who were otherwise faced with potential limb loss and for whom other graft materials were either unavailable or unsuitable. Because of the short period of investigation, no definitive conclusions can be drawn as to their efficacy.

In some instances a heroic operative approach is indicated as a last resort procedure in an effort to salvage a limb otherwise destined for amputation. Such a situation exists if ulceration or gangrene is present on the foot which has not responded to conservative therapy or has actually enlarged under the regimen and the runoff from the popliteal artery is poor, thus precluding the use of the conventional femoropopliteal graft. Under such conditions, careful pedal angiographic studies (Fig. 5.5)

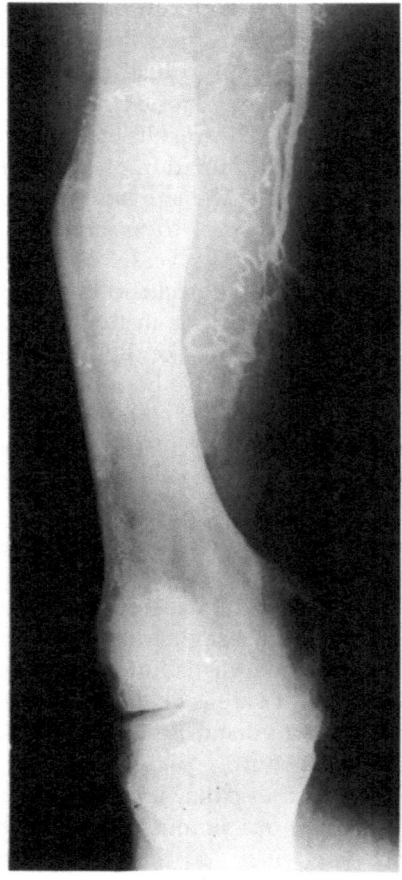 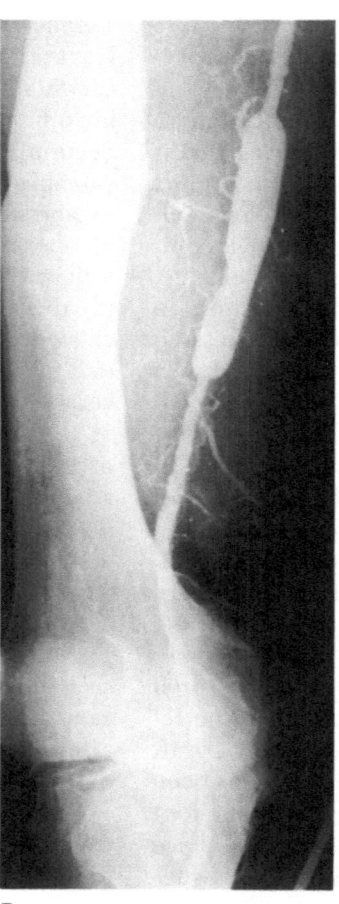

A   **B**

Fig. 11.7. **A** Complete occlusion of the superficial femoral artery due to arteriosclerosis obliterans. **B** Insertion of a reversed venous graft between patent segments of vessel by means of an end-to-end anastomosis. Popliteal artery is now visualized. From Abramson DI: Vascular Disorders of the Extremities. Hagerstown, Md, Harper & Row, 1974. Reproduced with permission.

are indicated in order to determine the degree of the occlusive process in the arteries of the foot. At times it may be necessary to perform the procedure while the patient is on the operating table by making an incision over the posterior tibial artery in the ankle [15]. (For a description of the techniques used in carrying out pedal angiography, see p. 70.)

If visualization of either tibial artery or even of the dorsal pedal artery is achieved, it may be feasible to use a long vascular graft for the purpose of anastomosing the lower segment of the superficial femoral artery with the patent vessel at the level of the ankle [44,48]. Even though such a procedure may only result in a temporary increase in local circulation, this may be sufficient to prevent progression of a necrotic lesion and facilitate demarcation of the gangrenous process or to promote healing of an indolent ulcer. In such a manner, the limb

may be preserved, even though a toe or toes may have to be sacrificed.

The most common operative means of treating aortoiliac arterial occlusive disease is the introduction of a Dacron or Teflon bifurcation graft. Because of the high head of pressure in the aorta and because the vessels below are usually patent (comprising an excellent runoff), there is a very good likelihood that the prosthesis will remain open for many years despite the fact that it is a foreign body. The coexistence of occlusive disease in the arterial tree in the lower limbs would reduce the possibility of such a prognosis unless attempts are simultaneously made to remedy this difficulty.

A number of conditions may adversely affect the success of even an autogenous graft in maintaining adequate circulation to a lower limb. These include technical operative errors; poor judgment in the choice of the candidate for the procedure (e.g., the insertion of a graft in the face of an inadequate runoff); spontaneous thrombosis of distal vessels due to the underlying pathology; proximal progression of the atherosclerotic process; and stenosis of the graft itself due to valve cusp fibrosis.

Although an autogenous graft is capable of conveying an increased amount of blood to distal tissues, thus reducing or even eliminating the state of ischemia, the pathologic process in the arterial tree is in no way affected by such a procedure. Hence, being invariably progressive in nature, the atherosclerotic changes continue to involve more and more of the proximal and distal arteries in the limb, reducing or even preventing blood flow through them. Actually, the only effective available mechanism for maintaining viability of tissues under such conditions is the growth of a collateral circulation in response to the state of chronic ischemia (see C-3, Chapter 10).

In the full evaluation of reversed saphenous vein grafts, it is necessary to consider the results of a long-term study of the procedure. It has been shown that if care is taken in the preparation and procurement of the prosthesis, in about 50 percent of cases, patency, as determined by arteriographic studies, will be maintained for up to 15 years [13]. The main late complications of patent anastomoses are graft degeneration, anastomotic false aneurysm, narrowing at the site of distal anastomosis, and infection [4].

E. Prognosis

1. Arteriosclerosis Obliterans

The outlook with regard to longevity in arteriosclerosis obliterans will, for the most part, depend upon the extent of atherosclerosis in critical organs in the body, such as the heart, brain, and kidneys. Only rarely does death occur because of involvement of the vascular tree in the lower limbs, as for example, when a major amputation is required in a patient who is a poor candidate for any type of anesthesia and surgical procedure.

The prognosis for intermittent claudication alone is good as far as maintenance of viability of the limb is concerned, a point of view which should be emphasized to the patient with this complaint, who ordinarily contemplates a sequence of events which includes subsequent gangrene of the foot and the need for a major amputation. However, life expectancy is considerably reduced in individuals with intermittent claudication for reasons already presented [33,40]. The cause of death is primarily a cardiovascular disorder and, much less often, cerebrovascular disease [7].

2. Arteriosclerosis Obliterans and Diabetes Mellitus

There is no question that the concomitant presence of diabetes mellitus untowardly affects the prognosis of the patient with arteriosclerosis obliterans. For example, it has been found that the 5-year survival rate in individuals suffering from both disorders was 54.4 percent, whereas in nondiabetics with arteriosclerosis obliterans, it was 75.7 percent [35]. Further support for this view was obtained by a study of 200 patients with arteriosclerosis obliterans alone and a similar number who also had diabetes [1]. In the first group, 92 percent demonstrated no signs of such trophic changes as ulceration and gangrene during the 5-year period of observation, the only treatment carried out in this group being meticulous care of the feet and abstinence from smoking. In the remaining 8 percent, ulcers and gangrene did develop. In the series of patients with arteriosclerosis obliterans associated with diabetes, despite a similar therapeutic program, 50 percent demonstrated trophic changes in the lower limbs and 25 percent of the entire series required an amputation of one or both lower extremities during the period of observation. Also of interest with regard to prognosis is the finding that more than one-half of all lower extremity amputations in the United States is performed on diabetic patients over the age of 55 years. However, it is necessary to point out, too, that the majority of diabetic patients with ischemic changes in the lower limbs die from other causes, generally complications of atherosclerosis in the heart, brain, and kidneys, without ever requiring an amputation. Of those who do, in about one-third of the cases, there is a well-healed and fully functional lower limb amputation at the time of death [5].

References

1. Abramson DI: Unpublished observations
2. Abramson DI: Vascular Disorders of the Extremities, 2nd ed, Hagerstown, Md., Harper & Row, 1974, pp 292–311
3. Abramson DI, Zayas AM, Canning JR, et al: Thromboangiitis obliterans: A true clinical entity. Am J Cardiol 12:107, 1963
4. Agrifoglio G, Costantini S, Zanetta M, et al: Infections and anastomotic false aneurysms in reconstructive vascular surgery. J Cardiovasc Surg 20:25, 1979
5. Baddeley RM, Fulford JC: A trial of conservative amputations for lesions of the feet in diabetes mellitus. Br J Surg 52:38, 1965
6. Barcroft H, Walker AJ: Return of tone in blood vessels of the upper limb after sympathectomy. Lancet 1:1035, 1949
7. Begg TB, Richards RL: The prognosis of intermittent claudication. Scott Med J 7:341, 1962
8. Bell ET: Incidence of gangrene of the extremities in nondiabetic and in diabetic persons. Arch Pathol 49:469, 1950
9. Campbell CD, Brooks DH, Webster MW, et al: The use of expanded microporous polytetrafluoroethylene for limb salvage: A preliminary report. Surgery 79:485, 1976
10. Cogan DG, Merola L, Laibson PR: Blood viscosity, serum hexosamine, and diabetic retinopathy. Diabetes 10:393, 1961
11. Dardik, H, Dardik I: Successful arterial substitution with modified human umbilical vein. Ann Surg 183:252, 1976
12. Dardik II, Ibrahim IM, Dardik H: Experimental and clinical use of human umbilical cord vessels as vascular substitutes. J Cardiovasc Surg 18:555, 1977
13. Dhall DP, Mavor GE: Long-term behavior of reversed saphenous vein grafts for advanced femoropopliteal disease. Surg Gynecol Obstet 146:241, 1978
14. Dormandy J, Widjetunge D, Barnes A: Clinical manifestations and management of leg ischaemia in diabetics. In Davis E (ed): The Microcirculation in Diabetes. Basel, Karger, 1979, p 95
15. Doscher W, Bole V, Babu S, et al: The determination of ankle or pedal level bypass by on-table angiography. Vasa 8:15, 1979
16. Dotter CT, Judkins MP: Transluminal treatment of arteriosclerotic obstruction: Description of a new technic and a preliminary report of its application. Circulation 30:654, 1964
17. Duff RS: Circulatory changes in the forearm following sympathectomy. Clin Sci 10:529, 1951
18. Eadie DGA: The management of arterial disease. Br J Hosp Med 3:337, 1970
19. Flasher J, White AE, Drury DR: Sympathetic denervation in the treatment of acute arterial occlusion. Circulation 9:238, 1954
20. Gillespie JA: Late effects of lumbar sympathectomy on blood flow in the foot in obliterative vascular disease. Lancet 1:891, 1960
21. Ireland JT: Small blood vessels disease in diabetes mellitus: With particular reference to the kidney. In Harcus AW, Adamson L (eds): Arteries and Veins. London, Churchill, Livingstone, 1975, p 143
22. Jarrett RJJ, Keen H: Diabetes and atherosclerosis. In Keen H, Jarrett RJJ (eds): Complications of Diabetes. London, Arnold, 1975, p 179
23. Koch G: Intraoperative angiography. J Cardiovasc Surg 16:359, 1975
24. Kontras SB, Bodenbender JG: Studies of the inflammatory cycle in juvenile diabetes. Am J Dis Child 116:130, 1968
25. Lundbaek K: Diabetic angiopathy: A specific vascular disease. Lancet 1:377, 1954
26. Lynn RB, Barcroft H: Circulatory changes in the foot after lumbar sympathectomy. Lancet 1:1105, 1950
27. Malins J: Clinical Diabetes Mellitus. London, Eyre & Spottiswoode, 1968, pp 267–268
28. Mayne EE, Bridges JM, Weaver JA: Platelet adhesiveness, plasma fibrinogen, and factor VIII levels in diabetes mellitus. Diabetologia 6:436, 1970
29. McGill HC Jr, Geer JC: The human lesion, fine structure. In Jones RJ (ed): Evolution of the Atherosclerotic Plaque. Chicago, Univ Chicago Press, 1963, p 65
30. McMillan DE: Disturbance of serum viscosity in diabetes mellitus. J Clin Invest 53:1071, 1974
31. O'Malley BC, Timperley WR, Ward JD, et al: Platelet abnormalities in diabetic peripheral neuropathy. Lancet 2:1274, 1975
32. Pareira MD, Handler FP, Blumenthal HT: Aging processes in the arterial and venous systems of the lower extremities. Circulation 8:36, 1953
33. Peabody CN, Kannel WB, McNamara PM: Intermittent claudication: Surgical significance. Arch Surg 109:693, 1974
34. Ross R, Glomset JA: Atherosclerosis and the arterial smooth muscle cell: Proliferation of smooth muscle is a key event in the genesis of the lesions of atherosclerosis. Science 180:1332, 1973
35. Schadt DC, Hines EA Jr, Juergens JL, et al: Chronic atherosclerotic occlusion of the femoral artery. JAMA 175:937, 1961
36. Scow RO, Blanchette-Mackie EJ, Smith LC: Role of capillary endothelium in the clearance of chylomicrons: A model for lipid transport from blood by lateral diffusion in cell membranes. Circ Res 39:149, 1976
37. Shepherd JT: Evaluation of treatment in intermittent claudication. Br Med J 2:1413, 1950
38. Silbert S, Lippmann HI, Gordon E: Mönckeberg's arteriosclerosis. JAMA 151:1176, 1953
39. Siperstein MD, Unger RH, Madison LL: Studies of muscle capillary basement membranes

in normal subjects, diabetic and prediabetic patients. J Clin Invest 47:1973, 1968

40. Spaulding WB: The prognosis of patients with intermittent claudication. Can Med Assoc J 75:105, 1956

41. Strandness DE Jr, Priest RE, Gibbons GE: Combined clinical and pathologic study of diabetic and nondiabetic peripheral arterial disease. Diabetes 13:366, 1964

42. Task Force Report: In: Arteriosclerosis. National Heart and Lung Institute. HEW Publ No (NIH) 72–219, June 1971

43. Thomas WA, Jones R, Scott RF, et al: Production of early atherosclerotic lesions in rats characterized by proliferation of "modified smooth muscle cells." Exp Mol Pathol 2:40 (Suppl 1), 1963

44. Tovar ME, Pérez Bustamante G: Femoro-tibial and femoro-peroneal bypass in the treatment of the ischemic lower limbs. J Cardiovasc Surg 15:360, 1974

45. Veith FJ, Moss CM, Fell SC, et al: Comparison of expanded PTFE and vein grafts in lower extremity arterial reconstructions. J Cardiovasc Surg 19:341, 1978

46. Williamson JR, Kilo C: Current status of capillary basement-membrane disease in diabetes mellitus. Diabetes 26:65, 1977

47. Wissler RW: Atherosclerosis: Its pathogenesis in perspective. In: Comparative Pathology of the Heart. Adv Cardiol 13:10, 1974

48. Zannini G, Spampinato N, Bracale CG: Revascularization of the distal arteries of the leg: Indications and results. J Cardiovasc Surg 15:554, 1974

49. Zeitler E, Grüntzig A, Schoop W: Percutaneous Vascular Recanalization. New York, Springer-Verlag, 1978

Chapter 12

Spontaneous Organic Occlusive Arterial Diseases

Part 2 Acute Arterial Disorders

This chapter deals with those occlusive arterial disorders which develop very rapidly and hence are invariably associated with the symptoms and signs of acute ischemia of at least the distal portions of the limbs (see Section B, Chapter 10). In this regard, they resemble the clinical picture of acute trauma to critical arteries (see Chapter 15).

A. Arterial Embolism

In arterial embolism, particulate matter of varying size becomes separated from its site of origin in the cardiovascular system, to enter the systemic circulation and cause total obstruction of an artery above a point at which the diameter of the vessel becomes smaller than that of the embolus. Because of the resulting sudden cessation of blood flow distal to the block, the condition can be considered a real emergency which requires immediate remedial measures if the viability of the involved structures in the limb is to be preserved. However, even with the introduction of the Fogarty balloon catheter technique, which is a relatively minor surgical approach, there is still a high operative mortality rate, probably related to the serious nature of the underlying cardiac diseases commonly found in patients prone to arterial

embolic episodes. Another possibility is the subsequent development of recurrent thromboembolic complications [5].

1. Sites of Origin of Arterial Emboli

In more than 80 percent of patients suffering from peripheral arterial embolism, the origin of the clotted material is in the heart. Other sources are rare and include aneurysms of the thoracic and abdominal aorta and of arterial trunks and thrombi forming on ulcerated atherosclerotic plaques or on sites of repeated minor trauma in peripheral arteries.

Valvular heart disease. Fairly common locations for the liberation of arterial emboli are diseased mitral and aortic semilunar valves. The cause for the development of the valvular excrescences or thrombi is either arteriosclerotic or rheumatic heart disease. Bacterial endocarditis superimposed upon the involved cusps may be responsible for the presence of infected emboli in the bloodstream.

Atrial disorders. In atrial fibrillation clots form in the left atrium due to incomplete emptying of the chamber by the feeble contractions of the atrial wall. The resulting stasis predisposes to the development of thrombi which then enter the left ventricle and are propelled into the bloodstream by the force of ventricular contraction. Atrial fibrillation may result from mitral valvular heart disease due to rheumatic fever, arteriosclerotic heart disease, hypertension, or rarely hyperthyroidism. A widely dilated, hypertrophied left atrium caused by mitral stenosis, even when contracting normally, may also be the source of arterial emboli because of the persistent pooling of blood in the enlarged chamber, particularly in its auricle.

Myocardial infarction. In at least one-half of fresh infarcts which have extended to the endocardium, mural clots line the involved surface of the left ventricle, with the result that in 10 to 20 percent of the patients, pieces of the material break loose to enter the bloodstream. In the great percentage of cases, the embolic episode takes place within the first 3 weeks after the onset of the condition. However, in some instances, the clot may lie dormant for many months and then become dislodged, to produce late peripheral arterial emboli.

Other abnormalities of left ventricle. The chamber of the left ventricle may be the source of peripheral emboli if it is widely dilated due to congestive heart failure or if an aneurysm has developed in its wall following an old myocardial infarct.

Aneurysms and thrombosis of the arterial tree. The cavity of an aneurysm of the abdominal aorta or of a main artery to a limb may also be the site of origin of arterial emboli, pieces of clot in the sac being separated from their source and entering the bloodstream. Other locations in which peripheral emboli may develop are a thrombosed segment or aneurysm of the poststenotic subclavian artery found in a neurovascular compression syndrome of the shoulder girdle (see B-4, Chapter 13) and a thrombosed popliteal artery.

Other less common conditions. Among infrequent causes for peripheral arterial emboli are left atrial myxoma and ulcerating atherosclerotic plaques in the abdominal aorta. From the latter debris is liberated, to enter the vessels supplying the lower limbs and then to occlude the terminal arterioles in the muscles and in the skin of the toes (atherothrombotic or cholesterol embolism) [1]. Pulmonary phlebitis associated with infections of the lungs and sarcomatous deposits in the lung parenchyma have also been implicated in the production of systemic emboli, as well as circulating fat particles (see C-3, Chapter 16). The use of artificial valve replacements may result in the deposition of aggregates of platelets and fibrin on the surface of the prostheses, followed by liberation of particulate material into the bloodstream [8]. Finally, thrombi may occasionally develop in the deep veins of the calf (phlebothrombosis) which then pass into the main venous system and through a patent foramen ovale into the peripheral arterial circulation (paradoxical embolus). This can only occur when the pressure in the right atrium is momentarily increased, as during defecation (Valsalva maneuver), thus causing reversal of the normal interatrial pressure gradient, which is from left to right atrium.

2. Sites of Occlusion

Peripheral emboli generally occlude arteries at their bifurcation where their caliber is suddenly narrowed or in the course of a vessel if there is a similar rapid reduction in lumen size. Such large arteries as the abdominal aorta are rarely obstructed except at their bifurcation (Fig. 12.1). At least two-thirds of all systemic arterial embolizations occurs in the limbs, the lower extremities being more frequently involved than the upper. At times, several vessels may be simultaneously obstructed if a soft embolus breaks on striking a bifurcation of a proximal main artery. The most common site of occlusion is the common femoral artery above the origin of the deep femoral artery (Fig. 12.2A). The others are affected in the following order of reducing frequency: popliteal (Fig. 12.2B), common iliac, brachial, bifurcation of the aorta, subclavian, external iliac, superficial femoral, posterior tibial, radial, ulnar, and anterior tibial arteries [4].

3. Clinical Manifestations

Symptoms. Generally, occlusion of a critical artery by an embolus is ushered in by the ab-

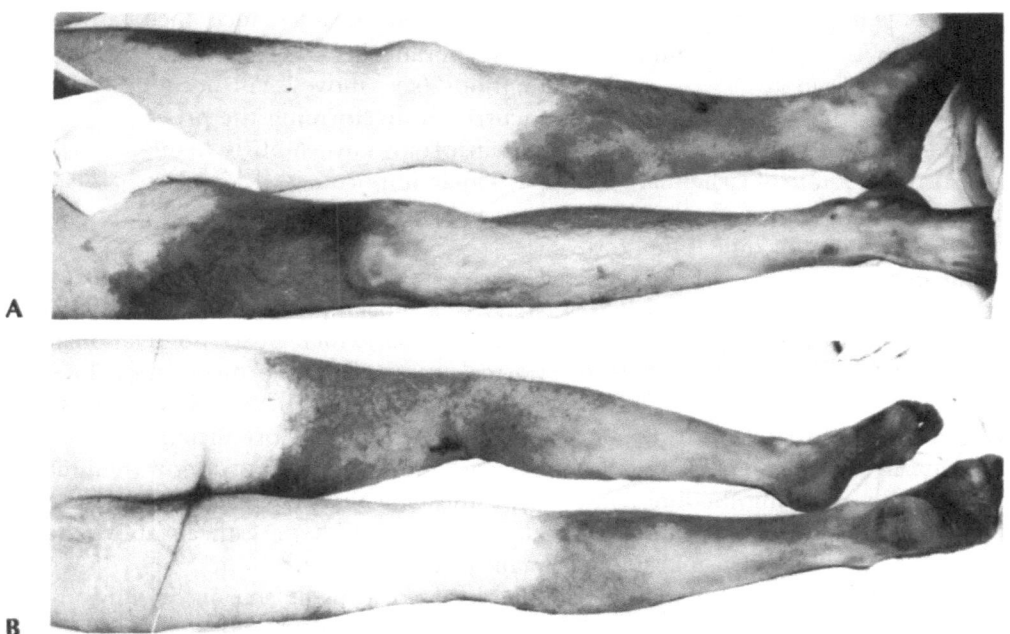

Fig. 12.1. Untreated saddle embolus occluding aortic bifurcation and causing gangrene of both lower limbs. **A** Anterior view. **B** Posterior view. From Abramson DI: Vascular Disorders of the Extremities. Hagerstown, Md, Harper & Row, 1974. Reproduced with permission.

rupt and dramatic onset of severe ischemic pain in the foot or hand, at times associated with a "dead" feeling and paresthesias in the digits. However, the onset may also be more insidious, manifested by only a slight aching or dull sensa-

tion, or the condition may even go clinically unrecognized. As the anoxia persists, the symptoms usually increase in intensity until the peripheral nerves become nonfunctioning, at which point a sense of numbness may replace

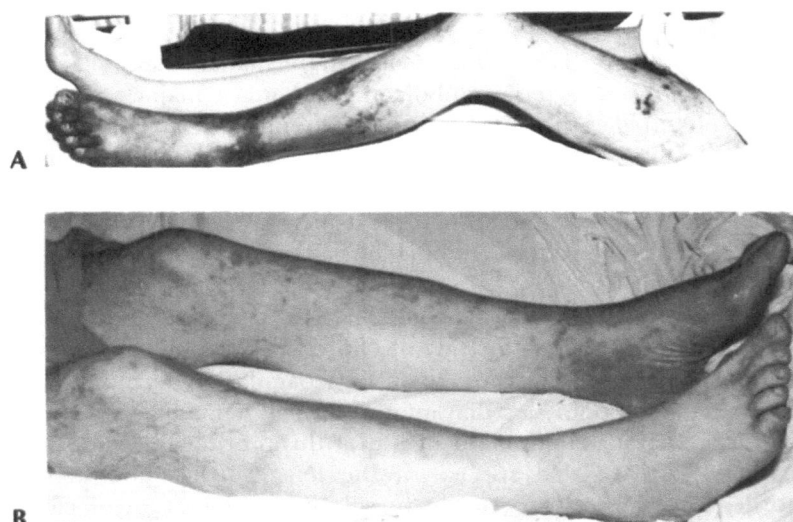

Fig. 12.2. Untreated emboli in arteries of lower limbs. **A** Occlusion of the left common femoral artery above the origin of the deep femoral artery. **B** Occlusion of the left popliteal artery at its bifurcation.

the pain; if the involvement is in the lower limb, the patient frequently describes a feeling akin to walking on a block of wood.

Vascular changes. These are generally clearcut and diagnostic of the state of ischemia. First the subpapillary venous plexuses in the distal portion of the extremity become empty of blood, resulting in intense pallor of the skin; however, there may be interspersed small islands of cyanosis, due to trapping of venous blood in portions of the cutaneous circulation as a consequence of vascular spasm on an ischemic basis. Since there is frequently also an associated vasospasm of the collateral circulation, very little blood is entering the limb, and hence venous outflow is likewise minimal, producing collapse of and barely visible superficial veins. Because of the reduced blood flow, the circumferences of the involved extremity appear smaller than those of the opposite normal limb. For the same reason, the amount of heat lost from the blood is small, and so the temperature of the skin falls rapidly and soon approximates that of the environment. This is particularly so in the distal portion of the limb, the skin of the digits demonstrating the greatest reduction. The change becomes much less prominent as the examining hand moves proximally up the limb. Generally this step may bring out a zone of demarcation between normal and reduced cutaneous temperature, information which has some value in grossly locating the site of obstruction of the main artery.

Due to the marked reduction in arterial inflow in the limb, pulses in the distal portions are absent, the same type of change being observed in the oscillometric readings obtained from various levels on the limb. Proximal to the involvement of the vessel, the amplitude of the pulsations may be somewhat reduced because of the associated superimposed vasospasm. Information obtained by palpation of pulses and by oscillometric studies is likewise helpful in locating the site of occlusion in the arterial tree. Also useful is the Doppler ultrasonic flowmeter which permits assessment of arterial flow velocity signals and segmental limb blood pressure (see D-2, Chapter 5). Arteriography is rarely necessary in order to make the diagnosis of arterial embolism and locate the site of occlusion, since such information can generally be collected using noninvasive methods (see above). Furthermore, the delay incurred in performing the procedure may result in progressive limb ischemia, which is of particular importance if viability of distal tissues is being threatened.

Neurologic changes. Among the diagnostic signs is a stocking-glove type of hypesthesia or anesthesia, which bears no relationship to normal anatomic nerve distribution but does resemble the sensory changes observed in hysterical patients. In most instances anesthesia is elicited in the distal portion of the limb and hypesthesia at the proximal levels. There may also be an area of hyperesthesia above the segment of reduced sensation.

Associated with the sensory findings may be signs of impairment in motor function. In the feet, they generally consist of difficulty or inability to move the toes and varying degrees of foot drop. In the upper limbs, there may be some reduction in the ability to move the fingers and a wrist drop, although usually such alterations are uncommon. The presence of motor impairment or loss in the distal portion of a limb signifies a much more marked degree of ischemia of nerve fibers than is the case for sensory changes alone, and hence such a situation indicates a much poorer prognosis with regard to limb viability.

4. Treatment

The basic principle in the management of acute arterial embolism involving a major vessel is the rapid restoration of pulsatile arterial blood flow to the involved limb. However, before discussing this aspect of therapy, it is necessary to mention several measures which may help reduce the incidence of arterial embolism.

Prophylactic steps. The general impression from a study of clinical reports is that the administration of anticoagulants during acute myocardial infarction may help retard the development of mural thrombi on the endocardial surface of the left ventricle and hence decrease the possibility of liberation of clots into the bloodstream. The various surgical procedures developed to deal with mitral stenosis may have a similar effect on the incidence of arterial embolism. Whether reestablishment of normal sinus rhythm in a patient with long-standing atrial fibrillation carries with it the risk of liberating pieces of clot from the left atrium has never been satisfactorily answered, and because of this uncertainty, there is a real question as to whether such a step should be performed. What appears to be more clear-cut is that the individual in whom there is a history of repeated transitions from one rhythm to another is in serious danger of liberating peripheral emboli. Therefore, in him the best policy is to maintain conditions present at the time of the first examination by means of appropriate medications.

Active medical therapy. If the clinical history suggests the possibility of a peripheral arterial embolism, the first step is to give the patient an intravenous injection of 7500 units of heparin. Following such a measure, time can now be spent confirming the diagnosis by physical examination, determining the approximate site of occlusion, and making the necessary surgical preparations for removal of the embolus, without the fear that in the interval, propagation of the process is occurring in branches proximal and distal to the obstruction. At the same time, the limb should be protected from injury by covering it with several layers of cotton padding to form a loosely fitting boot, and in the case of the lower extremity, the head of the bed is raised about 20 cm (8 in.) so as to increase local arterial inflow. It may also be necessary to give large doses of narcotics to control the pain. If there are definite signs of vasospasm, attempts should be made to remove it. Then the patient should be reexamined, since superimposed excess sympathetic tone may alter the physical findings, thus causing the observer to reach an erroneous conclusion regarding the site of organic occlusion.

Active surgical therapy. With the introduction of the Fogarty balloon catheter [3], there has been a radical change in the indications for embolectomy as therapy in arterial embolism. Because the instrument (usually a No. 6 size) can be inserted into an artery through an oblique arteriotomy under local anesthesia, the method is applicable to even very poor surgical risk and elderly patients, as well as others. It is simple, quick, and safe and should be utilized even in the case of noncritical arteries. However, the operation must generally be performed within 8 h after the onset of the acute occlusive episode. Otherwise, irreversible changes will occur in the tissues despite removal of the embolus because of propagation of a thrombus into the microcirculation.

The only exception to this rule is when the embolus is lodged at the aortic bifurcation. Because of the very serious consequences of allowing this condition to persist (Fig. 12.1), embolectomy should be performed even as late as 20 h after the occlusion. Such an approach may be successful in preventing gangrene of perhaps one lower limb. However, it is necessary to point out that such a course is not without some risk, since after a protracted period of ischemia of the muscles of both lower extremities, reestablishment of circulation may initiate the "revascularization syndrome" (see below).

Of greatest importance in achieving a successful result is the reestablishment of a good flow in the previously occluded artery and its distal branches. It is therefore necessary to remove not only the embolus, but also any thrombi which had formed at the site of obstruction and propagated distally and proximally in the segmentally blocked artery. This is accomplished by retrograde flushing of the vessel with heparin and inserting a Fogarty catheter into the smaller branches of the vascular tree.

It is necessary to point out, however, that reestablishment of the local circulation by a successful embolectomy is frequently not associated with rapid disappearance of all signs of ischemia, as might be expected. In fact, the return of normal skin color and normal skin temperature may not be observed for several days, probably until the superimposed local spasm of the artery initiated by the original condition is released. For the same reason, arterial pulsations may not be present for a similar period, although in some instances they are felt immediately after the operation.

Whether heparin should be given at intervals in the postoperative period in order to prevent subsequent thrombosis of the involved segment of artery is still a moot question. The objection to its use is the possibility of initiating bleeding in the operative site. However, this cannot be considered too serious a problem when a main artery in a limb has been used for the insertion of a Fogarty catheter, since bleeding under such circumstances can readily be identified and controlled. It would seem then that the advantages of administering heparin postoperatively far outweigh any possible associated risk, and hence the drug should be given for several days after operation, together with Coumadin or dicumarol. The explanation for instituting the latter step is found in the section "Later therapy," below.

Attention must be called to a revascularization syndrome which appears in patients in whom a successful embolectomy was performed but only after several days had elapsed following the acute episode. The abnormal changes, which are noted soon after local circulation is reestablished, consist of edema of voluntary muscles, hemoconcentration, hypovolemic shock, acidosis, myoglobinemia, and myoglobinuria, followed by oliguria or even anuria [7]. In the case of muscles contained in a rigid compartment, such as those in the anterior tibial compartment, the swelling may be so marked that extensive fasciotomies must immediately be performed in order to prevent irreversible damage and gangrene. The degree of metabolic alterations appears to be directly related to the amount of muscle mass previously made ischemic by the cessation of blood flow into the limb.

Therapy for patients with inadequate local circulation. For the individuals who were treated conservatively or in whom an embolectomy was unsuccessful in reestablishing blood flow through the involved artery, the viability of the limb will depend upon the previous role of the vessel in supplying the limb with blood and the functional state of the collateral circulation, provided one exists. In the case of obstruction of a noncritical artery, generally no trophic changes will appear, the only complaint being intermittent claudication and possibly some neuritic symptoms which usually diminish in intensity and then disappear several weeks or months afterward. No specific therapy is indicated under these circumstances.

If the artery that remains occluded had contributed significantly to the circulation of the limb, there may be some sequelae such as a foot drop requiring a foot-drop brace. However, if the main blood supply is lost, then invariably there will be necrosis of the foot. Under these conditions, anticoagulants should be discontinued and a major amputation carried out as soon as feasible.

Later therapy. In the case of the patients who have successfully recovered from the acute episode of arterial embolism without having developed any necrosis in the involved limb, the problem of how to prevent subsequent attacks of a similar nature must be dealt with.

If the source of the clots can be eliminated by surgical means, as through mitral commissurotomy, removal of the left atrial appendage, or repair of a left ventricular aneurysm resulting from a myocardial infarction, then such an approach should be given serious consideration. If the clots originate in an aneurysmal sac arising from the abdominal aorta or a main branch, a similar approach is indicated. Prevention of recurrence of paradoxical emboli arising in the deep veins of the leg requires ligation or plication of the inferior vena cava or the insertion of an intracaval umbrella filter (see E-4, Chapter 19).

When surgical intervention is not feasible, then at the time of discharge from the hospital heparin should be stopped, but the oral anticoagulant should be continued on an outpatient basis for the rest of the patient's life. It is realized that a number of objections can be raised regarding the practicability of such a plan, including the cost of repeated prothrombin time determinations (at least once every other week), the risks associated with protracted administration of anticoagulants, and the cost of medical supervision of the program. Nevertheless, the serious consequences of possible recurrence of peripheral arterial emboli if the therapeutic regimen is not carried out make almost imperative its institution in every patient in whom no other alternative approaches are available. (For other conditions which must be satisfied before initiating an outpatient anticoagulation program, see p. 291.)

Therapeutic program for atherothrombotic or cholesterol embolism. The initial treatment of microembolism differs from the regimen already described for large arterial emboli. There is a question as to whether heparin should be given, since this drug may prevent organization of a fibrin covering over the ulcerated vascular lesion from which the microemboli are arising and hence be responsible for recurrence of the condition. The proper therapeutic regimen consists of identifying the source of the emboli using angiography and then carrying out immediate surgical correction, whether this involves endarterectomy, insertion of an aortic bifurcation graft to replace an area of atherosclerotic ulceration in the abdominal aorta, or repair of an aneurysm of this vessel or its main branches [2].

Local treatment of ulcers or superficial gangrene of the toes is the same as for any other type of superficial necrosis. The lesions are aseptically treated, the gangrenous material is debrided when demarcation is apparent, and attempts are made to increase local blood flow. The latter involves the application of 2% nitroglycerin ointment (Nitrol ointment) to the base of the involved digits for 1 h, three times a day. Because of the good circulation that is generally present in the dorsal pedal and posterior tibial arteries, the possibility of obtaining complete healing of the lesions on the feet is excellent.

B.   Acute Spontaneous Arterial Thrombosis

1.   General Considerations

In spontaneous arterial thrombosis there is growth of a thrombus in situ, eventually completely occluding the lumen of the involved artery.

Etiologic factors.   A large number of agents may be responsible for thrombosis of arterial channels. Some of these are inflammatory in origin, such as thromboangiitis obliterans (see Section C, Chapter 11), polyarteritis nodosa and systemic lupus erythematosus (see Section C, Chapter 13), and mycotic arteritis; others are infectious (Fig. 12.3); while most are degenerative, typified by arteriosclerosis obliterans (see Section A, Chapter 11). There may also be a simple type of arterial thrombosis in which

little or no abnormal alterations occur in the walls of the affected arteries, as in essential thrombophilia [6]. Other conditions which may lead to spontaneous arterial thrombosis are cardiac arrhythmias, nephrotic syndrome, congestive heart failure, severe dehydration, prolonged immobilization, and increased coagulability of the blood secondary to administration of certain drugs, such as oral contraceptives.

Pathogenesis.   Spontaneous arterial thrombosis is generally the end result of a slowing of the systemic circulation and a loss of the axial stream in laminar flow pattern of the movement of the blood. This process ultimately results in complete stasis followed by occlusion of the vessel. Local changes responsible for such a sequence of events are atherosclerotic plaques producing stenosis of the vessel by encroachment upon its lumen; hemorrhage into the plaque, rapidly enlarging it; development of a clot on the surface of ulcerated plaques; arterial dissection causing projection of the involved side of the wall of the vessel into its lumen; and inward growth of clot in the cavity of an arterial aneurysm occluding the channel from which the lesion arises.

In certain infectious disorders, gangrene of a portion or of an entire digit may occur due to thrombosis of a digital artery or its branches, with the remainder of the arterial tree in the limb remaining normal. For example, this type of response has been reported in meningococcal (Fig. 12.3), staphylococcal, or streptococcal bacteremia, cholera, typhus fever, typhoid fever, trichinosis, and pneumonia. The etiologic agent may be exotoxins elaborated by the bacterial organisms which cause damage to the endothelium of the blood vessel. This change, together with the slowing of the bloodstream and the deposition of fibrin, may result in the initiation and growth of a thrombus that eventually obliterates the lumen of the involved artery.

2.   Clinical Manifestations

Findings associated with rapid arterial occlusion.   If obliteration of a critical artery occurs quickly, the clinical findings are, for the most part, similar to those observed in arterial embolism (see A-3, above), since in both condi-

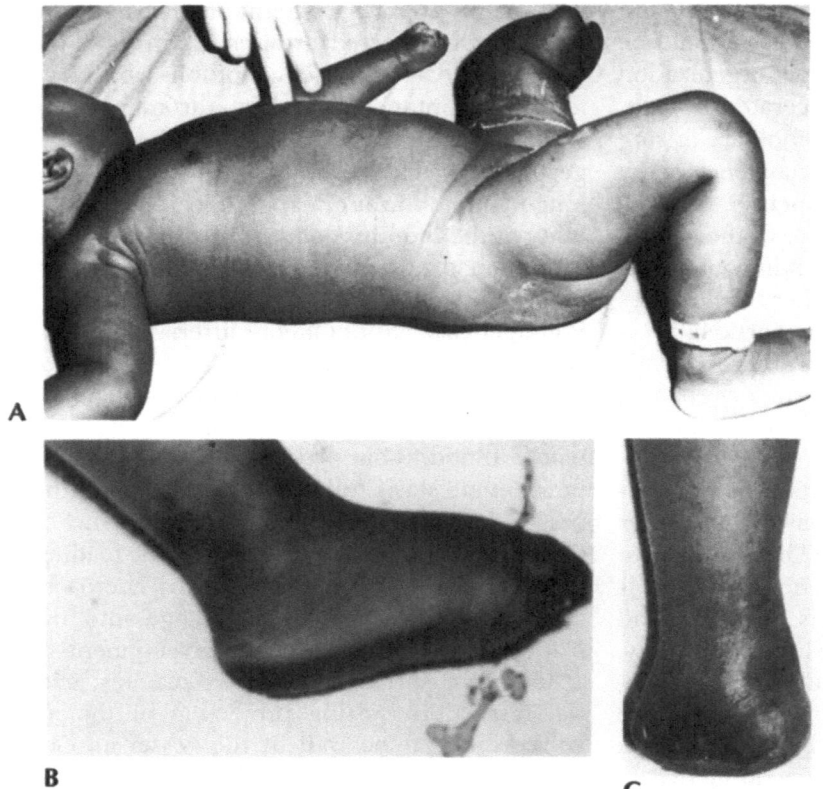

Fig. 12.3. Acute thrombosis of critical arteries as a result of meningococcic septicemia in infants. **A** Female, 1.5 years old, with gangrene of left foot, requiring a below-knee amputation. **B** Male, 1 year old, with gangrene of foot, requiring a Syme's amputation (**C**).

tions, initially marked ischemia of distal tissues exists. The abnormalities consist of pain in the distal portion of the limb, numbness, paresthesias in the digits, pallor, paresis or paralysis, coldness, absence of pulsations in distal arteries, and reduced or zero oscillometric readings. Arteriography is not necessary as a diagnostic tool.

If the rapidly forming thrombus is located in a diseased vessel, as in the case of arteriosclerosis obliterans, the severity of the clinical picture may quickly diminish because of the existence of a collateral circulation, previously developed in response to a chronic state of ischemia. After a delay, this secondary circulation assumes the function of delivering blood to the distal tissues, although generally not as efficiently as the normal vascular tree.

If the collateral vessels are poorly developed or if none is available, then the clinical picture of a rapidly forming arterial thrombus continues to resemble that of the untreated case of arterial embolism, even to the point of the appearance of necrosis of distal structures.

Findings associated with slow arterial occlusion. In most patients with arteriosclerosis obliterans, the obliterative process in the arterial tree in the lower limbs develops very slowly, so that an opportunity is afforded for the compensatory and simultaneous growth of collateral vessels; these then take over the function of supplying the tissues with blood. As a result, when complete occlusion of the main artery occurs, there may be no signs of ischemia of the skin, the only clinical indication of the presence of obliterative disease possibly being intermittent claudication. Hence, if the patient is leading a sedentary existence, he may only become aware of his condition when a routine examination reveals absent pulsations in the main arteries of the lower extremities.

If the pathologic process continues slowly until partial obliteration of the artery is present and then it is suddenly accelerated so as to cause complete occlusion, symptoms and signs of ischemia will appear, since suddenly thrusting the role of supplying the tissues with blood onto the available collateral circulation may find the latter temporarily inadequate for this task. However, after a short period of readjustment, the existing secondary arterial tree becomes efficient enough to cope with the situation and the symptoms and signs of acute anoxia disappear. This type of response is readily identified by the findings of decreased or absent arterial pulsations and corresponding changes in the oscillometric readings. However, nutritional circulation to the skin and its appendages appears adequate (see Chapter 6).

3. Differential Diagnosis

The clinical differentiation of arterial thrombosis from arterial embolism is of paramount importance, because the surgical approach to the two conditions is entirely different (see A-4, above, and B-4, below). In arterial embolism, there is generally an underlying cardiovascular condition which has the potential for liberation of particulate material into the general circulation (see A-1, above); such a situation does not necessarily exist in the case of arterial thrombosis. As a general rule, the degree of acute ischemia can be expected to be more marked in arterial embolism occurring in a limb with a previously normal arterial tree than in the case of a slowly developing arterial thrombosis, permitting the corresponding formation of some collateral circulation. Of importance in making the diagnosis of arterial thrombosis is a history of intermittent claudication in one or both lower limbs and of reduced or absent pulsations and oscillometric readings in them or the presence of such findings in the extremity not suffering from the acute occlusion. In arterial embolism, at least in the younger patient, no symptoms or signs of impaired local arterial circulation exist prior to the acute episode. Of course, in the elderly person, both arterial embolism and arteriosclerosis obliterans may coexist, thus making the identification of the cause of the local acute ischemia very difficult. A history of numerous sudden occlusions of arteries in other sites, such as the brain, spleen, and kidneys, generally indicates that the episodes of acute ischemia in the limbs are also on the basis of liberation of emboli into the bloodstream. However, it is necessary to point out that patients with arteriosclerosis obliter-

ans of the lower limbs, leading to sudden complete occlusion of critical arteries, frequently suffer from atherosclerosis in other vascular beds; this condition may lead to thrombosis with resulting clinical manifestations originating in such sites.

Rarely are the brachial artery and its two main branches occluded by spontaneous rapidly developing thrombi, the prevalent sites for such a process being the aortic bifurcation, the common and external iliac branches, and the arterial tree in the lower limbs. On the other hand, there is as much as a 15 percent incidence of peripheral arterial embolism involving the arterial tree in the upper extremities.

4. Treatment

When signs of severe ischemia are present, early treatment of spontaneous acute arterial thrombosis is similar to the therapeutic program for arterial embolism (see A-4, above), except that a thrombectomy is not performed. The reason for not attempting such a procedure is that on removal of the clot, a new one would invariably develop shortly thereafter. Furthermore, since the underlying mechanism is frequently atherosclerosis, subsequent repair of the artery could be difficult and, at times, impossible.

If it is considered imperative to reestablish circulation to a limb in order to prevent gangrene, then either a thromboendarterectomy or a reconstructive procedure should be carried out. The decision will rest on the same criteria discussed in D-2, Chapter 11, under the heading of restoration of arterial continuity with a graft. Arteriography is essential to assess the extent of the disease process, the degree of surgical reconstruction that is feasible, the adequacy of arterial inflow, and the status of the distal runoff.

References

1. Anderson WR, Richards AM: Evaluation of lower extremity muscle biopsies in the diagnosis of atheroembolism. Arch Pathol 86:535, 1968
2. Brenowitz JB, Gregory J, Edwards WS: Diagnosis and treatment of peripheral antheromatous emboli. J. Cardiovasc Surg 19:499, 1978

3. Fogarty TJ, Cranley JJ, Krause RJ, et al: A method for extraction of arterial emboli and thrombi. Surg Gynecol Obstet 116:241, 1963
4. Haimovici H: Peripheral arterial embolism: A study of 330 unselected cases of embolism of the extremities. Angiology 1:20, 1950
5. Hammarsten J, Holm J, Schersten T: Positive and negative effects of anticoagulant treatment during and after arterial embolectomy. J Cardiovasc Surg 19:373, 1978
6. Nygaard KK, Brown GE: Essential thrombophilia: Report of 5 cases. Arch Intern Med 59:82, 1937
7. Senn A, Althaus U: Revascularization syndrome after embolectomy. J Cardiovasc Surg 14:632, 1973
8. Washio M, Sakashita I, Nakamura C, et al: A new anticoagulant medication in cardiac valve replacement. J Cardiovasc Surg 19:455, 1978

Chapter 13

Clinical Entities with Both Vascular and Orthopedic Components

---

Part 1   Circulatory Disorders with Musculoskeletal Manifestations

---

Besides predominantly circulatory abnormalities, a number of vascular disorders also demonstrate significant changes in the skin and musculoskeletal structures of the limbs. This chapter deals with typical conditions which manifest such alterations.

A.   Posttraumatic Painful Vascular Disorders

In a number of functional vascular diseases, pain overshadows the other findings of sympathetic nervous system dysfunction. Examples of such a group of conditions are major causalgia, minor causalgia (causalgic states), post-traumatic vasomotor disorders (Sudeck's atrophy), and shoulder-hand syndrome. All of these entities are associated with alterations in the chemical constituents of the bones in the involved limb, contractures and other pathologic changes in the joints, and atrophy of the skin and voluntary muscles locally.

1.   Major Causalgia

Major causalgia is a vasospastic disorder which is characterized by local, agonizing, burning pain and extensive trophic changes in the integument.

Incidence and etiology.   Major causalgia is an important problem in the treatment of trauma since it occurs in about 2 percent of patients with peripheral nerve injury [30]. It most frequently follows trauma to median, ulnar, and sciatic nerves and is the result of an incomplete lesion, not transection. Injury to other nerves, such as the lower trunks of the brachial plexus and the popliteal and posterior tibial nerves, is also responsible for the appearance of major causalgia.

Typically, the disorder develops after penetrating wounds, although there are many other etiologic agents, such as fracture, a surgical procedure, application of a tight cast, a crush injury, contusion, a subcutaneous or intramuscular injection of a drug, and a third-degree burn.

Pathogenesis.   The mechanism responsible for the development of major causalgia has not been fully elucidated. Among the proposed theories is one which presupposes that there is a short-circuiting effect in the region of the injured segment of nerve which permits direct stimulation of sensory components in the latter by the continuous flow of sympathetic discharges. The afferent impulses initiated by such a process are transmitted to the thalamus where they are interpreted as pain. Another possibility is that the peripherally directed impulses from the artificial synapse cause liberation of neurokinin which produces the characteristic burning sensation. Finally, it has been suggested that infection in the wound or an irritable focus resulting from the trauma sets up an exaggerated state of activity in the spinal cord. The explanation for the widespread response following a localized stimulus is that reflex activation of even a single preganglionic fiber may result in synaptic contacts with as many as 32 postganglionic neurons.

There is no question that some of the findings noted in major causalgia are due to the superimposed state of disuse of the limb. The latter is a consequence of the fear of eliciting more pain with physical activity.

Clinical manifestations. Symptoms and signs of major causalgia may develop within several days of the time of injury (generally a war wound), or their appearance may be delayed for a number of weeks or even months. The most prominent complaint is the persistent, continuous, burning, violent pain, located in the involved hand or foot, especially the digits, the palm, or the sole of the foot. It is subject to exacerbations that may be provoked by emotional excitation, changes in environmental conditions, or cutaneous stimulation, such as contact with clothing or drafts of air. The symptoms originate at the site of injury and tend to spread over the full length of the limb, or they may even affect the entire side of the body.

The skin of the involved limb becomes shiny, red, thin, glossy, and devoid of wrinkles, and it no longer slides easily over the underlying structures but fuses with them. The muscles undergo fibrous changes and atrophy so that they are immovable; the joints become ankylosed. The bones show alterations, varying from slight generalized loss of density to the characteristic moth-eaten appearance of advanced osteoporosis. There may be tapering of the fingers, with the skin covering them becoming scaly and dry. Sudomotor and vasomotor disturbances are usually present in the later stage of the condition, manifested by hyperhidrosis, low skin temperature, increased respon-

siveness to cold, and cyanosis of the digits. Another finding is edema, in great part due to the dependent position and state of immobility in which the patient maintains the involved limb (Fig. 13.1). However, vasospasm may also contribute to the swelling by reducing local blood flow to all tissues, including the capillaries; the latter then become more permeable due to the resulting ischemia. The hair on the limb coarsens or disappears and the nails become brittle and ridged.

Major causalgia can be divided into three clinical states. In the first, reversible phase, there are manifestations of increased local blood flow, such as a high skin color, increased sweating, and soft-tissue edema, associated with the typical burning pain. In the second or dystrophic but still reversible stage, the pain becomes less, but the swelling extends to involve other tissues, at the same time changing its consistency to brawniness. The state of vasodilatation is replaced by one of vasoconstriction which is responsible for the findings already described. In the final or atrophic state, the changes are most marked in the integument, in the form of alterations in the skin, subcutaneous tissue, muscles, and joints, such abnormalities being irreversible. At this stage radiographic study generally demonstrates marked osteoporosis.

Treatment. The first approach to the management of major causalgia and other posttraumatic painful disorders is their prevention. This includes the care of those local lesions which could possibly act as a focus of irritation and thus initiate a reflex arc that produces and perpetuates a state of vasospasm. To accomplish such an aim, it is necessary to debride the wounds caused by trauma, remove foreign bodies, treat torn tendons, muscles, and ligaments surgically, evacuate hematomas, and adequately reduce and immobilize fractures. To control the associated pain, it may also be necessary to infiltrate hematomas in acute strain with procaine or even to produce regional nerve block. If there is obvious involvement of a major nerve, it may be necessary to expose the injured structure surgically, remove all traumatized soft tissues, and perform a neurolysis. Then the damaged portion of nerve is excised and end-to-end suture is carried out. Finally, attempts should be made to alleviate

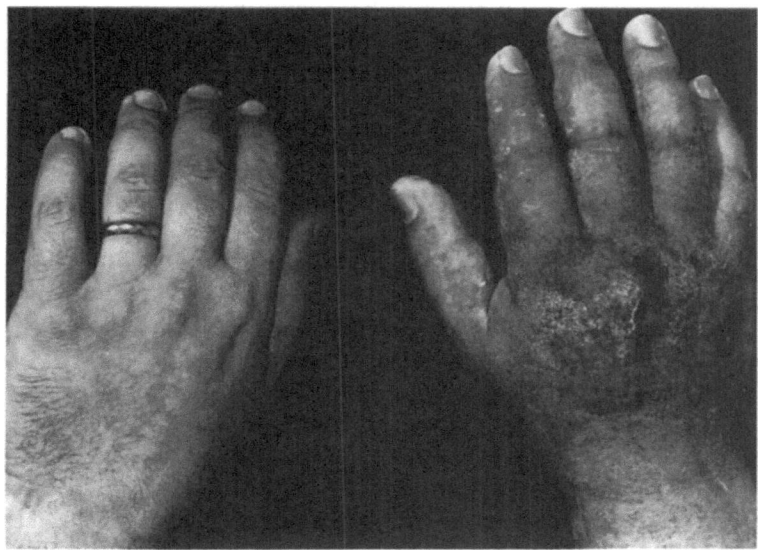

Fig. 13.1. Major causalgia produced by injury to the tissues of the right forearm, including partial transection of peripheral nerves. The predominant finding is swelling of the fingers and hand. The skin is scaly and dry.

fear and anxiety and to reassure the patient about the injury. This may reduce the possibility of a conscious or subconscious prolongation of a painful syndrome [16].

With regard to active therapy for major causalgia, it is essential to institute a program of exercises for the involved limb soon after the condition has developed, since, as already mentioned, disuse plays a significant role as an etiologic agent. However, such a measure must be preceded by attempts to control the pain, for otherwise there will be no cooperation on the part of the patient who is acutely aware of the fact that any movement aggravates the symptoms. Therefore, as preliminary steps, it may be necessary to use large doses of narcotics, steroids, or antiinflammatory drugs for this purpose. Also of value in this regard is repeated electric stimulation of the large A-delta fibers in the injured nerve proximal to the site of trauma for periods of 2 to 3 min, since this step may give relief from symptoms for several hours. The transcutaneous stimulating machine has likewise been used for this purpose.

Perineural infusion of the trigger areas with lidocaine (Xylocaine) may be effective in controlling the complaints. This is done by passing a large-bore needle through surgically prepared anesthetic skin, then inserting a flexible catheter through it, removing the needle, and leaving the catheter taped in place. In this manner, the areas of exquisite tenderness and pain

can be exposed to injections of 0.5 ml of 0.5% lidocaine with ephedrine every 3 h for several weeks. Only the sensory nerves are anesthetized by such a procedure.

If swelling is present, it is necessary to control this state before attempting a rehabilitative procedure. Complete bed rest with elevation of the affected limb may be required until the edema disappears. Then some type of elastic support is applied to prevent recurrence of the swelling, provided the patient will permit continuous application of pressure to the extremity. A salt-poor diet and oral diuretics may be used as adjunctive measures to maintain the limb edema-free.

The next step is to initiate a physical therapeutic program. In the case of the upper limb, traction and splints may be required if partial contractures are already present. Early treatment consists of gentle massage of the hand, followed by passive range of motion, and then directed active and resisted exercises of all the weak muscles. It is necessary to impress the patient with the need of repeating all the procedures by himself several times a day. Besides the local therapy, he should also be on a general conditioning program.

In the case of involvement of the lower limb, the patient should be encouraged to become ambulatory again as rapidly as possible, using crutches and canes at the beginning, but discarding them as soon as feasible. Weight bearing on the affected extremity is encouraged, and the patient is instructed in a proper gait, distributing his weight equally between the normal and the involved limb. Because of the beneficial effects of the buoyancy of water, walking in a pool may minimize the pain experienced on ambulation.

Together with a physical therapeutic program, attempts should be made to control vasospasm which is almost always present. To accomplish this, it may be necessary to perform daily paravertebral or stellate blocks for about a week. If, following each successive injection, there is a progressively increasing duration of benefit (which is significantly longer than the anticipated period of sympathetic anesthesia), there is a good possibility that such a procedure may be sufficient to produce permanent destruction of the existing reflex arc. On the other hand, if after a week's trial a satisfactory response is not noted, the treatment should be discontinued. In a limited number of patients, sympathectomy may be required in place of repeated paravertebral sympathetic blocks, as when there is immediate need for the elimination of excessive sympathetic tone. In others, alpha-receptor blocking agents, such as phenoxybenzamine (Dibenzyline), can be substituted as a means of controlling vasospasm.

Prognosis. Considerable deterioration of morale, emotional stability, and personality may be caused by major causalgia. In the more severe case, the patient assumes a defensive withdrawn attitude, his whole attention being focused on the agonizing pain in his involved limb. If left untreated for a prolonged period of time, the condition may even lead to drug addiction, chronic invalidism, and, at times, suicide. On the other hand, if the patient is intensively treated early enough, before irreversible alterations have occurred, there is an excellent possibility for restoration of normal function to the limb.

2. Posttraumatic Vasomotor Disorders (Sudeck's Atrophy)

Although injury to an extremity is generally followed by signs and symptoms which are readily explained on the basis of the trauma and the resultant dysfunction, in certain instances there are superimposed other changes which can only be accounted for on the assumption that some type of reflex vasomotor disorder has been initiated by the local tissue damage [21]. Involved in the reflex arc are the components of the sympathetic nervous system. Such a syndrome has been variously termed Sudeck's atrophy, acute atrophy of bone, posttraumatic osteoporosis, posttraumatic painful osteoporosis, traumatic arthritis, reflex nervous dystrophy, reflex sympathetic dystrophy, and, finally, posttraumatic vasomotor disorders (the designation adopted in this section).

Etiologic factors. The condition is unrelated to the extent or nature of the original trauma and may occur despite early competent treatment. It may appear after soft-tissue wounds, sprains, crushing injuries, simple or compound fractures of small or large bones, or as a consequence of infection.

Pathogenesis. In a sense, posttraumatic vasomotor disorders may be regarded as an excessive or abnormal response of an extremity to injury. A possible explanation for the development of the condition is that following trauma, overactivation of the central nervous system cell stations causes hyperactivity of the sympathetic nervous system reflex arcs; in turn, the resulting bombardment of impulses sets up a vicious cycle of reflexes, spreading upward, downward, and even across the spinal cord over an internuncial pool of many neuronal connections. At the same time, a constant circling of activity across the synapses perpetuates the various reflexes.

Among the structures involved in the process are the sympathetic motor neuron cells in the lateral horn of the cord which control vasomotor tone. As a consequence, vascular spasm is initiated in the microcirculation, which raises filtration pressure and results in the development of edema. The latter response is further accentuated by the increased capillary permeability due to the local state of ischemia, also produced by vasospasm. Augmented impulses likewise flow out of the pool to travel up the thalamic tract, causing an increase in the severity of the pain.

Clinical manifestations. The most common history elicited in posttraumatic vasomotor disorders is that of the sudden development of severe throbbing or burning, unrelenting pain in the affected hand or foot shortly after an injury, primarily experienced on weight bearing or during other types of physical activity. Other complaints are local tenderness and hyperesthesia. In some patients, the onset of the condition is insidious, and the pain is dull, aching, and diffuse in its distribution, being experienced at rest as well as with movement of the part or with emotional stimulation. On occasion, motor weakness may be present to the point of virtual paralysis.

Initially, the skin is warm, red, and dry. Pulses are bounding and oscillometric readings are high. Later, signs of increased sympathetic tone appear, in the form of reduced amplitude of peripheral pulses, decreased oscillometric readings, coldness and cyanotic rubor of the skin, and hyperhidrosis. Trophic changes vary, consisting mainly of atrophy of skin, subcutaneous tissue, muscles, joint structures, and bones. Edema occurs early in the inception of the condition (Fig. 13.2A). Transverse ridges appear on the nails.

During the initial phase, the patient may resist movement of the joints of the involved limb because of fear of eliciting pain, and so he maintains a guarded rigidity of the extremity. Later, after trophic changes have developed, mechanical alterations prevent return of function. The lack or delayed use of the limb, whether secondary to pain and vasomotor disturbances or to contractures of joints and atrophy of muscles and other structures, results in the most serious feature of posttraumatic vasomotor disorders—a functionless extremity.

Radiographic alterations. Changes in bone density appear rapidly (within 6 to 8 weeks) and frequently are extensive. Originally, spotty and cystic decalcification occurs in the bone beyond the location of the injury (patchy bone atrophy; osteoporosis), the foot and ankle being affected more often than the hand and wrist. Severe local pain is associated with the changes in the bone. Later, in the far-advanced case, a more diffuse process supervenes, resembling the generalized ground-glass appearance seen in disuse.

The alterations in the bone are induced in some manner by sympathetic nervous system reactions to external stimuli. According to one view [29], they result from the creation of a low pH in the vicinity of the involved bone due to the local irritation or trauma, a situation which promotes dissolution of mineral salts in the bone. Another proposal presupposes the existence of a sympathetic vasodilator mechanism which causes an increase in local blood flow, resulting in rapid removal of minerals from the bone, with production of progressive osteoporosis [16]. In this regard, an elevated oxygen saturation has been found in the veins of limbs affected by Sudeck's atrophy, an observation which has been attributed to increased arteriovenous shunting [2]. Finally, there appears to be good evidence that physical inactiv-

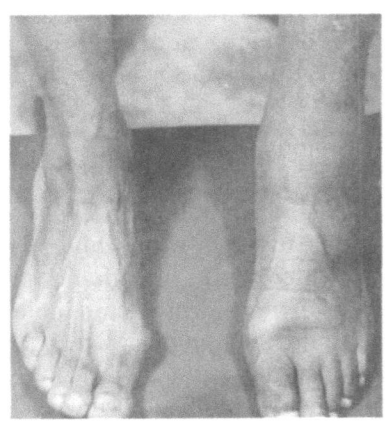 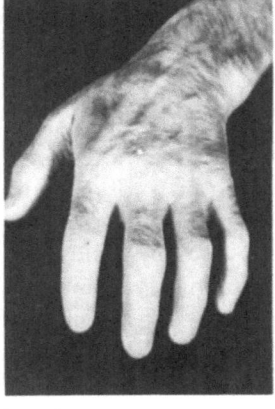

A   **B**

Fig. 13.2. **A** Posttraumatic vasomotor disturbance involving the left foot due to a soft-tissue injury. The prominent finding is edema, associated with other signs of increased sympathetic tone. **B** Shoulder-hand syndrome demonstrating stiffness, muscular atrophy, flexion deformity of the fingers, and trophic changes in the skin.

ity, resulting in disuse atrophy, also contributes to the abnormal changes in bone.

Treatment. The most important step in the therapeutic approach to posttraumatic vasomotor disorders is early institution of measures to restore normal function to the involved limb. As in the case of major causalgia (see A-1, above), the patient must understand the nature of the disorder to ensure cooperation in the treatment program, for initially the various steps may elicit pain, not infrequently, of a severe degree.

The physical therapeutic measures are similar to those outlined in the section on treatment of major causalgia (see above). Pain must be controlled by whatever means are effective, particularly when procedures to restore function are first initiated.

Most important in the treatment program is the repeated anesthetization of the efferent sympathetic pathways in order to interrupt sympathetic outflow. This can be accomplished either by continuous procaine ganglionic block or, infrequently, by ganglionectomy. In the case of the latter procedure, for the upper limb, the first to the fourth thoracic ganglia are decentralized, occasionally with simultaneous removal of the stellate ganglia, whereas for the lower limb, the first to the third lumbar ganglia are extirpated.

3. Shoulder-hand Syndrome

The shoulder-hand syndrome is a reflex neurovascular dystrophy affecting the shoulder and upper extremity and provoked by a number of different causes. Although the condition is believed by some workers to be related to posttraumatic vasomotor disorders [28], there are enough differences between the two to warrant presenting them as separate entities. The shoulder-hand syndrome has also been considered to fall into the category of minor causalgia.

Incidence and etiologic factors. The average age of patients developing the syndrome is about 63 years. Trauma to the upper limb, in the form of a sprain, a laceration, a fracture, or a tear of the rotator cuff, plays an important role in its development. However, there are a large number of other causative agents, such as cardiovascular disorders (including myocardial infarction and severe angina pectoris) and local tissue or regional lesions (including severe cervical disk degeneration and degenerative spondylosis). The syndrome has also been observed after hemiplegia and herpes zoster, among other disorders. It is of interest that whereas formerly the shoulder-hand syndrome was found in 10 to 20 percent of cases of myocardial infarction, it is much less frequent currently. The explanation for such a change may be the fact that there has been a liberalization of restriction of physical activity during the acute phase of myocardial infarction, in the form of the institution of a program of graded exercises.

Pathogenesis. In the shoulder-hand syndrome, the symptoms and signs presumably result from reflex stimulation of the sympathetic nerve supply. The afferent impulses are assumed to originate from some focus of irritation or from a site of injury in the limb, the heart, or the cerebral cortex [27]. In the case of myocardial infarction, the pathway probably involves the cardiac nerves, the impulses traversing this course to enter the cord at levels T1 to T4. With activation of the internuncial pool [15] at these locations in the cord by the strong impulses, there is a spread upward including stimulation of the anterior horn cells and downward to affect the sympathetic neurons of the lateral horn cells innervating the upper limb. As a consequence, disability of the shoulder muscles develops and signs of increased vasomotor tone appear in the hand.

Clinical manifestations. The abnormalities noted in the shoulder-hand syndrome consist of pain and tenderness in and limitation of motion of the shoulder, together with aching, paresthesia, swelling, increased sympathetic tone (cyanosis, coldness, hyperhidrosis), and limited mobility of the hand and fingers. Eventually the digits demonstrate stiffness, weakness, muscular atrophy, and flexion deformity (Fig. 13.2B). The assumption of a specific position is not required to precipitate an attack of pain, for symptoms are present at all times, even at rest. Such responses are in contrast with findings noted in neurovascular compression syndromes of the shoulder girdle (see Section B, below).

Shoulder-hand syndrome has been divided into several clinical stages. In the first, which lasts for about 3 to 6 months from the onset of the disability, the prominent findings are pain in the shoulder, loss of skin creases, non-pitting edema of the hand, and pain in this site. At the beginning, the cutaneous temperature and local blood flow are high, at which time the skin of the hand is colored pink or red. Later the hand becomes cyanotic or pale and the grip is weak. Trophic nail changes may be present, as well as x-ray findings of spotty or patchy ("ground-glass") osteoporosis of the head of the humerus, the carpus, and sometimes the phalanges. Stage 2 is typified by pain, stiffness, and limited movement of the involved limb, while complaints in the shoulder and swelling of the hand are generally absent. The hand is cold and the skin is thin and atrophic. The muscles also manifest atrophy, and the x-ray changes, first observed in stage 1, are present in an exaggerated form. After 6 to 9 months, the disorder progresses to the third or final stage in which digital contractures are prominent, associated with development of irreversible changes in the hand and permanent limitation of its mobility and similar alterations of the fingers and occasionally of the shoulder. The skin of the hand becomes smooth and glossy, and there is atrophy of subcutaneous tissue and intrinsic muscles. Local blood flow is diminished and cutaneous temperature continues to be low. Osteoporosis may now be observed in the bones of the entire limb. The fingers are generally fixed in flexion (clawhand) due to contraction of the palmar fascia, which resembles Dupuytren's contracture (see Section E, Chapter 14). In stage 3, the changes are frequently no longer capable of reversal and recovery cannot be expected.

In the case of myocardial infarction, the onset of the shoulder-hand syndrome occurs between 3 and 12 weeks following the acute episode. Either the left or the right upper limb, or both, may be involved. Generally the first manifestations are a painful shoulder and a sore, tender, swollen hand which becomes discolored and which initially is warmer than the opposite normal hand. The sequence of changes subsequently is similar to that described above.

Differential diagnosis. The shoulder-hand syndrome may simulate rheumatoid arthritis (see C-5, below), bursitis, periarthritis, acute arthritis, gout, and sclerodactylia. In the case of myocardial infarction, the symptoms of pain in the arm may be misdiagnosed as another episode of the original difficulty.

Treatment. The most important step in the management of the shoulder-hand syndrome is its prevention when conditions known to cause it exist. This involves alertness to the appearance of signs of neurovascular pain and reactions, institution of passive and active graded exercises of the limbs as prophylactic measures, local infiltration of tender points at the shoulder with procaine or hydrocortisone, and the avoidance of casts and of manipulation of parts in the presence of atypical pain or of findings of increased vasomotor tone.

The most effective active approaches to therapy for shoulder-hand syndrome involve the use of repeated stellate ganglion blocks and systemic administration of corticosteroids [26]. Generally the blocks, which are most helpful during the early phase of the disease, are given in the form of injections of 1% procaine solution, and as many as 14 can be used. However, if benefit beyond the duration of the anticipated therapeutic effect of the anesthetic does not become apparent after three or four treatments the program is discontinued. Corticosteroid medication is generally started with 30 mg of prednisone or prednisolone daily in divided doses. The amount is slowly reduced as improvement occurs.

To control the pain, 6 to 8 g of salicylates may be given daily in divided doses. If the symptoms are severe, codeine or other narcotics may have to be administered.

Another most important aspect of the treatment regimen is the institution of a physical therapeutic program, involving local heat and massage and passive assistive and active exercises of the shoulder and hand. This approach helps overcome the tendency to contracture and facilitates return of function. Treatment is continued until full range of motion is regained. At the same time, if at all possible, treatment of the cause of the shoulder-hand syndrome is attempted. Such orthopedic measures as shoulder manipulation under anesthesia and application of casts are not helpful and may even aggravate the symptoms.

Psychotherapy has been found to be of special benefit to those patients who manifest passivity and expect others to get them well, demonstrating no signs of motivation in counteracting the existing difficulties. In order to overcome such inertia, it may be necessary to offer repeated encouragement. If a definite emotional disorder is the basic etiologic factor, it may be necessary to have a psychiatric consultation and treatment.

Prognosis. The severity of the shoulder-hand syndrome is not always proportionate to the seriousness of the provocative agent. The disorder may resolve spontaneously at any time without residual changes or disability, or some of the contractures of the joints of the fingers may persist for many years. In general, the best results can be expected in those patients in whom the condition has been diagnosed early in its inception and active treatment begun immediately. Without therapy, the outcome is unpredictable.

In the case of the shoulder-hand syndrome associated with myocardial infarction, the disability is self-limited and the prognosis is usually good. The clawhand does not develop. Exercise of the shoulder and fingers soon after the onset of the attack of myocardial infarction and continued during the early stages of the shoulder-hand syndrome markedly reduces the severity of the latter [12].

4. Postamputation Fingers Syndrome

In some instances, following surgical removal of fingers, the stumps develop a cyanotic rubor and become sensitive to a low environmental temperature. Tenderness and burning pain are present locally and marked hyperesthesia exists. To this state has been given the designation, postamputation fingers syndrome, an entity which is included in the category of minor causalgia. No theory has been offered to explain the appearance of signs of severe vasomotor disturbance following a generally un-

complicated, relatively minor surgical procedure.

B. Neurovascular Compression Syndromes of the Shoulder Girdle

A number of neurovascular compression syndromes involving the upper limbs are known by such terms as neurovascular compression syndromes of the shoulder girdle, thoracic outlet syndrome, thoracic inlet syndrome, and shoulder girdle compression syndrome. The clinical manifestations found in these conditions result from intermittent compression of the brachial plexus and/or subclavian artery or vein either behind the scalenus anticus muscle, between the clavicle and the first rib, or beneath the pectoralis minor muscle.

The clinical entities included in the category of neurovascular compression syndromes of the shoulder girdle are the cervical rib, scalenus anticus, costoclavicular, hyperabduction, and scapulocostal syndromes. Since many of the symptoms and signs are common to all of them, it has been proposed that collectively they should be considered as a single clinical entity. However, opposed to this point of view is the fact that the basic mechanisms responsible for the various syndromes vary; moreover, the type of therapeutic correction of the conditions is not the same since each is dependent on the existence of a different specific causative agent. For these reasons and because the entities are well known by their individual names, they will thus be presented below.

1. Anatomic Considerations

Certain anatomic relationships are important in the understanding of the development of the different syndromes (Fig. 13.3). First is the fact that nerves, arteries, and veins must leave the thorax to enter the upper limbs through an outlet which is bounded by bone and muscle. Of these neurovascular structures, the subclavian artery takes a course which requires arching over the first rib, behind the scalenus anticus and in front of the scalenus medius muscle. It then passes under the subclavius muscle and the clavicle to enter the axilla be-

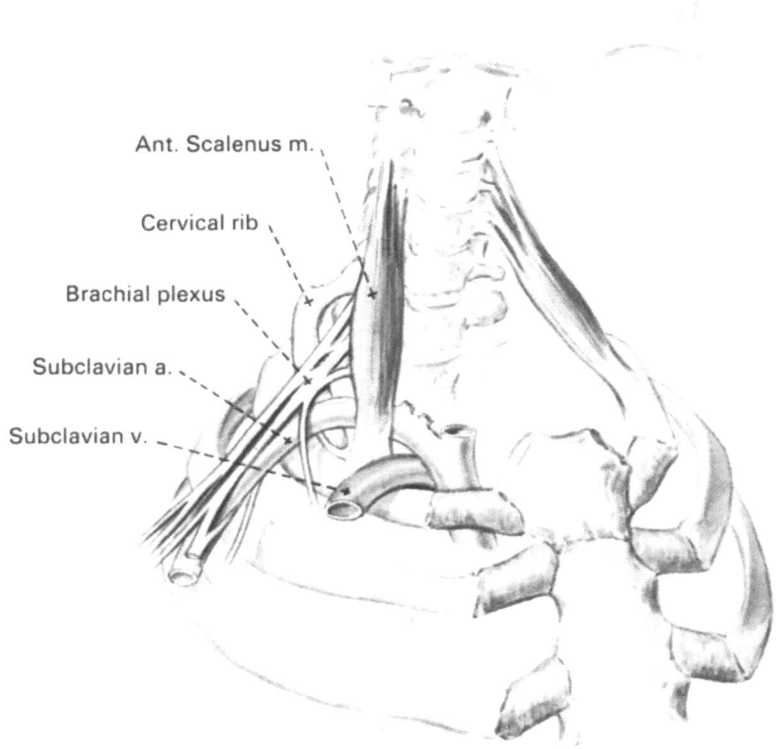

Ant. Scalenus m.

Cervical rib

Brachial plexus

Subclavian a.

Subclavian v.

Fig. 13.3. Normal anatomic relationships between the neurovascular structures and the scalenus anticus muscle in the neck. From Abramson DI: Diagnosis and Treatment of Peripheral Vascular Disorders. New York, Hoeber-Harper, 1956. Reproduced with permission.

neath the pectoralis minor muscle. The subclavian vein has a similar course except that it passes anteriorly rather than posteriorly to the scalenus anticus muscle.

The scalenus anticus muscle may play an important role in the production of compression of the neurovascular structures. It arises from the anterior tubercles of the transverse processes of the third to the sixth cervical vertebrae and descends vertically to be inserted into the inner border of the first thoracic rib (Fig. 13.3). When it contracts, as in respiration, it elevates the first rib. An anatomic relationship of significance is that the brachial plexus and subclavian artery pass behind the scalenus anticus muscle to its outer margin and then cross over the first rib.

Another structure which may contribute to the development of a neurovascular compression syndrome is a cervical rib (Fig. 13.3). This anomaly may take the form of a short osseous structure which extends just beyond the transverse process, with or without a free end, or it may be an almost complete or complete rib, with a true cartilage which unites with the cartilage of the first thoracic rib. Cervical ribs are found in the posterior triangle of the neck, a region which also contains the third portion of the subclavian artery, the subclavian vein, and the brachial plexus. When such structures are present, they tend to elevate the floor of the space between the scalene muscles and thus cause the brachial plexus to be displaced forward against the subclavian artery.

Finally, the vertebral fasciae may also play a role in the production of a neurovascular compression syndrome. The prevertebral fascia is a firm membrane located in front of the prevertebral musculature which binds down the splenius, levator scapulae, scalenus posticus, scalenus medius, and scalenus anticus muscles; the subclavian artery; and the three trunks of the brachial plexus, with accompanying loops of the cervical plexus. It is fixed to the anterior bodies of the cervical vertebrae and is attached to the clavicle. The postvertebral fascia is fixed to the ligamentum nuchal line of the occiput, the mastoid process of the temporal bone, and the inferior border of the mandible.

2. Clinical Manifestations

Symptoms and signs common to all neurovascular compression syndromes of the shoulder girdle. The severity of the clinical abnormalities associated with these entities depends upon the frequency, duration, and degree of pressure on the subclavian or axillary vessels and the lower cords of the brachial plexus. The symptomatology consists of pain in the fingers, hand, forearm, arm, and shoulder and paresthesias located in the area of distribution of C8 and T1. There may also be intermittent aching and numbness. In addition, signs of stimulation of the sympathetic nervous system are present in the hand, consisting of blanching, cyanosis, and increased sweating.

Cervical rib syndrome. This is one of the more common of the neurovascular compression entities of the shoulder girdle. In it the neurovascular structures are compressed primarily by an anomalous cervical rib and secondarily by the scalene muscles. The condition is more prevalent in women than in men and usually appears during the second to the fourth decades of life.

The local findings in cervical rib syndrome consist of tenderness, fullness, and a visible palpable deformity (the anomalous rib) in the supraclavicular fossa. Pressure to this area frequently elicits pain that radiates down the forearm along the course of the ulnar nerve; at times, there may be radial nerve distribution of the symptoms.

Clinical manifestations of compression of nervous elements are pain in the neck, shoulders, and upper limb; tenderness and heaviness of the arm; muscular weakness; atrophy of the thenar eminence and interossei muscles; and paresthesia and numbness in the hand. Sensory changes are the most common abnormalities.

Many of the symptoms are intensified by physical activity and are generally more severe at the end of the day when retiring. Such maneuvers as extension and lateral bending of the neck, rotation of the head, downward pull of the shoulders, and deep inspiration may produce referred pain.

Vascular changes and sympathetic overactivity take the form of coldness, duskiness, blanching, and hyperhidrosis of the hand and Raynaud's syndrome. With further compression and then destruction of the cervical sympathetic fibers in the trunks of the brachial plexus, a Horner's syndrome may develop. This consists of local loss of perspiration, constriction of the pupil, enophthalmos, and ptosis of the eyelid. Adson's maneuver, which is described below, is generally positive in cervical rib syndrome.

Scalenus anticus syndrome. This condition is also found primarily in women. Sensory disturbances are frequently noted, chiefly in the distribution of the ulnar nerve. Motor findings may be present but rarely as the only manifestation of the syndrome. There may be various signs of vascular abnormalities but no frank gangrene or ischemic changes. Otherwise, the clinical manifestations are similar to those of the cervical rib syndrome (see above) except for the absence of an osseous mass in the supraclavicular fossa. An associated finding may be a hypertrophied scalenus anticus muscle.

The Adson's maneuver, which is generally positive in scalenus anticus syndrome, consists of having the patient take a deep breath, hold it, and then rotate and hyperextend the head toward the affected side. If obstruction of the subclavian artery occurs with the maneuver, the pulse at the wrist becomes weak or disappears and the oscillometric readings at the level of the forearm either become very small or zero. If only partial occlusion is produced, a systolic bruit may be heard at the base of the neck, above the sternocleidal junction. It is necessary to point out, however, that too much reliance upon the results obtained with the Adson's maneuver is not justified.

Scapulocostal syndrome. This is a symptom complex consisting of unilateral involvement of the shoulder and the superior portion of the scapula, with radiation of pain patterns into the head and neck, the deltoid muscle, and the arm and hand. Common to the condition is the presence of "trigger points" at the superior vertebral angle of the scapula or at the base of its spinous process. Postural changes with round shoulderness and drooping of the shoulder girdle are the underlying etiologic factors in the scapulocostal syndrome. The condition may also result from an improper bed posture produced by the use of high pillows which causes the shoulders to sag and the head to be drawn to one side.

Costoclavicular syndrome. In this condition there is a reduction in the space between the clavicle and the first rib, causing compression of the neurovascular structures. Such a situation develops if the shoulders are forcibly retracted, as when carrying a heavy pack on the back. The symptoms are similar to those present in the cervical rib syndrome, consisting generally of pain, numbness, and swelling of the hand and weakness of the arm.

The costoclavicular maneuver is generally positive in the costoclavicular syndrome. The test consists of assuming the exaggerated military position with the shoulders drawn downward and backward. This narrows the costoclavicular space by approximating the clavicle to the first rib, thus compressing the neurovascular structures between them. If, as a consequence, considerable pressure is placed on the subclavian artery, radial artery pulsations at the wrist will either be reduced in amplitude or even obliterated, with reproduction of symptoms in the upper limb, particularly the hand. Again, as in the case of the Adson's maneuver (see above), damping of the pulse may be produced by the costoclavicular maneuver in many normal people. Such individuals do not have symptoms because in their usual posture, no pressure is exerted on the neurovascular structures. In contrast, in the patient with the costoclavicular syndrome, there is frequently a history of some type of injury, such as fracture of the clavicle, with subsequent compression of the subclavian vessels or brachial plexus.

Hyperabduction syndrome. This state is generally found in persons who sleep with their arms above their heads or assume this position at work (as, for example, people who rivet the under surface of airplane wings, paint ceilings, or spend time in repair pits under automobiles). The syndrome is caused by compression of the neurovascular structures by the hyperabducted position. The clinical manifestations consist of pain or aching in the hand, arm, or shoulder and numbness, paresthesia, swelling, and rubor of the hand. The hyperabduction maneuver, which involves elevation of the upper limb sideward beyond 90°, almost invariably produces obliteration of the pulse at the wrist. However, a similar response is noted in many normal individuals who do not have any symptoms or signs of the hyperabduction syndrome.

There are two potential sites of compression of the subclavian vessels and brachial plexus in the hyperabduction syndrome [32]. One is the point at which the neurovascular structures pass beneath the tendon of the pectoralis minor muscle and under the coracoid process and the other is the retroclavicular space between the clavicle and first rib, which is diminished to a variable degree by hyperabduction.

General diagnostic laboratory procedures. Roentgenograms of the chest, shoulder, and cervical spine are very helpful in determining the presence of a cervical rib. Antegrade arteriography (Fig. 13.4) is essential as a preliminary test if some type of surgical procedure is being contemplated for any one of the syndromes, since it offers an excellent opportunity to assess the arterial flow in the subclavian artery during the performance of the various clinical maneuvers (see above). In such a manner, the amount and significance of compression and obstruction of this vessel can be clearly determined. Also of importance is the fact that the data are collected under conditons which simulate the normal working routine, a situation difficult to reproduce on the operating table in the presence of sterile precautions.

Among other laboratory procedures is contrast venography, which is a valuable preoperative tool in the study of the patency of the subclavian vein with the upper limb being placed in positions which produce the symptomatology. Initially a record is taken with the arm by the side of the patient, followed by placing it in 120° abduction at the shoulder joint.

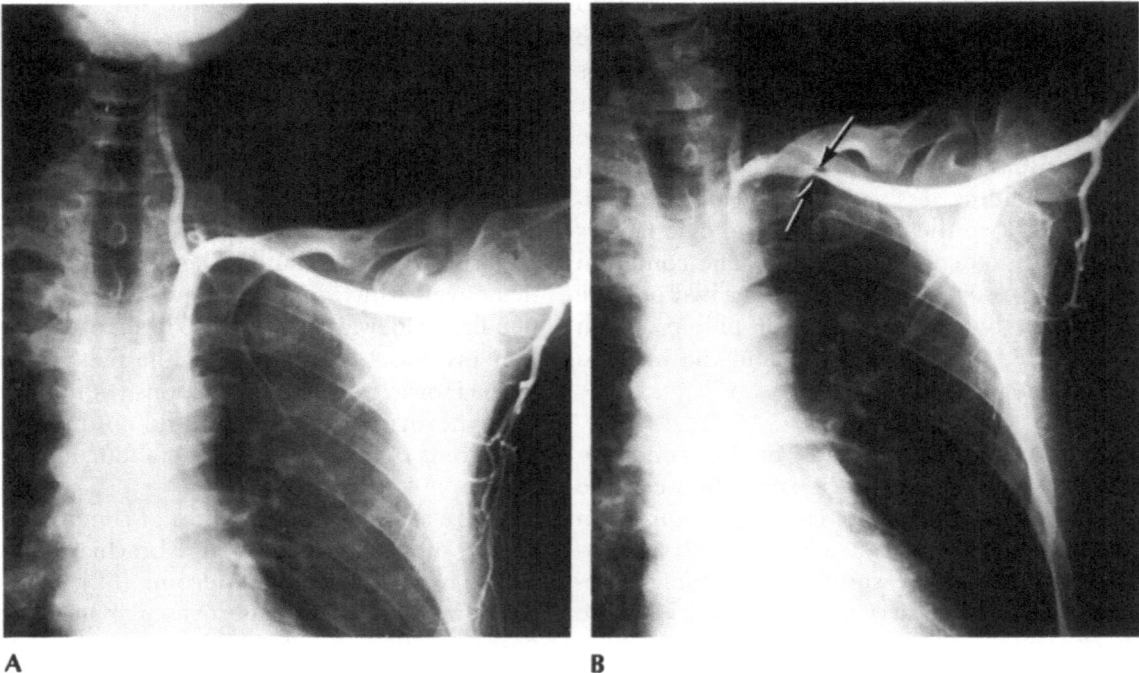

A   **B**

Fig. 13.4. Arteriograms of upper limb in a patient with a neurovascular compression syndrome. **A** Normal appearance of left subclavian artery. **B** Partial obliteration of the vessel *(arrows)* caused by the Adson's maneuver. From Abramson DI: Vascular Disorders of the Extremities, Hagerstown, Md, Harper & Row, 1974. Reproduced with permission.

Radiologic evidence of venous compression is present when there is narrowing of the axillary–subclavian vein in the region of the root of the neck, together with dilatation of the vessel proximal to the site of venous narrowing and signs of interference with movement of the radiopaque material through the vein. The main site of compression of the vessel is generally the space between the first rib and the clavicle, possibly due to the constrictive effects on the subclavian vein of the costocoracoid ligament and the subclavius muscle.

Also of great value in making a diagnosis of neurovascular compression syndrome of the shoulder girdle is the presence of a significantly reduced ulnar nerve conduction velocity measured across the outlet, i.e., from the neck to the hand. In contrast, the conventional way of obtaining the readings, using two points of reference located on the upper limb, may give normal results even in the presence of a definite neurovascular compression syndrome of the shoulder girdle.

3. Differential Diagnosis

Neurovascular compression syndromes of the shoulder girdle may mimic many conditions which produce symptoms and signs in the upper limbs.

Angina pectoris. Stretching or compression of neurovascular structures in the neck may cause complaints that are confused with those of coronary artery disease. Both conditions share the same dermatomal distribution of the pain: the heart, arms, and chest wall, which sites are innervated by afferent fibers situated in T2 to T5 segments of the spinal cord. The differentiation is made by eliminating the possibility of coronary artery disease using exercise stress testing and, on occasion, even coronary angiography. Also of importance is a reduction in ulnar nerve conduction velocity, observed in neurovascular compression syndromes, but not in angina pectoris. Electrocardiographic abnormalities are, of course, also very important in the differential diagnosis.

Paralytic brachial neuritis. This condition first produces aching or boring pain about the shoulder and extending to the neck or upper limb, which is aggravated by movement. Weakness or paralysis of the deltoid, supraspinatus, and infraspinatus muscles occurs several hours or days later, associated with atrophy and decreased reflexes. Sensory loss is slight.

Postural myoneuralgia. This condition [10], also known as acroparesthesia, tired arm syndrome, nocturnal dysesthesia, among others, consists of paresthesia and pain in the arms and hands, usually aggravated by rest and relieved by physical activity. It is most frequently observed in women suffering from severe cervical-thoracic scoliosis. The chief complaint of paresthesia may be present in any or all the fingers of either one or both limbs and may be accompanied by pain. It may also be referred to the head, neck, and thorax.

The symptoms are intermittent and generally chronic, and the attacks may last for minutes, hours, days, and even weeks. The discomfort is often associated with immobility, especially during the night. Daytime activity requiring long periods of elevation of the upper limbs usually exaggerates the nocturnal difficulties. There may be swelling of the hands, loss of strength, stiffness, and awkwardness in carrying out fine movements, especially early in the morning.

The most frequent sign in postural myoneuralgia is tilt of the shoulder girdle, which can usually be straightened at will. The spine may be curved laterally and the shoulders are often stooped. Radiographic examination may reveal structural scoliosis, hemivertebrae, or other bony abnormalities. Myalgia is most commonly found over the upper and middle thirds of the trapezius and the insertion of the levator scapulae, at the superior angle of the scapula. A significant sign is the appearance of a bruit over the subclavian artery, just below the clavicular midpoint, when the upper limb is gradually raised to abduct the humerus 90°, with the elbow flexed 90°.

Miscellaneous conditions. There are a number of other disorders which may mimic the neurologic manifestations found in the neurovascular compression syndromes of the shoulder girdle.

Among these are protruded cervical disks, cervical osteoarthritis, and cord tumors or exostoses of the laminae compressing various roots of the cervicobrachial plexus. Of importance as a differential point is that the neurologic manifestations of the compression syndromes are usually confined to involvement of the eighth cervical and first thoracic roots, whereas a protruded cervical disk usually affects C5 or C6. In the case of cervical arthritis, the involvement is generally more diffuse. Other conditions to be considered are anxiety tension states, carpal tunnel syndrome in the wrist, and inflamed or traumatized soft tissues in the form of bursitis, myositis, and fibrositis. However, these should offer no real difficulty in differentiation from neurovascular compression syndromes.

The vascular manifestations of the neurovascular compression syndromes of the shoulder girdle may be mimicked by conditions in which there is organic obstruction of the main arterial tree in the upper limbs, such as coarctation of the aorta, aortic arch disease, thromboangiitis obliterans, subclavian steal syndrome, and extrinsic compression of arteries by tumors. Since Raynaud's phenomenon may be part of the clinical picture of the different syndromes, Raynaud's disease must also be considered in the differential diagnosis.

4. Neurovascular Complications

Serious sequelae may result from chronic neurovascular compression syndromes, primarily as a consequence of permanent damage to the components of the brachial plexus or of abnormalities developing in the subclavian artery and vein. The principal etiologic factor is the persistent or repeated intermittent compression or stretching of these neurovascular structures. However, with regard to thrombosis of the subclavian artery (see below), there is a possibility that vasospasm of this vessel, initiated by irritation of sympathetic fibers in the trunks of the brachial plexus, is also responsible. Persistence of such a state almost invariably results in the development of a clot in the involved segment of vessel.

Thrombosis of subclavian artery. An occlusion of this vessel may or may not produce trophic changes in the hand, depending on both the rate at which the obstructive process progresses and the growth, efficiency, and extent of the collateral circulation which forms in response to chronic ischemia of distal tissues. With sudden acute anoxia of fingers, there may be signs of trophic disturbances even to the point of gangrene of the finger tips. Generally the latter change is observed in patients who have had symptoms for a long time before objective findings of a compromised arterial blood supply appear, although, on occasion, ischemic necrosis of the skin of the hand may be the initial indication of the presence of a cervical rib or a scalenus anticus syndrome. In the majority of patients, however, there is a slow occlusion of the subclavian artery, with the result that no nutritional lesions develop; instead, besides the symptoms mentioned above, pain may be experienced on exercising the muscles of the involved limb—the counterpart of intermittent claudication in the lower extremities.

Peripheral embolization. Another complication of neurovascular compression syndromes of the shoulder girdle is liberation of peripheral emboli which occlude distal arteries in the hand. These originate either in a thrombus, a poststenotic dilatation, or an aneurysmal sac, all usually located in the third portion of the subclavian artery.

A poststenotic dilatation is found distal to a partial occlusion of a segment of vessel, generally in patients with a complete cervical rib. It takes the form of persistent fusiform enlargement of the artery, but with its wall remaining grossly intact and without intimal disruption or intraluminal thrombosis. It is attributed to compression of the subclavian artery between the rib and the scalenus anticus muscle. The mechanism responsible for its production is probably as follows: When an artery becomes stenotic to the extent of about 50 percent of its normal lumen size, the resulting turbulence below the partial obstruction sets up vibratory waves or eddy currents which eventually lead to tissue fatigue of the vessel wall, followed by dilatation. The resulting increase in distensibility may be due to weakness of elastin fibers in the arterial wall [18]. Some correlation appears to exist between the amount of increase

in distensibility and the intensity of the murmur caused by the stenosis.

The poststenotic dilatation may be complicated by the development of an aneurysm in the site of involvement. In the latter type of lesion, localized weakening and disruption of the vessel wall occur, together with the formation of mural thrombi. The aneurysm is usually on the posterior surface of the artery, not infrequently in relation to exostosis on the first thoracic rib. The etiologic agent is some type of repeated mechanical trauma to the already dilated segment of subclavian artery. It is possible that the injury is sustained by a scissorlike action between the clavicle and the first rib, produced by respiration and shoulder movements [20].

Thrombosis of subclavian vein. When intermittent compression of the subclavian vein persists, eventually occlusion of this vessel will occur. Under such circumstances, the upper limb may become swollen and painful, and a prominent superficial venous network may develop on the arm and adjoining chest wall, the clinical manifestations being similar to those associated with primary thrombosis of the subclavian vein (see B-2, Chapter 18).

5. Treatment

Medical approach. The initial therapeutic regimen for neurovascular compression syndromes is medical, combined in some instances with psychiatric counseling. All patients should have a 4 to 12 weeks' trial of physical therapy [17]. This consists of radiant heat for 30 min, deep stroking and kneading massage to the neck and upper back to relieve muscle spasm, and corrective exercises to strengthen the muscles that elevate the shoulders and maintain good posture. The shoulders should be held in a neutral position—not too high or too low and not slumped forward or pushed backward. It should be stressed to the patient that he must make every effort to avoid positions or activities that aggravate his discomfort. If the scalenus anticus muscle is taut and tender, an injection of local anesthetic into it may bring relief from symptoms. A similar response may follow anesthetization of the stellate ganglion. At the same time, the patient must be reassured that the condition is not likely to progress or cause serious disability; this will help relieve some of the associated anxiety. Under such a conservative regimen, the great majority of individuals with mild to moderate symptoms and signs of neurovascular compression syndromes of the shoulder girdle will show significant clinical improvement in their condition.

Surgical approach. Before considering the possibility of some type of operative procedure, it is essential to weigh carefully the amount of incapacity and the patient's emotional stability. Moreover, it can be expected that satisfactory results from surgery will only be noted in people who preoperatively manifested clear-cut objective signs. Among the reasons for failure of surgical treatment in some patients is the difficulty in establishing a proper preoperative diagnosis, with the result that not all etiologic factors are dealt with during the operative procedure. Another is that some patients suffering from neurovascular compression syndromes may have strongly neurotic personality traits, a factor that adversely affects the outcome of surgery. Because of such complicating factors, operative intervention should only be utilized for the small percentage of individuals with serious involvement who have received no benefit from an intensive course of conservative management (see above).

The goal of surgical treatment is decompression of the neurovascular structures in the neck. This can be accomplished by skeletal traction or by removal of any of the following structures or a combination of them: bony anomalies and fibrotendinous bands; a segment of the scalenus anticus muscle; the clavicle; and the first rib. At the same time, it is mandatory to explore thoroughly the subclavian artery and vein and the nerve trunks in the area.

Skeletal traction is accomplished using a conventional skull traction apparatus and attaching weights (2.3 to 4.6 kg; 5 to 10 lb) at the free ends. Symptoms associated with the scalenus anticus syndrome and the scapulocostal syndrome may disappear within 6 to 8 h after traction is instituted; nevertheless, the procedure should be maintained for 10 days. Subsequently a cervical collar should be worn for 2 weeks, and heavy lifting should be avoided for at least the following month.

Resection of the distal portion of the scalenus anticus muscle is generally applicable to the scalenus anticus syndrome, provided this structure is found to be markedly hypertrophied [6]. The procedure may also be helpful in the cervical rib syndrome. However, if the rib is completely formed and is situated high in the neck, this structure should be removed at the same time; otherwise, it is left intact. Fibrous bands which might conceivably exert pressure on the vessels or the brachial plexus should be divided.

Claviculectomy is of value for selected patients with the costoclavicular syndrome [14]. Of importance is the fact that it can be utilized without producing functional derangement of the shoulder girdle. Complete removal of the periosteum is carried out at the same time so as to prevent regeneration, in some instances, in conjunction with anterior scalenotomy.

In the case of the costoclavicular syndrome, the costoclavicular space is effectively enlarged by extraperiosteal removal of the first rib alone or together with anterior scalenotomy. Relief can be expected in a large percentage of cases, particularly if the complaints are mostly neurologic. The decision to carry out the procedure should depend upon the results of the "finger-pinch" test [3]. This is performed at the time of operation in the following manner: The tip of the surgeon's index finger is placed alongside the subclavian artery and between the clavicle and first rib. If the finger is pinched when the patient's shoulder is forced backward and depressed, the test is considered positive and the first rib should be removed. The procedure does not deform or disable the patient.

Surgical treatment of complications. Therapy for the poststenotic dilatation of the subclavian artery or the superimposed aneurysm requires several approaches. First the cervical rib and the exostosis on the first thoracic rib must be surgically removed and the scalenus anticus muscle divided. Then direct arterial reconstruction must be performed after the involved segment of vessel is excised [20]. If the latter step is not carried out, the movement of the clavicle may dislodge other clots which invariably develop in the lesions months and years after control of the original difficulty. Such a situation is frequently followed by repeated episodes of peripheral embolization, eventually producing obliteration of critical vessels in the arm and forearm and possibly gangrene of the hand.

C. Connective Tissue Disorders

A number of the connective tissue (collagen) diseases are associated with significant structural changes in the integument, particularly the bones and joints. Aside from some general remarks concerning each entity, the discussion below is limited to the vascular and orthopedic changes in the limbs found in each of these conditions, together with the pathologic alterations.

1. Progressive Systemic Sclerosis

Progressive systemic sclerosis (generalized scleroderma) is a multisystem and multistage disease whose pathologic effects on skin, joints, heart, and kidneys are due to local vascular obstruction and collagen proliferation. The latter is laid down in concentric rings around blood vessels making up the microcirculation, as well as in nonvascular tissues such as the supporting structure of the skin.

Generalized scleroderma occurs in two forms: diffuse scleroderma and acrosclerosis. In the former, despite the absence of clinical vascular manifestations, the prognosis is poor, with death generally occurring within 2 years. Acrosclerosis usually follows a slow course, although at times it may be rapidly progressive.

Vascular alterations. A common finding in acrosclerosis is Raynaud's syndrome which may precede the cutaneous (Fig. 6.1D) and visceral changes by many years. Calcinosis cutis (see A-2, Chapter 9) is found late in the disease. Some patients develop telangiectasis of the face and trunk and occasionally angiomatous lesions on the mucous membranes which must be differentiated from Rendu-Osler-Weber disease.

Indolent ulcers, which are shallow and almost painless, are not infrequently found in acrosclerosis. In the upper limbs, the lesions are located on the tips of the fingers and, less often, on the elbows. In the lower limbs, they are present on the outer aspect of the legs above the external malleolus, on the toes, and on the knees. The associated typical alterations in the consistency of the skin, the loss of the normal wrinkling over the joints of the digits, and the poor therapeutic response should all be helpful in making the proper diagnosis. The rare ulcerations, as well as the superficial gangrene which is occasionally present, result from the existing local ischemic state, due both to a cutaneous angiitis and to a gradual compression of the cutaneous microcirculation by the firm adherence of the skin to the subcutaneous tissue. No impairment of blood flow is present in the main arterial tree.

Musculoskeletal manifestations. Patients with acrosclerosis suffer variable loss of function of the joints because of the pathologic changes in the overlying skin. Histologically, these consist of an increase in and a swelling of the collagenous connective tissue, with fragmentation and swelling of the elastic fibers in the cutis. The first clinical complaint is frequently joint swelling, associated with stiffness and pain. Hands and fingers are often edematous and puffy. Flexion deformities may occur, and at times a typical clawhand will develop.

2. Polyarteritis Nodosa

Polyarteritis nodosa is a generalized vascular disease affecting particularly medium-sized arteries in various portions of the body, associated with systemic responses. The cause of the difficulty has not been determined, although several theories have been suggested, among them the factor of hypersensitivity. However, the possibility has not been excluded that there is a hypersensitivity angiitis which resembles but is not identical with polyarteritis nodosa [4].

Pathologic alterations. Histologic changes are found in almost all tissues and organs, but particularly in the kidneys, heart, liver, and, less frequently, in the spleen, peripheral nerves, skin, and brain [13]. Typically, the gross changes are hemorrhage, thrombosis, infarction, and aneurysmal dilatation. The histologic changes consist of an acute arteritis, following which there are degeneration of the media and proliferation of the intima, partial obstruction of the lumen of the vessel, and then thrombosis. With loss of local blood supply, infarction occurs, the involved segment eventually being replaced by fibrous tissue. Hemorrhage or small aneurysms may develop as a result of complete or partial destruction of the vessel wall. Common findings are aggregations of neutrophilic and eosinophilic leukocytes, lymphocytes, plasma cells, and histiocytes within the wall of the vessel and surrounding it. Of diagnostic importance is the fact that inflammatory and reparative stages of the disease process are noted in the same histologic section.

Vascular alterations. The changes in the circulatory system may take the form of subcutaneous nodules along the course of peripheral arteries, representing aneurysmal dilatations. There may also be ischemic ulcerations at the tips of the digits or elsewhere, due to thrombosis of cutaneous arterioles. Raynaud's syndrome may be present.

Involvement of the nervous system. The peripheral nerves are commonly affected in polyarteritis nodosa, the pathologic change producing a clinical picture which resembles polyneuritis. In the upper limbs, there may be numbness and tingling, paresis of the extensor muscles of the wrists, and wrist drop; similar changes may be present in the lower limbs.

Musculoskeletal manifestations. Fairly frequent findings are fibrillation and atrophy of voluntary muscles, associated with pain, tenderness, and weakness. However, objective changes in the joints are not common.

Laboratory aids. An important diagnostic finding in polyarteritis nodosa is the presence in a single urine sample of albumin, blood, and various types of casts (red blood cell, oval fat body, fatty and waxy, and broad). Also of significance are a marked leukocytosis (as high as 50,000 per cubic millimeter) and an eosinophilia. The latter may not be present in every specimen of blood. Associated findings are a secondary anemia and an elevated sedimentation rate. At times a biopsy through inflamed tissues is necessary in order to make the diagnosis.

3. Systemic Lupus Erythematosus

Systemic lupus erythematosus is also a generalized disorder of the components of connective tissue, associated with characteristic skin eruptions, systemic responses, and visceral manifestations. The diagnosis of the condition may at times be difficult to make, since the clinical picture is protean, depending on the organ systems affected by the connective tissue changes. In recent years the incidence of the disease appears to be increasing, so that it can no longer be considered an obscure disorder. Although it was originally believed that systemic lupus erythematosus affected primarily young women, this view is no longer tenable since the condition is now found in both sexes at almost all ages.

Vascular manifestations. Alterations in the local circulation to the limbs in systemic lupus erythematosus are uncommon findings. Raynaud's syndrome may be present in about 10 percent of patients. Gangrene of the fingers and toes has been reported in about 1 percent of cases, the change probably following a vasculitis of medium-sized muscular arteries [7]. Petechiae with erythema may occur on the volar surface of the finger tips and about the nail folds. There may also be a true purpura due to a thrombocytopenic state or resulting from angiitis of the skin. Infarctive ulcers, which are also a consequence of cutaneous vasculitis, generally heal readily, although when deep tissues are involved, they may become indolent.

Musculoskeletal manifestations. Articular symptoms and signs, often in atypical or indeterminate form, are much more common findings in systemic lupus erythematosus than generally recognized [22]. Two important diagnostic clues are the frequent remissions and exacerbations, with few or no residual changes, and the discrepancy between severe arthralgias and inconspicuous physical and roentgenographic abnormalities. At times, however, radiographically detectable alterations are noted in the hands [31]. These consist of soft-tissue swelling and periarticular demineralization, findings which are nonspecific and of limited value in differentiation of the condition. Also described are periarticular calcification, acral sclerosis, and joint deformity without erosion. It is necessary to point out that the abnormal radiographic findings do not correlate significantly with the clinical manifestations of activity of the disease [31].

Among other musculoskeletal abnormalities is localized myalgia, associated with pain, stiffness, and swelling. Infrequently, avascular necrosis of the femoral head may develop, the symptoms of which are insidious, unpredictable, and predate the radiologic diagnosis by weeks or months. The possibility has been raised that steroid therapy for the control of systemic lupus erythematosus may play a role in the development of avascular necrosis of the femoral head. (For further discussion of this subject, see Section F, Chapter 14.)

Laboratory aids. Of importance in the diagnosis of systemic lupus erythematosus are the following: presence of LE cells, an abnormal creatinine clearance test, profuse proteinuria, cellular casts in the urine, and the changes observed with the antinuclear antibody test by indirect immunofluorescence. Currently the last procedure is being substituted for the LE cell investigation, since it is believed to be the best approach to screening patients with systemic lupus erythematosus. It is rarely negative in the presence of the disease, although it may be positive in a number of other conditions, such as progressive systemic sclerosis, rheumatoid arthritis, and chronic aggressive hepatitis. The existence of antinuclear DNA antibodies is further confirmation for the presence of systemic lupus erythematosus.

4. Dermatomyositis

Dermatomyositis is a primary inflammatory disease that affects skin or voluntary muscle, or both. The onset of clinical manifestations may be slow or rapid, the most obvious changes being muscular weakness and the appearance of cutaneous lesions. There is a high incidence of associated neoplasm.

Cutaneous and musculoskeletal alterations. In the acute phase of the disease, massive edema of the face and eyelids may be present, associated with mild to intense erythema and a violaceous color over the eyelids (heliotrope); later in the disease there is persistent symmetric erythema. Similar changes may also begin on the hands, forearms, and upper part of the thorax. The responses are particularly marked over the extensor surfaces of joints and over pressure points. With persistence of the chronic erythema, the skin becomes atrophic and indurated (Fig. 13.5A and B). Hyperpigmentation is also a common abnormality.

Muscular tenderness and aching in the limbs in dermatomyositis are more severe than in other connective tissue disorders. Almost specific for this condition is involvement of extraocular muscles, the diaphragm, muscles of the larynx and pharynx, and anal and vesical sphincters. Joint pain is common and flexion contracture may be observed; however, signs of inflammatory articular disease are lacking.

Calcinosis (see Section A, Chapter 9) is a relatively frequent finding in dermatomyositis, probably being due to damage to the panniculus adiposus. This state is noted principally in the limbs, especially about the joints, including the smaller articulations. Extensive deposits of calcium, when located near or in relation to large muscle groups, may cause interference with their ready contraction. At times, calcinosis may even occur within the muscles themselves, an alteration which is revealed by roentgenography. Extrusion of the calcific masses through the skin is associated with severe pain, frequently followed by the development of a nonhealing ulceration locally.

Vascular changes. Dermatomyositis is associated with Raynaud's syndrome in about 20 percent of cases. Telangiectasis is a not infrequent finding. Involvement of large arteries is not noted. However, gangrene and ulceration of finger tips may be present (Fig. 13.5C and D).

Laboratory aids. Of importance in the detection of dermatomyositis are electromyography, levels of serum transaminase, and biopsy of an affected muscle. Also helpful is the clinical evaluation of muscular function. Urinary creatine is high.

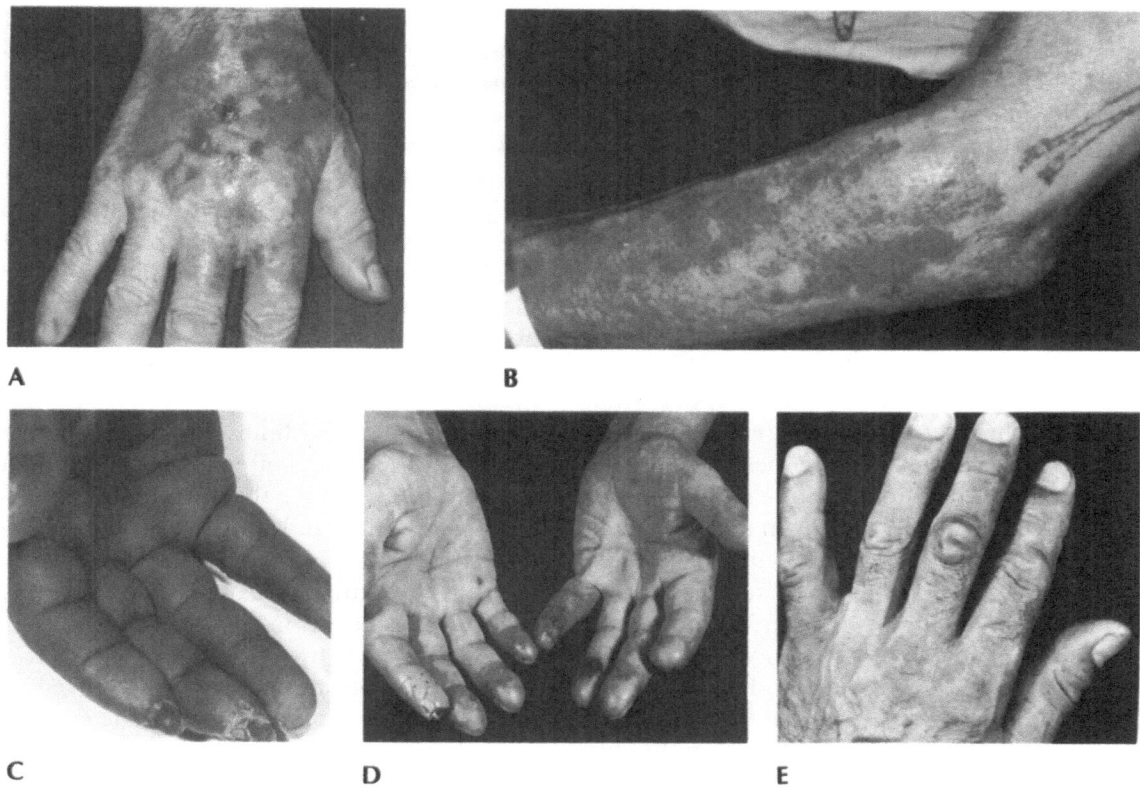

Fig. 13.5. Changes observed in connective tissue disorders. **A** and **B** Cutaneous eruptions over the dorsum of the hand and fingers and on the forearm in dermatomyositis. **C** and **D** Gangrene and ulceration of finger tips in dermatomyositis. **E** Subcutaneous nodule of rheumatoid arthritis.

5. Rheumatoid Arthritis

Inflammatory vascular lesions are common findings in rheumatoid arthritis, their presence being of considerable significance for several reasons. First, they may play a role in the pathogenesis of the disorder, and second they may constitute a morphologic link that relates rheumatoid arthritis to other connective tissue diseases [24]. The possibility that prolonged steroid therapy might be responsible for the activation of an angiitis in susceptible patients with rheumatoid arthritis has been proposed, but most of the pathologic evidence supports the view that vascular inflammation is an integral part of the disease [24].

Pathology. Arterial changes that accompany rheumatoid arthritis vary from slight inflammation to necrotizing arteritis histologically indistinguishable from polyarteritis nodosa (see

Section C-2, above). Most of the lesions probably are located in sites where they do not evoke symptoms or signs, but if the nervous system (particularly the peripheral nerves to the hands and feet) is affected, manifestations become readily apparent (see peripheral neuropathy, below).

Examination of striated muscle obtained by biopsy from patients with rheumatoid arthritis has revealed arteritic changes in very small arteries in approximately 10 percent of cases [25]. The histologic features of the inflammatory reaction are fairly constant, consisting primarily of infiltration of the adventitia, predominantly by large mononuclear cells. The lesions differ from those of polyarteritis nodosa principally in the absence of severe destruction of the arterial wall.

Vasculitis has been found in the articular tissues early in the course of rheumatoid arthritis [11,23]. Also reported is a marked diminution of the number of arteries supplying a joint region, followed by diffuse fibrosis and obliteration of muscular interspaces. There are inflammatory infiltrates, with a preponderance of plasma cells. Vascular proliferation is a common finding. The changes in the synovium can be correlated with the presence of clinically active joint disease; however, they are not specific for rheumatoid arthritis.

Arteritic lesions may also be noted in other parts of the body, including the heart, nerves, and infrequently in other viscera. Histologic examination of the subcutaneous nodules found in rheumatoid arthritis (Fig. 13.5E) generally reveals three distinct zones: a central area of necrosis; a palisade of elongated connective tissue cells arranged radially in a corona about the necrotic zone; and granulation tissue demonstrating chronic inflammatory cells surrounding the other two layers. Thrombosed vessels are usually observed in young nodules, which may be the explanation for the appearance of central necrosis in the lesions [1].

The histologic findings observed in the cutaneous ulcerations of rheumatoid arteritis resemble those present in the subcutaneous nodules (see above). There are also three distinct zones: a central layer of necrosis and fibrinous change; an intermediate layer of palisaded histiocytes, young fibroblasts, and small round cells; and an outer layer of fibrous connective tissue in which are found numerous altered blood vessels [5].

Clinical manifestations on a vascular basis. Rheumatoid arthritis is frequently associated with signs of vasospasm. However, there appears to be no consistent relationship between the location of the vascular signs and the site of the arthritic process. In fact, the possibility has been considered that the vasomotor disturbances in chronic rheumatoid arthritis and related conditions may be attributed to a systemic response, probably acting through the sympathetic nervous system. It is also believed that some of the vasospasm that exists in this entity is due to disuse, since the pain that is generally elicited whenever the affected limb is moved soon causes the patient to use it as little as possible. Probably as a result of all these mechanisms, the involved hands or feet in the patient with rheumatoid arthritis are cold, clammy, and somewhat cyanotic. The changes appear to be limited to the distal portions of the limbs, locations in which normally vasomotor tone is high.

An inflammatory vasculitis of the nerve trunks has been considered responsible for the peripheral neuropathy found in patients with rheumatoid arthritis [8,9]. The onset is usually insidious and not associated with exacerbation of the rheumatoid process. In some cases, however, it appears suddenly and in a severe form. Numbness or an intolerable burning pain in the toes and feet is an early symptom, being found in both lower limbs. Pressure from bedclothes or even socks often is unbearable. With extreme neuropathy, the neurologic changes affect the digits, and muscle weakness, especially in the grip and in the dorsiflexors of the feet, may accompany extensive sensory loss. The role of steroids in the development of peripheral neuropathy has not been clarified.

Purpuric spots and ecchymoses are frequent findings in rheumatoid arthritis. The cause for such changes is unknown, although the possibility has been raised that the response is allied to the vasculitis characteristic of connective tissue disorders. Administration of steroids as a treatment measure appears to accelerate somewhat the occurrence of the lesions. Rarely, extensive ecchymoses located on the limbs break down and ulcerate, with resulting indolent or slowly healing ulcers.

Subcutaneous nodules are present in about one-quarter of adult patients with rheumatoid arthritis, generally indicating a severe form of the disease. They are found lying freely in soft tissues over bony prominences or in sites subjected to repeated periods of pressure, such as at the elbow or the back of the heel.

Superficial ulcers may be found on both malleoli but more often on the lateral aspect. The lesions generally have a dirty base, are indolent, and are resistant to the treatment used for venous stasis ulcers. At times, arteritis of cutaneous and subcutaneous arteries is of such a severe degree that digital gangrene results [19].

Joint manifestations. These usually overshadow constitutional and extraarticular changes but tend to run a parallel course. Involvement is commonly symmetric and progressive. Deformities, contractures, ankylosis, and roentgen abnormalities are easily recognized.

D. Cold Injuries

There are a number of vascular disorders produced by exposure to cold which demonstrate orthopedic abnormalities later in their course. Among these are common frostbite, trench foot, immersion foot, and acute and chronic chilblain (acute and chronic pernio). Since trench foot and immersion foot are generally associated with warfare, the early stages of these disorders are never observed in clinical practice. However, patients suffering from the sequelae of trench foot may on occasion be seen by the orthopedist or the general practitioner, usually in a medical facility of the Veterans Administration. Acute chilblain and chronic chilblain are conditions rarely found in the United States, being present most often in England. On the other hand, common frostbite is observed in severe winter weather both in soldiers in combat and in the civilian population. For these reasons, the following section is devoted primarily to a discussion of this entity, with only a limited presentation of the sequelae of trench foot.

1. Common Frostbite

Common frostbite is a thermal injury which results from prolonged exposure to a much-below-freezing environmental temperature ($-17.8°$ C or less; $0°$ F or less). Contributing factors are wind velocity (which removes heat from the surface of the body), individual susceptibility to cold, impaired local arterial circulation, a poor state of general nutrition, and old age. In contradistinction to trench foot (see D-2, below), wetness does not play an important etiologic role.

Pathogenesis. Initially, exposure to cold produces marked and persistent vasoconstriction of the cutaneous arterioles and, to a lesser degree, of similar vessels in deeper tissues. This leads to a reduced local circulation and, consequently, ischemia of tissues; the latter state is aggravated by almost complete cessation of oxygen exchange due to the fact that dissociation of oxyhemoglobin is negligible at a low temperature. With extreme cold, there is actual solidification of fluid and tissues of the limb, with intracellular ice crystal formation.

When thawing occurs, the previous vasoconstriction is replaced by paralysis and dilatation of the cutaneous microcirculation, especially the capillaries (hyperemic stage). At the same time, the persisting ischemia produces damage to the capillary endothelium and increased permeability of this structure. As a consequence, there is marked transudation of plasma from the blood into tissue spaces, producing swelling of the affected structures.

Pathology. With loss of fluid from the blood, there is concentration of the red blood cells, producing a sludge of formed elements which fills the capillary lumens. After several days, the red blood cells become agglutinated to form real thrombi that obstruct local blood flow and lead to gangrene of the distal tissues. At the same time, the cold produces alterations in the walls of the larger blood vessels, consisting of early swelling and vacuolization of the intimal cells and proliferative changes. Such abnormalities cause further interference with local circulation and hence aggravation of the existing state of ischemia.

Clinical manifestations. Common frostbite can be divided into several clinical stages. The first or acute phase, which generally lasts for several weeks after exposure, is typified by freezing of the tissues, a short period of thawing followed by exudation, and then necrosis.

Initially, during the period of exposure, the affected parts become numb, occasionally preceded by a prickling sensation. At this time, the skin is waxy white and very cold. As thawing takes place and reactive hyperemia develops, the skin becomes red, warm, and swollen and blisters and blebs filled with yellow or blood-tinged fluid appear (Fig. 13.6A–C). Hemorrhages under the nails frequently give them a black appearance, and subsequently many of the affected structures are shed. Pulsations in the main arteries at levels proximal to the re-

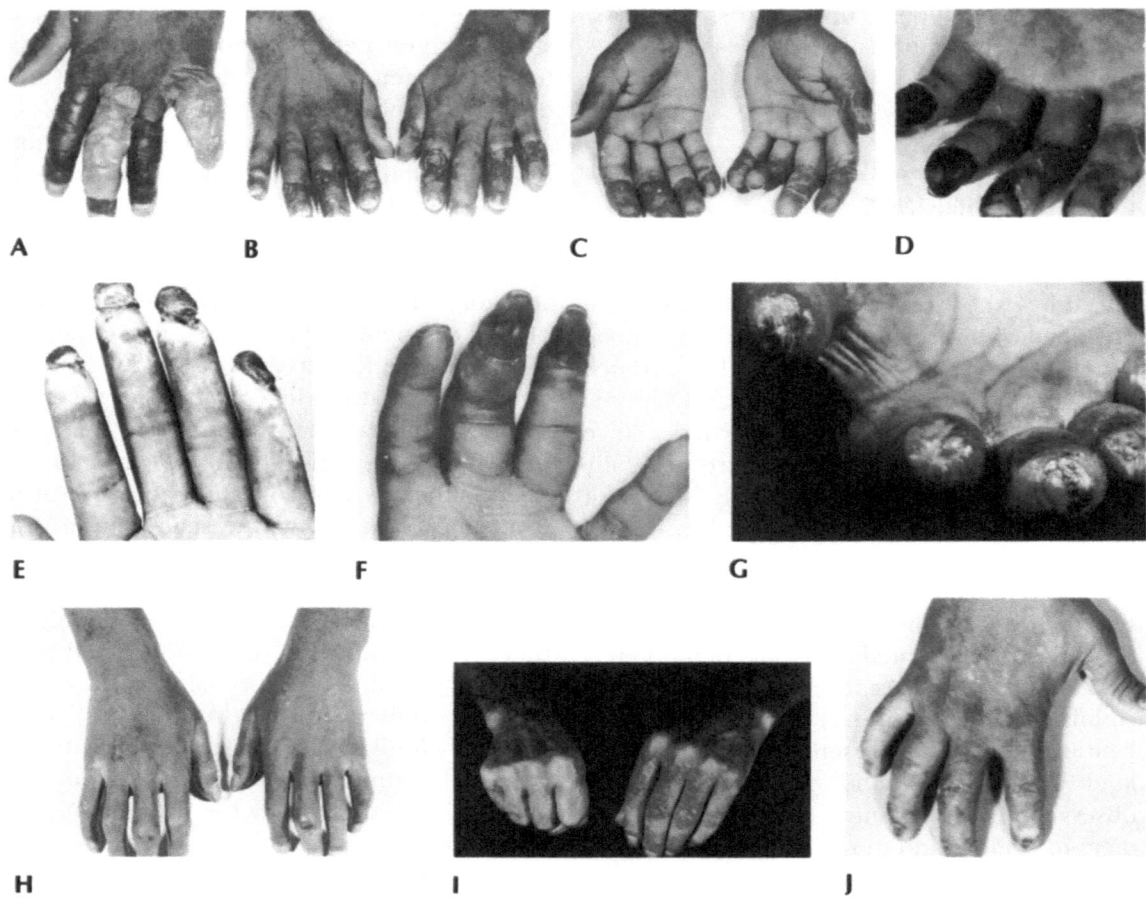

Fig. 13.6. Various stages of frostbite of the hand. **A–C** Changes occurring with thawing (development of blisters and then absorption of contents with wrinkling of overlying nonviable skin). **D** Necrosis of fingertips. **E** and **F** Separation of necrotic from viable tissue. **G** Surgical amputation of necrotic tissue. **H–J** Rigidity of hand and ankylosis of phalangeal joints.

gion of involvement are generally bounding and full.

Depending upon the severity of the existing local ischemia, the degree of trophic changes will vary. Necrosis of the skin is first noted in the distal segments of the limbs, i.e., the digits (Fig. 13.6D); the process may affect only the skin or all the tissues, including the phalanges. With longer exposure, the hand or foot proper will be similarly affected. However, the possibility of necrosis of deeper structures is less, with the destruction frequently being limited to the skin and subcutaneous tissue, a point to keep in mind when contemplating surgical removal of apparently nonviable structures.

In the second or subacute stage, there is sep-

aration of necrotic from viable tissues (Fig. 13.6E–F). The state of reactive hyperemia is replaced by a return of increased sympathetic tone, with the skin of the limb becoming cold, blue or pale, and excessively perspired. Increased sensitivity to cold is generally present. Neurologic abnormalities, in the form of a partial sensory loss (stocking-glove in distribution), appear; the greatest deficit is noticed in the digits, consisting of a reduction in light touch and fine temperature discrimination. Deep pressure and vibration sense are not affected.

Trophic changes become more apparent in the subacute stage. Cutaneous atrophy and sclerosis are common findings, particularly in previous sites of necrosis. The most marked changes are noted in the digits. These include thinning of the digital pulp pad, thickening and irregularity of the nails, and loss of normal wrinkling over interphalangeal joints due to firm attachment of the overlying skin to the subcutaneous tissue. Epiphyseal destruction in the distal and middle phalanges of digits, with shortening of involved bones, is not uncommon. The metaphysis may increase in breadth and the articular surfaces may be irregular.

In the chronic stage, necrotic tissue is no longer present, having been previously removed either by debridement or surgical amputation (Fig. 13.6G). Constant findings are rigidity of the foot or hand, ankylosis of the phalangeal joints, and exaggeration of the changes already existing in the digits (Fig. 13.6H–J). Vasospasm may become less marked or disappear, or it may persist for many months; Raynaud's syndrome may be noted on occasion. Pain in the areas of scarring and in the proximal portion of the limb becomes much more frequent and severe.

Treatment. Considerable differences of opinion exist regarding the initial therapy for frostbite. One approach is aimed at reducing the early swelling and reducing tissue metabolism by increasing the period of thawing and actually cooling the affected portions of limbs. Another program involves immediate thawing of the frozen part by immersion in a water bath at 43° C (110° F) for 20 min. However, it is necessary to point out that such a procedure causes rapid thawing of superficial tissues before deeply located frozen structures have had sufficient time to regain their function, with the result that the blood and lymph become liquid at a period when they still cannot be returned to the circulation. Also, this type of approach produces severe pain, much of which can be avoided by starting with cooled water and gradually raising the temperature. At no time should the limb be overheated, since the marked rise in metabolic needs, produced by the elevation in tissue temperature resulting from such a procedure, will invariably lead to extensive necrosis of poorly viable structures. This is so because the available local blood supply is not adequate to take care of the tissue requirements. In general, the highest level of

water temperature should not exceed body temperature.

Attempts have been made in the subacute stage to control the commonly found persistent intense vasoconstriction by removal of vasomotor tone using sympathetic blocking agents or, on occasion, even sympathectomy. However, the value of such an approach has not been fully determined, since vasodilatation is considered by some workers to be harmful when produced at this time, especially if the local circulation has not attained an adequate return to a near normal level of efficiency.

Another regimen which has been proposed is the early intravenous administration of heparin on the theoretical basis that this drug will prevent the formation of true agglutinative thrombi from the clumped erythrocytes, thus reducing the possibility of the development of severe ischemia and necrosis of tissue. However, such a measure appears effective in this regard only if initiated soon after exposure (within 16 h) and continued for at least 5 days. At present, a longer period of experimental and clinical study of heparin is necessary before a full evaluation of its efficacy in frostbite will be available.

Regardless of the approach taken for rewarming the frozen tissues, there is no question that once this is accomplished, the limbs are carefully cleansed with a mild antiseptic, cotton pledgets are placed between the digits to absorb the fluid from ruptured blebs or blisters and so minimize maceration, and the parts are covered with sterile dressings. In the case of the lower limbs, a cradle without lights is used to prevent the bedclothes from resting on them. For the upper limbs, a sterile towel or dressing is placed on the chest and abdomen to support the hands. The patient is given a tetanus-toxoid booster or a tetanus antitoxin injection, and a course of a wide-spectrum antibiotic (to prevent local infection).

A most important early step is the institution of a rehabilitative program even in the presence of bleb formation and necrotic tissue, conditions which would ordinarily be contraindications to such an approach. However, the only measure which is effective in controlling the rapidly forming ankylosis and contractures of the joints of the digits and atrophy of the small muscles of the hand or foot so commonly noted in frostbite is to prescribe and carefully supervise early exercises of the extremities. Otherwise, in the case of the upper limb, at least, a typical and useless clawhand will develop. The regimen consists of placing each joint of involved digits through a full range of motion a number of times every hour during the entire day.

As a general rule, extensive surgical removal of necrotic tissue should not be performed early in frostbite, since frequently the apparently necrotic structures are only superficially affected, a finding which initially may be difficult to determine. Later in the disease, when there is complete separation between viable and nonviable tissues (Fig. 13.6D–F) and the digits are mummified and completely necrotic, amputation of portions or of entire fingers or toes is indicated (Fig. 13.6G).

Once the necrotic tissue has been removed by repeated debridement or by surgery and healing is occurring in the involved sites, the rehabilitation program is intensified. In the case of involvement of the feet, ambulation is increased, with emphasis placed on a proper stance and gait. Following frostbite of the hands, the program of active exercise of the fingers is continued and enlarged so as to increase range of motion, improve muscle tone, and reduce the possibility of the development of a clawhand. If vasospasm persists, sympathetic blocking agents, like phenoxybenzamine hydrochloride (Dibenzyline), should be given orally. At times, sympathectomy is indicated to control the condition; this also helps heal indolent ulcerations in areas where necrotic tissue had been removed.

2. Sequelae of Trench Foot

Trench foot is most commonly seen in infantry soldiers following prolonged exposure of the feet to moderate cold (around 0° C; 32° F) and persistent dampness (contributed to by wet socks and wet footwear). That extensive destruction of tissue can occur under such circumstances is due to the fact that the transmission of the cold to deep tissues is enhanced by the associated moisture, since water has a high capacity for absorbing heat. In contrast with common frostbite (see D-1, above), at no time are structures actually frozen.

Clinical manifestations of later stages. As in the case of frostbite, the feet suffering from trench foot pass through a prehyperemic stage, a hyperemic stage, a posthyperemic stage, and finally, the stage of sequelae. The latter may persist for as long as 6 to 7 years after exposure. However, a suspicion regarding the severity of the symptoms always exists, since in every instance there is the matter of financial compensation from the government, in most cases based primarily on subjective complaints.

Generally the sequelae of trench foot consist

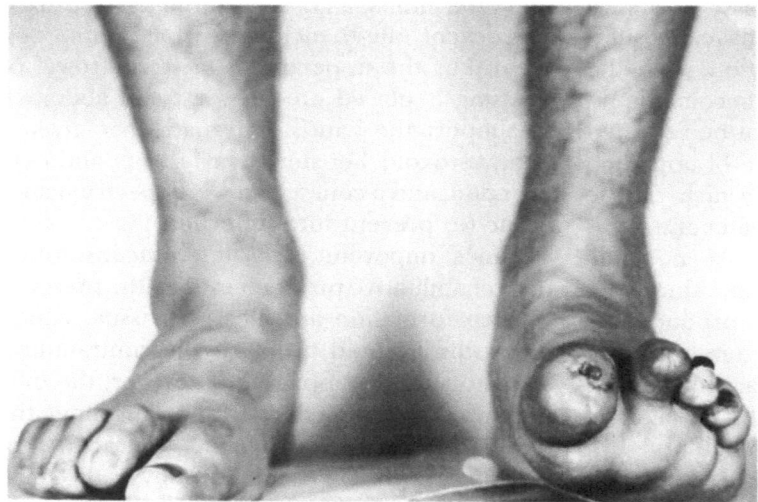

Fig. 13.7. Deformity of toes with dorsal displacement, a sequela of trench foot.

of symptoms and signs of excessive sympathetic activity and of peripheral nerve involvement. Irritation of the sympathetic nervous system may take the form of hyperhidrosis (at times, to an extreme degree), cyanosis, coldness, increased reactivity to cold, and swelling of the feet (noted usually in hot weather). Raynaud's syndrome may occasionally be present. As in the case of frostbite, atrophy of the small muscles of the feet (Fig. 13.7) and osteoporosis of the bones of the feet may be observed. The gait may not be normal, since the patient has a tendency to walk on the lateral edge of the feet with the toes extended, so as to minimize pain initiated by pressure to the plantar surface.

Treatment. The management of the sequelae of trench foot consists primarily of an intensive rehabilitative program. If bedridden, the patient should be made ambulatory as soon as possible without dependence upon crutches or canes. Exercises should be instituted which have as a goal the development of a normal stance and walking pattern, with the weight of the body placed equally on both lower limbs. At first, in order to minimize the discomfort and acute pain that such a program may initiate, the patient should be instructed to walk while in a pool of lukewarm water, to take advantage of the buoyancy effect. Another means of removing the weight from the sole of the feet is to attach a second heel to the shoe a short distance in front of the ordinary one so as to distribute pressure more equally. If the hyperhidrosis is of a very marked degree, thus increasing susceptibility to dermatophytosis and perpetuating this state, it may be necessary to perform a lumbar sympathectomy.

References

1. Bennett GA, Zeller JW, Bauer W: Subcutaneous nodules of rheumatoid arthritis and rheumatic fever: A pathologic study. Arch Pathol 30:70, 1940
2. Bolliger A: Gefässreaktionen und ihre Rolle bei der Entstehung des Sudeckschen Syndroms. Helv Chir Acta 1:61, 1954
3. Brintnall ES, Hyndman OR, Van Allen MW: Costoclavicular compression associated with cervical rib. Ann Surg 144:921, 1956
4. Churg J, Strauss L: Allergic granulomatosis, allergic angiitis, and periarteritis nodosa. Am J Pathol 27:277, 1951
5. Collins DH: Subcutaneous nodule of rheumatoid arthritis. J Pathol Bacteriol 45:97, 1937
6. De Palma AF: Scalenus anticus syndrome treated by surgery and skeletal traction. Am J Surg 76:274, 1948
7. Dubois EL, Arterberry JD: Gangrene as a manifestation of systemic lupus erythematosus. JAMA 181:366, 1962
8. Hart FD, Golding JR: Rheumatoid neuropathy. Br Med J 5186:1594, 1960
9. Hart FD, Golding JR, Mackenzie DH: Neuropathy in rheumatoid disease. Ann Rheum Dis 16:471, 1957
10. Johnson DA: Postural myoneuralgia: Integration of the acroparesthesia syndromes. Med Ann District of Columbia 27:6, 1958
11. Kulka JP, Bocking D, Ropes MW, et al: Early joint lesions of rheumatoid arthritis: Report of eight cases, with knee biopsies of lesions of less than one year's duration. AMA Arch Pathol 59:129, 1955
12. Leichlentritt KG: Prevention of shoulder-hand syndrome. Gen Practitioner 12:108, 1955
13. Logue RB, Mullins F: Polyarteritis nodosa: Report of 11 cases with review of recent literature. Ann Intern Med 24:11, 1946
14. Lord JW Jr: Surgical management of shoulder girdle syndromes: New operative procedure for hyperabduction, costoclavicular, cervical rib, and scalenus anticus syndromes. Arch Surg 66:69, 1953
15. Lorente de Nó R: Analysis of the activity of the chain of internuncial neurons. J Neurophysiol 1:207, 1938
16. Miller DS, de Takáts G: Post-traumatic dystrophy of the extremities: Sudeck's atrophy. Surg Gynecol Obstet 75:558, 1942
17. Nelson PA: Treatment of patients with cervicodorsal outlet syndrome. JAMA 163:1570, 1957
18. Roach MR: Changes in arterial distensibility as a cause of poststenotic dilatation. Am J Cardiol 12:802, 1963
19. Scott JT, Hourihane DO, Doyle FH, et al: Digital arteritis in rheumatoid disease. Ann Rheum Dis 20:224, 1961
20. Short DW: The subclavian artery in 16 patients with complete cervical ribs. J. Cardiovasc Surg 16:135, 1975
21. Shumacker HB Jr, Abramson DI: Posttraumatic vasomotor disorders: With particular reference to late manifestations and treatment. Surg Gynecol Obstet 88:417, 1949
22. Silver M, Steinbrocker O: The musculoskeletal manifestations of systemic lupus erythematosus: JAMA 176:1001, 1961
23. Sinclair RJG, Cruickshank B: A clinical and pathological study of sixteen cases of rheumatoid arthritis with extensive visceral involvement ("rheumatoid disease"). Q J Med 25:313, 1956

24. Sockoloff L, Bunim JJ: Vascular lesions in rheumatoid arthritis. J Chronic Dis 5:668, 1957

25. Sockoloff L, Wilens SL, Bunim JJ: Arteritis of striated muscle in rheumatoid arthritis. Am J Pathol 27:157, 1951

26. Steinbrocker O, Argyros TG: The shoulder-hand syndrome: Present status as a diagnostic and therapeutic entity. Med Clin North Am 42:1533, 1958

27. Steinbrocker O, Spitzer N, Friedman HH: The shoulder-hand syndrome in reflex dystrophy of the upper extremity. Ann Intern Med 29:22, 1948

28. Taylor JG: Sudeck's atrophy and the shoulder-hand syndrome. Proc R Soc Med 51:879, 1958

29. Turek SL: Orthopaedics. Principles and Their Application. Philadelphia, Lippincott, 1959, p 434

30. Webb EM, Davis EW: Causalgia: A review. California Med 69:412, 1948

31. Weissman BN, Rappoport AS, Sosman JL, et al: Radiographic findings in the hands in patients with systemic lupus erythematosus. Radiology 126:313, 1978

32. Wright IS: The neurovascular syndrome produced by hyperabduction of the arms. Am Heart J 29:1, 1945

Chapter 14

Clinical Entities with Both Vascular and Orthopedic Components

Part 2   Musculoskeletal Disorders with Circulatory Manifestations

This chapter is devoted to several orthopedic conditions in which local vascular alterations may be responsible, in part, for structural abnormalities or clinical manifestations.

A.   Anterior Poliomyelitis

A cold, blue, moist, at times edematous extremity may be present in the chronic stage of anterior poliomyelitis. As a result, the general impression has arisen that such a limb suffers from a reduction in blood supply. Whether this concept is true becomes an important point to establish, particularly if some orthopedic procedure is being contemplated.

1.   Local Blood Flow

In a study of the rate of peripheral blood flow in the paralyzed extremity using the venous occlusion plethysmographic method, it was found that in approximately one-half of the cases, the circulation in the affected limb was the same or even greater than that in the opposite normal side. In the other half, the readings were either somewhat or significantly reduced

[2]. However, in the latter, after the limb had remained in the plethysmograph for an hour or two and the patient had begun to relax, a definite increase in blood flow was observed, so that at the end of the experimental period, in only a small number of cases was a reduced blood flow still present. In all others the circulation in the paralyzed limb was now normal or even greater than that in the opposite control extremity.

2.   Local Cutaneous Temperature

Comparable data have also been obtained using cutaneous temperature determinations [2]. At first, reduced readings were recorded in the paralyzed extremity, in some instances as much as 5° C lower than those of the normal limb. However, with continued exposure to a warm environment, the figures gradually rose so that at the end of a 6-h experimental period, in most instances they were similar to those obtained from the opposite normal side. With subsequent exposure to a cold environment, there was an almost immediate drop in cutaneous temperature to the initial low level; a much less marked response was noted in the digits of the opposite normal extremity.

3. Factors Responsible for Vascular Changes

From available evidence, it can be concluded that in anterior poliomyelitis there are no structural changes in the local arterial tree which permanently reduce vascular lumen size. The finding that in a number of instances the blood flow and skin temperature readings in the paralyzed limb are initially reduced and then rise to normal levels when exposed to a physiologic environment indicates that the local sympathetic nervous system is hyperreactive to vasoconstricting stimuli. The marked drop in skin temperature on exposure to cold helps confirm this point of view. Another possible cause for the reduced cutaneous circulation is an insufficient stimulus and load placed on the local vascular tree, with the result that only small infantile arterial branches develop in the immobile limb [22]. Such a view is based on the belief that if a structure is inactive, its demand for blood supply is lowered and hence less circulation passes through the arteries. As a consequence, there is atrophy of the vascular tree. Regardless of the mechanism responsible for the alteration, there is no question that a sufficiently prolonged decrease in cutaneous circulation exists in the chronic stage of anterior poliomyelitis to be responsible for the not infrequent appearance of skin ulcers.

The finding of an increase in blood flow in the entire paralyzed limb in some patients, in the face of signs of reduced cutaneous circulation (cyanosis and low skin temperature), suggests that in such individuals there is an enhanced muscle circulation, possibly due to an abnormally high number of open vessels in the paralyzed muscle which are not responding normally to stimuli [15]. Also of interest in this regard is the arteriographic observation of an increased number of arteriovenous shunts in the muscles of the affected extremity [12].

The cause of the vasomotor disturbance in anterior poliomyelitis has not been completely explained. Pathologic changes have been reported in the intermediolateral cell columns in the cord [33,34], from which the efferent sympathetic preganglionic fibers arise, and it is conceivable that irritation of these nerve tracts might produce increased vasomotor tone in the cutaneous vessels of the paralyzed limb. Another possibility is that vasospasm exists as a result of disuse of the limb [36,38,44].

4. Conclusions

It would appear, therefore, that the affected extremity in the later stages of poliomyelitis demonstrates signs of hypertonus limited to the cutaneous vessels and that there is no proof for the existence of structural alterations in the arterial tree. On the basis of such a view, the question of an operative procedure in this type of case can be viewed in a much more favorable light, since vasospasm can be temporarily removed by blocking the sympathetic pathway through paravertebral sympathetic block and peripheral nerve block. A much longer period of absent vasomotor tone, with the appearance of a warm, pink limb, can be produced by sympathectomy.

B. Cerebrovascular Disorders

1. Adult Hemiplegia

It has generally been accepted that alterations in normal vascular reactions do occur in the affected limb in hemiplegia, but the changes noted by the various workers have not fallen into any consistent pattern. This is probably due to the fact that the location of the lesion in the reported cases was probably not in the same portion of the brain and also that the patients were studied at different times in the paralytic state.

With regard to the arterial blood pressure in the upper limb, some evidence has appeared to indicate that the readings are lower than normal in the flaccid state and higher in the later spastic period; other data have indicated the reverse. At the same time, there are a number of investigators who believe that the changes in blood pressure in the affected extremity are in no way related to the state of tonus of the muscles.

Concerning the peripheral circulation, it has been found that in the acute stage of hemiplegia there is an elevation of several degrees centigrade in skin temperature in the affected limb, as compared with the opposite side, whereas in the chronic state the paralyzed extremity is cooler than normal.

Utilizing oxygen arteriovenous differences, it has been noted that the blood flow in the paralyzed arm is greater than on the normal side [19]. However, a correlation has not been found between the magnitude of the increase in circulation in the affected extremity and the extent of paralysis, its duration, the state of muscle tone, and the blood pressure alteration. Similar studies on the lower extremities do not show as significant a difference in blood flow between the paralyzed and normal side as exists in the upper limbs.

Actual blood flow readings have been obtained with the venous occlusion plethysmographic method, and in most instances the circulation in the paralyzed and the normal hand has been found to be the same; on occasion it has been noted to be increased on the affected side, but in no instance has there been a decreased blood flow [1]. In the forearm, however, in approximately one-half the cases, a reduction in circulation has been observed on the paralyzed side, whereas in the remaining instances the readings have been normal or greater than those obtained from the opposite unaffected limb. In the leg, in most cases the blood flow has been found to be normal or increased in the paralyzed extremity.

A number of experimental studies favor the view that destruction of the pyramidal tracts in their course through the brain produces alterations in normal vasomotor control of the vessels in the affected limb, possibly through a release of cortical vasoconstriction. However, there is also evidence to the contrary [47] indicating that lesions of the cerebral hemisphere do not in any way affect the functional capacity of the blood vessels in the hemiplegic limb to constrict in response to a sensory stimulus or to a fall in blood temperature. Regardless of the differing views, it can still be stated that there may be changes in local blood pressure, cutaneous temperature, and at times blood flow in the paralyzed limb. It is also necessary to point out that some of the manifestations of vasospasm, as in the case of anterior poliomyelitis (see Section A, above), are due to the associated dependency, disuse, and inactivity of such a limb.

The finding that for the most part the circulation in the paralyzed limb is not significantly compromised is of value with regard to its orthopedic management, particularly if some type of operative procedure is being considered. Not infrequently the involved extremity suffers from such complications as ingrown toenails, calluses and corns, traumatic arthritis of the knee joint, changes in the hamstring muscles, and contracture of the tendo Achillis requiring heel and cord lengthening, and generally surgical treatment is attempted with much trepidation. Although such a view appears to have little basis in fact, it is still necessary to point out that atherosclerosis, a common cause of cerebral artery occlusion and hemiplegia, may at the same time be present in the arterial tree of the lower limbs, in the form of arteriosclerosis obliterans (see Chapter 11). Hence, it is essential to rule out such a possibility before attempting any operative procedure on a paralyzed lower limb.

2. Infantile Spastic Hemiplegia (Cerebral Palsy)

An interesting feature of infantile spastic hemiplegia is the reduced size of the affected limb, the latter being both shorter and thinner than the corresponding normal extremity. The cause of this growth disturbance is not known, although the possibility has been raised that it is due to an alteration in local circulation.

In regard to the above view, actual blood flow measurements, using venous occlusion plethysmography, have been made on paralyzed and normal legs in children with cerebral palsy, and it has been found that the local circulation is generally lower in the involved extremity [29]. However, no distinct relationship appears to exist between the decrease in size of the paralyzed limb and the reduction in blood flow.

C. Pulmonary Hypertrophic Osteoarthropathy

Pulmonary hypertrophic osteoarthropathy is a syndrome characterized by proliferation at the distal ends of long bones of the limbs, joint manifestations (in the form of local soft-tissue swelling, synovitis, pain, and tenderness), clubbing of the fingers, and sometimes gynecomastia.

1. Etiologic Factors

Of the two types, one, primary or idiopathic hypertrophic osteoarthropathy, typically occurs in men, often with a familial history [26]. Development of the disorder is complete between the ages of 13 and 22 years, without later significant changes.

Secondary hypertrophic osteoarthropathy is seen most frequently in chronologic relationship to various intrathoracic diseases and generally recedes when the cause is treated. The most commonly associated clinical entities are chronic pulmonary disorders, particularly the slow-growing epidermoid and well-differentiated bronchogenic carcinoma [25]. Another group is cyanotic congenital heart disease.

Although clubbing of the fingers is a constant finding in typical chronic hypertrophic pulmonary osteoarthropathy of the larger joints, this type of abnormality may also develop separately. Because of such a possibility, the tendency to refer to all cases of clubbing of the fingers as being part of the clinical picture of pulmonary hypertrophic osteoarthropathy is misleading and should be discarded.

The actual cause of pulmonary hypertrophic osteoarthropathy is unknown, although a number of theories have been proposed to explain the findings. One is a possible underlying endocrine imbalance; in another, the neurogenic concept, it is proposed that a reflex neural arc exists, involving vagal afferent fibers with transmission through the vagus nerve [20]. Support for the latter view has been obtained through the results of vagal section in five patients with bronchogenic carcinoma and hypertrophic osteoarthropathy, prompt symptomatic relief being obtained following the operation [20]. Originally, the liberation of toxins was also considered to be an etiologic factor.

Finally, the suggestion has been made that ferritin, a vasoactive polypeptide, may be involved in the response. In this regard, it has been shown that such a substance is present in both arterial and venous blood in patients with clubbing and hypertrophic osteoarthropathy and only in venous blood in a nonclubbed control group [23,24]. Normally, ferritin is metabolized in the lungs; therefore its presence in arterial blood in patients with hypertrophic osteoarthropathy suggests that in them, it passes through pulmonary shunts unaltered and is thus available for the production of vasodilatation of arteriovenous anastomoses in the fingers [7].

2. Pathophysiology

Clubbing of fingers. The characteristic deformity of the terminal phalanges in clubbing is due to an increase in number and caliber of blood vessels locally, together with hypertrophy and hyperplasia of the surrounding tissue bed [37]. The response is a complex one in which capillary pulse pressure, hypoxia, and other factors play a role.

The anatomy of the microcirculation is altered. The arterial arcades of the terminal bony phalanges demonstrate an increase in blood flow, while the capillaries are wide and elongated, with no pulsations noted in them.

Most of the physiologic evidence indicates that the blood flow to the entire limb in pulmonary hypertrophic osteoarthropathy is increased [21], this type of change being particularly marked in the digits [39,40]. However, based on the rate of absorption of radiosodium from the clubbed fingers [23] and on the finding of small arteriovenous oxygen and carbon dioxide differences [7], the conclusion has been reached that actually the nutritional blood flow through the capillary bed is relatively decreased. All these findings suggest the presence of open arteriovenous anastomoses in the digits which shunt blood away from the capillary circulation, thus decreasing local blood flow to the tissues and producing reduced tissue oxygen tension. This, in turn, could be responsible for the clubbing.

Changes in long bones and joints. It has been found experimentally in dogs that when the pulmonary artery is anastomosed to the left atrium, periosteal bone formation, comparable to that of pulmonary hypertrophic osteoarthropathy, is produced [40]. Such a change has been linked to the resulting enhanced cardiac output, which causes an increased blood flow to the bones, including a greater source of oxygen available to the marrow. Also of importance in this regard is the finding that, conversely, when the supply of oxygen to bone cells is cut off, synthesis of new organic matrix ceases [48]. Such information may cast some light on the mechanisms responsible for the periosteal proliferation noted in long bones in hypertrophic osteoarthropathy.

It has been suggested that the joint effusions and pain in this condition are merely a manifestation of increased vascularity rather than of a true inflammatory process [28], a point of view which has some clinical support.

D. Paget's Disease of Bone

Paget's disease of bone (osteitis deformans) is one of the most frequently encountered chronic progressive bone disorders. It affects chiefly those skeletal structures possessing a rich arterial circulation and hematopoietic marrow, and it is characterized by deformity of the external bony contour and of the internal architecture. The major defect is primary resorption of bone.

1. Incidence

The condition is found in about 3 to 5 percent of the general population above 40 years of age. In hospitalized individuals, the incidence is about one in 30,000 patients. Men are affected twice as often as women. The disorder is fairly common in the United States, Australia, Germany, New Zealand, and South Africa, but it is rare in India, Japan, the Middle East, and the Scandinavian countries. The most common site of involvement is the pelvis, followed by the femur, skull, tibia, lumbosacral spine, dorsal spine, clavicle, and ribs. Only rarely are the hands and feet attacked.

2. Etiologic Factors

The finding that there is a direct correlation between the magnitude of the increase in circu-

lation to the involved bone and the degree of destructive activity (see D-3, below) has focused attention on vascular mechanisms as a possible cause for Paget's disease of bone. However, such an approach has not been productive in solving the problem. One theory which has been advanced is that the augmentation in local blood flow is a consequence of an elevated metabolic rate of the affected bone, a point of view which is supported by the finding that when steroid therapy is given, there is a reduction in osseous circulation, and at the same time the level of serum alkaline phosphatase falls. There is no convincing evidence that extensive arteriosclerosis is involved in the production of the disease or that the development of arteriovenous fistulae in the affected bone is an etiologic factor. Current speculation deals with the possibility that an autoimmune inflammatory process exists or that there are aberrations of hormone secretion, possibly involving calcitonin. It has also been proposed that Paget's disease of bone is a neoplastic or a connective tissue disorder. Recent studies demonstrating nuclear inclusion bodies in the osteoclasts of bones involved in the disorder suggest a possible "slow virus" cause.

3. Pathogenesis

During the period of bone destruction in the involved limb, there is a greatly increased local blood flow [17,18]; in fact, a direct relationship appears to exist between the magnitude of the circulatory response and the degree of resorptive activity. Also of importance is the finding that spontaneous remissions in Paget's disease are associated with reductions in the magnitude of the osseous circulation. In the active stage, the periosteal blood supply is particularly raised (a three- to fourfold augmentation), the change being limited to the affected areas of bone [17]. At the same time, there appears to be a decrease in circulation to the distal portion of the limb. That the rise in osseous blood flow is not due to local arteriovenous shunting has been proved by hemodynamic studies using the intravenous injection of 15- to 30-μm particles [45]. The marked vascularity of the bone is probably responsible for the increase in cardiac output found in Paget's disease, a direct correlation being present between the magnitude of the change and the severity of the local bone involvement.

4. Pathology

Histologic examination of involved bones reveals an excess of osteoblasts in the spongy bone, surrounded by osteofibrosis which extends into the marrow. The normal haversian systems are replaced by a mosaic of cement lines and the trabeculae become coarser. The pathologic process begins as a destruction of bone in the haversian canals and spreads to the endosteal and periosteal surfaces of the cortex. The result is resorption of bone at the endosteal surface and proliferation of bone in the connective tissue adjacent to the periosteal surface, the new bone fusing with the underlying cortical bone.

The increased availability of calcium, particularly during periods of physical inactivity, may be responsible for metastatic calcification which often affects arteries (producing Mönckeberg's sclerosis) and heart valves, as well as other structures.

5. Clinical Manifestations

Generally the onset of Paget's disease is insidious, with no appearance of symptoms or signs. In fact, frequently its presence is detected when radiographs are taken for some other purpose or when there is an unexplained elevation of alkaline phosphatase. Only occasionally is there extensive involvement of the skeleton (generalized Paget's disease), producing progressive enlargement of the skull, kyphosis, and thickening and bowing of the long bones. In most instances, the condition is present in limited areas. For this reason, it is considered to be a nonmetabolic bone disorder.

The initial clinical finding may be swelling or deformity and bowing of a long bone, generally in the lower limbs, or an increase in hat size. An associated change is a high temperature of the skin overlying the involved structure, which evidently is a reflection of the increased local osseous blood flow (see D-3, above). Deformity of the vertebrae or skull may cause impingement on spinal or cranial nerves or compression of brain tissue, producing such findings as headache and deafness; compression by the expanding bone in the limbs results in skeletal pain. Symptoms due to movement of the involved portions of the body are related, in part, to the structural abnormality of the bone and, in part, to local inflammation. In the presence of extensive disease of skeletal structures, the associated increase in cardiac output may be sufficient to place a great enough load on the heart that ultimately cardiac reserve is exhausted and heart failure ensues [3].

6. Radiographic Changes

Characteristically in Paget's disease, there are radiolucent areas in the involved bone, reflecting the osteolytic process, and dense, coarsely striated areas, representing compensatory bone formation. Such findings are particularly noted in the pelvis, spine, femur, and skull. In the long bones, the process generally starts at one end and spreads to the other. The progression along the cortex occurs in the form of an advancing wedge of involvement [31], usually identifiable on x-ray by the V-shaped radiolucent area behind the wedge; the affected cortex is thick and radiopaque, resembling finely porous pumice stone [31]. When the process affects the entire bone, bowing results, associated with widening and thickening of the cortex. Because the newly formed bone lacks a functional structure, fissure fractures are common. Due to misalignment of joints, varying degrees of degenerative arthritis may be present.

The radiographic findings in osteogenic sarcoma superimposed on Paget's disease consist of smaller or larger, irregular, mottled or uniform areas of radiolucency, set against a background of bone altered by the original disorder [31]. Occasionally there may be radiopaque flecks of ossification within the sarcoma. The tumor may arise from the fibrous substratum of bone affected by Paget's disease.

7. Laboratory Aids

A very important laboratory indicator of the presence of active Paget's disease is an increase in serum alkaline phosphatase. Such a response reflects hyperfunction of osteoblasts and a high rate of bone formation [6]. However, it is necessary first to rule out pathologic changes in the liver which may also produce a rise in alkaline phosphatase. In most cases of active Paget's disease, serum alkaline phosphatase levels are increased 4 to 100 times the normal amount. With the King-Armstrong method, the procedure most commonly used, normal values may range between 5.0 and 13.0 units.

A rise in 24-h urinary excretion of hydroxyproline is also of diagnostic importance since such a change indicates a greater resorption of bone matrix, specifically collagen, the main source of the amino acid in the urine. An increase in the amount of this substance therefore reflects the rate of the skeletal destructive process. In the normal adult, the average rate of hydroxyproline excretion is less than 50 mg per 24 h, whereas in active Paget's disease, the quantity rises to 100 to 200 mg per 24 h. Although some patients with extensive Paget's disease have excessive turnover of calcium with increased urine calcium excretion, in most instances serum calcium and phosphorus levels are normal.

Bone scans are likewise useful in Paget's disease, since they determine the extent and activity of the disease and may detect areas of involvement not seen radiographically. The procedure measures the increased uptake of bone-seeking isotopes by the lesions. In the early stages of the disorder, scans will generally be positive because both the processes of bone resorption and compensatory bone formation affect a large mass of bone. However, in the quiescent phase, when sclerotic bone lesions are present, they may be negative because of the low rate of bone turnover [8]. Of importance in bone scanning is the fact that the basically symmetric skeleton provides a means of comparison between abnormal and corresponding normal areas [8].

8. Complications

Pathologic fractures of weakened long bones may complicate Paget's disease. At times they may be the first indication of the presence of this condition. The lesions occur spontaneously or after slight trauma and are usually transverse fissure fractures rather than complete ones. They develop on the convex side of the curved bone, due to the mechanical bowing and the altered bone architecture, and penetrate the cortex for varying depths. Sites of predisposition are the upper third of the tibia and the subtrochanteric region of the femur.

The most serious complication of Paget's disease is osteogenic sarcoma, a condition which is found in about 5 to 10 percent of patients with extensive and severe skeletal involvement. In the milder type of Paget's disease, the incidence falls to 2 to 3 percent. An early finding in osteogenic sarcoma is localized pain accompanied by bony enlargement. The tumor may be found in any affected bone, with a predilection for the upper limbs and the skull. (For the radiographic changes in osteogenic sarcoma, see D-6, above.)

9. Treatment

Although a number of medications have recently been proposed as therapy in osteitis deformans, only one, calcitonin, has thus far been approved by the FDA for such use. This drug is a small polypeptide hormone secreted by the ultimobranchial gland of fish, amphibia, reptiles, and birds. In mammals, it is formed by the parafollicular cells found chiefly in the thyroid gland.

A definite physiologic role for calcitonin in normal calcium homeostasis has not been established. Among the possibilities suggested is that the hormone acts to prevent a surge in blood calcium that would ordinarily occur during the intestinal absorption of dietary calcium. Another theory which has been postulated is that calcitonin plays a homeostatic role in skeletal remodeling. Theoretically, it is possible that the hormone induces an increase in the rate of bone formation and a decrease in osteoclastic bone resorption, thus contributing to the development of a positive skeletal balance.

The activity of the hormone is expressed in British Medical Research Council (MRC) units and is defined as the ability to lower plasma calcium in the rat as compared to a standard. Synthetic salmon calcitonin (Calcimar) is available commercially, each vial containing 400 MRC units. An adequate dosage schedule consists of a starting dose of 100 MRC units/day injected subcutaneously or intramuscularly, followed by as little at 50 units three times a week once the patient's condition has stabilized.

The therapeutic effect from a course of calcitonin consists of symptomatic improvement which has been reported to be maintained for as long as 1 year [5]. Significant changes are relief of bone pain in a matter of weeks, an increase in the patient's mobility, a fall in the elevated skin temperature over the site of the lesion, reduction in severity of symptoms from cord compression due to vertebral involvement, and a decrease in cardiac output in patients with high output. X-ray examination has demonstrated the formation of normal-appearing new bone in the involved structure at the same time that abnormal bony changes regress.

The chief advantages of salmon calcitonin are that it rarely exhibits primary toxicity, side effects are mild and infrequent, and radiologic improvement in bone lesions can be demonstrated relatively soon. However, it does have the disadvantage of requiring parenteral administration; moreover, a significant proportion of patients receiving the agent will develop antibodies to the foreign protein in it, thus rendering the drug ineffective in some cases.

Among other drugs which have been proposed for the treatment of Paget's disease of bone is disodium etidronate, which is included in a group of chemicals known as diphosphonates. Since it has only recently been approved for use by the FDA, the available clinical information regarding its efficacy is limited. It appears to be less effective than salmon calcitonin, but it is more convenient to administer since it can be given orally and it is less expensive. However, its use has been associated with increased bone pain early in the course of treatment and with high dosages, spontaneous fractures may occur.

Mithramycin (Mithracin), a cytotoxic agent, has shown promising early results, but the necessity for intravenous administration and such side effects as nausea, possible bone marrow suppression, and liver damage may rule out its use in Paget's disease of bone. Among other drugs which have been proposed as therapy

is dactinomycin (actinomycin D, Cosmegen), which like mithramycin is an RNA inhibitor. All of these chemicals have in common an ability to prevent calcium resorption from bone.

Attempts have also been made to reduce blood flow to the involved bone, on the basis that the increase in local circulation found in Paget's disease is responsible for the pathologic alterations in bony structure (see D-3, above). Among the medications used for this purpose is epinephrine by intravenous administration [17]. However, the marked reduction in osseous blood flow is transitory, and so the approach is unsuitable for prolonged treatment or for proper evaluation.

E. Dupuytren's Contracture

Dupuytren's contracture, an overgrowth of the normal palmar fascia, is probably a hereditary disorder which is most prevalent in men over 40 years of age. An early finding is a small mass near the distal palmar crease opposite the ring finger; this is followed by hypertrophy of the tissues, to produce a subcutaneous contracting band which becomes palpable in the line of the palmar fascia.

1. Etiologic Factors

Among the numerous causative agents which have been proposed for this condition are toxic substances (alcohol, nicotine, lead) and particularly osteochondritic changes in the cervical portion of the vertebral column, producing compression of the contents of the intervertebral foramina. Other frequent etiologic factors are a hereditary tendency and trauma. It is possible that Dupuytren's contracture is a complex process in which several causative agents operate.

2. Vascular Manifestations

There appears to be a definitely altered reaction of the sympathetic nervous system in Dupuytren's contracture [41]. This takes the form of reduced vasomotor response to noxious stimuli in the involved hand and a lack of uniformity of the pulse wave, with a tendency toward decreased amplitude. The vasomotor reactivity continues to diminish as the severity of the anatomic alterations increases.

F. Avascular (Aseptic) Bone Necrosis

1. Definition

Avascular or aseptic bone necrosis results from death of subchondral bone, followed by osseocartilaginous sequestration and adjacent secondary osteosclerosis. When small areas of bone are involved (a segment of femoral head or a condyle), the designation osteochondritis dissecans is given to the process. In children the changes occur in the capital epiphysis of the femur (Legg-Calvé-Perthes disease; osteochondritis deformans juvenilis).

2. Etiology

The cause of avascular bone necrosis is unknown, although in some instances trauma has been implicated as the etiologic agent. For example, in the case of a medial femoral neck fracture, it has been shown by arteriography that if the superior capsular branches of the medial circumflex femoral artery leading to the femoral head are also destroyed by the injury or if the distal branches of this vessel are occluded, invariably femoral head necrosis will follow [13,27,46]. Subcapital (intracapsular) and, less frequently, intertrochanteric fractures may also be associated with avascular bone necrosis.

However, there are a number of other situations in which the cause for avascular bone necrosis is not apparent. This condition may be associated with such systemic disorders as sickle-cell anemia [14], Gaucher's disease, neoplasms, and systemic lupus erythematosus (see C-3, Chapter 13). Also, it may arise spontaneously [42].

3. Pathogenesis and Pathology

The precipitating factor is an obliteration of the blood supply to the epiphysis, followed by

a state of reactive hyperemia, as demonstrated in the radiograph by the appearance of osteoporosis [16]. During the healing stage, as new blood vessels grow into the area, bone repair takes place. Since the resulting structure is soft, continued pressure on the surface may produce flattening of the bone and irregularities in the contour of the articular surfaces; such alterations are subsequently responsible for the appearance of adaptive changes.

4. Clinical Manifestations

The most common entity in this group is Legg-Calvé-Perthes disease which occurs in children between the ages of 4 and 12 years, with a greater incidence among boys. Only rarely is bilateral involvement of the capital femoral epiphysis present. Generally there is complete healing after a period of years, with usually good anatomic restoration of the femoral head. The main initial finding is a limp with or without pain; this may disappear for periods of time and then return. If no attempt is made to treat the condition, as by the use of a cast or removal of the weight of the body from the involved joint by some other means, deformity of the hip may follow; in part, this may be due to the subsequent development of degenerative arthritis.

The general pattern which suggests the presence of aseptic necrosis is persistent localization of pain to one joint on motion. Rest completely relieves the symptom, in contrast to the usual discomfort of rheumatoid arthritis which is constant. If there is knee involvement, initial unilateral swelling with effusion may be present, but with no increase in cutaneous temperature of the overlying skin. When the hip is affected, the painful limp is localized to one side with radiation of pain down the thigh, occasionally associated with spasm of thigh muscles.

5. Laboratory Aids

Roentgenographic changes are usually observed soon after onset of symptoms. The early manifestation is demarcation of necrotic bone from viable bone, with no decalcification being seen in the former since it no longer has a blood supply. As a result of the secondary osteoporosis in the adjacent viable bone (due to reactive hyperemia), the necrotic segment of bone by comparison appears increased in density on the radiograph.

Since necrosis of the femoral head occurs in about one-third of the cases of fracture of the neck of the femur (especially with the fracture in poor position) [10], it is essential when these conditions exist to make every effort to detect the early presence of such a complication. For this purpose, the use of radioactive phosphorus (^{32}P) has been proposed [4]. However, subsequent investigation with this diagnostic technique has revealed that an error would have been made in about 10 percent of the cases of the uptake of radioactive phosphorus had this test been relied on to decide whether a femoral-head prosthesis should have been inserted previously [11]. Another problem with the procedure is that it is difficult to obtain data from the weight-bearing portion of the femoral head. Because of such objections, other diagnostic approaches have been proposed, among which is the use of ^{24}Na as a preferable isotope for determining the blood supply of the femoral head and, therefore, its viability [35]. Injection of radiopaque dyes into the femoral head, to visualize the veins and to estimate the degree of intactness of or damage to the circulation to this structure, has also been suggested [30,32].

6. Treatment

Aside from physical means to eliminate or reduce weight bearing on the affected limb, attempts have been made to revascularize the necrotic femoral head with bone grafts [43]. Satisfactory results have been reported in 75 percent of the patients treated by drilling and bone-grafting of the femoral head [9].

References

1. Abramson DI, Fierst SM, Flachs K: Unpublished observations
2. Abramson DI, Flachs K, Freiberg J, et al: Blood flow in extremities affected by anterior poliomyelitis. Arch Intern Med 71:391, 1943
3. Alpert S: Cardiovascular complications of Paget's disease: A case report. Ann Intern Med 48:871, 1958
4. Arden GP, Veall N: The use of radioactive phosphorus in early detection of avascular necrosis in the femoral head in fractured neck of femur. Proc R Soc Med 46:344, 1953
5. Avramides A, Flores A, De Rose J, et al: Paget's disease of the bone: Observations after cessation of long-term synthetic salmon calcitonin therapy. J Clin Endocrinol Metab 42:459, 1976
6. Barry HC: Paget's Disease of Bone. Edinburgh, Livingston, 1969, pp 3, 95, 105, 141
7. Bashour FA: Clubbing of the digits: Physiologic considerations. J Lab Clin Med 58:613, 1961
8. Blumhardt R, Nusynowitz ML: A guide to bone scanning. Am Fam Physician 9:153, 1974
9. Bonfiglio M, Bardenstein MB: Treatment by bone-grafting of aseptic necrosis of the femoral head and non-union of the femoral neck (Phemister technique). J Bone Joint Surg 40A:1329, 1958
10. Boyd HB: Avascular necrosis of the head of the femur. In: Instructional Course Lectures, American Academy of Orthopaedic Surgeons, Vol 14. Ann Arbor, Edwards, 1957, p 196
11. Boyd HB, Calandruccio RA: Further observations on the use of radioactive phosphorus (P^{32}) to determine the viability of the head of the femur: Correlation of clinical and experimental data in 130 patients with fractures of the femoral neck. J Bone Joint Surg 45A:445, 1963
12. Braibanti T: Die Arteriographie der Extremitäten bei den Folgen der Heine-Medinschen Krankheit. Fortschr Geb Röntgenstrahlen Nuklearmed 89:277, 1958
13. Brünner S, Christiansen J, Kristensen JK: Arteriographic prediction of femoral head viability in medial femoral neck fractures. Acta Chir Scand 133:449, 1967
14. Chung SMK, Ralston EL: Necrosis of the femoral head associated with sickle-cell anemia and its genetic variants: A review of the literature and study of thirteen cases. J Bone Joint Surg 51A:33, 1969
15. Dohn K: Functional plethysmography in disturbances of the circulation following poliomyelitis. Acta Orthop Scand 22:337, 1952–1953
16. Dubois EL, Cozen L: Avascular (aseptic) bone necrosis associated with systemic lupus erythematosus. JAMA 174:966, 1960
17. Edholm OG, Howarth S: Studies on the peripheral circulation in osteitis deformans. Clin Sci 12:277, 1953
18. Edholm OG, Howarth S, McMichael J: Heart failure and bone blood flow in osteitis deformans. Clin Sci 5:249, 1945
19. Ellis LB, Weiss S: Vasomotor disturbance and edema associated with cerebral hemiplegia. Arch Neurol Psychiat 36:362, 1936
20. Flavell G: Reversal of pulmonary hypertrophic

osteoarthropathy by vagotomy. Lancet 1:260, 1956

21. Ginsburg J: Observations on the peripheral circulation in hypertrophic pulmonary osteoarthropathy. Q J Med 27:335, 1958

22. Goetz RH, Du Tort JG, Swart BH: Vascular changes in poliomyelitis and the effect of sympathectomy on bone growth. Acta Med Scand 152:56 (Suppl 306), 1955

23. Hall GH: The cause of digital clubbing: Testing a new hypothesis. Lancet 1:750, 1959

24. Hall GH, Laidlaw CD: Further experimental evidence implicating reduced ferritin as a cause of digital clubbing. Clin Sci 24:121, 1963

25. Harper FR, Patterson LT: Osteoarthropathy in carcinoma of the lung. Arch Surg 70:643, 1955

26. Hecht A: Idiopathic hypertrophic osteoarthropathy. NY State J Med 65:3038, 1965

27. Herndon JH, Aufranc OE: Avascular necrosis of the femoral head in the adult: A review of its incidence in a variety of conditions. Clin Orthop 86:43, 1972

28. Holling HE, Brodey RS: Pulmonary hypertrophic osteoarthropathy. JAMA 178:977, 1961

29. Holt KS: The calf blood flow in normal children and in children with cerebral palsy. Clin Sci 22:363, 1962

30. Hulth A: Injection of contrast medium in the head of the femur at intracapsular fractures of the neck of the femur: A method of studying the remaining vascular supply of the capital fragments. Acta Soc Med Upsal 59:41, 1953

31. Jaffe HL: Metabolic, Degenerative, and Inflammatory Disease of Bones and Joints. Philadelphia, Lea & Febiger, 1972, Chap 10

32. Jergesen F: Osteography of the femoral head. J Bone Joint Surg 38A:435, 1956

33. Kottke FJ, Stillwell GK: Studies on increased vasomotor tone in the lower extremities following anterior poliomyelitis. Arch Phys Med 32:401, 1951

34. Kozák P: Circulatory changes of the paretic extremities after acute anterior poliomyelitis. Arch Phys Med Rehabil 49:77, 1968

35. Laing PG, Ferguson AB Jr: Sodium-24 as an indicator of the blood supply of bone. Nature 182:1442, 1958

36. Lewis T, Pickering GW: Circulatory changes in the fingers in some diseases of the nervous system with special reference to the digital atrophy of peripheral nerve lesions. Clin Sci 2:149, 1936

37. Lovell RRH: Observations on the nature of clubbed fingers. Clin Sci 9:299, 1950

38. Martin P, Lynn RB, Dible JH, et al: Peripheral Vascular Disorders. Edinburgh, Livingstone, 1956

39. Mendlowitz M: Some observations on clubbed fingers. Clin Sci 3:387, 1938

40. Mendlowitz M, Leslie A: The experimental simulation in the dog of the cyanosis and hypertrophic osteoarthropathy which are associated with congenital heart disease. Am Heart J 24:141, 1942

41. Paletta FX, Adams J, Avery W: Vasomotor reactivity in Dupuytren's contracture. J Appl Physiol 10:455, 1957

42. Patterson RJ, Bickel WH, Dahlin DC: Idiopathic avascular necrosis of the head of the femur: A study of fifty-two cases. J Bone Joint Surg 46A:267, 1964

43. Phemister DB: Treatment of the necrotic head of the femur in adults. J Bone Joint Surg 31A:55, 1949

44. Redisch W, Tangco FF: Peripheral Circulation in Health and Disease. New York, Grune & Stratton, 1957

45. Rhodes BA, Greyson ND, Hamilton CR Jr: Absence of anatomic arteriovenous shunts in Paget's disease of bone. N Engl J Med 287:686, 1972

46. Théron J: Superselective angiography of the hip: Technique, normal features, and early results in idiopathic necrosis of the femoral head. Radiology 124:649, 1977

47. Uprus V, Gaylor JD, Williams DJ, et al: Vasodilatation and vasoconstriction in response to warming and cooling the body: A study in patients with hemiplegia. Brain 58:448, 1935

48. Vaes GM, Nichols G Jr: Oxygen tension and the control of bone cell metabolism. Nature 193:379, 1962

49. Wilson GM: Local circulatory changes associated with clubbing of the fingers and toes. Q J Med 21:201, 1952

Chapter 15

Vascular Complications of Musculoskeletal Disorders Produced by Trauma

---

Part 1 Injury to Main Blood Vessels

A. General Considerations

1. Approach to the Dual Problem

Since fractures of the bones of the extremities, dislocations, and sprains may be associated with injury of neighboring vascular channels, it is always necessary to consider the possibility of the coexistence of the two types of disorders when planning the therapeutic approach to the orthopedic problem. Some workers believe that because of the relatively greater seriousness of the circulatory condition, its control takes precedence over the repair of the musculoskeletal difficulty [24]. Others, however, are of the opinion that a fracture, for example, should be handled first through stabilization by an appropriate form of internal fixation [4]. There are certain disadvantages to the latter approach since the insertion of internal fixating devices adds to the period of ischemia of the limb which may thus be critically prolonged. Moreover, the procedure contributes to further soft-tissue disruption and venous stasis, both of which may adversely affect the viability of the extremity. On the other hand, if vascular surgery is performed first, extreme care must subsequently be exercised in skeletal fixation to prevent a second injury to the involved artery. If feasible and practical, perhaps the dilemma could be resolved through a combined cooperative approach by an orthopedic and a vascular surgical team.

2. Types of Vascular Injuries and of Causative Agents

Arterial injuries fall into several categories: those which are caused by direct trauma of vascular structures, resulting in acute arterial insufficiency (Fig. 15.1); those which are secondary to stretch, angulation, compression, or spasm; and those which develop later as a consequence of damage to the walls of vessels, such as false arterial aneurysms and acquired arteriovenous fistulae.

Direct effects of trauma. Acute ischemia of distal tissues may result from penetrating wounds that produce severance, laceration, perforation, contusion, or disruption of the intima of a critical artery and from external compression of a vessel by a hematoma. Nonpenetrating or blunt trauma may have a similar effect by causing contusion followed by thrombosis of the artery or by producing an intramural hemorrhage or disruption of the intima.

Iatrogenic lesions. In recent years, because of the increasing use of diagnostic and therapeutic procedures requiring puncture of the arterial

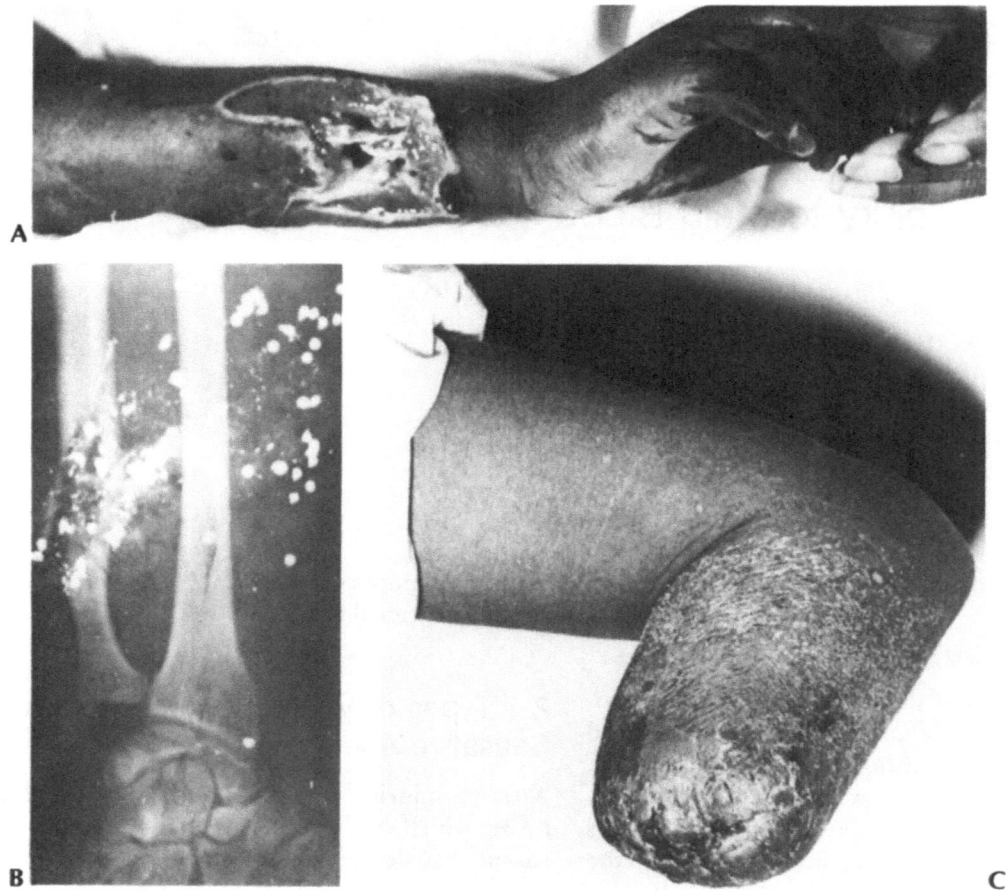

Fig. 15.1. Trauma to radial and ulnar arteries at the wrist, due to a shotgun blast. **A** Gangrene of hand. **B** X ray of forearm demonstrating the pellets. **C** Amputation of distal portion of forearm.

tree, the incidence of iatrogenic arterial injuries has increased significantly. Such lesions are generally seen in the femoral and radial arteries because these superficial vessels are readily accessible for performing such procedures as heart catheterization, angiography, and puncture and cannulation for monitoring blood gas levels and blood pressure. The types of resulting arterial injuries consist of false aneurysm, acquired arteriovenous fistula, severe local spasm followed by thrombosis, and dissection and laceration of the wall of the vessel [1].

3. Common Sites for Vascular Trauma

There are a number of locations where a fracture of a long bone alone or associated with a dislocation has a great tendency to produce injury to vascular structures. In general, deep, relatively fixed arteries, such as those found about main joints, are more prone to such a possibility than are other vessels. For example, the popliteal artery is firmly attached at the upper end of the popliteal space by the tendinous arch of the adductor magnus muscle and distally by the soleus and gastrocnemius arches. This anatomic relationship, together with the direct contact of the vessel with the posterior portion of the knee joint, explains its liability to injury (Fig. 15.2B and C). Fractures of the femur, both of the shaft and intertrochanteric, may be associated with trauma to the deep femoral artery and its accompanying vein. When there is an injury to the lower end of the femur, the superficial femoral (Fig. 15.3B) or the pop-

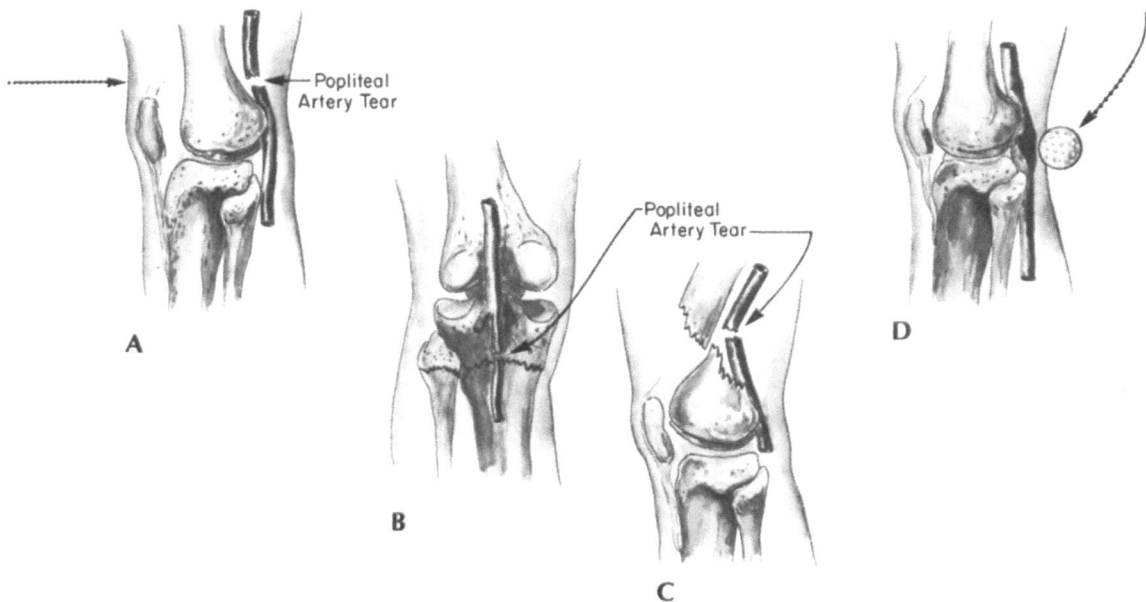

Fig. 15.2. Schematic presentation of various types of popliteal artery injuries. **A** Tear of vessel due to a blow over the patella causing a backward thrust of the femur. **B** Tear of vessel due to fracture of the upper portion of the tibia. **C** Tear of vessel due to supracondylar fracture of the femur. **D** Thrombosis of vessel due to trauma to the popliteal space from a driven golf ball.

liteal artery (Fig. 15.2C) may be affected, whereas a fibular fracture endangers the posterior tibial, the anterior tibial, or the peroneal artery. With a fracture of the ankle, there is the possibility of damage to the lower segment of the posterior tibial artery (Fig. 15.3C) and its vein.

In the upper portion of the body, fracture of the clavicle may produce aneurysmal dilatation, thrombosis, or transection of the subclavian artery. Rupture or thrombosis of the axillary artery may follow anterior dislocation of the shoulder or fracture of the neck of the humerus (Figs. 15.3A and 15.4). The brachial vessels are vulnerable to supracondylar fracture of the humerus, as well as to fracture-dislocation of the elbow joint [13]. Fractures of the ulna or radius may cause laceration or spasm of the ulnar or radial arteries (Fig. 15.5).

Fractures of the pelvis, especially if multiple, have been associated with laceration of iliac arteries, uncontrollable hemorrhage, and ultimately shock and death. Also there may be neurovascular complications, including sensory deficits in the lower limbs, foot drop, and weakness of the entire extremity. (For the control

of hemorrhage in pelvic fractures, see B-4, below.)

4. Role of Contrast Angiography in Vascular Injuries

The question of when contrast arteriography (see Section E, Chapter 5) should be utilized in vascular trauma has not been fully answered. It is the opinion of some vascular surgeons that all penetrating injuries in the vicinity of major arteries should be explored immediately rather than first performing an arteriogram. Others, however, believe that a surgical procedure should never be carried out following trauma without having available the information derived from angiography.

Contraindications to use of angiography. Neither of the above viewpoints appears to apply to all situations. For example, if there are clearcut signs of severe arterial ischemia and absent pulses in the distal portion of the limb following trauma to a segment of limb in which a critical artery is located, or if there is profuse

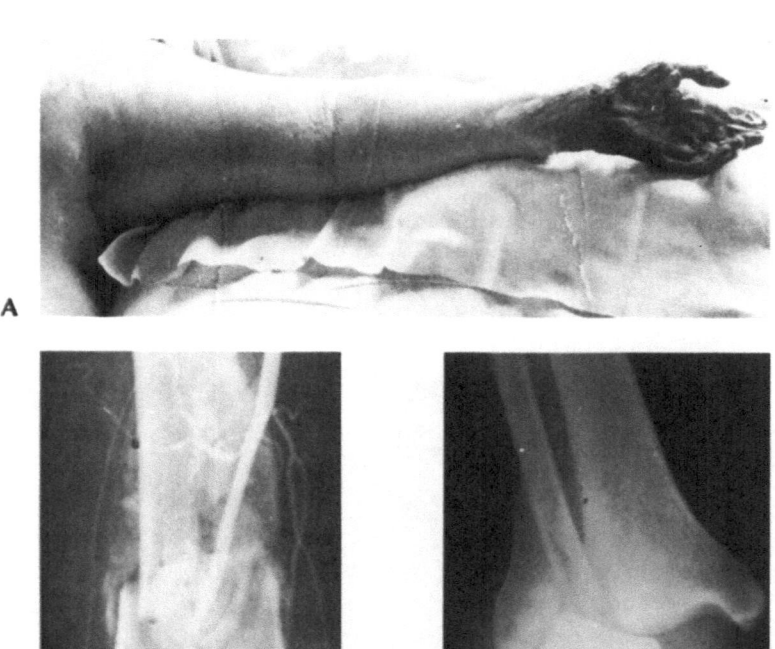

Fig. 15.3. Vascular trauma incurred with fracture of long bones. **A** Fracture of neck of humerus causing partial severance of the axillary artery and repeated episodes of local bleeding, followed by infection of the hematoma, thrombosis of the vessel, and gangrene of the hand. **B** Comminuted supracondylar fracture of the femur, causing thrombosis of the lower portion of the superficial femoral artery, as visualized by arteriography. **C** Fracture dislocation of the right ankle, causing a tear of the posterior tibial artery and gangrene of the foot requiring subsequent below-knee amputation.

hemorrhage or a pulsating hematoma with or without an associated bruit, both types of findings point toward immediate surgical exploration without the need for first performing such a time-consuming procedure as arteriography. Nor is this measure indicated when the injury is some distance removed from the location of any critical artery, the local hemorrhage is readily controlled, and signs of ischemia of distal tissues are absent or minimal. Under such circumstances, the possibility of trauma to important vascular structures is very slight, and therefore angiography and surgical intervention should not be contemplated.

Indications for use of angiography. Arteriography is a valuable diagnostic tool when the clinical changes are equivocal (as, for example, if signs of ischemia are of a mild degree but pulses are absent in the hand or foot) and there is difficulty in evaluating the extent of the hemorrhage or in determining whether the trauma could conceivably have injured a critical artery. Under such circumstances, arteriography may demonstrate an intact arterial tree, thus avoiding unnecessary surgical intervention, or a vascular injury may be identified, requiring immediate operative exploration. The procedure is very helpful in defining the location and extent of the arterial injury and in deciding upon the most practical approach to the problem. It is particularly useful in distinguishing a hematoma from soft-tissue swelling.

Precautions in interpreting changes in the angiogram. It is necessary to point out, however, that the information derived from arteriography may at times be misleading. For example,

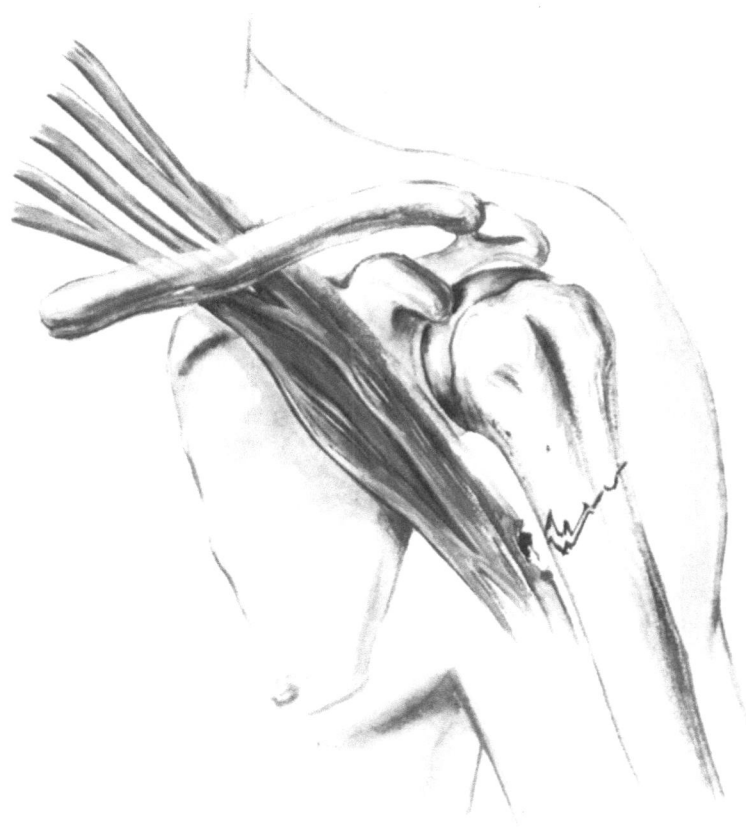

Fig. 15.4. Schematic presentation of laceration of the axillary artery associated with a fracture at the junction of the neck and shaft of the humerus.

a severely contused or lacerated artery possessing an intact wall will not be identified by such a means. Therefore, a negative angiogram does not always constitute a contraindication to surgical exploration, especially if the clinical evidence supports the possibility of the existence of an arterial lesion. Another point to consider is the fact that arteriography gives no information in a situation in which venous bleeding of a degree to warrant surgical intervention is present.[1]

5. Role of Venography in Vascular Injuries

Since not infrequently the accompanying vein is injured at the same time that the artery is traumatized, a study of the venous system by

means of contrast venography (see C-2, Chapter 7) is frequently indicated. The procedure should also be carried when the possibility exists that the trauma is limited to venous channels, with the result that no signs of ischemia of tissues are noted, and still the patient's life may be in danger due to bleeding from the severed vessel.

6. Essential Measures for Preservation of the Limb

Long-bone fractures are almost invariably associated with some degree of local arterial damage. This may take the form of injury to the nutrient or periosteal arteries, which is usually disregarded in the initial phase of treatment of the fracture although it is significant with regard to fracture healing. The trauma may also cause interruption of circulation through a large or medium-sized artery with the result

---

[1] Isotope angiography with ^{99}Tc-pertechnetate has been proposed as a means of reducing the number of contrast angiograms required as a screening procedure in determining whether arterial injury exists.

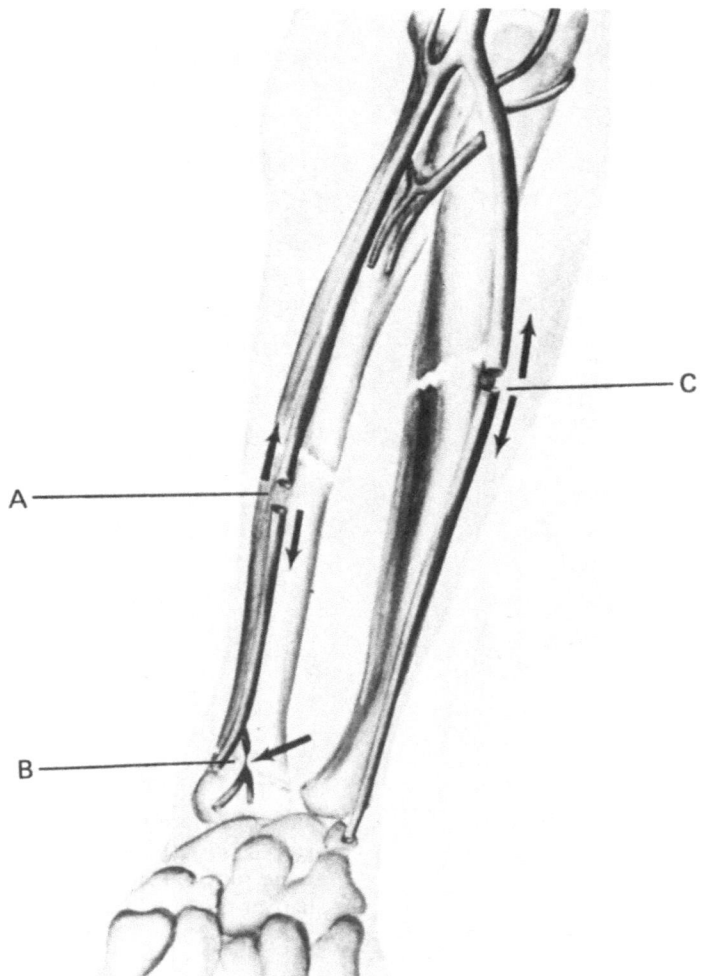

Fig. 15.5. Schematic presentation of types of vascular lesions associated with fractures of the forearm. **A,** fracture of the radius causing laceration of the radial artery; **B,** spasm of the radial artery at the wrist caused by fracture of distal segment of bone; **C,** fracture of the ulna at its midpoint associated with laceration of the ulnar artery.

that the viability of the limb is placed in jeopardy (Fig. 15.3A).

In those instances in which the local circulation is compromised, the salvage rate will depend basically on a number of factors: early recognition of the vascular difficulty; definitive diagnosis, frequently based on arteriography (see A-4, above); early exploration (without first resorting to such temporizing measures as periods of prolonged observation, fasciotomies, trials of vasodilators and anticoagulants, or paravertebral sympathetic blocks); and an aggressive operative approach including arterial reconstruction in order to reestablish circulation through the traumatized artery. Surgical measures are carried out in spite of the possibility of converting a simple fracture into a com-

pound one, with great care being taken to decontaminate the area through which the arterial repair is to be done.

7. Factors Impeding an Appropriate Therapeutic Program

Associated soft-tissue damage (requiring extensive debridement), hematoma formation, the fracture itself, hypovolemic shock or hypotension due to blood loss, and limitations to observation of the state of the limb imposed by casts and dressings untowardly affect the institution of a proper therapeutic program for the vascular difficulty. If there are any questions regarding the existence of vascular complications, then the type of cast applied for closed fractures should permit inspection of the digits. Where a massive wound or external fixation is involved, a bivalved cast should be used so that the limb can readily be examined at frequent intervals.

B. Laceration or Severance of a Main Artery

1. Etiology

Trauma to an artery in the limb may result in laceration or complete division of the vessel. Either type of injury is generally followed by marked ischemia of distal tissues and serious hemorrhage. The most extensive bleeding occurs when the artery is only partially severed (Fig. 15.3A), since in such circumstances the small intact bridge of vascular tissue prevents contraction of the proximal end of the cut vessel and normal retraction into the surrounding tissues. With a totally severed artery, hemorrhage is less marked. The injury may be caused by sharp objects (a razor, a knife, or an ice pick), high-velocity missiles, blunt instruments, or fragments of fractured bone. Commonly the superficial femoral artery is traumatized since it is located close to the surface of the limb and is not well protected by bony structures.

2. Pathogenesis

The type of bleeding which occurs following laceration or severance of an artery depends upon whether the skin has been penetrated by the causative agent. If it has, then the hemorrhage will be external. Otherwise, bleeding into the surrounding soft tissues will occur, with the production of a hematoma. In the case of the latter, the buildup of pressure within the mass may compress or even obliterate the lumen of the involved artery, thus preventing further hemorrhage.

3. Clinical Manifestations

The symptoms and signs of laceration or severance of a main artery depend upon the quantity of blood lost and the degree of ischemia of the distal tissues in the involved limb. If there is external bleeding and blood loss is great, the patient will develop the manifestations of hypovolemic shock. The production of a hematoma may result in lesser signs of such a state. With regard to local changes in the affected limb, the symptoms and signs closely resemble those of sudden occlusion of an important artery by an embolus (see A-3, Chapter 12).

4. Treatment and Prognosis

Therapy for laceration or severance of a main artery has a twofold aim. One is to combat the state of shock and to restore the normal blood volume by preventing further bleeding and replacing the lost blood. Bleeding should be controlled by pressure and not with a tourniquet, since the latter occludes collateral circulation as well and increases the existing ischemia. Such a measure also encourages distal thrombosis. The other step is to reestablish the local circulation of the involved limb by reconstructive methods if necessary and thus maintain viability of the tissues. Although at no time should the patient's life be placed in jeopardy in an attempt to save a devascularized limb, still, if feasible, prompt repair of all arterial injuries should be carried out. Such a measure generally prevents prolongation of acute ischemia and hence the onset of gangrene. Also, it reduces the incidence of traumatic false aneurysms and arteriovenous fistulae. Whenever possible, the companion vein, if also traumatized, should be repaired at the same time (see Section I, below). The need for postoperative anticoagulants does not exist if a forceful circulation has been reestablished.

Failure of arterial reconstruction may be due either to delay in attempting the procedure, postoperative edema with arterial compression, or technical difficulties resulting in anastomotic thrombosis. The type of wound also affects salvage rate. Blunt trauma generally produces more extensive soft-tissue injury than is caused by sharp penetrating objects and hence the prognosis is much poorer. In such circumstances the wound must be debrided so that all remaining soft tissue is assuredly viable; otherwise infection commonly supervenes. However, radical debridement frequently results in inadequate remaining tissue to cover the site of vascular reconstruction, and as a consequence, secondary hemorrhage and thrombosis may follow unless some type of protective measure is instituted.

In the presence of a fracture of the pelvis, signs of severe internal bleeding require heroic treatment. This consists of open exploratory pelvic laparotomy and ligation or repair of traumatized vessels. In this regard, selective aortography, with insertion of the catheter into a branch of the hypogastric artery, may be useful in identifying the involved channels [15, 30,31]. With this approach, it may then be possible to inject autologous clotted blood or Gelfoam (gelatin) strips into the lacerated vessel to produce arterial embolization, thus bringing about control of distal hemorrhage. In most patients blood replacement is necessary to counteract the shock state.

C.   Acute Vascular Spasm

Acute vascular spasm (traumatic vasospasm) is another complication of trauma to a limb, although in recent years it has been given less importance as a causative factor in the production of local ischemia of tissues. The response may be noted not only in the injured vessel but frequently in the entire arterial bed in the extremity. It may last for hours or even days and it may produce irreversible changes in the skin, nerves, muscles, and joints of the limb.

1.   Etiology

Acute vascular spasm may be caused by a blunt blow to the limb, a fracture of long bones (Fig. 15.5), manipulation of the artery during a surgical procedure, crushing injuries, or a gunshot wound in proximity to the vessel but not directly affecting it. The condition must be differentiated from arterial contusion which likewise does not result in either external or internal bleeding.

2.   Pathogenesis

The mechanism responsible for spasm of a large artery is active contraction of the circular muscular fibers in the wall of the vessel. Two types of arterial spasm exist: neurogenic and myogenic.

In the case of neurogenic arteriospasm, a reflex arc is established which includes the sympathetic nervous system as the efferent arm, the trigger mechanism which initiates it being the irritated segment of artery. The spasm follows from an increase in number and intensity of the vasoconstrictor impulses originating in the vasomotor center and reaching the neuroeffector organs (α-receptor endings) in the walls of the involved vessel and its branches. The resulting marked contraction of the vascular circular muscle fibers causes almost complete or complete obliteration of the arterial lumen.

In the case of myogenic arteriospasm, the initiating factor is also some type of irritation of a segment of artery, but the exact mechanism responsible for the change is not clear. It is possible that the intense contraction of the circular muscle fibers in the vessel wall represents a response of sensitized vascular tissue to circulating vasopressor substances. What is accepted is the fact that myogenic spasm is not dependent upon the integrity of the sympathetic nervous system.

The difference between neurogenic and myogenic spasm is manifest after removal of vasomotor tone by any of the clinically available means. This results in an almost immediate marked improvement in the appearance of the limb in the case of neurogenic arteriospasm, whereas if myogenic vasospasm exists, there is no therapeutic effect. However, it is necessary to point out that if neurogenic vasospasm persists for a relatively long time before excessive vasomotor control is removed, the latter measure may no longer produce reversal of the abnormal clinical changes, due to two possible mechanisms: permanent damage to nervous tissue from persistent anoxia and thrombosis of the segment of involved artery because of pathologic alterations in the intima of apposing portions of vessel wall.

3.   Clinical Manifestations

Initially the findings in neurogenic and myogenic vasospasm are the same since in both states there is a markedly reduced local circulation resulting from obstruction to blood flow in the artery feeding the distal tissues. Pain is usually severe, being located in the digits and possessing characteristics of neuritic involvement.

There is a decrease in cutaneous temperature beginning at the level of the arterial spasm or slightly above this point and extending over the remainder of the limb distally. The skin becomes very pale with cyanotic mottling in some areas as a result of trapping of blood in the cutaneous venules. Neurologic signs are prominent, consisting of foot drop or wrist drop, paralysis of the intrinsic muscles of the foot or hand, and a stocking-glove type of anesthesia or hypesthesia. The peripheral pulses become greatly reduced or even impalpable, and oscillometric readings are decreased or absent.

The subsequent clinical course depends upon whether the vasospasm can be removed before irreversible changes in the skin and peripheral nerves occur. If this can be accomplished readily, the abnormal findings soon recede and the limb assumes a normal appearance. On the other hand, if the vasospasm persists, this may be followed by necrosis of distal tissues if the affected vessel is a critical one.

4. Treatment

Neurogenic arteriospasm. Therapy consists of means to produce temporary paralysis of vasomotor control over the peripheral arteries. For this purpose, repeated paravertebral sympathetic blocks, continuous spinal or caudal anesthesia, and the use of sympathetic blocking agents are indicated. Also of adjunctive value are the intraarterial administration of papaverine sulfate, oral whiskey, and reflex vasodilatation.

Myogenic arteriospasm. Attempts should be made to eliminate the causative agent, as by reducing a fracture to remove pressure of bony fragments on the involved artery, evacuating collections of blood clot, and splinting the injured limb to minimize pressure on irritable vascular elements. Attempts to remove vasomotor tone, as mentioned above, are ineffective, thus revealing the true nature of the condition.

If there is still no change in the clinical picture, more heroic procedures are indicated. These include careful surgical exposure of the artery, which is then covered by warm saline dressings, and local application of myovascular relaxants, such as a warm 2.5% solution of papaverine sulfate [10] or a warm 1% solution of procaine sulfate. If relaxation of the artery does not occur in a period of 10 to 15 min, the wound should be loosely closed, leaving a fine polyethylene tube in contact with the vessel for future installations of a 1% solution of papaverine at intervals until circulation is restored. In some cases it may be necessary to strip the adventitia of the involved segment of artery (periarterial sympathectomy), followed by forcibly stretching the lumen of the vessel by injecting warm saline under pressure after the involved portion is temporarily isolated between bulldog clamps. Finally, if this procedure fails to remove the spasm, transection of the contracted segment of artery should be performed and then an end-to-end anastomosis or insertion of a segment of venous graft carried out.

D. Traumatic Arterial Thrombosis

Traumatic arterial thrombosis may occur either in a healthy or a diseased artery following injury to the vessel.

1. Etiologic Factors

Mechanisms producing rapid occlusion. One group of causative agents consists of fracture, a blunt blow, shell fragments, or a bullet. In each instance there is a sudden, direct contusion of the artery, producing rupture or rolling up of the intimal layer and possibly the media, but no destruction of the continuity of the vessel wall. Following such an injury, platelets and debris from the blood tend to be deposited on the involved site, with the result that they act as a nidus for further accumulation of material until complete filling of the lumen occurs.

Mechanisms producing slow occlusion. Much more frequently traumatic arterial thrombosis follows moderate and indirect pressure to the exterior of an artery, applied intermittently and transiently over a protracted period. This causes injury to the intima and a gradual growth of thrombus at the site of trauma until complete obstruction of the vessel lumen is produced. The location of such a lesion is generally close to a joint or between bone and the tendinous insertion of a muscle.

The anatomic location of the popliteal artery is such that, besides direct trauma from dislocation of the knee joint or fracture of the long bones of the lower limb, this vessel may be damaged by repeated contractions of surrounding muscles, in its course through the fibromuscular canal at the level of the upper border of the femoral condyles. Thrombosis of the superficial femoral artery in its passage through the adductor canal may occur because of repeated compression by similar forces.

2. Clinical Manifestations

The symptoms and signs of traumatic arterial thrombosis depend upon the type of agent producing the original intimal injury. If a strong blow or a fracture is the cause, resulting in extensive damage and rapid development of a thrombotic process, the clinical picture will be similar to that of an acute arterial embolism or a rapidly developing spontaneous arterial thrombosis (see Sections A and B, respectively, Chapter 12). In the presence of repeated mild trauma to an artery, resulting in a slow buildup of a thrombus, the signs and symptoms will resemble the clinical picture usually associated with a chronic occlusive arterial disorder (see B-1 and B-2, Chapter 11). In fact, if the process develops very slowly, the compensatory collateral circulation may be adequate enough to prevent the appearance of any abnormal manifestations.

3. Treatment

In the acutely developing traumatic arterial thrombosis, the first step in therapy is removal of the precipitating agent. A dislocation should be reduced and a hematoma evacuated, and if fragments of bone are present, muscle must be interposed. Attempts to perform a thrombectomy are generally of no avail since rethrombosis almost inevitably results. Hence, if the vascular injury is extensive, excision of the segment of injured vessel, followed by end-to-end anastomosis or insertion of a venous graft, is indicated. If there is superimposed vasospasm, attempts should be made to remove this by repeated paravertebral sympathetic blocks or, in the case of the lower limb, also by continuous spinal or caudal anesthesia.

In the slowly developing traumatic arterial thrombosis, again attempts should be made to remove the causative agent if possible. If complete occlusion has occurred, the treatment is the same as described above, provided the affected artery is a critical one.

E. Traumatic Arterial Aneurysm

1. Etiology and Pathogenesis

Traumatic arterial aneurysm (false aneurysm; pulsating hematoma) is a pulsatile mass arising from or located in a segment of artery. It results from an injury to the vessel wall, generally due to sharp penetrating missiles (Fig. 15.6), certain surgical procedures, fracture of long bones (Fig. 15.7), and hypodermic needles, although blunt trauma and even an osteochondroma of the femur associated with severe physical exertion may also be responsible for such a lesion.

A traumatic arterial aneurysm generally develops as a result of actual perforation of the wall due to injury to all coats of the vessel, followed by bleeding into the surrounding tissues. The clotted material is then covered only by a wall of fibrin, and the interior of the sac thus formed communicates with the vessel through the original site of rupture (false aneurysm). On occasion, trauma to an artery results in the formation of a true aneurysm in which the continuity of the vessel wall is still intact, but dilatation has occurred due to weakness, thinning, and stretching of the muscle coat. This type of lesion may develop if the injury has resulted in the destruction of only the outer layers of vessel.

Frequent sites for the production of a traumatic arterial aneurysm are the femoral (Fig. 15.6) and brachial arteries, although almost all vessels in the limbs are so situated that they

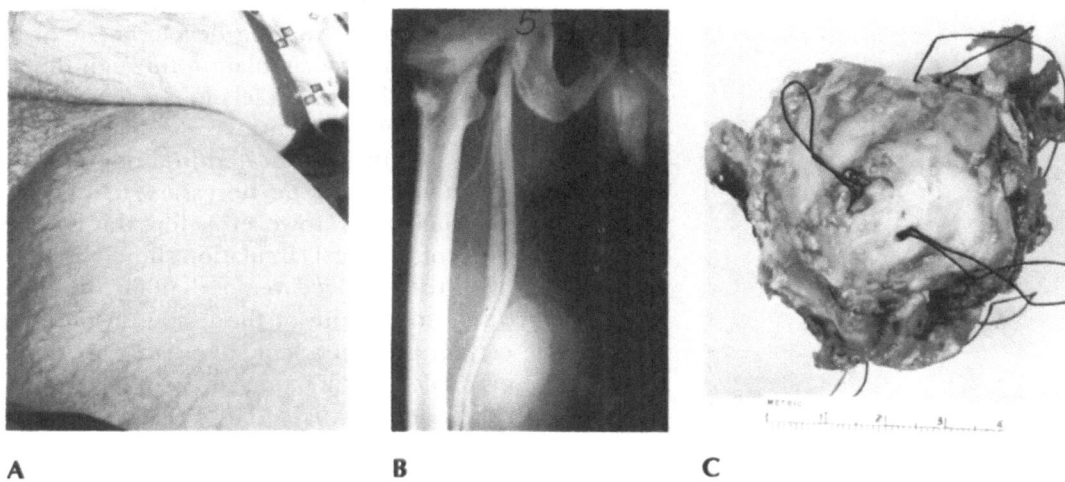

A   B   C

Fig. 15.6. **A** Aneurysm of superficial femoral artery following trauma caused by shell fragments. **B** Visualization of superficial femoral arterial aneurysm by arteriography. **C** Aneurysm removed and arterial circulation reestablished using a venous graft.

also may be similarly affected. Fusiform dilatations of the subclavian artery may be found in long-standing cervical rib and scalenus anticus syndromes (see p. 194). Repeated blunt trauma to the palm of the hand may produce aneurysms of the palmar arteries (see G-1, below).

2. Clinical Manifestations

The development of a traumatic arterial aneurysm is not associated with any clear-cut complaints. Pain may be present in the area of involvement due to compression of neighboring nervous structures by an expanding lesion. The patient may also become aware of the presence of a pulsatile mass following a local injury. If the aneurysm is large and is located in a confined space, as in the case of the popliteal fossa, symptoms may be more marked.

Examination generally reveals the presence of an expansile mass (Fig. 15.6A) synchronous with the heartbeat. A thrill can be felt and a systolic bruit heard over the lesion, unless the sac is filled with clot; under the latter circumstances, these clinical findings may be difficult to elicit or may even be absent. Signs of reduced arterial circulation in the distal portion of the limb are minimal, since once the sac has formed and is filled with blood, the circulation through the arterial channel becomes rees-

tablished at about the previous level of efficiency. Of course, if the clot in the sac grows and projects into the lumen of the artery, reducing its size, then indications of local impairment of blood flow will become evident.

Because of lack of clear-cut clinical manifestations of the uncomplicated, stable traumatic arterial aneurysm, generally the diagnosis is not made unless areas of previous trauma are routinely examined for the presence of pulsatile masses and possibly bruits.

3. Complications

There is a tendency for a traumatic arterial aneurysm to enlarge with time, resulting in the appearance of such serious complications as liberation of pieces of clot from the cavity of the sac with occlusion of distal arteries; thrombosis of the aneurysm and of the adjoining portion of vessel; thrombosis of the associated vein as result of continuous and increasing compression by the growing aneurysmal sac; pressure on neighboring peripheral mixed nerves, with the production of bizarre neurologic symptoms and signs; and internal or external hemorrhage, due to disruption of the wall of the lesion as the latter enlarges.

Most of the above complications may cause loss of limb and even life. Furthermore, with their appearance, the possibility of performing

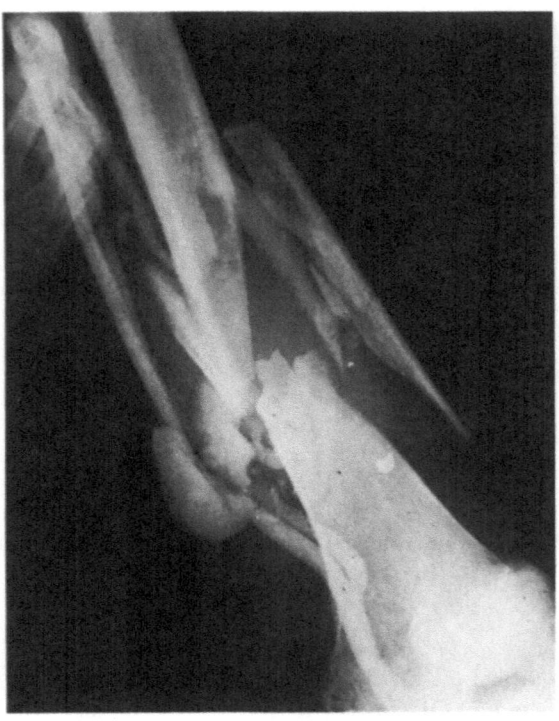

Fig. 15.7. Supracondylar comminuted fracture associated with the development of an aneurysm of the superficial femoral artery; a supracondylar amputation was subsequently carried out.

a successful reconstructive procedure on the original lesion is very slight. Hence, the great need for early recognition of traumatic arterial aneurysm is evident.

4. Treatment and Prognosis

Therapy for traumatic arterial aneurysm is surgical, although rarely is it a matter of emergency except when the lesion is rapidly progressing in size or serious complications are developing.

If a critical artery is affected, the approach is excision of the lesion and reestablishment of local circulation, either by end-to-end anastomosis or by insertion of a venous graft (Fig. 15.6). If pulsations were previously present in the distal segment of the involved vessel, necrosis of the limb may develop unless such a step is carried out. The reason for this possibility occurring is that the existence of an arterial aneurysm is associated with an adequate blood

supply to the tissues locally, and hence the stimulus required for the development of an effective secondary circulation through the ingrowth of collateral vessels (a chronic state of ischemia) is not present.

If the aneurysm is located in a nonessential artery, it may only be necessary to perform aneurysmectomy. However, before this is done, the state of the local circulation should be studied with the involved vessel digitally occluded proximal to the site of the lesion, in order to be certain that an adequate circulation would be available after ligation of the artery.

If the aneurysm is so large that its removal might produce damage to the surrounding nerves and secondary arteries, it is advisable to carry out an endoaneurysmorrhaphy. All vessels feeding it are ligated and then the lesion is separated from its parent vessel and left undisturbed in the wound. This is followed by reestablishment of the continuity of the artery through the use of a venous graft.

F. Acquired Arteriovenous Fistula

1. Etiology and Types

Another clinical entity which may follow trauma to an extremity is an acquired arteriovenous fistula, a condition in which there is an abnormal communication between a large artery and companion vein. Several different types may develop: a simple direct connection between the two vessels; an aneurysmal dilatation between them; an aneurysmal sac arising from the artery which, in turn, is joined to the corresponding vein at approximately the sac level; and entrance of both vessels into a common aneurysmal sac through a single orifice. Fractures of long bones (Fig. 15.8C), among other etiologic factors, may be responsible for the production of the lesion.

2. Clinical Manifestations

Pathophysiology. The clinical picture of an acquired arteriovenous fistula is generally much more characteristic than that associated with a traumatic arterial aneurysm. This is so because the introduction of a secondary circula-

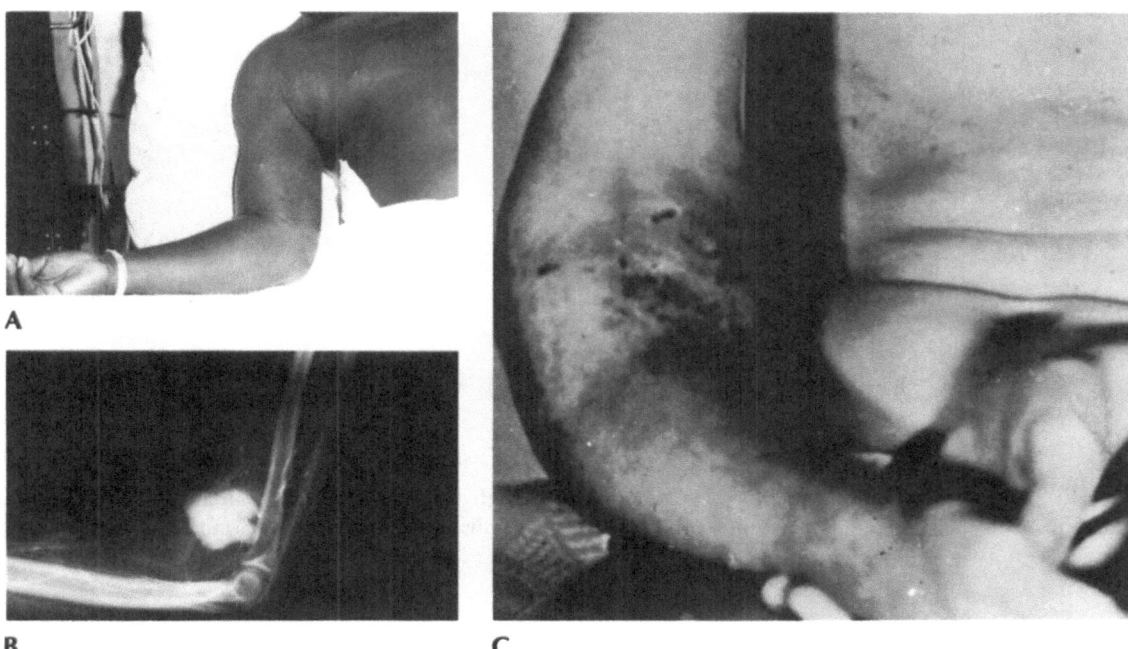

Fig. 15.8. Arteriovenous fistulae. **A** Injury to upper limb, producing a brachial arteriovenous fistula. **B** Arteriogram in same patient as in **A,** demonstrating the lesion and the immediate filling of the veins with contrast material. **C** Brachial arteriovenous fistula at elbow associated with a supracondylar fracture of the humerus. Before appearance of the lesion, there were numerous episodes of bleeding and of aspiration of hematomas.

tion, consisting of the artery feeding the fistula, the lesion itself, and the collecting vein, produces profound hemodynamic disturbances in the peripheral arterial and venous circulations and the heart. Blood seeks the pathway of least resistance, with the result that the abnormal arteriovenous communication, providing such a route, is responsible for the constant shunting of blood away from the high arteriolar and capillary resistance of the distal arterial bed into the large veins proximal to the lesion, in which the intraluminal pressure is normally very low. In a sense, there are now two systems of circulating blood, each competing for the available blood volume. To compensate for such a situation, a significant increase in circulating blood volume develops, with a consequent greater load placed on the heart by the augmentation in venous return, eventually resulting in congestive heart failure.

Symptoms. After the initial effects of the original injury have disappeared, the patient may begin to experience pain in the vicinity of the lesion, probably due to compression of nervous elements by the distended sac. At times, a shaking, throbbing, or even humming sensation may be present in the limb.

Local signs. In all instances there is a pulsatile mass in the vicinity of the original injury (Fig. 15.9) which varies in size. A thrill is generally palpated over the lesion, and a murmur is invariably heard which is continuous, with accentuation during systole. These physical findings are due to the passage of blood from the artery, through the communication, into dilated venous channels both in systole and diastole; the systolic intensification of the bruit results from the higher pressure present in the fistula in the period of time the heart is contracting. If the lesion has developed rapidly, the skin over it may be taut, thinned out, and red. Total digital obstruction of the main arterial channel feeding the fistula causes the latter to collapse.

Due to the marked shunting of blood through the fistulous tract, there is reduced circulation to distal tissues, which manifests it-

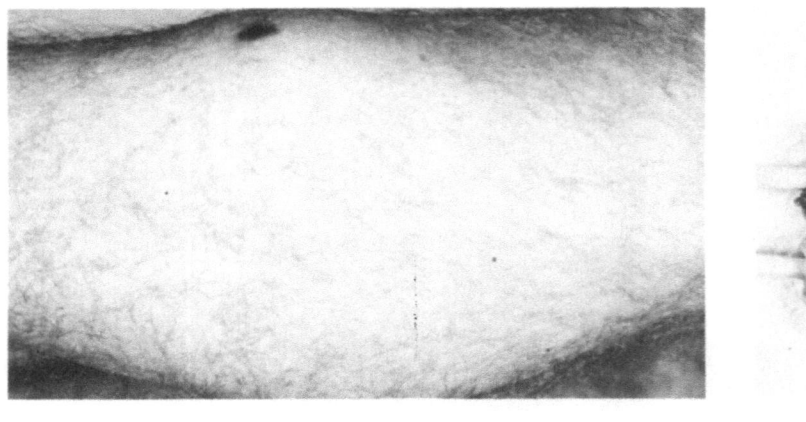
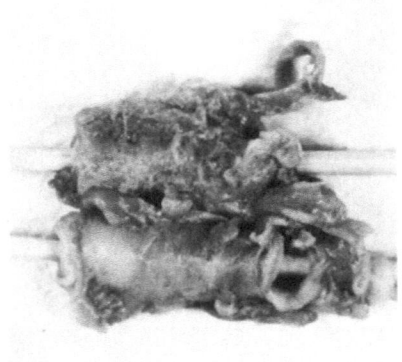

A   **B**

Fig. 15.9. Femoral arteriovenous fistula produced by a high-velocity projectile bullet. **A** Enlargement of thigh produced by lesion. **B** Fistula removed and reestablishment of arterial circulation accomplished using a venous graft.

self in the form of a low cutaneous temperature. At the same time, the skin above the level of the lesion has a higher than normal skin temperature because of the large quantity of blood passing into the large, tortuous, and varicose cutaneous veins proximal to the lesion. Associated with these findings are reduced or absent pulsations and oscillometric readings below the level of the fistula. Because of the greater movement of blood through the large veins, the circumference of the segment of the limb at and above the level of the lesion is greater than that of the opposite normal side (Fig. 15.9A). However, there is no increase in the length of the involved extremity, in contrast with a congenital arteriovenous fistula (see B-2, Chapter 21), unless the lesion developed before puberty.

Systemic changes. There is generally a rise in pulse rate, associated with a widening of pulse pressure due primarily to a fall in diastolic blood pressure. If the proximal segment of the artery feeding the lesion is occluded digitally, a transient rise in blood pressure and a slowing of the heart rate result (positive Branham's bradycardiac sign); the magnitude of the changes is directly related to the quantity of blood which ordinarily passes through the fistulous tract between artery and vein.

Diagnostic laboratory procedures. In the longstanding case, an increase in the size of the

ventricular chambers of the heart is noted by x ray, and the electrocardiogram demonstrates a left heart strain pattern. Circulating blood volume is definitely increased, while the oxygen content of venous blood obtained from above the level of the fistula is invariably high. A study of the velocity wave form, using the Doppler probe (see D-2, Chapter 5), is of value, since in the presence of an arteriovenous fistula, there is an increased forward flow of blood, especially during diastole. In contrast, in the resting normal limb, the forward flow in the latter period is negligible or absent. The Doppler probe can also be used to demonstrate the low blood pressure in arteries distal to the fistulous tract. If there is still question regarding the diagnosis, arteriography generally clearly visualizes the fistulous tract and outlines the arterial tree and the large venous channels proximal to the lesion (Fig. 15.8B).

3. Complications

Systemic changes. As has been mentioned before, the most serious complication of an untreated acquired arteriovenous fistula is congestive heart failure. If the lesion is small and some distance from the heart, the possibility of this state developing is minimal. However, with a large communication, the alterations in hemodynamics will generally be of sufficient magnitude to place a gradually increasing load on the heart that cannot be compensated for, particularly in the individual in the fifth to the seventh decade of life. As a consequence, clinical symptoms and signs of congestive heart failure will develop. Usually upper limb arteriovenous fistulae are better tolerated than those in the lower extremities. Although this difference has been attributed to the smaller size of the former, some experimental evidence has also been advanced to indicate that fistulous flow is decreased as the location of the communication is raised above the level of the heart.

Local changes. Because of the persistence of a high venous pressure in the limb below the level of the fistula, signs of chronic venous stasis, such as ulcers around the ankle, pigmentation, and changes in the consistency of the skin, develop. At times, intermittent claudication in the calf muscles may be present if the fistula is located in the superficial femoral or popliteal artery.

4. Treatment

As in the case of traumatic arterial aneurysm, acquired arteriovenous fistula of the major vessels of the limb requires surgical therapy, for otherwise impaired function of the heart will eventually result. Although in the past quadruple ligation was the procedure of choice, currently early excision of the lesion followed by arterial reconstruction is considered to be most effective. Through such a step, vascular repair is facilitated, blood loss is reduced, and systemic responses are avoided. Because end-to-end anastomosis generally results in a high incidence of arterial thrombosis, the insertion of an autogenous venous graft is used most often (Fig. 15.9B). Usually no attempt is made to reestablish venous flow and instead the cut ends are ligated.

G. Arterial Abnormalities of the Hand Resulting from Trauma

1. Palmar Artery Aneurysm

Etiology and location of lesion. A palmar artery aneurysm usually has a traumatic origin and may follow repeated contusions of the palm

or a single severe blow to this site [27]. The condition can also result from idiopathic or mycotic processes.

The most common location for a palmar artery aneurysm is the unprotected segment of superficial ulnar artery lying between the distal border of the volar carpal ligament and the palmar aponeurosis (on the hypothenar eminence) [27]. The hooklike process of the hamate bone is adjacent to the vessel and probably acts as an anvil, intensifying the effect of repeated trauma. In this location the artery is covered only by skin, subcutaneous tissue, and a few fibers of the palmaris brevis muscle. Another, less frequent, site for a palmar artery aneurysm is the base of the thenar eminence. Here the radial artery, unprotected by fascia, courses over the scaphoid and along the edge of the trapezium and base of the thumb, to enter the palm between the heads of the first dorsal interosseous muscle; it then joins the deep palmar arch.

Signs and symptoms. The clinical manifestations of an ulnar artery aneurysm consist of the presence of a tender, spongy, pulsatile mass over the ulnar aspect of the palm, at the base of the hypothenar eminence, and diminution of light touch and pin-prick sensation in the fourth and fifth fingers (ulnar nerve neuropathy). Pain may be present on movement of the digits. Of diagnostic significance is collapse of the lesion and disappearance of symptoms on digital obliteration of the ulnar and radial arteries at the wrist. Generally no thrills or bruits are present over the aneurysm. Coolness or cyanosis of the fourth or fifth fingers generally indicates that a secondary thrombotic process is developing in the aneurysm and in the artery from which it arises. Rarely is arteriography necessary to make a diagnosis of an ulnar artery aneurysm in the hand.

In the case of a radial artery aneurysm, the pulsating mass is found at the base of the thenar eminence. The lesion is often painful or tender and, if present for any period of time, generally contains a partially organized thrombus in its sac.

Treatment consists of resection of a segment of the involved artery and primary reanastomosis utilizing microvascular technique or the insertion of a reversed venous graft. Whether such an approach should always be followed is debatable. It has been suggested, however, that aneurysmal resection and ligation alone may lead to vascular insufficiency in the hand, despite the excellent collateral circulation present in the palm [11].

2. Hypothenar Hammer Syndrome

Etiology. Hypothenar hammer syndrome is a term given to occlusion of the superficial palmar branch of the ulnar artery. It is related to the repetitive use of the hand as a hammer in the course of daily work [14].

Signs and symptoms. The clinical manifestations of hypothenar hammer syndrome consist of rest pain, numbness, hypesthesia, paresthesia, coldness, cold sensitivity, Raynaud's syndrome, ischemic petechiae, and nonhealing ulcerations in the affected fingers [14,25]. At the wrist, ulnar artery pulsations may be absent and the ulnar confirmatory test and its modification (see A-3, Chapter 5) are positive for occlusion of the artery or its main branch.

Therapy. This consists of avoidance of further trauma to the hand, abstinence from smoking, and protection from injury. For the control of Raynaud's syndrome, phenoxybenzamine hydrochloride (Dibenzyline) may be helpful in decreasing the hyperresponsiveness to cold. If the ulcerations do not respond to conservative therapy, upper thoracic sympathectomy is indicated. Surgical exploration and removal of a portion of the ulnar artery may be necessary on occasion.

H. Compartmental Syndromes

A compartmental syndrome is defined as a condition in which increased pressure within a closed unyielding fascial space may cause the local circulation to be compromised to the point that the viability and function of the enclosed tissues are placed in jeopardy. Although most often found in several sites in the lower limbs (particularly the anterior tibial compartment), compartmental syndromes may also occur in the forearm and elsewhere. The different types are discussed below.

1. Anterior Tibial Compartmental Syndrome

The anterior tibial compartmental syndrome is a condition in which the soft tissues comprising the anterior tibial compartment in the leg become ischemic and then necrotic unless immediate steps are taken to reestablish local circulation.

Anatomic considerations. The anterior tibial compartment is an almost closed chamber formed by the tibia, the interosseous membrane, the lateral compartment, and the anterior crural fascia, each structure contributing an unyielding wall. It contains the extensor hallucis longus muscle, the extensor digitorum longus muscle, and the tibialis anterior muscle (Fig. 15.10). The latter structure receives its blood supply solely from the anterior tibial artery, whereas the other two muscles have a dual source (see A-1, Chapter 2). The anterior tibial artery runs in the anterior compartment in its course to the foot, accompanied by its venae comitantes and the anterior tibial nerve.

Etiologic factors. Anterior tibial compartmental syndrome can be produced by a number of unrelated conditions. Its inclusion in this chapter rests on the fact that among these is trauma to the lower limbs. Such an agent may be responsible for the appearance of the syndrome if, as a consequence, thrombosis or laceration of the superficial femoral artery or the proximal segment of the anterior tibial artery or its muscle branches ensues. For example, the entity has been reported following a crushing force to the anterior tibial compartment, as exerted by an automobile bumper. It has also occurred after surgical repair of a muscle hernia of the anterior tibial compartment [35], following a tibial tubercle transplant for chronic recurrent patellar displacement (Fig. 15.11) [34], and after vascular reconstructive procedures [7,12]. Another etiologic mechanism is unaccustomed severe physical exertion involving the muscles of the lower limbs [3,9].

Anterior tibial compartmental syndrome may likewise be found in association with medical conditions, unrelated to trauma. Among these are embolism to the popliteal or anterior tibial artery [6], toxemia of pregnancy, the nephrotic

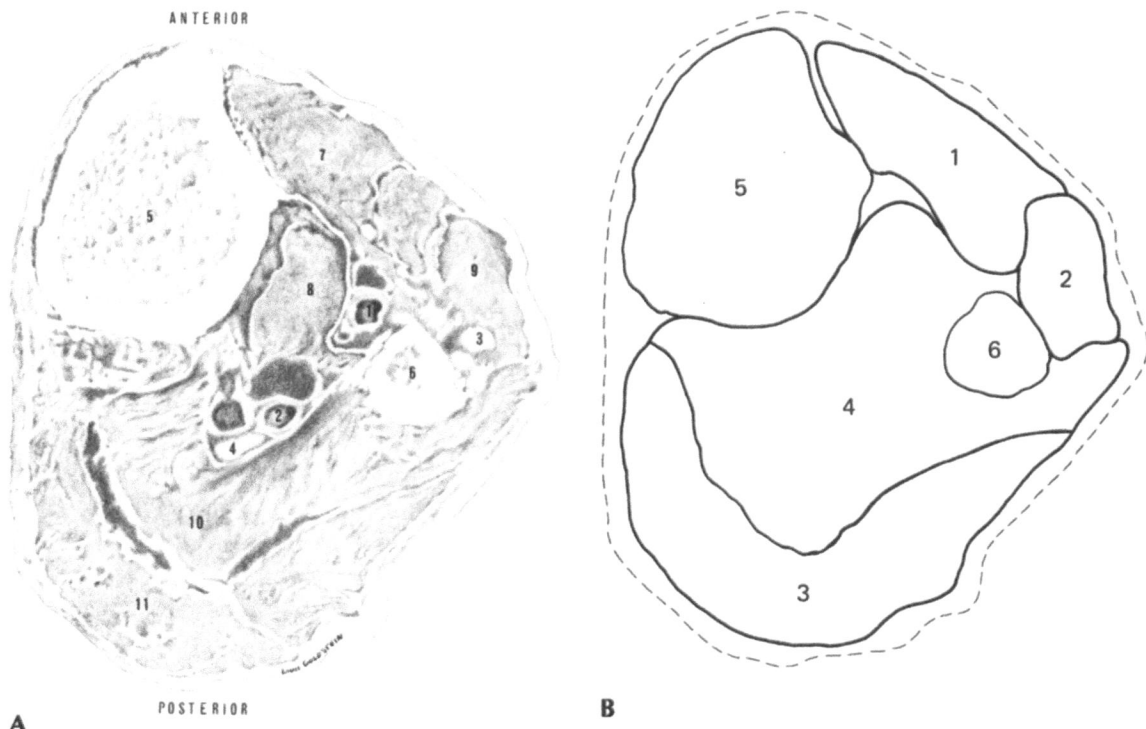

Fig. 15.10. Anatomic relationships of the compartments of the lower limb to other structures. **A** Cross-sectional drawing of middle portion of the leg. *1*, Anterior tibial artery; *2*, posterior tibial artery; *3*, peroneal nerve; *4*, tibial nerve; *5*, tibia; *6*, fibula; *7*, tibialis anterior muscle; *8*, tibialis posterior muscle; *9*, peroneus longus muscle; *10*, soleus muscle; *11*, gastrocnemius muscle. **B** Schematic outline indicating the location of the various compartments in cross section. *1*, Anterior tibial compartment; *2*, lateral compartment; *3*, superficial posterior compartment; *4*, deep posterior compartment; *5*, tibia; *6*, fibula.

syndrome [29], carbon monoxide poisoning, postoperative shock, and severe circumferential burns on a leg. Moreover, it may occur after prolonged periods of severe local arterial insufficiency, as produced by pressure bandaging [8] or tight casts, at times appearing even after the ischemia has been relieved.

Pathogenesis. The anterior tibial compartmental syndrome is generally due to cessation of blood flow through the upper segment of the anterior tibial artery. First there is swelling of the structures in the osseous compartment and then a rise in tissue pressure, thus causing an even more severe compromise of the local blood supply. Such changes are followed by greater capillary permeability due to ischemia and a further increase in edema formation. As a result, anoxia of tissue develops to the point of total loss of viability. Arterial spasm has also

been considered to be an important factor in the production of the syndrome (Fig. 15.11).

Clinical manifestations. Early in the inception of anterior tibial compartmental syndrome, severe pain suddenly develops over the muscle mass comprising the anterior tibial compartment, associated with intense rubor, cyanosis, or reddish-purple discoloration of the overlying skin and an increase in local cutaneous temperature. Subsequently the skin may become glossy and then necrotic, and the muscles locally may become edematous, hard, and tender on palpation. Pain is aggravated on plantar flexion of the foot. Soon the pulse in the dorsal pedal artery disappears, whereas that in the posterior tibial artery remains unaffected unless an embolus to the popliteal artery is the causative agent. Of diagnostic importance is the fact that, despite the signs of a severe

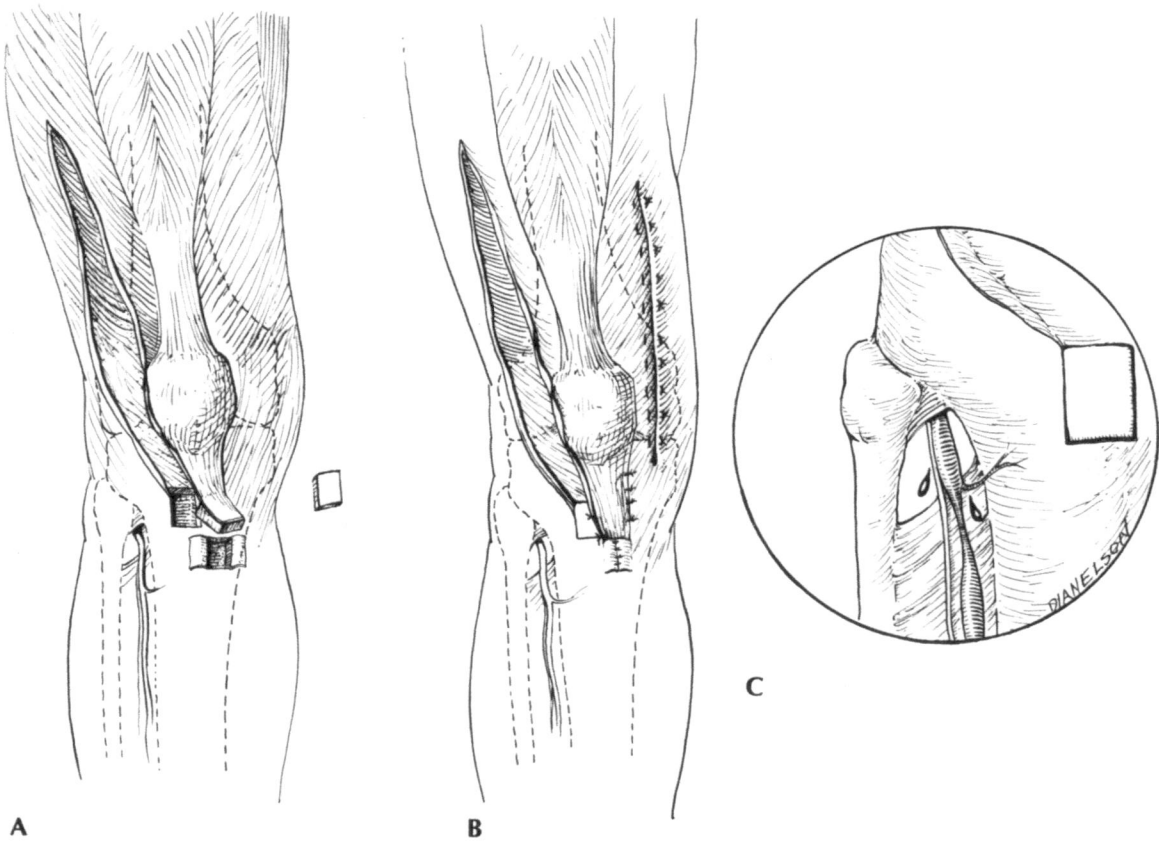

Fig. 15.11. Schematic drawing demonstrating how an anterior tibial compartmental syndrome could follow a transplant of the patellar ligament and tibial tubercle. **A** Two bone incisions. **B** Transplantation of tendon and bone medially. **C** Spasm of upper segment of anterior tibial artery produced by trauma incurred during surgery.

degree of ischemia of the tissues in and over the anterior tibial compartment, the distal structures, including the foot, generally demonstrate an adequate circulation. Associated findings are such systemic responses as a low-grade fever and a moderate leukocytosis.

Neurologic findings consist of weakness of the muscles in the anterior tibial compartment and then foot drop (caused by paralysis of the anterior tibial, extensor hallucis longus, and extensor digitorum longus muscles), together with inability to dorsiflex the toes. Associated with signs of motor impairment, there may be a sensory deficit in the form of anesthesia in the cutaneous distribution of the anterior tibial and deep peroneal nerves.

Differential diagnosis. The clinical picture of anterior tibial compartmental syndrome may resemble that of a number of different entities.

In the case of acute cellulitis and osteomyelitis of the leg, the systemic manifestations are much more pronounced than in anterior tibial compartmental syndrome and the ability to dorsiflex the foot and to move the toes is usually preserved. In contrast, the latter function is lost in anterior tibial compartmental syndrome.

Tenosynovitis of the tendons of the anterior tibial muscle or of the long extensors of the toes often develops under conditions similar to those associated with anterior tibial compartmental syndrome. However, characteristic crepitus may be felt or heard, and the loss of function is minimal. In stress fracture, another condition which may mimic anterior tibial compartmental syndrome, pain and tenderness are located over the bone and not elsewhere. Moreover, the condition can be identified by conventional x ray and tomography.

In shin splints, which is seen following athletic exertion in the untrained individual, pain and tenderness are associated with induration and swelling of the pretibial muscles. The complaints can generally be controlled by rest, elevation, and cold packs, whereas in anterior tibial compartmental syndrome, the pain is frequently so intense that it does not respond to even large doses of narcotics. Another distinguishing point is that the common finding of induration of the structures in the anterior tibial compartment is not noted in shin splints, although there are signs of local inflammation, such as rubor of the skin and an increased cutaneous temperature. Of interest in this regard is the view that shin splints may be a mild form of anterior tibial compartmental syndrome.

Among neurologic conditions which may resemble anterior tibial compartmental syndrome is common peroneal nerve compression in the vicinity of the neck of the fibula. This may occur as a result of application of tight bandages or of a rigid cast, hematoma formation from extensive reconstruction of the knee, or improper leg positioning for fracture of the hip. The condition may also be found in elderly or unconscious patients if their lower limbs are maintained in eversion against an unyielding mattress for a protracted period of time. Compression of the common peroneal nerve may be associated with abnormal electromyographic changes, a reduction in sensory and motor nerve conduction velocity, foot drop, sensory loss, and trophic alterations in the foot, but no symptoms or signs of impairment of local arterial circulation. In contrast, the physical findings in anterior tibial compartmental syndrome invariably reflect the presence of a marked reduction of blood flow to the affected site.

Treatment. In most instances, therapy in anterior tibial compartmental syndrome is immediate fasciotomy of the entire structure in order to prevent paralysis and necrosis of the affected muscles [23]. The incisions must be extensive and the whole compartment must be exposed; short incisions will generally only result in herniation of the muscles through them, producing strangulation of these structures. With complete decompression of the compartment, there may be a considerable return of local circulation and, at times, even of pulsations in the dorsal pedal artery. Functional recovery is dependent upon how rapidly decompression is carried out after onset of the condition.

If necrosis cannot be prevented, then it is necessary to remove all of the devitalized tissue up to the interosseous membrane and tibial surface and cover the defect with split-thickness skin grafts. Rapid production of granulation tissue can be achieved by penetrating the medullary cavity of the tibia and producing fine channels at spaced intervals with a drill. If necrosis of soft tissue is extensive, an above-knee amputation may have to be carried out.

Sequelae. In those instances in which the untreated or improperly treated syndrome does not progress to necrosis, almost invariably a foot drop results, a situation which can be controlled to some extent with a foot-drop brace. However, in other cases, the changes produced by the period of ischemia are much more serious, with fibrous replacement of necrotic muscles occurring. In such circumstances, the patient may be unable to dorsiflex the foot properly and so has difficulty in walking. Another sequela of anterior tibial compartmental syndrome is a condition which is the counterpart of Volkmann's ischemic contracture in the upper limb (see Section E, Chapter 22). This may result in equinovarus deformity and clawing of the toes, producing an almost useless foot.

2. Lateral Compartmental Syndrome

Anatomic considerations. The lateral (peroneal) compartment of the leg contains the peroneus longus and peroneus brevis muscles (Fig. 15.10). These structures receive numerous vascular branches from the peroneal artery, as well as those arising from the anterior tibial artery. As a result, they are in a much less precarious state following occlusion or laceration of the anterior tibial artery than is the tibialis anterior muscle under similar circumstances (see H-1, above).

Etiologic factors. The lateral compartmental syndrome may be caused by a direct blow to the upper fibular area, producing destruction of the nutrient vessels to the peroneal muscles. As a consequence, necrosis of these structures may develop.

Clinical manifestations. The symptoms of lateral compartmental syndrome consist primarily of pain located on the upper portion of the lateral aspect of the leg [21]. Swelling and tenderness are also found in this location.

Treatment. The therapeutic approach is similar to that for the anterior tibial compartmental syndrome and consists of early decompression of the compartment and release of the abnormal pressure to which the tissues have been subjected. In some cases fibulectomy may be necessary to accomplish such a goal [5]. This measure has the added advantage that if improvement is not noted, deep incisions can then be made into the anterior, deep posterior, and superficial posterior compartments through the bed of the resected shaft of the fibula. In the event that decompression cannot be accomplished by surgical means, a varus and equinus foot deformity, with loss of foot eversion, may result.

3. Superficial Posterior Compartmental Syndrome

Anatomic considerations. The superficial posterior compartment of the leg contains the gastrocnemius, soleus, and plantaris muscles (Fig. 15.10) [26]. These structures receive their blood supply from branches of the posterior tibial and peroneal arteries.

Etiologic factors. Superficial posterior compartmental syndrome may be caused by a dissecting popliteal cyst (Fig. 18.2), rupture of a popliteal arterial aneurysm, or a direct blow to the calf musculature.

Clinical manifestations. The symptoms and physical findings in the superficial posterior compartmental syndrome are similar in all regards to those of the anterior tibial compartmental syndrome except that they are located on the posterior surface of the leg. If the response is extensive, then the posterior tibial artery may go into spasm, with eventual loss of pulsations distally and secondary contracture of the intrinsic plantar musculature of the foot. Trauma to the gastrocnemius and soleus

muscles may also result in equinus deformities due to contracture of these structures.

Treatment. In the case of the superficial posterior compartmental syndrome, therapy also consists of decompression.

4. Deep Posterior Compartmental Syndrome

The deep posterior compartmental syndrome of the leg has only recently been described as a separate entity, due, in part, to the fact that it is rarely noted alone [16]. In most instances there is also involvement of one or several other compartments in the lower limb, with the result that the more dramatic response to them generally masks its presence.

Anatomic considerations. The deep posterior compartment, in its proximal portion, is bounded by the tibia, interosseous membrane, fibula, and transverse crural septum (Fig. 15.10). The upper end of the compartment consists of the origin of the soleus muscle, while distally the boundaries converge around the flexor hallucis longus, flexor digitorum longus, and tibialis posterior muscles as they taper toward their musculotendinous junctions [16]. Each of these three muscles is encased in its own epimysium.

Also enclosed in the deep posterior compartment are the posterior tibial and peroneal arteries which run almost parallel to each other and are the blood supply for the surrounding muscles and the tibia. Accompanying them are their respective venae comitantes. The posterior tibial nerve, which is found lateral to the posterior tibial artery, innervates all of the muscles in the compartment.

Etiologic factors. The most common cause of deep posterior compartmental syndrome is fracture of the tibia and fibula, usually at the middle or distal third. The fact that the posterior tibial artery supplies nutrient vessels to the tibia at the level of the middle third of the bone may be the explanation for the high incidence of vascular injuries associated with tibial fractures. The peroneal vessels lie immediately medial to the fibula where they also are susceptible to laceration when a fracture of this bone occurs, or if some type of surgery is being performed on it. Trauma to soft tissues in the compartment, major venous occlusion, injuries about the knee, and fracture of the tibial plateau, ankle, calcaneus, or talus may all be responsible for the development of the deep posterior tibial compartmental syndrome.

Clinical manifestations. The most common symptom of the deep posterior compartmental syndrome is severe pain locally, although at times it may be mild. The most important signs of the condition are plantar hypesthesia in the distribution of the posterior tibial nerve, weakness of toe flexion, pain on passive toe extension, and tenseness of the tissues in the area between the tibia and triceps surae in the distal medial part of the calf [16].

Differential diagnosis. Deep posterior compartmental syndrome must be differentiated from conditions in which trauma has produced neuromuscular damage, from local arterial occlusion, and from deep venous thrombophlebitis (phlebothrombosis).

Treatment. To prevent sequelae from the deep posterior compartmental syndrome, decompression of the compartment should be performed as early as possible. Otherwise the patient will be left with plantar hypesthesia, weakness or contracture of the tibialis posterior and long flexors of the toes, and claw toes. Prompt diagnosis and treatment also minimize the complications of fasciotomy. The compartment must be opened by incising the limiting fascia through a medial, lateral, or posterior approach, the medial one having certain advantages over the others [16]. If the fasciotomy does not adequately release the swollen muscles, then the epimysium surrounding each one may also have to be incised.

5. Other Compartmental Syndromes

Volar compartmental syndrome of the forearm. This relatively rare entity may be responsible for serious deformities of the limb, both functionally and cosmetically.

The condition is caused either by direct trauma to soft tissues following fractures of the radius and ulna, by injury of the blood supply to the forearm in the vicinity of the elbow, by arterial embolic episodes, by dialysis treatment, and by arterial puncture in patients on anticoagulants. In recent years, self-injection of drugs by addicts has also been reported to produce the condition, with resulting ischemia, necrosis, such deformities as a clawhand, and contracture of the wrist and hand. Caffey's syndrome [2] may cause the forearm compartmental syndrome through vascular compression by the cortical hyperostosis of the radius or ulna, a situation requiring fasciotomy of the volar fascia in order to maintain viability of involved structures.

In contrast with anterior tibial compartmental syndrome, the clinical picture in volar compartmental syndrome is not as dramatic in development because the efficiency of the collateral circulation around the elbow joint is generally of a degree to permit adequate nutrition to be brought to the tissues. Nevertheless, at times Volkmann-like ischemic contractures may occur.

Miscellaneous compartmental syndromes. Among other compartmental entities are those involving the gluteal area [20], the plantar surface of the foot, and the thenar space of the hand. All of these are produced by trauma, which causes vascular compression and local swelling, tenderness, and marked pain. Incision over the affected site relieves the pressure and allows for reestablishment of blood flow through the peripheral arteries. By means of such a measure, ischemic necrosis is avoided, with the result that normal function may return.

6. Determination of Interstitial Fluid Pressure

The one finding which is common to all compartmental syndromes is a local elevation of tissue pressure. Hence, attempts to determine whether such a state exists are helpful in both early diagnosis and immediate treatment of these conditions. A simple means of obtaining the desired data consists of placing a small needle into the muscle compartment and measuring the pressure directly with a mercury manometer or transducer [32]. A somewhat more complicated approach involves the use of the wick catheter technique which provides accurate and reproducible figures [18,19]. Another approach consists of infusion of fluid into the muscle at a rate of 0.7 ml/day and measuring the pressure necessary to accomplish this [17].

Tissue pressure readings in the normal recumbent person have been found to have a range between 4 [18] and 12 mmHg. It is the opinion of some workers [19] that a fasciotomy should be performed whenever the figures rise to 30 mmHg or higher, whereas others believe that such a procedure is indicated only if there is an elevation to 40 to 50 mmHg [17] or if the readings increase to within 10 to 30 mmHg of the diastolic level [33].

In most patients a compartmental syndrome can be identified clinically, and documentation of an elevated intracompartmental pressure merely helps to confirm the diagnosis. However, there are several groups of patients in whom difficulties are encountered in eliciting or interpreting the physical findings, and in them these readings are essential, especially in regard to determining whether fasciotomy should be performed [19]. Among such individuals are uncooperative or unreliable persons, unresponsive people (drug addicts suffering from an overdose), and patients with fractures or contusions demonstrating a nerve deficit.

I. Injury to Major Veins

The subject of trauma to main veins (which occurs in about 10 percent of arterial injuries) is one that has not been extensively investigated. Although it is true that such a situation does not have the serious connotation attributed to arterial damage, still it may be of sufficient importance to be responsible for loss of viability in a limb with a precarious arterial circulation and even in a previously normal extremity [22,28]. For example, if no attempt is made to reestablish blood flow through a severed collecting vein in the lower limb and instead it is ligated, a clinical entity similar to that produced by an iliofemoral thrombophle-

bitis (see A-3, Chapter 18) will develop. The resulting swelling of the limb and the marked rise in venous pressure may be sufficient initially to impede arterial inflow and thus further exaggerate an already existing ischemia of tissues. This is particularly true in the case of damage to the popliteal artery and vein [22,28].

If at all feasible, lateral suture repair of lacerated veins is preferred to ligation of the vessels. Grafts to bridge venous defects are not advisable since the vein will generally not remain patent. In any event, prompt surgery, regardless of the type, is essential in order to control bleeding and avoid the production of an arteriovenous fistula (see Section F, above).

References

1. Boontje AB: Iatrogenic arterial injuries. J Cardiovasc Surg 19:335, 1978
2. Caffey J: Infantile cortical hyperostoses. J Pediatr 29:541, 1946
3. Carter AB, Richards RL, Zachary RB: The anterior tibial syndrome. Lancet 2:928, 1949
4. Doty DB, Treiman RL, Rothchild PD, et al: Prevention of gangrene due to fractures. Surg Gynecol Obstet 125:284, 1967
5. Ernst CB, Kaufer H: Fibulectomy–fasciotomy: An important adjunct in the management of lower extremity arterial trauma. J Trauma 11:365, 1971
6. Freedman BJ, Knowles CHR: Anterior tibial syndrome due to arterial embolism and thrombosis. Br Med J 5147:270, 1959
7. Gitlitz GF: The anterior tibial compartment syndrome: A complication of a femoropopliteal bypass procedure. Vasc Dis 2:122, 1965
8. Husni EA, Ximenes JOC, Hamilton FG: Pressure bandaging of the lower extremity: Use and abuse. JAMA 206:2715, 1968
9. Kennedy JC, Roth JH: Major tibial compartment syndromes following minor athletic trauma. Am J Sports Med 7:201, 1979
10. Kinmonth JB: The physiology and relief of traumatic arterial spasm. Br Med J 1:59, 1952
11. Kleinert HE, Burget GC, Morgan JA, et al: Aneurysms of the hand. Arch Surg 106:554, 1973
12. Ledgerwood AM, Lucas CE: Massive thigh injuries with vascular disruption: Role of porcine skin grafting of exposed arterial vein grafts. Arch Surg 107:201, 1973
13. Linscheid RL, Wheeler DK: Elbow dislocations. JAMA 194:1171, 1965
14. Little JM, Ferguson DA: The incidence of the hypothenar hammer syndrome. Arch Surg 104:684, 1972

15. Margolies MN, Ring EJ, Waltman AC, et al: Arteriography in the management of hemorrhage from pelvic fractures. N Engl J Med 287:317, 1972

16. Matsen FA III, Clawson DK: The deep posterior compartmental syndrome of the leg. J Bone Joint Surg 57A:34, 1975

17. Matsen FA III, Mayo KA, Sheridan GW, et al: Monitoring of intramuscular pressure. Surgery 79:702, 1976

18. Mubarak SJ, Hargens AR, Owen CA, et al: The wick catheter techniques for measurement of intramuscular pressure: A new research and clinical tool. J Bone Joint Surg 58A:1016, 1976

19. Mubarak SJ, Owen CA, Hargens AR, et al: Acute compartment syndrome: Diagnosis and treatment with the aid of the wick catheter. J Bone Joint Surg 60A:1091, 1978

20. Owen CA, Woody PR, Mubarak SJ, et al: Gluteal compartment syndrome: A report of three cases and management utilizing the wick catheter. Clin Orthop 132:50, 1978

21. Reszel PA, Janes JM, Spittell JA Jr: Ischemic necrosis of the peroneal musculature, a lateral compartment syndrome: Report of case. Proc Staff Meet Mayo Clin 38:130, 1963

22. Rich NM, Jarstfer BS, Geer TM: Popliteal artery repair failure: Causes and possible prevention. J Cardiovasc Surg 15:340, 1974

23. Rorabeck CH, Macnab I, Waddell JP: Anterior tibial compartment syndrome: A clinical and experimental review. Can J Surg 15:249, 1972

24. Rosental IJ, Gaspar MR, Gjerdrum TC, et al: Vascular injuries associated with fractures of the femur. Arch Surg 110:494, 1975

25. Schatz IJ: Occlusive artery disease in the hand due to occupational trauma. N Engl J Med 268:281, 1963

26. Scott, WN, Jacobs B, Lockshin MD: Posterior compartment syndrome resulting from a dissecting popliteal cyst: Case report. Clin Orthop 122:189, 1977

27. Smith, JW: True aneurysms of traumatic origin in the palm. Am J Surg 104:7, 1962

28. Sullivan WG, Thornton FH, Baker LH, et al: Early influence of popliteal vein repair in the treatment of popliteal vessel injuries. Am J Surg 122:528, 1971

29. Sweeney HE, O'Brien GF: Bilateral anterior tibial syndrome in association with the nephrotic syndrome: Report of a case. Arch Intern Med 116:487, 1965

30. Tadavarthy SM, Knight L, Ovitt TW, et al: Therapeutic transcatheter arterial embolization. Diagn Radiol 111:13, 1974

31. van Urk H, Perlberger RR, Muller H: Selective arterial embolization for control of traumatic pelvic hemorrhage. Surgery 83:133, 1978

32. Whitesides TE Jr, Haney TC, Harada H, et al: A simple method for tissue pressure determination. Arch Surg 110:1311, 1975

33. Whitesides TE Jr, Haney TC, Morimoto K, et al: Tissue pressure measurements as a determinant for the need of fasciotomy. Clin Orthop 113:43, 1975

34. Wiggins HE: The anterior tibial compartment syndrome: A complication of the Hauser procedure. Clin Orthop 113:90, 1975

35. Wolfort FG, Mogelvang LC, Filtzer HS: Anterior tibial compartment syndrome following muscle hernia repair. Arch Surg 106:97, 1973

Chapter 16

Vascular Complications of Musculoskeletal Disorders Produced by Trauma

Part 2   Fat Embolism

With the increase in the number of patients suffering from major trauma who are seen in emergency rooms of community and general hospitals, fat embolism has become a fairly common clinical entity. Because of its close relationship to fractures of long bones, this disorder is of special interest and concern to the orthopedic and the general surgeon, particularly since it is associated with a high morbidity and mortality [7].

A. General Considerations

1. Incidence

The frequency of fat embolism is very difficult to determine. Of importance in this regard is the fact that fat particles of sufficient size to lodge in and temporarily occlude capillaries or vessels of larger caliber may be present in the bloodstream without producing clinical manifestations. Only when enough of the pulmonary capillary bed is obstructed by such emboli to interfere with proper oxygenation of blood is the underlying difficulty diagnosed.

Men are more commonly affected than · women, probably because there is more trauma associated with the type of work performed by the former. In general, fat embolism is seen more often in adults than in children, a finding which may be a reflection of the greater amount of fat and less hematopoietic tissue found in the bone marrow of older people.

Following severe fractures, the incidence of clinically evident fat embolism is approximately 10 percent. Under such circumstances, the condition is most common in the second and third decades of life, when long-bone fractures are frequent, and in the sixth and seventh decades, when the incidence of fractures of the hip is high.

2. Etiology

In the past it was the general opinion that the most frequent causative agents in fat embolism were skeletal trauma and surgical procedures, with the result that this disorder became an almost exclusive orthopedic or surgical problem. However, at present it is of interest to other disciplines of medicine, having been found in association with a large number of diverse and varied diseases, states, or situations. Among these are soft-tissue trauma, decompression sickness, fatty metamorphosis of the liver, severe burns, inadvertent intravenous injection of oily radiographic media during lymphangiography, the use of film-type oxygenators in cardiopulmonary bypass procedures, during corticosteroid therapy, in chronic alcoholism, in pancreatitis, and in sickle-cell anemia crises with bone marrow infarction. Various other types of infection, intoxication, and metabolic disturbances have also been associated with fat embolism.

B. Pathogenesis

The source of the embolic fat in fat embolism has not as yet been clarified. In this regard, two major theories have been proposed: the mechanical and the physiochemical.

1. Mechanical Concept

The mechanical theory, supported by clinical investigations and studies of experimentally produced fractures, postulates that fat particles in bone marrow are liberated into tissue spaces by the disruption of their cellular envelopes, the responsible mechanism being severe trauma to long bones. The free fat is then forced into local veins which have also been injured. The fact that veins of the haversian canals of the bone substance are prevented from collapsing by their osseous walls facilitates the movement of the fat into the systemic venous circulation. A contributing factor to the disruption of a large number of fat cells and the resulting liberation of free fat is the grinding action of bony spicules and trabeculae.

2. Physiochemical Concept

Because the mechanical theory cannot explain the development of fat embolism in the absence of trauma, it is necessary to consider other causative factors. One which has definite experimental and clinical support is based on metabolic changes mediated through physiochemical means. It postulates that in an as yet unexplained manner, the physical state of the normal lipids in the blood is altered, with the result that there is an increased tendency for the small emulsified chylomicra to coalesce and form fat droplets, followed by subsequent embolization of these particles. The increase in platelet adhesiveness found in trauma, infec-

tion, and metabolic disturbances (all conditions in which fat embolism occurs) evidently contributes to the aggregation of the fat globules.

Studies in animals using radioactive iodine have demonstrated that even in the case of trauma, the fat absorbed from a site of injury is not the only source of embolic fat [8]; tissue injury may also initiate changes in the physiochemical state of blood, thus altering the emulsion stability of the blood lipids. The lipid-mobilizing hormone is also activated by trauma, an increase in blood lipid concentration thereby resulting. All these factors may be involved in fat embolism.

3. Role of Fat Particles in Causation of Clinical Manifestations

Once in the systemic venous circulation, the free fat particles are trapped in the capillary bed of the pulmonary system. There they cause mechanical blockage of the microcirculation, leading to A-V shunting and alveolar hypoperfusion, and an increased resistance to pulmonary blood flow. The latter change is associated with a rise in pulmonary artery pressure and dilatation of and strain on the right ventricle.

Later there is hydrolysis of the neutral fats to glycerol and free fatty acids through the action of lipase present in lung tissue. As a result of the injurious effect of the fatty acids on the cells of the bronchi and bronchioles, there is disruption of alveolar-capillary membranes, together with curtailment of surfactant activity, edema formation, hemorrhage, and alveolar collapse. A contributing factor to further reduction in pulmonary function is the adhesiveness of large numbers of platelets to fat emboli. These then break down, with the release of serotonin, the latter producing local vasoconstriction and bronchoconstriction.

In those instances in which the ability of the pulmonary vascular bed to contain the fat in the venous blood is overwhelmed, systemic embolization occurs. The rise in pulmonary artery pressure elongates the pliable fat droplets and forces them to pass through the venules into the pulmonary veins and then into the systemic circulation where they are again arrested in terminal capillaries, this time of the brain, kidneys, liver, and skin. Hence, local ischemia is produced in these organs, resulting in the appearance of the constitutional manifestations of fat embolism (see C-3, below).

C. Clinical Manifestations

In those patients in whom skeletal trauma is the cause of fat embolism, the symptoms and signs of the condition may appear within a few hours following the injury to as long as 4 days afterward. Generally the manifestations become apparent after a lucid latent period of about 48 h. The fulminating cases, associated with severe multiple injuries, are rarely diagnosed clinically before death occurs. Likewise, many mild states of fat embolism are frequently overlooked because of an unclear clinical picture. A sense of awareness regarding such a possibility should make the diagnosis much less difficult to reach, especially since the early findings are fairly typical. The character of the symptoms and signs will depend largely upon which organ or organs are suffering from reduced local circulation.

1. Constitutional Changes

The syndrome of fat embolism generally begins suddenly with a rise in temperature to 38.5 or 39° C (101.3 or 102.2° F), a significant tachycardia with the heart rate increasing to 140 beats/min or higher, and tachypnea, with a respiratory rate of 30 to 50 respirations/min. Blood pressure may be unchanged or it may fall. Venous pressure generally rises.

2. Manifestations of Pulmonary Bed Involvement

The clinical findings due to obstruction of the pulmonary capillary bed by fat emboli consist of stertorous breathing, dyspnea, cough, wheezes, and rales at the base of the lungs. Cyanosis of the nail beds and lips may be present. Such changes are not specific for the condition and resemble those observed in pulmonary embolism (see Section B, Chapter 19) and acute cor pulmonale.

3. Manifestations of Systemic Embolization

Although numerous organs may be affected in systemic fat embolism, cerebral symptoms predominate. The patient may develop disorientation, drowsiness, obstreperousness, confusion, and, less often, delirium, coma, and decerebrate rigidity, without any apparent pattern of appearance or progression. Other neurologic findings are abnormal pupillary reflexes, spasticity, increase or decrease in deep-tendon reflexes, incontinence, and convulsions. In the fulminating case, the patient is usually conscious immediately after the extensive trauma, but he soon becomes stuporous and comatose. Death from irreversible shock occurs 1 to 3 days after the injury. The basis for the symptoms and signs of cerebral fat embolism may, in part, be generalized hypoxia due to inadequate oxygenation of the blood in the pulmonary vascular bed and, in part, local hypoxia which follows occlusion of cerebral arterioles by the emboli.

Among other organs affected by systemic fat embolism, resulting in clinically significant findings, are the kidneys and the liver. In fatal cases, renal glomeruli may be the site of extensive lipid deposits. However, in most instances there are generally sufficient patent channels in the glomerular tufts so that signs of renal failure are not present. Supporting such a view is the finding that patients who have recovered exhibit no evidence of impaired renal function as demonstrated by the concentrating ability of the kidneys.

4. Petechial Rash

A common diagnostic feature in fat embolism is the appearance of brown petechiae on the second or third day after trauma to a long bone. They may be as small as 1 mm in diameter and are frequently overlooked as normal skin pigmentation. Their location is generally across the root of the neck; in the axillae, conjunctivae, and fundi; on the anterior chest wall; and less often on the abdominal wall and the flanks, extending onto the thighs. The rash is transient, with the lesions fading rapidly in one area at the same time that new crops are appearing elsewhere. Such changes occur during the first week after injury. It is believed that the abnormality results from a form of thrombocytopenic purpura [4] and not from obstruction of cutaneous vessels by fat emboli. However, some workers [7] have found fat in the superficial dermal capillaries in biopsy specimens of the skin about the petechiae, an observation not confirmed by others [4]. It has been suggested [4] that when petechiae are not noted in a suspected case of fat embolism, the application of a positive or negative pressure to the skin using a petechiometer should be performed. Such a step can provoke an abnormal response since there is an increase in capillary fragility in this condition (positive Rumpel-Leede phenomenon).

D. Diagnostic Laboratory Tests

1. Alterations in Constituents of Blood and Urine

In the early stage of fat embolism, there is a decrease in the hemoglobin level that is generally greater than that which can be explained by blood loss from other areas. Also during this period, in about half the cases, free fat is noted in the urine (using Sudan 3 staining). In fact, during the acute phase, the fat globules may be observed floating on the surface of the urine specimen provided the bladder is completely emptied.[1] Such findings persist for about 4 days after the injury and rapidly decline thereafter. The serum lipase is usually elevated by the fourth day, a response that indicates an increased production of pulmonary lipase required for hydrolyzing the neutral fat into fatty acids and glycerol in the pulmonary bed. Early and repeated measurements of arterial blood gases (P_{O_2} and P_{CO_2}) are essential in evaluating the degree of hypoxia, since the substitution of clinical means for this purpose generally is inaccurate and misleading. Consistently there is a significant drop in P_{O_2} with levels as low as 40 mmHg being reported.

---

[1] Percutaneous renal biopsy with proper staining of the specimen is useful in demonstrating free fat in the vascular tree of the kidney.

2. Electrocardiographic Alterations

Changes in the electrocardiogram associated with fat embolism do not always appear immediately but may be noted 24 to 48 h after injury. They are due to the greater load placed on the right side of the heart because of alterations in the pulmonary vascular bed, and they reflect myocardial ischemia and/or acute cor pulmonale. The abnormalities consist of tachycardia, prominent S waves in lead I, and large Q waves in lead III, with a shift of the transition zone to the left. Nonspecific S-T alterations may also be present, as well as inversion of the T waves.

3. Roentgenographic Alterations

Changes in the chest roentgenogram are noted within several hours or a few days after trauma and resolve in a short period of time. They consist of patchy fluffy infiltrates of various degrees of severity ("snowstorm" appearance); the distribution tends to be perihilar, nodular, or basal. The alterations resemble those seen in pulmonary edema. The pulmonary vessels are usually not engorged.[2]

E. Differential Diagnosis

Although no difficulty should be encountered in making a diagnosis of fat embolism in the patient with both pulmonary and cerebral findings, in the case of others with less marked and characteristic manifestations, there is need for differentiation from several similar types of clinical entities.

1. Intracranial Bleeding

When cerebral symptoms and signs predominate, it is necessary to rule out intracranial bleeding, especially if there is a history of a relatively free interval after an injury, followed by progressively deepening coma. In fat embolism, there may be numerous bizarre neurologic findings, including twitching and even

---

[2] Another important diagnostic tool is fundoscopic examination, since this may reveal refractile bodies within retinal vessels when fat embolism exists.

convulsions, but because of the diffuse nature of the condition, no localizing signs are present; this is in contrast with the situation present in the case of intracranial bleeding. Of course, it is always necessary to consider the possibility that the two conditions coexist, particularly if severe trauma precedes the onset of the clinical manifestations.

2. Chronic Alcoholism

In the chronic alcoholic, who appears to have a predilection for fat embolism, a differentiation may have to be made between the latter condition and delirium tremens. In both states there may only be cerebral signs of restlessness followed by delirium. A therapeutic response to drugs used in delirium tremens, such as prochlorperazine (Compazine) or chlorpromazine (Thorazine), may be a helpful differential point.

3. Cardiac Injury

In the patient who primarily manifests cardiopulmonary symptoms and signs, it may be necessary to rule out cardiac contusion. In both fat embolism and injury to the heart, there may be dyspnea and precordial distress, but in cardiac contusion the rapid, deep, stertorous breathing is not present and the cerebral signs do not progress beyond restlessness and anxiety. Of help as a diagnostic aid are the changes in the electrocardiogram. In the case of cardiac contusion, there are changes in the form of S-T segment elevations and T wave inversions, indicating injury of heart muscle. In fat embolism, either there is no change in the record or nonspecific S-T segment alterations are present (see D-2, above).

4. Pulmonary Embolism

The differentiation of fat embolism from pulmonary embolism (see Section B, Chapter 19) is generally not difficult. Following an injury, symptoms and signs of fat embolism are seen within the first 1 to 6 days, whereas in pulmonary embolism they are rarely present before the tenth day. Moreover, systemic manifestations, such as cerebral abnormalities, are usually not noted in pulmonary embolism except in the very severe type in which there is a shock state.

F. Treatment

1. Prophylaxis

Local treatment of fracture. At all times care should be taken in the manipulation of the fracture. If the patient is to be transported in an ambulance, the injured limb should be carefully and correctly splinted, followed by definitive reduction and immobilization of the fracture as soon as feasible. However, the use of intramedullary rods or skeletal traction for fixation of a fractured femur should be delayed until vital signs have improved and stabilized. In the case of multiple fractures, placing tourniquets above the injuries so as to increase local venous pressure has been proposed as a useful measure, since presumably the amount of fat entering veins from the site of trauma is thereby decreased. However, it is necessary to point out that the resulting compression of the soft tissues may by itself produce a minor degree of fat embolism. Moreover, the value of the procedure has not been satisfactorily proven.

Hypertonic glucose therapy. The institution of such a program has been reported to have eliminated fat embolism, with serum determinations of cholesterol, free fatty acids, and total lipids showing a decrease following intravenous administration of the medication [5].

Ethanol administration. Another proposed prophylactic measure is the intravenous administration of dextrose-alcohol mixtures or the oral use of alcohol in patients with fractures of the hip and elsewhere [1]. Such an approach is considered to suppress the elevation of the serum lipase which frequently occurs under these circumstances, thus slowing the hydrolysis of the neutral fat emboli to a toxic form. However, the clinical evidence at present is not clear-cut enough to permit any conclusion regarding the efficacy of the medication as a preventive measure in fat embolism.

Heparin therapy. This approach has been utilized for fat embolism, since heparin, besides its effect on the coagulation mechanism, also has a lipid-clearing action on the blood. The mode of administration is similar to that utilized in the treatment of deep venous thrombosis in the lower limbs (see p. 271); the medication is given for a period of 3 days. Again, no true evaluation of this regimen as a prophylactic agent is available. Moreover, it is important to point out that heparin therapy is associated with certain serious complications when utilized for patients with fractures of long bones. First, there is a good possibility of hemorrhage developing in the site of injury. Second, the medication has a detrimental effect upon fracture union, causing delay in this process.

2. Active Treatment

Since the significant abnormal alterations in fat embolism are hypovolemia, hypoxia, excessive catecholamine release, and a tendency to platelet aggregation, the therapeutic approach should be directed toward control of such changes.

General measures. Among these are included maintenance of an airway, resuscitation from shock, and the parenteral administration of fluids. Specific therapy is directed at lowering the plasma lipid value and improving the microcirculatory flow patterns.

Aggressive oxygen therapy. This approach is considered to be one of the most effective measures in the control of the clinical manifestations of fat embolism. The rationale for such a step is an attempt to correct the severe arterial hypoxia which regularly accompanies the condition, as established by repeated measurements of P_{O_2} and P_{CO_2} in arterial blood. In this manner, adequate oxygenation of the blood is maintained.

Oxygen therapy is begun by using a mask and endotracheal or a cuffed tracheostomy tube and assisted respiration [9]. At first a known volume of 100% oxygen concentration is given at a controlled rate (usually 20 to 30 times/min) for approximately 30 min. Then this is reduced to 40 to 60% to avoid oxygen toxicity during prolonged administration. A favorable response to such a program is indicated by an increase in the arterial P_{O_2} to 350 to 450 mmHg. Therapy is continued until it is established by means of repeated arterial punctures and through trial and error that a normal level of oxygenation of the blood can be achieved without additional oxygen or mechanical assistance.

Dextran 40. Low molecular weight dextran has been used in fat embolism since it has a beneficial effect upon the microcirculatory flow. It reduces intravascular aggregation of red blood cells, increases the fluidity of the blood by its hypertonic effect, improves capillary flow, raises tissue perfusion, and exerts a siliconizing effect on injured walls of blood vessels. The medication is given intravenously in the amount of 500 ml every 12 h [2,3].

High-dose steroids. This approach may succeed when other therapeutic programs have failed. However, it is reserved for severely ill patients since there is a definite risk associated with the administration of large amounts of corticosteroids. The treatment program consists of an initial intravenous dose of 125 mg of methylprednisolone sodium succinate (Solu-Medrol; A-MethaPred), followed by 80 mg every 6 h for 3 days. Definite improvement can generally be expected within 12 to 24 h, the first change being a rise in P_{O_2}, followed by a reduction in pulse rate and clearing of the x-ray findings in the chest. Later the neurologic abnormalities slowly disappear.

G. Prognosis

About 20 percent of all fatalities following fractures of long bones are considered to be due to fat embolism. The high morbidity and mortality of this condition are, in part, directly related to the degree of pulmonary involvement [6]. However, systemic embolization to the brain, causing a rapid onset of cerebral signs and the appearance of coma, portends an even graver prognosis.

With effective therapy, generally the time required for reversal of neurologic findings and a return to a healthy state of consciousness is directly proportional to the length of the period during which the changes were present. The alterations in the lungs usually disappear sooner than the cerebral manifestations.

The mortality rate from fat embolism varies from 2 to 15 percent. However, autopsy studies appear to support the impression that fat emboli in the lungs of patients dying after severe injuries are quite common. How important a factor they are in causing or in contributing to death of the patient is not known.

References

1. Adler F, Lai SP, Peltier LF: Fat embolism: Prophylactic treatment with lipase inhibitors. Surg Forum 12:453, 1961

2. Bergentz SE: Studies on the genesis of posttraumatic fat embolism. Acta Chir Scand (Suppl) 282:1, 1961

3. Evarts CM: Emerging concepts of fat embolism. Clin Orthop 33:183, 1964

4. Garner JH, Peltier LF: Fat embolism: The significance of provoked petechiae. JAMA 200:226, 1967

5. Horne RH, Horne JH: Fat embolism prophylaxis: Use of hypertonic glucose. Arch Intern Med 133:288, 1974

6. Peltier LF: Fat embolism: A pulmonary disease. Surgery 62:756, 1967

7. Sevitt S: Fat Embolism. London, Butterworths, 1962, p 192

8. Szabó G, Serényi P, Kocsár L: Fat embolism: Fat absorption from the site of injury. Surgery 54:756, 1963

9. Wertzberger JL, Peltier LF: Fat embolism: The importance of arterial hypoxia. Surgery 63:626, 1968

Chapter 17

Vascular Complications of Musculoskeletal Disorders Produced by Trauma

---

Part 3   Factors Responsible for Deep Venous Thrombosis and Measures for Their Control

---

Under certain conditions (see Section A, below), the efficiency of the various mechanisms which maintain the fluidity of the circulating blood is impaired, with the result that intravascular thrombosis occurs. Since the movement of blood is considerably slower in the venous than in the arterial system, there is a much greater tendency for this abnormal state to develop in veins, particularly of the lower limbs. Although retarded blood flow by itself cannot initiate intravascular coagulation, such a situation does facilitate the thrombotic process once it has developed [45]. The different factors responsible for the initiation and propagation of venous thrombi and means to combat them are discussed in this chapter.

A. Predisposing Factors to Venous Thrombosis

1. General Considerations

Among the causes of venous thrombosis are those first proposed by Virchow, namely, damage to venous endothelium, slowed venous blood flow (venous stasis), and changes in the composition and coagulability of the blood. Of these, only venous stasis is readily identifiable.

Changes in the venous endothelium are assumed rather than positively proved, since by the time pathologic examination can be performed, it is not clear as to whether this type of abnormality preceded or followed thrombosis. Alterations in the coagulability of blood are also difficult to determine or, in fact, to ascertain whether they even exist [46].

2. Direct Trauma

Thromboembolic disease is a common complication of injury to tissues, particularly if a fracture or joint trauma has been sustained and the patient is elderly [39]. In the case of fracture of the tibia, direct injury, rupture of the deep crural veins, or compression of the deep venous plexuses by an increase in subfascial pressure may be responsible for the formation of venous thrombosis [28].

What makes the whole problem of trauma to a limb even more serious is the fact that less than one-third of the injured individuals with definite laboratory evidence of deep venous thrombosis (as demonstrated by routine venography) can be expected to manifest obvious clinical signs of this state [10]. Moreover, the time of onset of the condition following an injury is difficult to determine. For example, although nearly one-half of the cases of pulmonary embolism occurs within 2 weeks after the trauma, fatal attacks can still develop for as long as 3 or 4 months afterward [38]. In the case of hip fracture, in only one-half of the elderly patients who ultimately suffer from deep thrombophlebitis are signs of this condition noted within 3 weeks of the injury [36]. Some available data appear to suggest that clot formation may precede clinical manifestations by several weeks and that the thrombotic process may even be initiated soon after trauma is sustained.

With regard to hip fractures, other factors may contribute to intravascular clotting. Among these is the fact that most of the patients are of an advanced age and require protracted periods of immobilization in the treatment of their difficulty. As a result, thrombus formation may occur not only in the injured limb but also in the opposite normal one [10].

3. Physical Effort or Strain

Besides direct injury to the tissues of the lower limbs, physical exertion, without external trauma, may be responsible for deep venous thrombosis in these sites [6]. Among the causative agents are lifting heavy objects, twisting a knee, sitting-up exercises, squatting, a misstep while climbing stairs, jumping, landing after a fall, the "step-up test," and running. The response may be noted in active healthy persons, as well as in others. In the upper limbs, effort or strain may be responsible for thrombosis of the axillary or subclavian vein (see B-1, Chapter 18).

Several factors play a role in the production of deep venous thrombosis following physical effort or strain. One is an increase in intraabdominal pressure resulting from fixation of the diaphragm and contraction of the abdominal musculature, as occurs during voluntary straining, lifting, or jumping. As a consequence, there is a rise in venous pressure in the inferior vena cava and the iliac and iliofemoral veins, any local weak point in the venous system of the lower limbs thus being exposed to a bursting force.

Another etiologic agent is muscular contraction in the limb. In most situations of effort, the large flat muscles of the calf and the quadri-

ceps group of the thigh contract simultaneously, the former sharply compressing the main veins of the calf against the posterior surface of the tibia. This causes venous blood to be pumped forcibly through the relaxed muscular compartment surrounding Hunter's canal. Violent or repeated muscular contraction, when added to the high venous pressure factor, may exert a bursting force of enough magnitude to contuse the thin-walled veins, bruise their vasa vasorum, or, in association with a muscle tear, rupture a venous branch at its point of origin [6]. Such positions as prolonged kneeling or squatting may produce considerable distension of the venous tree distally because of the resulting venous angulation in the popliteal space, and if sudden contraction of the calf muscles is then carried out, the combined effect may be responsible for trauma to or even rupture of a venous channel.

4. Mechanisms Initiated by Surgical Procedures

A large number of factors have been implicated in the development of postoperative deep venous thrombosis. Among these are shock, hypotension, trauma to veins, infection and its consequences, dehydration and increased blood viscosity, slowing of the bloodstream (particularly in the microcirculation), pathologic changes in vascular endothelium, and alteration in the lipids and proteins of the blood. During the early postoperative period, a decrease and later an increase in the number of platelets have been noted, together with a rapid rise in fibrinogen concentration and in factor VIII activity; an associated finding is a reduction in both plasminogen concentration and spontaneous fibrinolytic activity. Such changes have been considered to be related to the trauma resulting from the operative procedure. However, there is no evidence to indicate that they are directly responsible for clinically evident thrombosis; predisposing factors must also be present [48].

5. Venous Stasis

Venous stasis, which plays a very important role in the development of deep venous thrombosis in the lower limbs, results from physical inactivity, immobilization of a limb as by a cast, other therapeutic measures which inadvertently interfere with venous outflow, and varicosities. It may also be present in patients with congestive heart failure and in pregnant women (in whom there is external pressure on pelvic veins). Venous stasis is a common finding in paraplegic, quadriplegic, and hemiplegic lower extremities, since such limbs are generally held in dependency without the ability to contract local voluntary muscles.

6. Prolonged Mechanical Compression of Calf

Injury to the intima of veins may develop from protracted pressure exerted by the weight of a leg on the vessels in the calf muscles, as during an operation or in the postoperative period when the patient lies on his back immobile for fear of initiating pain. The collapse of the veins produces a situation in which their intimal folds remain in close contact with each other, eventually leading to irritation and other conditions conducive to thrombus formation. Long train, automobile, or airplane trips, with the lower limbs in dependency for protracted periods, may also cause trauma to deep veins and predispose to venous thrombosis due to prolonged pressure of the edge of the seat against the vascular structures. A similar type of response is noted in elderly individuals who, for various reasons, are forced to sleep in reclining chairs. The factor of prolonged dependency with the development of venous stasis, which also exists under these circumstances, contributes to the tendency toward venous thrombosis.

7. Contraceptive Agents

The role of contraceptive drugs in the production of venous thrombosis remains unsettled. Some workers believe that there is an increased risk of deep venous thrombosis [19] (from six to nine times greater [42]) in women on the drug than in control persons. Such a view is supported by a number of experimental studies. For example, antithrombin III activity, which normally constitutes a natural protective barrier against intravascular clotting [43], is reduced. Also of interest is the finding that women on contraceptive drugs require a greater than usual dose of anticoagulants to maintain prothrombin activity at a therapeutic level of depression [37]. Such a response has been interpreted as indicating that the use of the medication increases the rate of formation of intravascular fibrin [30].

Women on contraceptive drugs have been found to have elevations in factors VII and X, but such changes have not been interpreted as indicating a greater tendency to thrombosis [18]. Attention has likewise been called to the fact that similar alterations are quite pronounced in the last trimester of pregnancy when the incidence of thromboembolic disease is actually decreased [18].

With regard to the effect of estrogens on the fibrinolytic systems, the results are again not clear-cut. There is general agreement that the plasminogen level is raised, but there also seems to be an elevation of the antiplasmin level. Plasminogen activator in the venous wall decreases in quantity, while soluble fibrin and platelet aggregability increase. The administration of estrogen is likewise associated with an increase in fibrinogen, prothrombin, and factors V, VIII, and IX, besides the factors mentioned above.

All that can be stated at present, therefore, is that while not themselves thrombogenic, the estrogens aggravate the severity of a thrombotic stimulus, this response, in part, being due to a decrease in the inhibitory activity of antithrombin III. Moreover, the extent to which a thrombotic challenge is intensified is dose-related and reflected by the extent to which antithrombin III inhibitory activity is depressed [46].

8. Hematologic Disorders

Certain diseases of the blood favor blood coagulation. One of these, polycythemia vera, probably has such an effect through the greater number of red blood cells found in this disorder, as well as through the rise in platelets and other formed elements. Another condition is severe anemia, in which there is a more marked than normal clot retraction, resulting in the expression of large quantities of serum containing a high concentration of thrombin. Such a response may account for the rapid growth of clot found in this condition.

9. Neoplastic Infiltrations

Metastasis of carcinomatous cells may be associated with invasion of veins locally, followed by thrombosis of the involved vessels. Occlusion generally occurs as soon as the adventitia is affected, although in some instances this process is delayed until the tumor has reached the lumen of the vein. Aside from a direct effect, the presence of neoplastic growths, particularly of the pancreas, is associated with an increased coagulability of the blood. Such a situation may result from destruction of tissue by the infiltration of cancerous material, this being followed by liberation of substances which, on being absorbed, raise the clotting tendency of the blood.

10. Aging Process

Old age is an important predisposing factor in venous thrombosis. This may be related to the fact that various degenerative and neoplastic diseases and hip fractures are much more common in the elderly than in younger people. Another factor is that older persons are frequently subjected to such operations as prostatectomy, herniorrhaphy, and gynecologic procedures, which are associated with a relatively high incidence of deep venous thrombosis; this, in part, is due to an exaggerated postoperative period of immobility.

11. Gestation and Puerperium

Pregnancy and the postpartum period are not infrequently followed by episodes of deep venous thrombosis. Some of the factors which may play a role in this regard are changes in coagulability, injuries due to delivery, vascular damage after traumatic operative procedures, and, in the case of pregnancy, venous stasis resulting from pressure of the enlarging uterus on the pelvic veins.

12. Miscellaneous Factors

Among other states conducive to venous thrombosis are obesity and a previous thromboembolic episode. There is little question that

the patient who has already suffered one attack of thrombosis of either a superficial or a deep vein is an excellent candidate for another episode of intravascular clotting if conditions exist which predispose to such a response. Finally, various infectious diseases, including typhoid fever, influenza, acute rheumatic fever, and pneumonia, are also associated with venous thrombosis.

B. Development of a Venous Thrombus

1. Morphologic Characteristics of a Clot

A thrombus is composed of layers of amorphous material derived from platelets, alternating with irregular deposits of packed fibrin and of clot (red blood cells trapped in a looser fibrin network). When formed in moving blood, it is made up of a head, a body, and a tail. The head consists of masses of agglutinated platelets, together with numerous white blood cells, a few red blood cells, and a small quantity of fibrin interspersed between individual platelets. The body, which enlarges laterally as well as longitudinally, is made up of fibrin and formed elements of the blood. As it grows, it may eventually fill the lumen of the vessel and occlude it. When this occurs, there is more or less fixation of the body of the clot to the wall, the degree and extent of attachment depending upon the amount of inflammatory reaction initiated by the foreign body. The tail is composed primarily of fibrin rather than platelets, with many red blood cells trapped in the interstices. In contrast with the body of the clot, the tail is not attached to the wall of the vessel, since it grows longitudinally before enlarging laterally. Because it is friable, it is readily broken off, to become the source of pulmonary emboli.

2. Mechanisms Involved in Clot Formation

There is little question that platelet aggregation is an early stage in the production of a thrombus, but what the mechanism is that triggers the process is not entirely clear. The view has been advanced that some platelets possess a quality of "stickiness" or adhesiveness and that when they collide with sufficient force, they may adhere to each other and form a small platelet nidus. In the presence of an abnormal increase in circulating platelets, this process may be enhanced. It is also possible that a locally generated substance, like adenosine diphosphate or thrombin, is responsible for making normal platelets sticky, thus initiating the process of thrombus formation.

Although normal circulating platelets do not adhere to intact healthy endothelium, damage to the inner lining causes them to do so, provided there is exposure of subendothelial collagen.[1] Whether intensely sticky platelets can adhere to normal or slightly damaged endothelium has not been clarified; nor is it certain how often venous endothelial damage occurs. However, once the platelets are adherent either to each other (aggregated) or to the wall, a number of biologically active compounds, including adenosine diphosphate, adenosine triphosphate, serotonin, calcium, and pyrophosphate, are released from them (release reaction), and these, unless washed away or neutralized, will cause further increase in stickiness of the platelets locally and growth of the aggregation. The finding that oral anticoagulants depress factors II, VII, IX, and X and thus decrease the incidence of clinical venous thrombosis supports the view that one or more of these factors contribute to fibrin deposition in the clot, probably a late event in thrombus formation.

Endothelial injury or alterations of a degree to initiate thrombosis may result from forces as severe as the trauma of surgery or as minimal as the changes which follow stressful daily situations [27]. Such substances or states as endotoxins, viral infections, antigen-antibody complexes, epinephrine, homocystinuria, and anoxia have all been implicated as causes of endothelial injury.

C. Measures for the Prevention of Deep Venous Thrombosis

1. General Considerations

In patients who are potential candidates for deep venous thrombosis (particularly the elderly when required to remain at complete bed rest for protracted periods of time and people who are undergoing a major surgical procedure), an important aspect of the treatment program is prophylaxis.[2] Ideally, the approach to such a task should be simple, safe, effective, applicable to all individuals, and inexpensive. Unfortunately, such a goal has not as yet been satisfactorily achieved. However, a large number of avenues have been explored, and the search for effective and universally acceptable prophylactic measures against intravascular clotting still continues.

Solution of the problem of venous thrombosis is especially important to the orthopedic surgeon because of the relatively high incidence of the condition found in patients with fractures or in those being treated for degenerative diseases of skeletal structures. For example, total hip reconstruction has a mortality rate from pulmonary embolism of 1 to 2 percent [20], a figure which is unacceptable for an elective operation. However, a finding which decreases the seriousness of the situation somewhat is the observation that adequate prophylactic measures established early enough have been shown to reduce substantially the high incidence of deep venous thrombosis following the procedure.

2. Means to Control Venous Stasis

In bedridden patients and in those who have been subjected to a major operation, every effort should be made to counteract pooling of blood in the venous system of the lower extremities.

Physical measures. Frequent planned and supervised voluntary movements of the legs

---

[1] It is necessary to point out that considerable evidence is now available to indicate that the endothelial cell can no longer be viewed as a passive participant in thrombosis. It appears to be emerging as a complex entity which has metabolic and functional roles of equal importance to those of the platelet in the process of clot formation [7].

[2] It is apparent that any attempt to prevent the development of a thrombus in the deep veins of the lower limbs or elsewhere will likewise have a similar effect on the incidence of pulmonary embolism.

should be carried out during the entire period of bed confinement. The regimen should include active flexion and extension of the feet, legs, and thighs and movement of the feet against some type of resistance. To facilitate matters, an apparatus has been devised to regulate both the degree and frequency of leg exercises that can be carried out in bed [12].

In the case of a surgical procedure, while the patient is still under a general anesthetic, the lower limbs should be passively exercised by repeatedly dorsiflexing and plantar flexing the feet. Such a measure has the advantage of being easily controlled and, at the same time, the intensity of the contractions is not affected by any muscle relaxants given to the patient or by the degree of anesthesia.

Precautions should be taken to avoid obstruction of venous return. The use of pillows under the knees is contraindicated, since this enhances the already existing interference to the movement of blood out of the limb resulting from anatomic relationship of the structures in the popliteal space. Placing the patient in Fowler's position and applying tight abdominal dressings should be avoided, for such measures reduce venous outflow by raising the intraabdominal pressure. At the same time, abdominal binders restrict the motion of the diaphragm which also contributes to venous stasis.

Repeated deep breathing helps reduce venous stasis in the legs, since it increases venous return from these sites, the mechanism being an exaggeration of that operating with normal inspiration. Therefore, as soon as a surgical patient regains consciousness, he should be instructed to take 12 or 15 deep breaths every hour during the day. In this regard, it is necessary to limit the use of sedatives, for otherwise there may be some depression of respiration.

Since a certain amount of vasoconstriction of the peripheral vessels is generally associated with the immediate postoperative period, it is advisable to counteract such a tendency. This is accomplished by the application of heating pads or diathermy to the abdomen, to produce indirect vasodilatation in the extremities, or by direct warming of the limbs using a thermostatically controlled heat cradle (provided a normal arterial circulation exists locally). Either measure will cause an increased rate of blood flow

through the arterioles and capillaries and hence through the venous bed. This more rapid circulation will facilitate the return of blood to the heart and thus prevent venous stasis.

If feasible, the legs should be elevated approximately 15° by raising the foot of the bed about 15 cm (6 in.), at the same time being careful not to produce a hump in the mattress at the level of the break in the bed. In the case of the surgical patient, such a step should also be carried out during the operation if possible and in the recovery room. In this manner, venous outflow from the lower limbs is facilitated and venous stasis controlled. This measure has been found especially effective in reducing the incidence of deep venous thrombosis in patients being treated for fracture of the hip [16]. However, it does impose an added burden on the heart which might cause dyspnea at rest in elderly patients with threshold cardiac function.

In the case of a limb held immobile by application of a rigid cast, instructions should be given to the patient to make a practice of contracting the muscles in the involved extremity. Although no apparent movement will result (isometric contractions), the tensing of the muscles will help facilitate the movement of lymph and blood out of the limb and thus reduce venous stasis. Coincident with this step, the patient should exercise the opposite normal extremity so as to maintain muscle tone reflexly in the involved limb and increase local blood flow as a result of the greater cardiac output produced by the exercise. Also of value is the use of an electrically operated muscle stimulator (see below) to produce passive isometric muscular contractions. It is necessary to point out, however, that such a measure may produce painful sensations.

Elastic compression appliances. For many years the routine use of elastic (Ace) bandages on the lower limbs has been advocated as a prophylactic measure in individuals 45 years of age and older who have undergone an operative procedure or are bedridden. The bandages are placed around the extremities immediately after surgery, beginning with the toes and extending upward to the groin. In this manner, stagnation of blood in the superficial veins is obviated, and, at the same time, shunting into the deeper vessels occurs, with an acceleration of flow.

However, there are several disadvantages to the use of elastic bandages. One is the inability to apply them so that they continuously maintain the uniform compressibility that is required for effective use. Therefore, they must be repeatedly rewrapped during the course of the day. Another problem is that unless they are applied with the proper tension, they will be either too tight and have a tourniquet effect (thus interfering with venous return) or too loose (which will not cause collapse of the superficial veins and control venous stasis). Moreover, there is no definitive evidence available to support the view that the application of elastic bandages prevents postoperative venous thrombosis.

In recent years a much more common practice has been to supply the patient with elastic stockings (antiembolism stockings) in place of compression bandages. Some of these produce the same amount of pressure to the entire limb, whereas others have a built-in gradient of pressure, averaging 18 mmHg at the ankle, tapering to an average of 10 mmHg at the knee and 8 mmHg at the midthigh.

A definite disadvantage to the use of antiembolism stockings is that in most hospitals very little attempt is made by nursing personnel to give a patient ones which fit his legs. As a result, too much pressure may be applied to some sites and too little to others, thus causing discomfort. What generally happens then is that the stockings are discarded if there is no close supervision of the patient's activities. Also important is the fact that if a poorly fitting stocking is worn, it does not cause sufficient collapse of superficial veins to control venous stasis, a situation which may be conducive to intravascular clotting. This is supported by the observation that the application of the standard stocking has no prophylactic value [34], although the use of graded compression stockings appears to be somewhat more effective in this regard [17]. Another objection to the routine use of antiembolism stockings is that they predispose to heel ulcers and prevent proper care of the skin of the legs, both of which may have serious implications if the pa-

tients are elderly and have some degree of local arterial insufficiency and a clouded sensorium.

Intermittent calf compression. An inflatable, pressurized plastic boot has been used to prevent venous stasis before, during, and after an operation. The apparatus is fitted over the patient's foot and reaches up to the knee, and it inflates for 12 s of each minute to an air pressure of 40 mmHg (supplied by a pneumatic pump). The external compression is considered to empty the venous system without interfering with arterial inflow. The clinical results with the inflatable boot have been varied; some surgeons report a definite reduction in venous thrombosis and pulmonary embolism whereas others have noted equivocal results. In general, it can be stated that it may have a place as a prophylactic measure, especially in patients for whom anticoagulants are contraindicated. However, full evaluation of the method must await much more clinical data than are available at present. A contraindication to its use is the presence of severe arterial insufficiency and ischemia in the limb to be treated.

A modification of the procedure consists of the application of pneumatic leg sleeves or leggings, connected to a power source that uses compressed gases and ambient air at a pressure up to 45 mmHg; the apparatus sequentially squeezes both calves and thighs simultaneously every 120 s. According to some clinical reports [33], the technique reduces the incidence of postoperative thrombosis by over 75 percent, even in patients suffering from malignant disease who are generally considered to be in the very high risk category (the reduction achieved being about 90 percent). The value of the method is that it increases pulsatility of venous outflow from the leg veins rather than mean blood flow. In addition, there is some evidence that it raises the fibrinolytic activity of the blood in surgical patients [2].

Electric stimulation of calf muscles. This approach is used during the operation on the basis that thrombosis of the deep veins of the leg may have its inception in the period of general anesthesia [4]. Support for such a belief is the finding that the volume flow rate in the veins is halved during this interval [5].

The method consists of using a galvanic current to produce intermittent contraction of the calf muscles in the anesthetized patient. Reversal of polarity with each pulse ensures absence of tissue ionization. Two electrodes, enclosed in pads soaked in saline, are applied to the back of each leg, one at the ankle and the other at the knee; the voltage is adjusted to produce brisk calf-muscle contraction throughout the operation. Use of the procedure after the patient has recovered from the anesthetic is generally not practicable since the electric stimulation may produce discomfort.

3. Means to Reduce Blood Coagulability

Precautions associated with the operative procedure. During surgery, care should be taken to minimize trauma to neighboring nonvascular structures since destruction of tissues may be followed by changes in the blood plasma which predispose to increased coagulability.[3] Dehydration should be counteracted by intravenous infusion of 5% glucose solution or isotonic saline solution, in order to reduce the viscosity of the blood.

Prophylactic low-dose heparin administration. In recent years a large number of reports have appeared supporting the view that small subcutaneous doses of heparin have a beneficial effect on reducing the incidence of venous thrombosis detected by laboratory means [13,21,47]. This is so despite the fact that the quantity of the drug routinely used is so low that it can have little direct antithrombin action. The rationale for such a program is based on the fact that a much smaller concentration of heparin is required to prevent thrombin formation than is necessary to inhibit propagation once a clot has developed. Moreover, even in the small doses utilized, the drug helps prevent platelet aggregation [29] and acts indirectly to form a complex with a naturally occurring plasma inhibitor, termed antithrombin III, anti-factor X^a, or heparin cofactor. As a result of this latter type of reaction, the ability of antithrombin III to inactivate factors IX^a, X^a, XI^a, and thrombin is greatly potentiated [22,44,49]. By its inhibiting action on factor X^a, particularly, heparin prevents the conversion of prothrombin to thrombin. Such a response can occur without any significant prolongation of the partial thromboplastin time or whole-blood clotting time, thus making it possible to induce an antithrombotic effect without seriously impairing hemostasis.

The regimen for the subcutaneous administration of heparin in surgical patients is as follows: Two hours before operation 5000 units are given subcutaneously, followed by 5000 units every 12 h for 7 days thereafter or until the patient is fully ambulatory. Another regimen consists of 5000 units every 8 h postoperatively. The injection of the low dose of the drug does not require monitoring, unlike its use in larger amounts. (For a discussion of intravenous administration of heparin as active therapy in deep venous thrombosis, see p. 271; in pulmonary embolism, see p. 288.)

A study of the available clinical data relating to the prophylactic effect of small amounts of heparin on the incidence of deep venous thrombosis does not result in the formulation of a clear-cut concept of the efficacy of the drug in this regard. Even the international multicenter trial [31], involving 4300 patients over the age of 40 years scheduled for major surgery, has been criticized on several grounds, including the fact that it was not a double-blind study, that not enough patients were utilized to prove unequivocally that subcutaneous heparin saves lives, that no arrangements had been made for review by independent observers unaware of the treatment patients received, and that diagnostic criteria were not uniform, among others. Nevertheless, this investigation is critical because if the conclusions which have been drawn are accepted, they will serve as as basis for further study of the usefulness of subcutaneous heparin in the prevention of venous thrombosis and pulmonary embolism for many years to come.

It is necessary to point out that there are

---

[3] Aside from the effect on the coagulation mechanism, trauma can also be responsible for damage to vascular elements in the operative field, particularly the veins, which may lead to thrombosis. Therefore special precautions must be taken to protect them. Manipulation and forced stretching of these structures should be avoided, and knee crutches and leg holders should be well-padded; restraining straps should not be too tight. Also of great importance in the application of a cast for the management of a fracture is to minimize pressure in the vicinity of a main vein.

certain limitations and exceptions to the routine prophylactic subcutaneous administration of small doses of heparin. For example, such an approach is of little value in the case of a number of orthopedic procedures, especially repair of femoral fractures and reconstructive surgery of the hip and knee. In the case of total hip replacement for osteoarthritis, the incidence of venous thrombosis is not significantly reduced unless the dose of 5000 units is given three times a day instead of two times, but as a result bleeding also increases in frequency [8]. The regimen is not recommended in the case of eye or brain surgery, spinal or epidural anesthesia, radical mastectomy, or prostatectomy.

Subcutaneous administration of heparin may be responsible for several types of untoward responses. One is the rare production of a bleeding diathesis in patients with a low level of antiheparin activity, which manifests itself as ecchymosis, blood loss sufficient to require transfusion, or even lethal hemorrhage. Another is a significantly greater incidence of wound hematomas than would be expected in a control group [11,31].

Prophylactic oral anticoagulant therapy. Because older patients in need of orthopedic surgical treatment are especially prone to thromboembolic complications (mainly because of the necessarily long periods of immobility), oral anticoagulants, such as warfarin sodium (Coumadin) and dicumarol, have been advised as a routine prophylactic measure for them. However, the dosage has to be meticulously controlled by frequent laboratory tests, since the ratio between the effective and the toxic quantity is small. As a result, this approach has not attracted many advocates, particularly because of fear of hemorrhage, as for example, into a fracture site. Although the latter is a definite possibility, still there are some workers [23,40,41] who believe that the derived benefit, in the form of a significant reduction in postoperative thromboembolism, more than compensates for the development of such a complication, even though a serious one. It would appear, therefore, that the general rejection of prophylactic oral anticoagulants in the postoperative period warrants reexamination and reevaluation.

Prophylactic dextran therapy. The reluctance of orthopedic and general surgeons to utilize oral anticoagulants during the postoperative period has led to the initiation of other avenues of investigation for a prophylactic agent against venous thrombosis. Among those proposed for this purpose is the administration of glucose polymer dextran [14,24], which achieves its therapeutic effect by simultaneously inhibiting vascular stasis and platelet adhesiveness, two mechanisms essential to thrombus formation. However, there is no block of fibrinogen-fibrin conversion as occurs with the use of antithrombogenic agents of the anticoagulant type. The dextrans have been found to decrease the episodes of pulmonary embolism significantly [3,24] but not the incidence of clinical and isotopically detectable deep-vein thrombosis in the legs. The explanation may be that since they are not anticoagulants they cannot be expected to affect the initial thrombosis. At the same time, however, they may prevent the growth of large thrombi which are the cause of serious pulmonary embolism. In this regard, it has been noted that dextran-treated patients postoperatively show little change in total platelet count, a 30 percent decrease in platelet adhesiveness, and an 11 percent fall in plasma fibrinogen [3]. In contrast, in control postoperative patients, the platelet count rises by 35 percent, the platelet adhesiveness increases by 13 percent, and the plasma fibrinogen becomes greater by 16 percent. The dextrans also expand plasma volume and decrease blood viscosity, enhance the microcirculation, and coat erythrocytes and endothelial walls.

The dextrans have been used in total hip replacement and fractures of the pelvis, hip, and femoral shaft, with a resulting reduction in the incidence of thromboembolic episodes [3], although not consistently so [35]. The medication is given as follows: During the operation the patient receives 200 to 500 ml of 10% dextran 40 (Rheomacrodex; low molecular weight dextran) in either saline solution or 5% glucose. In the next 6 to 8 h, 500 ml are given, followed by 500 ml daily for the first 3 days postoperatively and every other day thereafter until the patient becomes ambulatory.[4]

---

[4] Six percent dextran 700 (Macrodex), although widely used in Europe as a prophylactic agent against venous thrombosis, does not presently have regulatory approval by the FDA for this purpose in the United States.

Although wound hematomas may not be as frequent as when an oral anticoagulant or subcutaneous heparin is used, dextran administration may be responsible for several serious complications. Aside from the fact that anaphylactic reactions and hypotension may appear, the use of dextran may be associated with precipitation of pulmonary edema in elderly patients with reduced cardiac reserve, due to the increased plasma volume resulting from the hypertonicity of the drug. It is also important to point out that the quantity of dextran tolerated by different people varies considerably, and hence the dosage must be individualized. This caution is particularly important in the case of the patient who has some reduction in kidney function and in whom the possibility of renal failure must be seriously considered. For example, dextran 40 produces hydropic changes in the proximal tubular cells which may be followed by complete obliteration of the lumen of the tubules.

Other prophylactic medications. As already mentioned in B-2, above, when the release reaction occurs in vitro, adenosine diphosphate is liberated from platelets, this response leading to greater platelet aggregation. Recently it has been found that aspirin prevents such a response and thus inhibits further aggregation of platelets and their adherence to sites of damaged endothelium. Because of this type of reaction, the drug is being used as a prophylactic agent in potential candidates for deep venous thrombosis. Much more extensive clinical investigation is required, however, before a definite conclusion regarding its efficacy can be reached. Still, evidence is present that in certain orthopedic procedures, such as total hip replacement, the prophylactic use of this drug produces a statistically significant protection against venous thrombosis [15]. Of interest is the finding that such a therapeutic effect is noted only in male patients. Supporting data for the value of aspirin in orthopedic patients is a report dealing with a small number of patients undergoing reconstruction of the knee; daily doses of 3600 mg of the drug resulted in significantly better results than when smaller amounts were used [26].

Another antiplatelet agent, dipyridamole (Persantine), has been advocated for maintain-

ing patency of shunts used for renal dialysis, with reported encouraging results. When aspirin in amounts of 1 g daily is also given, this appears to potentiate the action of dipyridamole, permitting a reduction in the dosage of the latter from 400 to 100 mg daily [32]. Such a combination helps reduce the incidence of hypotension and other side effects of dipyridamole. Sulfinpyrazone (Anturane) has been used as an antiplatelet agent on the basis that it may be a competitive inhibitor of cyclooxygenase in platelets, thus preventing synthesis of prostaglandin endoperoxides and thromboxane A_2 [1].[5] Another possibility is that the drug acts to stabilize the erythrocyte membrane and so prevent a leak of adenosine diphosphate.

Several snake venom extracts, which are available in Europe but not in the United States, have been used in the prevention of venous thrombosis. They include Venacil, Reptilase, and Defibrase. These drugs rapidly decrease fibrinogen content; they also have a weak platelet-aggregating effect but no influence on the platelet count. They have been reported to cause fewer side reactions (including bleeding) than other anticoagulants.

Discontinuation of contraceptive agents. Despite the differences of opinion that exist regarding the role of contraceptive agents in the production of venous thrombosis (see A-7, above), certain prophylactic measures are still warranted. In patients with a hereditary predisposition to intravascular clotting or who give a history of venous or arterial thrombosis or arterial embolism, the medications are contraindicated, since the possibility of thrombosis is increased by their administration. Because contraceptives are responsible for a temporary development of hypercoagulability in catheterized blood vessels, they should be discontinued 2 weeks before performing angiography. The same rule applies to elective surgery, for otherwise transitory hypercoagulability will occur during the operation or in the subsequent

---

[5] Prostaglandin endoperoxides are labile substances which have been shown to induce platelet aggregation as well as the platelet release reaction when added to human platelet–rich plasma [25]. Thromboxane A_2, which is formed from prostaglandin endoperoxides, is also capable of causing platelet aggregation and serotonin release.

week, or at both times. In the case of an emergency operation on a patient who is receiving contraceptives, the administration of postoperative anticoagulant therapy should be seriously considered. Since statistical studies have revealed a higher incidence of death from thromboembolism after the use of contraceptives in women who smoke than in those who do not [9], abstinence should be followed while the patient is receiving the drug.

References

1. Ali M, McDonald JW: Effects of sulfinpyrazone on platelet prostaglandin synthesis and platelet release of serotonin. J Lab Clin Med 89:868, 1977
2. Allenby F, Boardman L, Pflug JI, et al: Effects of external pneumatic intermittent compression on fibrinolysis in man. Lancet 2:1412, 1973
3. Atik M, Harkess JW, Wichman H: Prevention of fatal pulmonary embolism. Surg Gynecol Obstet 130:403, 1970
4. Browse NL, Negus D: Prevention of postoperative leg vein thrombosis by electrical muscle stimulation: An evaluation with ^{125}I-labelled fibrinogen. Br Med J 3:615, 1970
5. Clark C, Cotton LT: Blood-flow in deep veins of leg: Recording technique and evaluation of methods to increase flow during operation. Br J. Surg 55:211, 1968
6. Crane C: Deep venous thrombosis in the leg following effort or strain. N Engl J Med 246:529, 1952
7. Day HJ: Platelet and endothelial cell participation in hemostasis and thrombosis. In Mielke CH Jr, Rodvien R (eds): Mechanisms of Hemostasis and Thrombosis. Miami, Symposia Specialists, 1978
8. Dechavanne M, Saudin F, Viala JJ, et al: Prévention des thromboses veineuses. Succes de l'héparine ã fortes doses lors des coxarthroses. Nouv Presse Med 3:1317, 1974
9. Frederiksen H, Ravenholt RT: Thromboembolism, oral contraceptives, and cigarettes. Public Health Rep 85:197, 1970
10. Freeark RJ, Boswick J. Fardin R: Posttraumatic venous thrombosis. Arch Surg 95:567, 1967
11. Gallus AS, Hirsh J. O'Brien SE, et al: Prevention of venous thrombosis with small, subcutaneous doses of heparin. JAMA 235:1980, 1976
12. Goldsmith HS: Thromboembolic disease: Emphasis on prevention. Med Times 96:774, 1968
13. Gordon-Smith IC, Grundy DJ, Le Quesne LP, et al: Controlled trial of two regimens of subcutaneous heparin in prevention of postoperative deep-vein thrombosis. Lancet 1:1133, 1972
14. Gruber VF: Dextran and the prevention of postoperative thromboembolic complications. Surg Clin North Am 55:579, 1975
15. Harris WH, Salzman EW, Athanasoulis CA, et al: Aspirin prophylaxis of venous thromboembolism after total hip replacement. N Engl J Med 297:1246, 1977
16. Hartman JT, Altner PC, Freeark RJ: The effect of limb elevation in preventing venous thrombosis. J Bone Joint Surg 52A:1618, 1970
17. Holford CP: The effect of graduated static compression on isotopically diagnosed deep vein thrombosis of the leg. Br J Surg 63:157, 1976
18. Hougie C: Thromboembolism and oral contraceptives. Am Heart J 85:538, 1973
19. Inman WH, Vessey MP, Westerholm B, et al: Thromboembolic disease and the steroidal content of oral contraceptives: A report to the Committee of Safety of Drugs. Br Med J 2:203, 1970
20. Ivins JC, Benson WF, Bickel WH, et al: Arthroplasty of the hip for idiopathic degenerative joint disease. Surg Gynecol Obstet 125:1281, 1967
21. Kakkar VV, Field ES, Nicolaides AN, et al: Low doses of heparin in prevention of deep-vein thrombosis. Lancet 2:669, 1971
22. Kakkar VV, Spindler J, Flute PT, et al: Efficacy of low doses of heparin in prevention of deep-vein thrombosis after major surgery: A double-blind randomized trial. Lancet 2:101, 1972
23. Kistner RW, Smith GV: Ten-year analysis of thromboembolism and dicumarol prophylaxis. Surg Gynecol Obstet 98:437, 1954
24. Kline A, Hughes LE, Campbell H, et al: Dextran 70 in prophylaxis of thromboembolic disease after surgery: A clinically oriented randomized double-blind trial. Br Med J 2:109, 1975
25. Malmsten C, Hamberg M, Svensson J, et al: Physiological role of an endoperoxide in human platelets: Hemostatic defect due to platelet cyclo-oxygenase deficiency. Proc Natl Acad Sci USA 72:1446, 1975
26. McKenna R, Bachmann F, Galante J, et al: Prospective trial of aspirin and phlebo-dynastat in the prevention of thrombo-embolic disease. Blood 48:977, 1976
27. Mustard JF, Packham MA: The role of blood and platelets in atherosclerosis and the complications of atherosclerosis. Thromb Diath Haemorrh 33[3]:444, 1975
28. Nylander G, Semb H: Veins of the lower part of the leg after tibial fractures. Surg Gynecol Obstet 134:974, 1972
29. O'Brien JR, Etherington M, Jamieson S, et al: Platelet function in venous thrombosis and low-dosage heparin. Lancet 1:1302, 1972
30. Pilgeram LO, Ellison J, Von dem Bussche G: Oral contraceptives and increased formation of soluble fibrin. Br Med J 3:556, 1974

31. Prevention of fatal postoperative pulmonary embolism by low doses of heparin: An international multicentre trial. Lancet 2:45, 1975

32. Renney JTG, O'Sullivan EF, Burke PF: Prevention of postoperative deep vein thrombosis with dipyridamole and aspirin. Br Med J 1:992, 1976

33. Roberts VC, Cotton LT: Prevention of postoperative deep vein thrombosis in patients with malignant disease. Br Med J 1:358, 1974

34. Rosengarten DS, Laird J, Jeyasingh K, et al: The failure of compression stockings (Tubigrip) to prevent deep venous thrombosis after operation. Br J Surg 57:296, 1970

35. Rothermel JE, Wessinger JB, Stinchfield FE: Dextran 40 and thromboembolism in total hip replacement surgery. Arch Surg 106:135, 1973

36. Salzman EW, Harris WH, De Sanctis RW: Anticoagulation for prevention of thromboembolism following fractures of the hip. N Engl J Med 275:122, 1966

37. Schrogie JJ, Seigel D, Corfman PA: Letter. JAMA 220:416, 1972

38. Sevitt S: Anticoagulant prophylaxis against venous thrombosis and pulmonary embolism. In Sasahara AA, Stein M (eds): Pulmonary Embolic Disease: Proceedings of the Symposium. New York, Grune & Stratton, 1965, p 265

39. Sevitt S, Gallagher NG: Prevention of venous thrombosis and pulmonary embolism in injured patients. Lancet 2:981, 1959

40. Sevitt S, Innes D: Prothrombin-time and thrombotest in injured patients on prophylactic anticoagulant therapy. Lancet 1:124, 1964

41. Skinner DB, Salzman EW: Anticoagulant prophylaxis in surgical patients. Surg Gynecol Obstet 125:741, 1967

42. Vessey MP, Doll R: Investigation of relation between use of oral contraceptives and thrombo-embolic disease. Br Med J 2:199, 1968

43. von Kaulla E, von Kaulla KN: Clinical hypercoagulability as reflected by the kinetics of thrombin generation and antithrombin III activity. Proc IX Congress. Internat Soc Hematology, Mexico, 1962. Basel, Karger, 1964, p 133

44. Walsh PN, Biggs R: The role of platelets in intrinsic factor-Xa formation. Br J Haematol 22:743, 1972

45. Wessler S: The role of stasis in thrombosis. In Sherry S, Brinkhous KM, Genton E, Stengle JM (eds): Thrombosis. Washington, DC, National Academy of Sciences, 1969, p 461

46. Wessler S: The current status of the hypercoagulable state. In Joist JH, Sherman LA (eds): Venous and Arterial Thrombosis. New York, Grune & Stratton, 1979, p 23

47. Williams HT: Prevention of postoperative deep-vein thrombosis with perioperative subcutaneous heparin. Lancet 2:950, 1971

48. Ygge J: Changes in blood coagulation and fibrinolysis during the postoperative period. Am J Surg 119:225, 1970

49. Yin ET, Wessler S, Stoll PJ: Biological properties of the naturally occurring plasma inhibitor to activated factor X. J Biol Chem 246:3703, 1971

Chapter 18

Vascular Complications of Musculoskeletal Disorders Produced by Trauma

---

Part 4 Clinical Manifestations of Deep Venous Thrombosis

Thrombosis of the deep venous system, particularly in the lower limbs, is a problem of great importance to the orthopedic and general surgeon. Because of its close association with pulmonary embolism (see Chapter 19), it may alter the entire outlook of a relatively benign illness or an operative procedure. Even if pulmonary embolism does not develop, occlusion of a main venous channel by itself will considerably prolong the postoperative course and convalescent period. Moreover, in many instances, it may be followed by the disabling sequelae of the postphlebitic syndrome which can restrict the patient's physical activity for months or even years (see Chapter 20). It is therefore essential always to be aware of the possibility of the existence of deep venous thrombosis, so as to be in the favorable position of recognizing the condition early in its inception and instituting appropriate therapy immediately.

A. Thrombosis of Deep Veins of the Lower Limbs

1. Definition of Terms

An attempt has been made to divide acute thrombosis of the deep veins of the lower ex-

tremities into two clinical types, a step which has not met with universal acceptance since the criticism has been offered that such differentiation is without physiologic or anatomic basis. However, it would seem reasonable to accept the view that clinically, at least, one should distinguish between occlusion in small deep veins—phlebothrombosis—and a similar process in a large venous collecting channel in the lower extremity—popliteal or iliofemoral thrombophlebitis—although remaining cognizant of the possible errors that might arise because of the close association between the two conditions.

2. Clinical Manifestations of Phlebothrombosis

The abnormal clinical changes in phlebothrombosis may frequently be ambiguous, meager, and fragmentary, with the result that the conclusions reached are only provisional.

Constitutional responses. Among these is a slight and simultaneous increase in temperature, pulse, and respiratory rates (for which there is no obvious reason) in an individual who has been at complete bed rest for some

263

time or is convalescing from an operative procedure. Such findings may be associated with apprehension, restlessness, and a feeling of impending disaster or sometimes an ill-defined sensation of something being wrong. At times, no symptoms exist.

Local symptoms and signs. The presence of localizing complaints or findings in the calf, combined with the above-mentioned systemic reactions, gives support to the diagnosis of phlebothrombosis. A very important symptom is an aching or cramplike pain in the calf at rest. Among the physical findings are a positive Homans' sign (see B-2, Chapter 7); tense or spastic calf muscles; the presence of an indefinite mass between the bellies of the gastrocnemius muscle; and pain in the lower portion of the leg on passive extension of the foot and plantar flexion of the toes. On occasion, there may be some findings indicating increased sympathetic tonus, such as cyanosis of the foot, coolness of the skin, and hyperhidrosis. Another diagnostic sign is a slight increase in the

circumference of the calf, frequently determined only by measurement, although obvious edema of the leg and foot is generally not present, except possibly at the ankle. Moreover, the venous pressure in the superficial veins, as determined by the state of distension of the vessels on elevation of the limb, is not increased. (For the other, less common, clinical diagnostic signs of phlebothrombosis, see B-3, Chapter 7.)

Diagnostic laboratory aids. Since the symptoms and signs of phlebothrombosis are frequently not diagnostic of the condition, the examiner must usually resort to laboratory procedures to confirm its presence. In this regard, contrast venography is considered the most accurate test (Fig. 18.1), but it has definite disadvantages, particularly the fact that it is invasive. Radioactive fibrinogen studies and radionuclide venography are also very effective in diagnosing fresh thrombi in the deep venous plexuses of the muscles of the calf. On the other hand, a number of noninvasive proce-

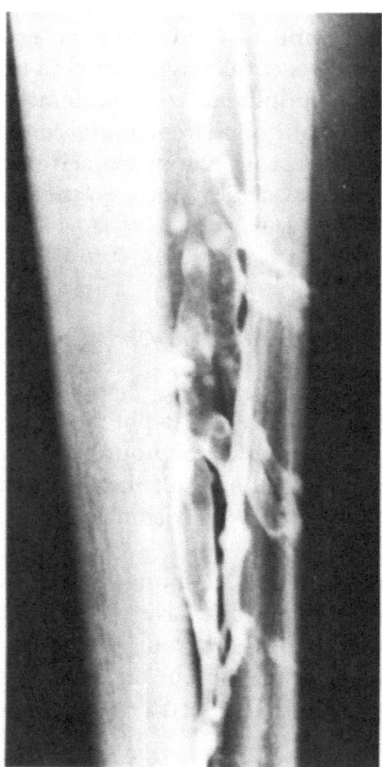 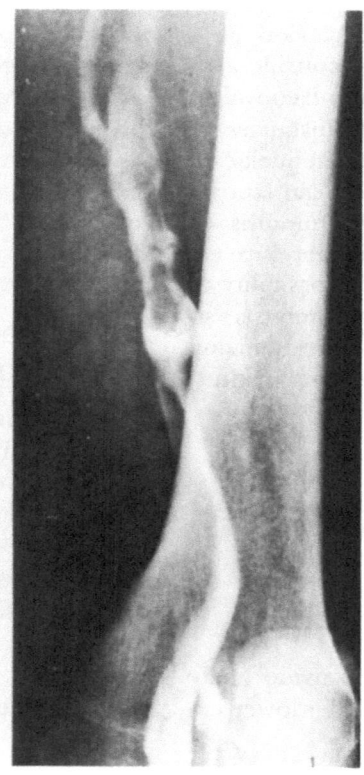

A   **B**

Fig. 18.1. Changes in the venogram indicating the presence of thrombi in the deep venous plexuses of the calf and in collecting veins. **A** Thrombi in the tibial veins seen as filling defects, which persist in an otherwise well-opacified vessel in two successive films without any alteration in shape and location. **B** Partially occluding thrombi in the popliteal and superficial femoral veins, seen as well-defined translucent areas surrounded by a rim of contrast medium. From Kakkar VV, Flanc C, O'Shea MJ, et al: Treatment of deep-vein thrombosis with streptokinase. Br J Surg 56:178, 1969. Reproduced with permission of John Wright & Sons, Bristol, England.

dures, such as impedance plethysmography, mercury strain-gauge plethysmography, the phleborheograph, and the Doppler ultrasonic technique, are primarily of help if the thrombus has already propagated into the lumen of large collecting veins and has occluded these channels. (For the advantages, disadvantages, and relative value of the different laboratory tests for detecting the presence of phlebothrombosis, see C-6 Chapter 7.)

Differential diagnosis. A large number of clinical entities may mimic phlebothrombosis. Among these is a *popliteal (Baker) cyst,* a benign disorder which may be part of the clinical picture of rheumatoid arthritis or other types of arthritis of the knee joint. It results from the development of an abnormal communication between the gastrocnemius–semimembranosus bursa and the knee joint, in response to an elevated intraarticular pressure; the lesion then fills with effusion to form a cyst. Rupture or dissection of the latter is followed by extravasation of the cyst fluid into the compartments of the calf, thereby producing local symptoms and signs [10].

The first manifestations of ruptured popliteal cyst are pain, tenderness, and swelling of the calf in a patient with existing pain or swelling of the knee; at times there may also be edema of the ankle. Homans' sign is positive and deep pressure in the calf elicits pain. However, the differentiation from phlebothrombosis is readily made by an arthrogram (using ^{131}I serum albumin or contrast medium), which visualizes the presence of the communication arising from the knee joint (Fig. 18.2), and by venography, which reveals a normal main deep venous system in the leg, with no signs of occlusion of the venous plexuses in the calf muscles.

Muscle strain may also produce symptoms and signs which resemble those of phlebothrombosis. These include stiffness, pain, and disability located in a lower limb. The condition is due to hematoma formation, with the symptoms becoming most severe 4 to 24 h after the precipitating bout of physical effort or period of strain. In contrast, the clinical picture of phlebothrombosis following trauma to the calf, for example, usually develops no sooner than from 2 to 7 days after the injury; this is because a relatively long period of time is required for the slowly

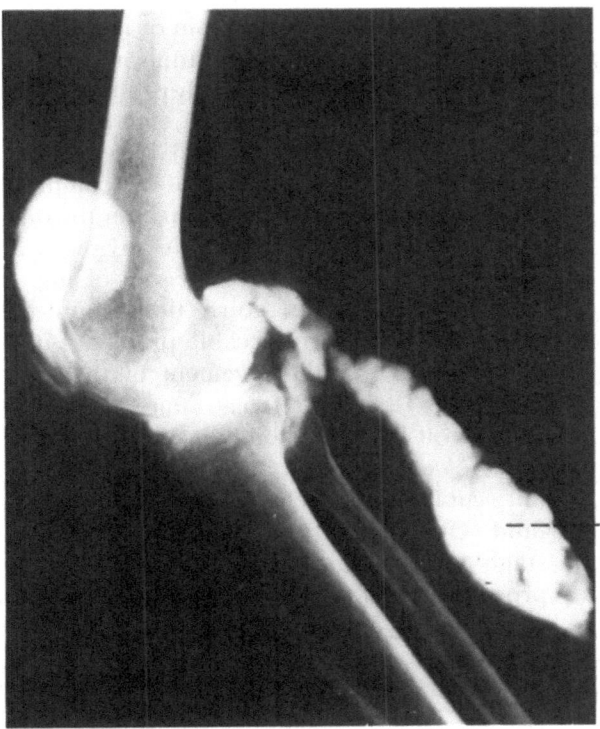

— Cyst filled
with dye injected
into joint cavity

Fig. 18.2. Arthrogram demonstrating chronic dissection of a popliteal (Baker's) cyst. Cyst filled with dye injected into joint cavity. From Abramson DI: Vascular Disorders of the Extremities. Hagerstown, Md, Harper & Row, 1974. Reproduced with permission.

forming thrombus to grow sufficiently large to cause blockade of the deep venous plexuses. Moreover, in the case of a muscle tear or hematoma formation, generally several days later ecchymosis gradually appears in the skin overlying the lesion or distally around the ankle, a finding never noted in phlebothrombosis. Homans' sign is of no diagnostic importance since it will be positive in both muscle strain and phlebothrombosis. At all times, it must be kept in mind that the two conditions can and do coexist.

Tennis leg may likewise be mistaken for phlebothrombosis. In this condition, generally produced when stress falls heavily on the foot as in stepping from a high curb, the gastrocnemius avulses from its aponeurotic sheet, which, in turn, separates from the underlying aponeurosis of the soleus muscle [4]. The condition may also follow a tear of the plantaris tendon. The clinical manifestations are sudden pain in the calf, the appearance of a medial bulge, and inability to bring the heel down to the floor or to stand on the toes. The calf is extensively swollen and is tender from its middle portion to the malleolar level. Flexion of the knee to a right angle and full plantar flexion of the foot result in distal movement of the gastrocnemius to its former position, with loss of the medial bulge of the muscle. This type of response is an important differential point from phlebothrombosis, in which such a maneuver has no effect on the swelling and contour of the posterior portion of the calf. Furthermore, in tennis leg, there is a history of the onset of symptoms and signs immediately after some type of injury to the calf.

Muscle hernia (myocele) is a protrusion of a muscle through a defect in the overlying fascial sheath, usually in the anterior tibial compartment, without involvement of the muscle substance itself, in contrast to muscle strain in which a hematoma forms in the muscle (see muscle strain, above). In almost every case of muscle hernia, a history of direct or indirect trauma is elicited. The clinical manifestations are due to the fact that the herniated muscle is forced through an unyielding ring of fascia, producing pain, incarceration, and, at times, strangulation [9]. However, if the fascial split is extensive enough to allow the muscle to herniate and regress freely, there may be no mani-

festations except for the noticeable mass. Unless adhesions develop, the diagnosis can easily be made by having the patient use the involved muscle, causing it to be depressed and allowing the fascial covering to be palpated. When the tibialis anterior and peroneus longus muscles are involved, the differentiation of muscle hernia from phlebothrombosis must be considered. However, the fact that the external mass disappears on contraction of the affected muscle readily identifies the condition.

3. Clinical Manifestations of Popliteal or Iliofemoral Thrombophlebitis

Constitutional responses. In contrast with phlebothrombosis, systemic reactions in popliteal or iliofemoral thrombophlebitis are quite prominent, thus contributing significantly to early diagnosis. Among these are fever, up to 38.9° C (102° F), tachycardia, mild malaise, leukocytosis, and a high sedimentation rate.

Local manifestations of iliofemoral thrombophlebitis. The complaint first noted in the acute stage of iliofemoral thrombophlebitis (phlegmasia alba dolens) is pain in the involved limb, located either along the course of the affected vessel and in the groin or in the whole extremity. At times the symptoms may be very severe. Tenderness is generally present in Scarpa's triangle and in the groin, and any movement of the limb is associated with a marked exaggeration of the intensity of the complaint.

Usually swelling appears soon after the onset of the pain, although at times it may occur before. Depending upon the degree of impairment of local venous return, the amount may vary from a barely noticeable pretibial pitting edema to massive involvement of the entire limb (Fig. 18.3A).[1] The extremity may appear cyanotic at first but rapidly becomes white because of compression and collapse of the minute cutaneous vessels produced by the edema fluid. Other important findings in the acute stage of iliofemoral thrombophlebitis are prominence and distension of the superficial veins due to the increased venous pressure.

---

[1] If the thrombus is located in the popliteal vein, the symptoms and signs (including the edema) are similar but limited to the leg and foot.

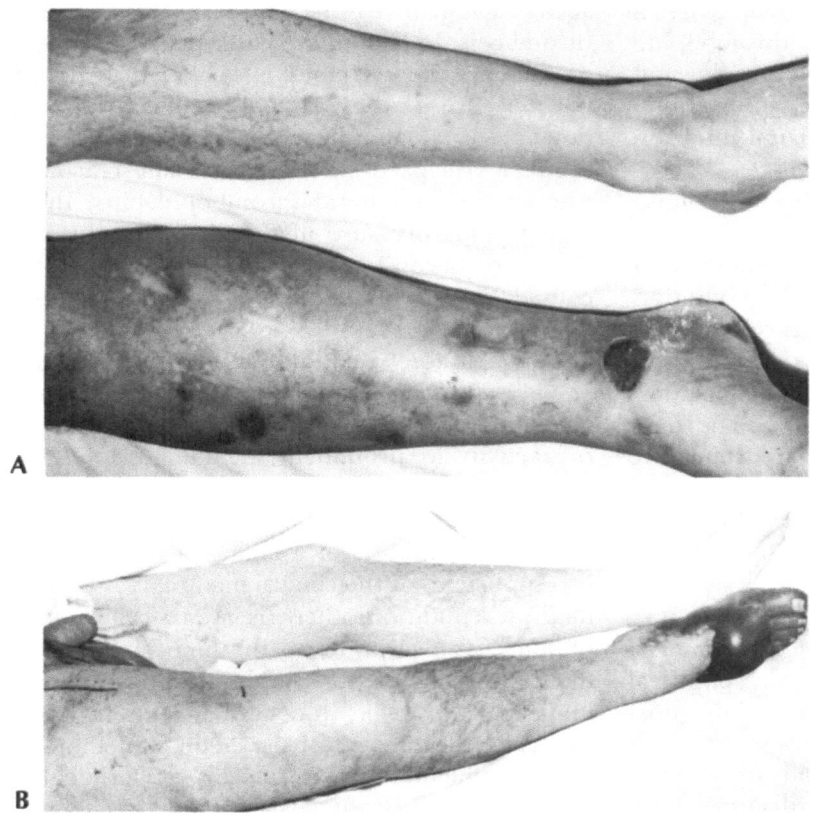

Fig. 18.3. Acute iliofemoral thrombophlebitis. **A** Marked swelling of right foot, leg, and thigh (phlegmasia alba dolens), with some superficial ulceration. **B** Extensive thrombosis of iliofemoral vein and its main tributaries, producing phlegmasia cerulea dolens with bullae and venous gangrene of the foot. From Abramson DI: Diagnosis and Treatment of Peripheral Vascular Disorders. New York, Hoeber-Harper, 1956. Reproduced with permission.

Such changes generally indicate either thrombosis above the level of the femoral vein, placing the major burden of venous drainage on the great saphenous vein and its tributaries, or occlusion of the mouth of the great saphenous vein where it enters the femoral vein, this also increasing the pressure in the superficial system distally. It must be pointed out, however, that the distension of the superficial veins may not readily be discernible because of the masking effect of the edema. (For the pathogenesis of edema formation following occlusion of a main collecting vein, see p. 109.)

Phlegmasia cerulea dolens. This condition is an acute fulminating form of iliofemoral thrombophlebitis which is characterized by severe circulatory disturbances in the involved limb due to massive occlusion of the local deep venous system. An important diagnostic point is the deeply violaceous or cyanotic hue of the skin, with purpuric areas or petechial lesions scattered over the entire extremity. The swelling is marked, which may be the cause for the frequent appearance of cutaneous blebs or bullae filled with serum or blood (Fig. 18.3B). Excruciating local pain is generally present. Pulsations in the arteries of the foot are distant or may even be absent. At times there may be actual necrosis of the foot (venous gangrene) (Fig. 18.3B), which may require an amputation.

The cause of the condition is not known, although there is no question that a marked interference with venous return exists, due to complete obstruction of both the main venous channel and its tributaries, followed by hindrance to arterial inflow. An associated reflex vasospasm further increases the ischemia of the tissues in the limb. The release of serotonin (a vasoconstrictor agent) through platelet breakdown [1] has also been implicated.

Clinical manifestations of suppurative iliofemoral thrombophlebitis. Although the great majority of patients exhibit no signs of bacterial invasion in iliofemoral thrombophlebitis (nonsuppurative iliofemoral thrombophlebitis), in the occasional case, suppurative thrombophlebitis exists [8]. Such a situation may follow pelvic manipulation (intrauterine insertion of radium), postabortal or postpartum infection, a difficult delivery, or a pelvic abscess.

In acute suppurative iliofemoral thrombophlebitis, the clot obstructing the vein is infected. As a result, the systemic responses are very marked. At the onset of the condition, there is generally a high, spiking, relapsing fever, associated with chills and other signs of a serious blood-borne infection, including rapid heart and respiratory rates. The local findings in the involved limb are similar to those noted in nonsuppurative iliofemoral thrombophlebitis. Signs of abscess formation may be found in the pulmonary bed due to liberation of infected emboli.

Diagnostic laboratory aids. Since the clinical manifestations of iliofemoral or popliteal thrombophlebitis are so clear-cut and diagnostic, only rarely is it necessary to resort to such procedures as contrast venography or radionuclide venography to make the diagnosis and identify the site of occlusion of the vessel. If verification is necessary, such noninvasive procedures as Doppler ultrasonic technique and impedance and strain-gauge plethysmography are helpful. In the case of suppurative iliofemoral thrombophlebitis, roentgenograms of the chest are indicated.

Differential diagnosis. Because of the superimposed vasospasm not infrequently observed in acute iliofemoral thrombophlebitis, the latter may manifest certain clinical characteristics which resemble those seen in *arterial embolism* and a rapidly forming *arterial thrombosis* (see A-3 and B-2, respectively, Chapter 12). For example, the pulsations in the foot may be reduced or even absent, with comparable alterations in the oscillometric readings. Moreover, the skin is cool and pale. Also, in the case of phlegmasia cerulea dolens, venous gangrene and other nutritional disturbances may be present, mimicking the changes observed in marked arterial impairment. The most important difference between the two types of conditions is the enlargement of the limb by edema fluid in iliofemoral thrombophlebitis and the lack of

such a change in arterial embolism and arterial thrombosis. In fact, in the latter two disorders, if anything, the extremity is smaller than normal because of the markedly reduced blood flow into it. Furthermore, the superficial veins are in a collapsed state for the same reason, whereas in iliofemoral thrombophlebitis, the high venous pressure in these vessels causes them to become prominent, provided, of course, such a finding is not masked by the edema.

A comparable situation exists in the case of *posttraumatic painful vascular disorders* (see A-2, Chapter 13), in which signs of sympathetic overactivity are prominent, including coldness, pallor, and pitting edema. As a result, superficial examination may lead to the mistaken belief that thrombosis of a main collecting vein is responsible for the clinical picture. However, in these conditions there is always a history of some type of injury to the limb preceding the appearance of the symptoms and physical findings. Moreover, the swelling rarely approaches the degree observed in iliofemoral thrombophlebitis, and its onset is very gradual, in contrast to the rapid accumulation of edema fluid observed in the latter condition. At no time is an increase in venous pressure, resulting in distension of the superficial veins, noted in posttraumatic painful vascular diseases, whereas this is a prominent finding in acute thrombosis of a collecting vein.

There should be no problem differentiating *superficial benign thrombophlebitis* (see A-1, Chapter 7) from sudden occlusion of a main collecting vein in a limb. Of paramount importance is the fact that this condition is never associated with any swelling of the involved extremity, whereas in iliofemoral thrombophlebitis, varying degrees of edema of the foot and leg or of the entire lower limb are consistent findings. Moreover, systemic changes do not occur with superficial benign thrombophlebitis, whereas these are almost invariably a part of the clinical picture of occlusion of a main collecting vein. Nor are there signs of an increase in pressure in the uninvolved superficial vessels of the limb. At the same time, there are obvious signs of an inflammatory process in the surface veins, a finding which is absent in occlusion of main collecting veins.

On occasion, the *postphlebitic syndrome* (see

Section B, Chapter 20) has been mistaken for acute iliofemoral thrombophlebitis. However, in patients suffering from this condition, a history is almost always elicited of an acute episode of iliofemoral thrombophlebitis occurring years before. Moreover, there are signs of a prolonged, chronic state of venous stasis, in the form of pitting and nonpitting edema, secondary varicosities, induration and brawniness of the skin of the lower portion of the leg, brown pigmentation around the ankle, and, at times, stasis dermatitis and stasis ulceration. Finally, the postphlebitic syndrome is not associated with any systemic responses, such as a rise in temperature, an increase in cardiac and respiratory rates, or an elevation of the sedimentation rate. On the other hand, signs of persistent venous stasis are not noted in acute iliofemoral thrombophlebitis and constitutional changes are invariably present. At times it may be necessary to resort to venography, so as to demonstrate a block in the main collecting vein, with bridging collaterals, to make the diagnosis of the postphlebitic syndrome.

When *acute cellulitis* with lymphangitis is located in a lower limb, the clinical manifestations may resemble those of iliofemoral thrombophlebitis. However, the systemic responses are generally greater than those of nonsuppurative iliofemoral thrombophlebitis, although not as marked as those of the rare suppurative type. The swelling of acute cellulitis may be considerable in amount but it is nonpitting and limited to the area of local involvement. This is in contrast with that of iliofemoral thrombophlebitis in which the edema encompasses the entire circumference of the limb, usually being pitting in type and uniform. A most important distinction is that the swelling of acute cellulitis is associated with other local signs of inflammation, such as rubor of the skin, elevated skin temperature, bounding pulses in the foot, and lymphangitis and regional lymphadenitis. On the other hand, as already indicated, iliofemoral thrombophlebitis manifests signs of increased sympathetic tone, including pallor or cyanosis of the skin, a low cutaneous temperature, reduced or absent pulsations in the foot, and hyperhidrosis. Finally, in acute cellulitis, the venous pattern on the surface of the limb is normal, whereas in thrombosis of a main collecting vessel, the superficial

veins are distended and prominent and demonstrate a high venous pressure. (For a differentiation of the edematous limb of iliofemoral thrombophlebitis from the swollen extremity noted after prolonged compression by a cast, see A-1, Chapter 22.)

B. Primary Thrombosis of Axillary and Subclavian Veins

1. Incidence and Etiologic Factors

Primary thrombosis of axillary and subclavian veins, also designated as effort thrombosis of the axillary and subclavian veins, is a relatively rare condition, constituting 1.3 to 1.7 percent of the total cases of venous thrombosis throughout the body [3].

The cause of primary thrombosis of the axillary and subclavian veins may be compression of the vessels by neighboring structures. The most common site for such a response to occur is the space between the first rib and the clavicle [13] where the subclavian vein is vulnerable to constrictive forces exerted by the costocoracoid ligament and the subclavius muscle. Other possible sites include the space between the pectoralis minor tendon and the coracoid process [13] and that formed by the anterior scalenus muscle, the subclavius muscle, and the first rib.

Generally the precipitating factor is some type of heavy physical effort involving the upper limb and including marked abduction of the shoulder and, less often, extreme adduction; at times, a direct blow to the arm may act as an initiating factor.

2. Clinical Manifestations

Constitutional responses. In contrast with iliofemoral thrombophlebitis, the systemic reactions noted in primary thrombosis of the axillary and subclavian veins are minimal. The temperature and pulse rate are normal, and only rarely are the white blood count and sedimentation rate increased.

Symptoms and signs. The identification of the condition is based on the following: the sudden

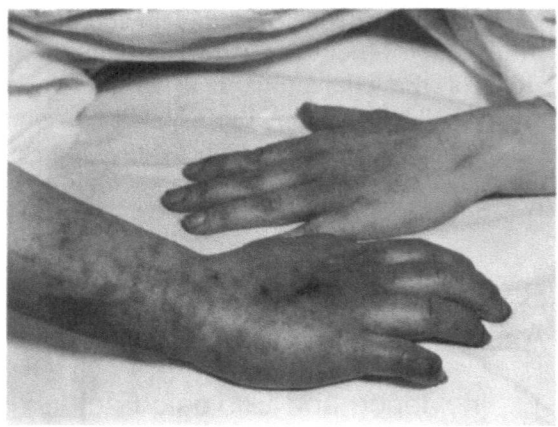

Fig. 18.4. Acute primary thrombosis of right subclavian vein. Massive edema is present in hand and forearm which extends up the arm, although not noted in the figure.

appearance of swelling of an upper extremity (Fig. 18.4) in an otherwise normal individual; pain in the involved limb; palpation of a thrombosed axillary vein in the axilla; distension of superficial veins on the forearm and hand which is not affected by elevation of the limb; and the appearance of a rich superficial collateral venous circulation extending from the involved arm onto the anterior chest wall, a finding which is readily visualized by infrared photography (Fig. 18.5). In addition, the fingers may be cyanotic and cold.

Differential diagnosis. Not infrequently it may be difficult to differentiate primary thrombosis

of the axillary and subclavian veins from occlusion of these vessels secondary to other disorders. Among the latter are polycythemia, cachexia, congestive heart failure, mediastinal tumors, and aneurysms of the ascending aorta causing compression of the innominate vein. Thrombosis of the axillary vein may also result from the intravenous administration of irritating hypertonic or sclerosing solutions, hyperalimentation therapy, passage of an indwelling catheter into the superior vena cava, and intimal injury due to local trauma. Metastasis of primary carcinoma to the axillary lymph nodes may invade the axillary vein or exert extrinsic compression on it. Furthermore, a radical mastectomy may cause direct trauma to the vessel. Local infection may likewise play a role in the initiation of the thrombotic process in the collecting vein. Other mechanisms which may be responsible for such a result are scar tissue formation consequent to radical mastectomy, alteration in the course of the axillary vein following removal of the pectoral muscles, and compression of this vessel as a complication of a neurovascular compression syndrome of the shoulder girdle (see Section B, Chapter 13).

Among other conditions which may mimic primary thrombosis of the axillary and subclavian veins is secondary lymphedema, generally due either to repeated episodes of cellulitis followed by lymphangitis and lymphadenitis or to radical mastectomy. A congenital arteriovenous fistula of the upper limb (see Section B, Chapter 21) causes an increase in both length and circumference of the extremity, whereas

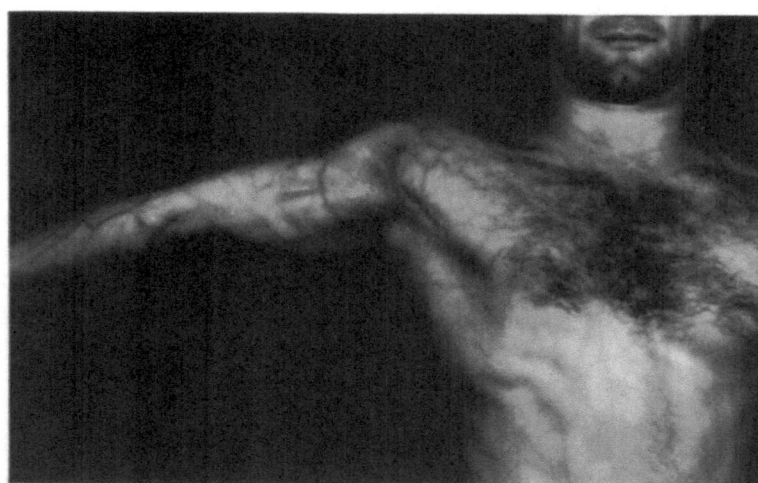

Fig. 18.5. Right subclavian vein thrombosis. The superficial venous collateral network on the arm and anterior chest wall is made more prominent with infrared photography.

an acquired arteriovenous fistula (see Section F, Chapter 15) usually only produces an enlargement in the circumference of the limb. The onset of the swelling of the arm in all three of the above conditions is slow, and in each instance clear-cut clinical findings identify the underlying entity.

C. Active Therapy for Deep Venous Thrombosis

1. Treatment of Phlebothrombosis

Therapy for phlebothrombosis consists of placing the patient at bed rest with no bathroom privileges and instituting anticoagulant therapy. The foot of the bed is elevated 12.5 to 17.5 cm (5 to 7 in.). (For a discussion of the physical measures used in the prevention of deep venous thrombosis, see C-2, Chapter 17.)

Heparin therapy. Continuous intravenous infusion of heparin has a definite advantage over intermittent injection through an indwelling catheter primarily because the number of major bleeding episodes are significantly less. This is due to the achievement of a more uniform and more or less constant effect on the clotting mechanism. On the other hand, bolus heparin may result in periods of inadequate, as well as excessive, anticoagulation.

The main disadvantage of the continuous sustaining infusion of heparin is the requirement for some flow-regulated device to ensure that the patient receives the proper dose of the drug at a constant rate. Use of an ordinary intravenous drip may result in the administration of a high concentration at times, with resulting serious consequences. For this reason, the method requires greater nursing and medical attention than does intermittent therapy. Close control of the rate of delivery of the solution may be achieved using a Harvard pump. The solution of 5% glucose in water or the isotonic salt solution in the infusion system should contain 20,000 units of heparin for each 1000 ml of fluid, and the flow is so regulated that 20 to 25 drops are entering the vein each minute. The aim of heparin therapy is to maintain a constant activated partial thromboplastin time (APTT) at 1.5 to 2.5 times the control value. To accomplish this, it is necessary to repeat the test at least every 12 h.

If adequate laboratory monitoring is not available, the intermittent bolus injection is probably safer since under such circumstances it is less likely to lead to dangerous accumulations of heparin in the circulation. A practical schedule consists of the intravenous administration of the medication (by way of an indwelling catheter) in doses of either 5000 units every 4 h or 7500 units every 6 h over the 24-h period. The method has the advantage of being much less confining to the patient than is a continuous infusion and also it is less costly.

Regardless of the method of administration, at all times, the possibility of bleeding from an operative site or elsewhere must be kept in mind. Generally this complication, which occurs in 6 to 8 percent of heparinized patients, can be reduced by avoiding all antiplatelet drugs such as aspirin and all intramuscular, intravenous, and arterial punctures. Also, in the case of the elderly, it is advisable to modify the heparin dose. Moreover, all unexplained symptoms such as back pain should be investigated to rule out the possibility of bleeding at a remote site. Frequent testing for the occurrence of thrombocytopenia likewise decreases the possibility of bleeding episodes.

When hemorrhage is already present, the first step in its control is the immediate discontinuation of the heparin. If this does not produce the desired response after a short period of observation, it may be necessary to give protamine sulfate intravenously to neutralize the coagulation defect. Only the smallest effective quantity of the drug should be used, since an excess may actually bring on an increased state of coagulability in the blood. The amount depends on how much time has elapsed since the last injection of heparin. If it is found necessary to give protamine sulfate immediately after administration of heparin, 1.0 to 1.5 mg will be needed for every 100 units of the anticoagulant injected; if 30 min has passed, then only 0.5 mg will be required to neutralize 100 units of heparin.

In general, heparin should not be given to patients in whom any one of the following states or situations exists: ascorbic acid deficiency, capillary fragility, a hemorrhagic diathesis, severe hypertension, cerebrovascular hemorrhage, bacterial endocarditis, recent surgical procedures on the brain and spinal cord, and obstructive jaundice and severe liver disease. Caution should be used when administering the drug to patients with extensive denudation of the skin, ulcerative lesions of the gastrointestinal and genitourinary tracts, drainage tubes in operative wounds, and tubes in the renal pelvis or the common bile duct. Special care must be taken if heparin is to be given following prostatectomy if the indwelling catheter is still in place or the urine continues to be bloody. The drug should be used with caution during pregnancy and in the immediate postpartum period. However, it does not appear to pass the placental barrier and hence provides no undue risk to the fetus. A complication of heparin which may appear in orthopedic patients with joint pathology is bleeding into or around the joint space. (For the effect of protracted heparin therapy on bone healing and on the production of osteoporosis, see C-1, Chapter 23.)

The question of whether the patient with phlebothrombosis should receive an oral anticoagulant together with heparin while in the hospital, in preparation for an outpatient regimen of a coumarin, has not been fully resolved. Some investigators hold the opinion that if signs or symptoms of activity in the calf muscles still persist shortly before discharge from the hospital is being contemplated, then Coumadin or dicumarol should be given during the last week of hospitalization while the patient is still on heparin and then the coumarin should be continued at home for the next several months. On the other hand, if at the time of discharge the process in the calf shows signs of complete subsidence, there does not appear to be an adequate basis for the introduction of an oral anticoagulant unless significant signs and symptoms of chronic pulmonary or cardiac disease coexist.

2. Treatment of Iliofemoral and Popliteal Thrombophlebitis

Preliminary medical measures. The first therapeutic approach to iliofemoral and popliteal thrombophlebitis is an attempt to reduce ve-

nous stasis by placing the patient at bed rest with no bathroom privileges and elevating the foot of the bed 12.5 to 15.5 cm (5 to 7 in.). Care should be taken to maintain the involved limb extended rather than flexed at the knee, in order to facilitate venous return through the popliteal space. At the same time, acute flexion of the hip should be avoided.

Removal of vasospasm should be accomplished by the application of local heat using a thermostatically controlled cradle, provided of course, that a normal arterial circulation exists in the lower limbs. The affected extremity is wrapped in large moist towels from the groin to the toes and the surrounding temperature is maintained around 35° C (95° F). Not only does this procedure inhibit excessive sympathetic tone, but it also tends to counteract the associated periphlebitis. It is generally utilized for at least the first week (during which period the pain and swelling are most marked).

Anticoagulation program. Of paramount importance is the institution of anticoagulant therapy as soon as the patient is placed at complete bed rest, so as to inhibit propagation of the thrombus proximally into the mouths of large tributaries and distally into main channels in the thigh and leg. Since an immediate effect is desired, heparin is given intravenously in a manner already described (see C-1, above). At the same time, a slow-acting oral anticoagulant, like Coumadin or dicumarol, is administered. The combined medication is generally continued for 5 or 6 days, until the prothrombin activity is reduced to a therapeutic level (a prothrombin time which is double the control reading). At this point, heparin is discontinued and the patient is maintained on Coumadin or dicumarol for the remaining period of hospitalization. On discharge, the slow-acting anticoagulant is stopped.

It is necessary to point out that during the period that both heparin and a coumarin are being given, blood for a prothrombin time determination should be drawn just before the next intermittent intravenous injection of heparin, at a time when the concentration of the latter in the body is the lowest. Otherwise, any significant amount of this drug in the bloodstream may raise the readings and thus mislead the physician in his attempt to control the oral anticoagulant. If heparin is being administered continuously in an intravenous drip, it is much more difficult to obtain prothrombin times that are of value.

In case bleeding is noted with oral anticoagulant therapy, either from an operative site or from other parts of the body, the medication is immediately discontinued, and blood loss and prothrombin times are monitored. If the readings indicate that the state of coagulability of the blood is returning to normal, no further measures are taken. On the other hand, if the bleeding persists and the prothrombin times remain high or even increase, then phytonadione, a synthetic vitamin K analogue, is given intramuscularly (Konakion; Mephyton) or intravenously (Aquamephyton) in doses of 2.5 to 10.0 mg or more. The coagulant effect of the drug can be expected in 1 to 2 h after administration, in the form of an improvement in the prothrombin time.

Although the list of absolute and relative contraindications to the use of heparin (see C-1, above) applies in general to oral anticoagulants as well, it is also necessary to consider the possibility of renal insufficiency since coumarins are excreted by the kidneys. Hence, a reduction in kidney function may result in a rapid rise in concentration of the drugs in the bloodstream and the appearance of bleeding. In patients with right heart failure and hepatic congestion or hepatitis, the reaction to the usual dosage of an oral anticoagulant may be intensified, sometimes to the extent of inducing a dangerous degree of prothrombinopenia. The coumarins, in contrast to heparin, are contraindicated during pregnancy since they pass through the placental barrier and may cause a bleeding tendency in the fetus, a complication which may be responsible for cerebral hemorrhage during delivery. Moreover, there is some evidence that the coumarins may cause fetal malformations, particularly of the facial bones and other osseous sites.

Also of importance in the administration of oral coumarins is the fact that other drugs interact with them, either by causing potentiation of their action or by having an inhibiting influence. In the first group fall the antiplatelet medications or those which interfere with or antagonize the action of vitamin K, such as aspirin and salicylates. Among those that enhance the effectiveness of oral anticoagulants are phenylbutazone (Butazolidin), Chloramphenicol (chloromycetin), tetracycline, neomycin, sulfisoxazole (Gantrisin), quinine and quinidine, clofibrate (Atromid-S), anabolic steroids, oxyphenbutazone (Tandearil), diazoxide (Hyperstat), allopurinol (Zyloprim), methylphenidate hydrochloride (Ritalin), indomethacin (Indocin), chloral hydrate, and phenytoin sodium (Dilantin). Barbiturates, corticosteroids, oral contraceptives, glutethimide (Doriden), ethchlorvynol (Placidyl), meprobamate (Miltown), griseofulvin, and cholestyramine (Questran) all antagonize or inhibit the action of the coumarins. It is apparent that if the patient is receiving any of these drugs, their effect must be taken into consideration when initiating an anticoagulation program.

Use of fibrinolytic agents. Now that streptokinase (Streptase) and urokinase (Abbokinase) have become available commercially in adequate quantities (see E-3, Chapter 19), there is a better opportunity for a true evaluation of their therapeutic effects in deep venous thrombosis of the lower limbs. It has been claimed that in the case of recent major thrombotic occlusions (less than 3 to 4 days old), the clot will be completely or partially lysed by fibrinolytic drugs, with rapid subsidence of edema and tenderness in the groin and along the course of the affected vessels. Although by no means proved, the evidence suggests that early dissolution of the clot preserves valvular function and avoids the postphlebitic syndrome. The fact that they are very costly (especially urokinase) and that a high incidence of hemorrhage (see E-3, Chapter 19) is associated with their administration detracts significantly from their value as a conventional therapeutic approach to popliteal and iliofemoral thrombophlebitis.

Therapy for phlegmasia cerulea dolens. To prevent the appearance of nutritional disturbances in this state, more heroic therapeutic measures may be necessary. One of these is immediate thrombectomy (see below) to counteract the existing very high venous pressure. Also early administration of fibrinolytic drugs (see above and E-3, Chapter 19) has been advised in the hope that the lysing effect on the extensive thrombotic process will help reduce the existing venous pressure and reestablish venous return.

Therapy for suppurative iliofemoral thrombophlebitis. In the presence of an infected thrombus, measures must be taken at once to prevent liberation of septic material into the bloodstream so as to arrest the development of fatal pulmonary embolism. The first step is to obtain cultures of the blood collected at 10-min intervals and to carry out sensitivity studies on the bacterial growth, so as to be able to administer appropriate antibacterial agents. Until such information is available, the patient is given massive doses of a wide-spectrum antibiotic. After 24 h of intensive therapy with the proper antibacterial agent, his condition is reevaluated. If it is definitely improved, then the same regimen is continued. If not, the possibility of ligation of the inferior vena cava (see E-4, Chapter 19) should be seriously considered, together with maintenance of the antibacterial therapy.

Surgical approach. Currently there is considerable controversy regarding the value of surgical procedures in the management of the early stage of nonsuppurative iliofemoral thrombophlebitis. Although it is generally agreed that the treatment of choice is a medical program including anticoagulant therapy, several operations have been advocated as alternative or ancillary therapeutic approaches.

Among the surgical measures that have received clinical trial is thrombectomy. This involves the removal of a thrombus from the iliofemoral vein, followed by the administration of heparin. The goal is to preserve the venous valves located in the segment of occlusion and prevent ambulatory venous hypertension and disabling sequelae associated with the postphlebitic syndrome (see Section B, Chapter 20).

The success of the operation appears to be directly related to the interval between the onset of the thrombotic process, as determined clinically, and the extraction of the clot. If this is longer than 6 days, no benefit can be expected from thrombectomy, since a fresh thrombus will almost inevitably develop on the original site of obstruction. Another contraindication to the procedure is the presence of visceral carcinoma. Also it should not be performed in patients who are not candidates for postoperative anticoagulants or who will not be able to become ambulatory after a proper period of bed rest. Signs of prior venous thrombosis noted at the time of surgery are an indication for terminating the procedure without attempting to remove the thrombus.

For the most part, thrombectomy should only be considered for patients with clinical manifestations of extensive thrombosis of the deep venous system, as in the case of phlegmasia cerulea dolens (see above), in which even minimal improvement in venous outflow might help prevent venous gangrene and thus preserve the viability of the limb. In the usual type of iliofemoral thrombophlebitis, such a procedure is not indicated because in most instances the early institution of appropriate medical therapy (see above) will be sufficient to prevent the appearance of the postphlebitic syndrome.

Venous thrombectomy is not without dangerous complications. The incidence of pulmonary embolism following the procedure is reported to be about 3 percent. Because of such a possibility, the insertion of a serrated clip into the inferior vena cava through an abdominal approach has been proposed as a supplemental step to thrombectomy [12]. Other disadvantages may be a considerable loss of blood during the operation and wound infection in a relatively large number of patients [6]. Most important in the evaluation of the procedure are venographic studies indicating that early rethrombosis and later recanalization with destruction of valvular function still occurred in almost all patients so treated [2,5]. However, another investigation reports that excellent long-term results were obtained in 82 percent of the patients and satisfactory ones in 14 percent, the authors concluding that thrombectomy is an efficient treatment of iliofemoral thrombophlebitis [7].

Ambulation program. With the disappearance of all edema and subsidence of all signs of active inflammation (fall of sedimentation rate, white blood cell count, and temperature to normal and absence of tenderness in the groin and along the inner aspect of the thigh), the patient is placed on a routine of exercises in bed, preparatory to ambulation. First he is encouraged to move his toes, provided this step does not cause too much discomfort, and then the degree of physical activity is gradually increased during the period of bed rest.

Before the ambulation program is begun, the patient is measured for an elastic stocking with a built-in gradient of pressure, which extends up to the midthigh and is held in place with a garter belt. Since the garment takes approximately a week to fabricate, in the interval an elastic bandage is substituted. The ambulation program consists of 15-min periods of walking, at the start of each of which measurements of the limb are made at several levels before the bandage is applied. After termination of the exercise, the patient is returned to bed and another set of readings is obtained. If the results are the same as the control figures, then the 15-min periods of walking are gradually increased in number during the day, with no standing or sitting being permitted. If there are no signs of return of edema on such a program, the patient is ready for discharge from the hospital. With proper early treatment, a week of ambulation is an adequate testing period. At home, the patient is instructed to follow carefully the regimen outlined in Table 18.1 and in Section A, Chapter 20.

Table 18.1. General Home Care Directions for Patients Who Have Recovered from a Clot in a Main Vein.

1. Since the acute attack in the main veins has subsided, you are now allowed to be up and around, with gradual return to normal activity. A daily schedule of noncontact light athletics, especially swimming, is advisable.
2. You may soon notice that there is some return of swelling in your leg, particularly around the ankle, at the end of the day. This is no cause for alarm, but still it must be controlled by carefully following the directions listed below.
3. You must apply the elastic stocking, which was made to your order while you were in the hospital, before you get out of bed in the morning. In order to be able to do this, you will have to keep the stocking near at hand and you must take your shower or bath the night before. You must wear the stocking during the entire day, only taking it off when you retire. A new one should be ordered when the one you have becomes worn or loose. It is best to have two stockings, so that the one you have worn can be washed each evening.
4. At all times you should sleep with the foot of the bed elevated 6 in. by raising both feet of the bed on the appropriate thickness of books, blocks, or bricks. Placing your legs and feet on pillows or raising the end of the mattress is not an acceptable substitute.
5. During the course of the day, elevate your lower limbs whenever possible. If a bed or couch is not available, lie on the floor and place your lower limbs on the back of a chair which has been turned over so that the back forms a 45° angle with the floor. Don't sit with the legs hanging down for any period of time and try to stand as little as possible. Walking is preferable to all positions except lying down with the legs elevated.
6. On long train, plane, or automobile rides, it is essential for you to walk around for at least 5 minutes every hour.
7. Avoid exposure of the involved limb to strong sunlight. Don't wear any tight or constricting garment, socks which contain elastic tops, or circular garters on the legs, since they may interfere with the movement of blood out of the limb.
8. Avoid constipation and control your weight.
9. Try to keep the skin of the leg in healthy condition and avoid injury through cutting, bruising, or scratching it. If the skin is dry and scaly, apply a lotion containing lanolin to it daily. However, do not apply the cream on or between the toes. Avoid athlete's foot by always wearing shoes or slippers in the house, carefully drying and powdering between toes after a bath or shower, and changing socks or stockings daily. Use one of the common fungicidal powders for application between toes, especially after using a public shower.
10. See your physician if the swelling does not disappear or becomes greater or if you have injured or broken the skin on the leg or foot.
11. Finally, if the swelling is no longer present, see your physician before discarding the elastic stocking.

If, at the beginning of the ambulation program, there is a return of swelling on walking for 15-min intervals, it can be assumed that a longer period of bed rest is necessary to allow for the formation of a more efficient collateral circulation. The only way to determine when the latter state has been reached is to expose the patient to trial periods of ambulation, followed each time by measurement of several circumferences of the limbs to ascertain when swelling no longer occurs.

3. Treatment of Primary Thrombosis of Axillary and Subclavian Veins

Active therapy for primary thrombosis of the axillary and subclavian veins is, for the most part, nonspecific: bed rest, elevation of the upper limb on pillows or by means of a sling suspended from a Balkan frame, and the application of warm, moist dressings. At the same time, the patient should be encouraged to move his fingers to promote movement of lymph and blood out of the limb; such a measure also improves local arterial circulation and reduces the possibility of propagation of the thrombus into other segments and tributaries of the axillary and subclavian veins. On occasion, operative removal of the clot or bypass of the obstruction has been utilized.

The question of whether anticoagulants should be given has not fully been resolved. However, since cases of pulmonary embolism have been reported following thrombosis of the axillary and subclavian veins [11], it would appear advisable, on general principles, to give heparin and Coumadin at least during the acute stage and then discontinue heparin after several days and the oral anticoagulant on discharge from the hospital.

With loss of swelling of the limb, the patient then becomes ambulatory. He is instructed to use the involved arm in a normal fashion during the course of daily activities but to avoid excess strain. At first, the limb is placed in a sling, and a fabricated elastic sleeve is worn to prevent the reaccumulation of edema. After a week

of ambulation, the patient is discharged from the hospital. It is important to emphasize to him that at no time should he permit the veins in the involved limb to be used for the introduction into the body of any sclerosing or irritating solutions like contrast media. In some patients, despite adequate early therapy, such sequelae as swelling, prominent superficial veins, and easy fatigability of the involved limb may persist.

References

1. Anlyan WG, Hart D: Special problems in venous thromboembolism. Ann Surg 146:499, 1957
2. Barner HB, Willman VL, Kaiser GC, et al: Thrombectomy for iliofemoral venous thrombosis. JAMA 208:2442, 1969
3. Coon WW, Willis PW III: Thrombosis of axillary and subclavian veins. Arch Surg 94:657, 1967
4. Fahrni WH: Tennis leg. Can J Surg 7:157, 1964
5. Karp RB, Wylie EJ: Recurrent thrombosis after iliofemoral venous thrombectomy. Surg Forum 17:147, 1966
6. Lansing AM, Davis WM: Five-year follow-up study of iliofemoral venous thrombectomy. Ann Surg 168:620, 1968
7. Lindhagen J, Haglund M, Haglund U, et al: Iliofemoral venous thrombectomy. J. Cardiovasc Surg 19:319, 1978
8. Munster AM: Septic thrombophlebitis: A surgical disorder. JAMA 230:1010, 1974
9. Schechter DC, Waddell WR, Coppinger WR: Muscle hernia: Twenty personal observations. Am Surg 29:483, 1963
10. Schmidt MC, Workman JB, Barth WF: Dissection or rupture of popliteal cyst: A syndrome mimicking thrombophlebitis in rheumatic diseases. Arch Intern Med 134:694, 1974
11. Swinton NW Jr, Edgett JW Jr, Hall RJ: Primary subclavian-axillary vein thrombosis. Circulation 38:737, 1968
12. Van de Berg L: Venous thrombectomies and partial interruption of the vena cava in 125 cases of thrombophlebitis. J Cardiovasc Surg 19:143, 1978
13. Wright IS: Neurovascular syndrome produced by hyperabduction of the arm. Am Heart J 29:1, 1945

Chapter 19

Vascular Complications of Musculoskeletal Disorders Produced by Trauma

Part 5 Pulmonary Embolism with or without Pulmonary Infarction

A. General Considerations

1. Incidence

Despite the progress which has been made in recent years in the prevention and treatment of pulmonary embolism, this condition continues to be a major, potentially fatal complication of a large number of states and disorders. Therefore, as in the case of deep venous thrombosis, it is imperative at all times to be aware of such a possibility, so as to be able to identify its early presence. This is particularly true in the case of patients prone to intravascular clotting, such as the elderly and those undergoing orthopedic or gynecologic surgery or suffering from cardiac conditions or malignant neoplasms.

In support of the above is the observation (based on a screening procedure using the radioactive fibrinogen test) that more than one-third of patients with myocardial infarction, more than half of those with cerebrovascular accidents, and almost one-third of general surgery patients can be expected to harbor thrombi in the deep veins of the lower limbs, a situation conducive to liberation of clots into the venous circulation with subsequent occlusion of branches of the pulmonary artery. Pul-

monary embolism is also a significant cause of morbidity and mortality in burn patients, being present to the extent of 29 percent of all persons admitted to a burn unit of a hospital; moreover, it may be responsible for death in such individuals in 43 percent of cases [2]. This condition has likewise been found in 49 to 60 percent of people dying after fracture of the femur or tibia; in 27 percent of those succumbing after a fracture of the pelvis; and in 14 percent, after fracture of the spine [11].

2. Pathogenesis

Since the pulmonary bed is located at the termination of the venous circulation, it acts as a natural filter for particulate matter in the bloodstream which is larger than the formed elements. Although there are many opportunities for venous clots to form during a lifetime, most that do are evidently small and hence are handled by the fibrinolytic system located in the lungs; as a result, they produce no clinical manifestations. When venous thrombi occlude the larger vessels or when great numbers of small ones obstruct minor branches of the pulmonary artery, then their presence is recognized by the symptoms and signs they elicit. But even under such conditions, they are responsible for obvious clinical changes only if a significant segment of the pulmonary vascular tree is already compromised.

The fact that small pulmonary arteries can become obstructed with the production of a minimum of symptoms is due to the great reserve possessed by the pulmonary circulation, namely, the ready distensibility of the small vessels and the presence of large numbers of bronchial-pulmonary arterial vascular anastomoses which, although ordinarily not functioning, can quickly respond when needed. Through the latter, blood can pass from gradually enlarging bronchial arteries into the pulmonary circulation distal to the obstruction.

Reflex vasoconstriction of unaffected pulmonary arteries contributes to the seriousness of pulmonary embolism. In fact, if the vasospasm is marked, it may cause death, even in the face of occlusion of vessels which are not of major importance.

3. Source of Emboli

Most of the emboli responsible for pulmonary embolism form in the deep venous system of the lower limbs. Although generally originating in the venous plexuses in the muscles of the calf and, less often, of the foot, they frequently develop into clinically important clots only when they propagate into the venae comitantes of the posterior and anterior tibial arteries and the main collecting channels (popliteal and superficial femoral veins), but not necessarily occluding them. There is also good anatomic evidence that the femoral vein itself may be the primary seat of thrombosis in a high percentage of cases. Other sites from which emboli may arise are pelvic, prostatic, and, occasionally, axillary and subclavian veins and the right atrium and right ventricle. On dislodgment from their source, the thrombi are liberated into the bloodstream, to be transported to the pulmonary arterial bed where they obstruct orifices of vessels having a smaller diameter.

4. Pathology

The morphologic changes depend upon the size of the vessel or vessels occluded and the state of the secondary vascular tree in the lungs. In the case of obstruction of blood flow through the pulmonary artery or its main branches (Fig. 19.1), the resulting alteration in pulmonary artery dynamics may be so marked that the patient will not survive long enough to permit infarction of lung tissue. Also, if the emboli are multiple but minute, occluding only terminal pulmonary arteries, the lung parenchyma may show very few pathologic changes. Even in the case of obstruction of major vessels, pulmonary infarcts are observed in only about 10 percent of patients

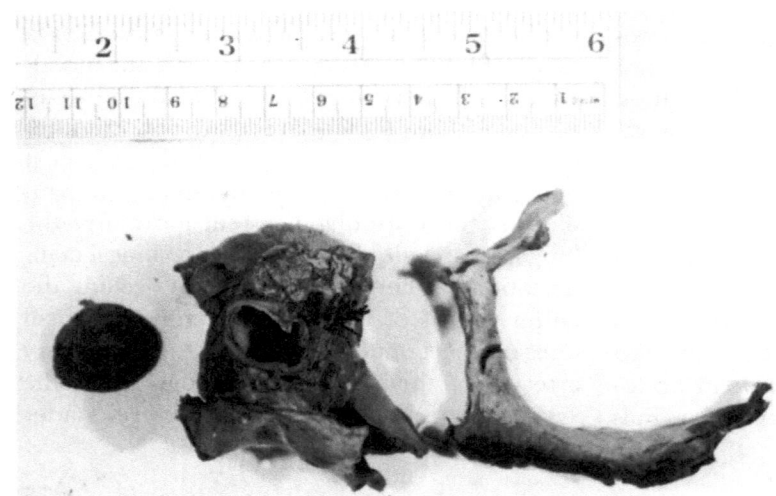

Fig. 19.1. Fragment of clots removed from main pulmonary arteries at autopsy.

[13,14]. Such lesions generally occur if there is obstruction of the smaller muscular arterial segments, particularly in sites where two or more pleural surfaces are in contact.

The relatively low incidence of pulmonary infarcts can probably be attributed to the fact that lung tissues receive blood supply from bronchial, as well as from pulmonary, arteries, and, in the presence of previously normal lung parenchyma, the circulation from the former is generally adequate by itself to take care of the metabolic needs of the structures (see A-2, above) and thus prevent necrosis from developing. However, if there is a preexisting compromised collateral circulation to the lungs or a high bronchial venous pressure, then a superimposed occlusion of a critical pulmonary artery by an embolus may result in death of lung parenchyma.

Pulmonary infarcts may vary in diameter from 0.3 to 10.0 cm and are usually multiple; most of them are located in the lower lobes, especially in the costophrenic angles. Histologically, in the early stage, marked congestion of capillaries is noted and the alveolar spaces are filled with red blood cells and debris. On about the third day, the alveolar wall becomes necrotic and there is a breakdown of the free red blood cells. During the second week after the acute episode, organization occurs. If the extent of the original injury is minimal, in some instances the whole process may be terminated by resolution within 4 days from the onset of the acute infarction.

B. Clinical Manifestations

Not infrequently there is a poor correlation between the severity of the symptoms and signs of pulmonary embolism, on the one hand, and the size of the emboli and of the vessels they occlude, on the other. This is due to the great reserve capacity of normal lung, with the result that if less than half the vascular bed is obstructed, the clinical manifestations may still be minimal, provided there is no previous underlying pulmonary disease. Greater interference with pulmonary blood flow generally produces severe insufficiency, which, in turn, is responsible for the development of symptoms and signs. Another factor which may blur

the clinical picture is the degree of effectiveness of the fibrinolytic system in the lungs themselves in lysing small pulmonary emboli. For all these reasons, pulmonary embolism is frequently not recognized on the basis of presenting signs and symptoms alone, and hence heavy reliance is placed on laboratory aids (see below) for its detection.[1]

Nonmassive pulmonary embolism. Early findings in this state are dyspnea (in about 80 percent of cases); tachypnea; a dry, nonproductive cough; and rales at the bases, together with accentuation and transient splitting of the pulmonary second sound. Other less common signs and symptoms are apprehension, pleural pain (in about 50 to 60 percent of cases), sweating, tachycardia, gallop rhythm, dizziness, and syncope. Hemoptysis, regarded as a constant finding in the past, actually is relatively infrequent (in 27 percent or less of patients with clinical embolism). Because of the associated reflex bronchoconstriction, audible wheezing may occur over the affected area. A low-grade fever and a moderate increase in leukocytes and sedimentation rate are usually present early in the disorder. Cyanosis is not a common finding in nonmassive pulmonary embolism, although oxygen desaturation is noted in most patients (see below).

Massive pulmonary embolism. If a main branch of the pulmonary artery or this vessel itself is occluded by a nonseptic embolus, the clinical picture is very dramatic. The patient frequently presents with anxious facies and apprehension of a degree greater than would be expected on the basis of objective signs. However, very quickly thereafter the symptoms and physical findings become very marked in the form of labored breathing and air hunger, cyanosis, severe substernal pain, tachycardia, a rapidly falling blood pressure to a shock level, and a corresponding rise in jugular venous pressure. Pulmonary edema may also develop. If heroic medical or surgical therapy is not effective in reestablishing blood flow in the pulmonary arterial bed, death may ensue.

---

[1] In patients not in shock it appears advisable to attempt venography, for if the deep venous system in the lower limbs is entirely normal, pulmonary embolism is unlikely to be the cause for the clinical manifestations.

If the patient survives the initial stage of the disorder, fever, cough, and localized pleuritic chest pain may appear. In about 20 percent of cases there is hemoptysis which persists for 2 to 3 weeks. Signs of right heart failure may be present, manifested by epigastric discomfort from liver engorgement and a high central venous pressure.

Pulmonary infarction. When the area deprived of pulmonary blood flow is large and the bronchial circulation is insufficient to maintain viability of lung parenchyma, then the findings of pulmonary infarction will become apparent. These consist of knifelike pleuritic chest pain, which calls forth chest splinting and restriction of breathing, associated with hemoptysis.

Multiple small pulmonary emboli. Even more difficult to detect than sudden occlusion of a moderate-sized pulmonary artery by an embolus are the multiple showers of small clots that occur repeatedly over months and years without clear-cut evidence of pulmonary embolism. Generally, only after right ventricular overload and pulmonary hypertension become apparent is this possibility given serious consideration. In the past, patients with these findings were thought to have primary pulmonary hypertension, but pathologic examination of the lungs of such individuals has led to the conclusion that the clinical picture is due to multiple pulmonary emboli developed over extended periods.

C. Laboratory Aids

1. Chest Roentgenography

Changes in the chest x ray are helpful but not always reliable diagnostic signs of pulmonary embolism; in fact, at times the film may be normal, or radiolucency rather than opacity may result from the occlusion of a branch of the pulmonary artery. Highly suggestive but infrequently present are prominent pulmonary arteries and a localized reduction or lack of vascular markings in the area of the lesion, in conjunction with radiolucency in the same site. Other, nonspecific abnormalities are infiltrates, elevation of the diaphragm, and pleural effusion. Fleischner lines, which are atelectatic streaks distal to the sites of small bronchial obstructions, may be found reaching to the pleural surface but rarely to the hilus and never crossing an interlobar fissure. In the absence of other conditions causing small bronchial obstruction (pneumonia, asthma, chronic bronchial disease), such abnormalities should arouse suspicion of pulmonary emboli. If pulmonary infarction is present, chest radiography may disclose the area of involvement as a truncated cone whose apex is directed toward the hilus and whose base is on a pleural surface [12]. More frequently, only a transient abnormality is seen on the roentgenogram, perhaps evidence of "incomplete infarction."

2. Electrocardiography

The changes in the electrocardiogram observed in pulmonary embolism are not specific, and at times the record may even be normal. Most often only sinus tachycardia and nonspecific T-wave and S-T–segment changes are the only findings. Infrequently noted, but highly suggestive of the diagnosis, are inverted TV_1-V_4; transient, incomplete right bundle branch block; right ventricular hypertrophy; transient S_1, Q_3, or S_1, S_2, S_3; and tall and peaked P waves in leads II, III, and a VF. More commonly, such nonspecific changes as premature contractions, left axis deviation, and low QRS voltage in the limb leads are present.

3. Radioisotopic Pulmonary Perfusion Scanning

Basis for test. Pulmonary perfusion scanning, a widely used and sensitive method, is based on the principle that when macroaggregated human albumin particles (10 to 50 μm in diameter), tagged with either ^{131}I or ^{99m}Tc, are injected into a peripheral vein, they will temporarily be trapped in the capillary bed of the lungs, thus reflecting the distribution of the blood from the right side of the heart in the pulmonary parenchyma. With an external scintillation counter applied immediately after injection, the resulting perfusion pattern can be detected. The procedure is easily performed and is completed within about 15 min. After approximately 90 to 120 min, the particles in the lungs are broken down to molecular albumin, which now is capable of passing through the pulmonary capillaries into the systemic circulation. The material is then metabolized by the reticuloendothelial system, mainly in the liver and spleen. The previously attached isotope is rapidly excreted by the kidneys, but in the case of ^{131}I, this occurs only if the thyroid gland is protected by a preliminary dose of iodides.

In sites in which blood flow is impeded, accumulation of radioactive material does not take place, a finding which is demonstrated on the scan as areas of absent perfusion (Fig. 19.2). The abnormal changes are generally found along the lateral and basal portions of the lung fields, appearing as crescent-shaped defects (Fig. 19.2B). To derive the greatest benefit from the test, lung perfusion should include a posterior oblique and two lateral views, as well as an anterior view.

Adverse reactions. In the presence of severe underlying vascular disease of the pulmonary arterial bed, circulatory difficulties may follow the transient occlusion of the pulmonary capillaries by the large albumin particles. Otherwise, the possibility of developing a reaction to the injected material is slim, since the particles are in such relatively small numbers that only 1 of every 250,000 pulmonary arterioles is temporarily blockaded [12]. The incidence of radiation hazards is also very low.

Application of method. Since the test is generally safe to carry out and thus can be frequently repeated, it allows for improved diagnostic accuracy and better evaluation of therapeutic procedures. Moreover, it is suitable for screening of large numbers of potential candidates for deep venous thrombosis. In fact, it has been suggested that the test should routinely be performed preoperatively in high-risk surgical patients, particularly those undergoing arthroplasty or pelvic operations, so as to have available a base line study in the event of subsequent appearance of symptoms in the chest. A very important advantage of the method is that the changes in the scan closely reflect the abnormalities occurring in the lung parenchyma, so that repeated testing at intervals of 5 to 7 days

may frequently demonstrate dramatic alterations or at times a normal pattern in areas of previously absent perfusion (Fig. 19.2C). The latter type of response may be observed even after only 30 percent of the luminal diameter of the involved vessel is restored. Since false-negative photoscanning in pulmonary embolism is extremely rare, a completely normal result obtained early in the inception of the condition with a technically adequate test practically rules out such a clinical diagnosis. Of course, emboli not large enough to cause a perfusion defect could still be present, but, at the same time, these would not produce any significant clinical problems. The main contribution of pulmonary perfusion scanning is that it provides information regarding the state of terminal arteries, arterioles, and capillaries of the pulmonary vascular bed.

Limitations of method. It is necessary to point out that reduced vascularity in the lungs, as determined by perfusion photoscanning, is not specific for pulmonary embolism. Similar changes may be found in some cardiac states and in a number of pulmonary conditions, such as pneumothorax, bulla, atelectasis, asthma, bronchitis, a patch of pneumonia, pleurisy, and a lung tumor. Hence, to exclude false-positive interpretations, the results of the scan may have to be correlated with data obtained with other tests, including standard x-ray examination, lung ventilation scanning, pulmonary angiography, serum enzymes, and arterial oxygen tension, all described below. The gallium-67 lung scan is a useful noninvasive adjunctive aid in diagnosing a suspected pulmonary embolism in the presence of a pulmonary infiltrate, since in this test, radioactivity concentrates in areas of inflammation and not it sites of uncomplicated embolization. Also, to distinguish emboli from pneumonitis, isoproterenol hydrochloride (parenteral Isuprel) can be used to reverse the vasoconstriction that causes the perfusion defect in the latter.

4. Lung Ventilation Scanning (Ventilation-Perfusion Lung Scanning)

In order to differentiate perfusion scanning defects produced by pulmonary embolism from

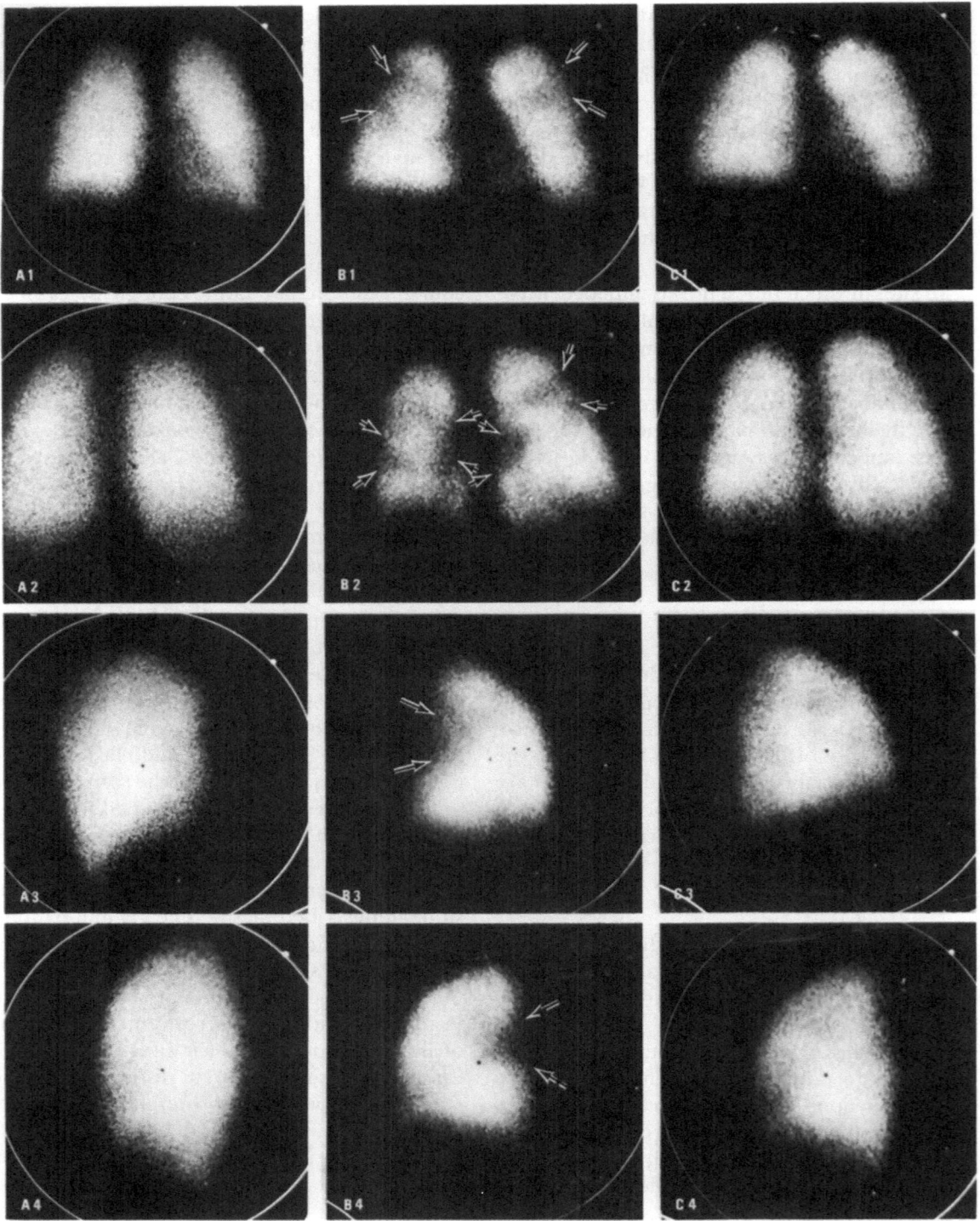

Fig. 19.2. Radioisotopic pulmonary perfusion (lung) scanning. **A** Perfusion pattern in a normal subject. *A1,* Anterior view. Area of reduced perfusion in lower portion of left lung is a normal finding, being due to compression of parenchyma by the heart. *A2,* Posterior view; *A3,* right lateral view; *A4,* left lateral view. **B** Scan of a patient with multiple pulmonary emboli, their location being indicated by arrows. *B1,* Anterior view. Areas of reduced perfusion in upper portion of right and left lungs. *B2,* Posterior view. Areas of reduced perfusion noted in both lung fields. *B3,* Right lateral view. Area of absent or reduced

those associated with other types of lung pathology (generally of a chronic type), it may be necessary to perform lung ventilation scanning using radioactive gas (xenon-133 or xenon-127) introduced through a closed system. Ventilation in those areas with perfusion defects due to pulmonary embolism has been shown generally to be normal, whereas in cases in which similar perfusion defects are produced by tumors, pneumonia, and obstructive lung disease, the ventilation scans are abnormal in the same sites. However, it is necessary to point out that in the patient with underlying lung pathology who subsequently develops a pulmonary embolism, there may be defects in both the perfusion scan and in the ventilation scan. Under such conditions, only if the abnormal findings obtained with each test are located in different areas of the lung field would they be of significance in confirming the existence of both disorders. Even then, other diagnostic procedures should be performed in order to establish the presence of pulmonary embolism beyond doubt.

5. Arterial Oxygen Tension

Hypoxemia, as indicated by a low oxygen tension in arterial blood (below 80 mmHg), is a very important diagnostic point in pulmonary embolism; at the same time, however, it is necessary to point out that a similar situation may exist in a large number of other disorders. Another fact to be considered is that although normal P_{O_2} values (greater than 80 mmHg) exclude an extensive involvement, they do not necessarily rule out the presence of pulmonary embolism, since in 10 to 15 percent of patients with this condition the readings remain unchanged. In those individuals demonstrating a low P_{O_2}, the hypoxemia may persist for approximately a week even when appropriate treatment has been instituted. It has been suggested that the mechanism responsible for the reduced oxygen tension in arterial blood is an increased release of smooth-muscle–active substances from the platelets, resulting in pulmonary arteriovenous shunting, bronchoconstriction, and microatelectasis. Typically the change in P_{O_2} is associated with a lowering of the arterial carbon dioxide tension to below 40 mmHg, owing to the alveolar hyperventilation that usually occurs.

6. Enzyme Changes

Abnormalities in the levels of enzymes in the blood are somewhat helpful in the differential diagnosis of pulmonary embolism, particularly if significant infarction is also present, although they are rarely conclusive. In the uncomplicated case, serum lactic dehydrogenase (LDH) activity is generally increased, whereas serum glutamic oxaloacetic transaminase (SGOT) remains unchanged. In about half the cases, serum bilirubin rises during the first few days of the illness. The fact that changes in enzymes can be determined only after several serial readings detracts from their value as an early diagnostic aid. Moreover, the alterations are not always present.

7. Pulmonary Angiography

Technique. With the conventional approach, pulmonary angiography is performed by catheterizing an antecubital vein following a cutdown, and, under fluoroscopic control, passing the catheter tip into the right ventricle; at this point, the contrast medium (Renografin-76) is injected (selective pulmonary angiography).[2] Such a procedure provides detail and definition of the ossified pulmonary vascular tree (Fig. 19.3).

With percutaneous injection of the contrast medium into one of the peripheral veins, a less

[2] Cineangiography, a recently developed type of angiography, is more helpful than conventional angiography when the diagnosis of pulmonary embolism is equivocal.

perfusion along posterior border. *B4,* Left lateral view. Area of absent perfusion noted along posterior border. **C** Lung scans on the same patient as in **B,** performed 2 weeks later. For the most part, the areas of reduced or absent perfusion previously noted are no longer present in all of the views. From Abramson DI: Vascular Disorders of the Extremities, Hagerstown, Md, Harper & Row, 1974. Reproduced with permission.

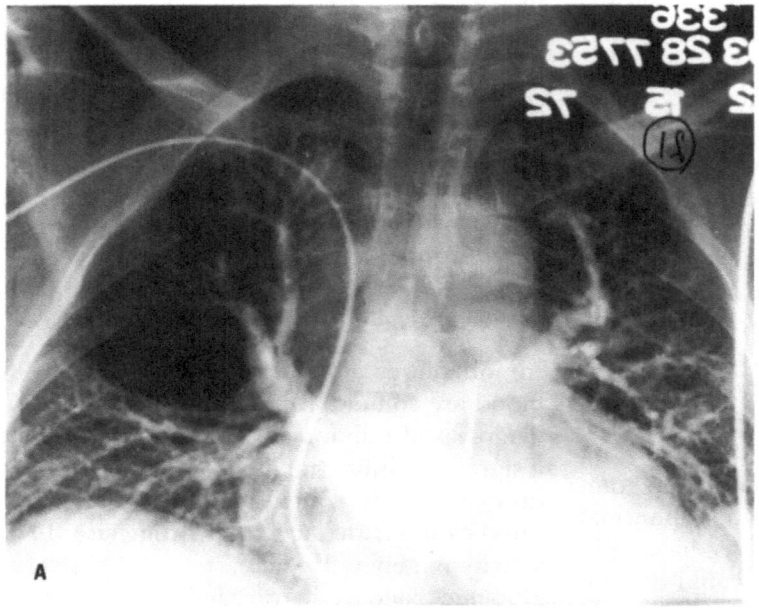

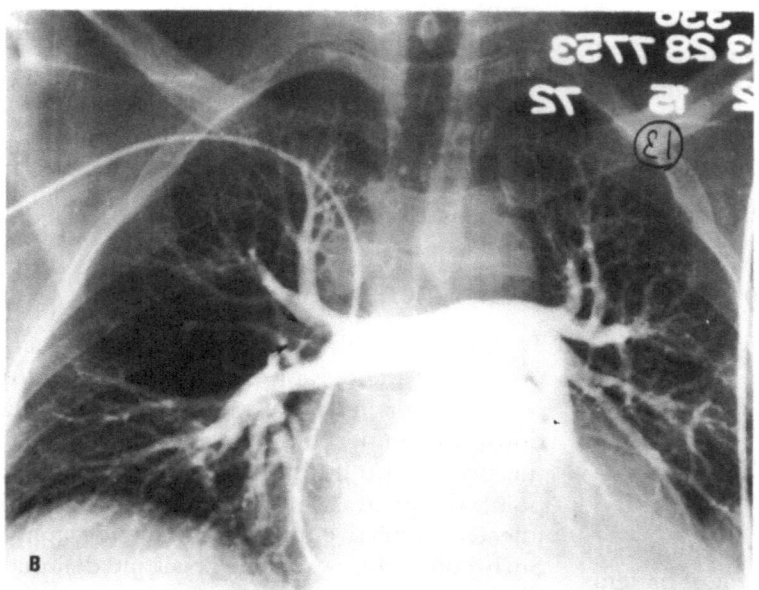

Fig. 19.3. Pulmonary angiograms demonstrating occlusion of a main branch of the right pulmonary artery by an embolus. **A** Only a few visualized vessels are present in the midportion of the right lung field. Normal extensive vascularization is noted in the left lung field. **B** Another film on the same patient demonstrating a partial filling defect (arrows) in the right branch of the pulmonary artery. From Abramson DI: Vascular Disorders of the Extremities, Hagerstown, Md, Harper & Row, 1974. Reproduced with permission.

clear-cut visualization of the pulmonary arterial tree is obtained. However, such an approach can be done expeditiously and with less preparation and manipulation of the patient, which are important points to consider in the case of an acutely ill individual. Moreover, the method obviates venous cutdown, catheterization, and fluoroscopy and reduces the possibility of dislodging thrombi or emboli from the

superior vena cava, the right side of the heart, and the pulmonary artery.

Another means of performing nonselective pulmonary angiography is through the insertion of a catheter into the femoral vein, which is then passed into the right atrium. The procedure is considered to be safer than selective pulmonary angiography. Besides giving information regarding the state of the pulmonary arterial bed, it also allows for evaluation of the inferior vena cava and iliac veins. However, it is important to mention that when unilateral pelvic thrombophlebitis is suspected, the opposite femoral vein should be catheterized. With all procedures, simultaneous electrocardiographic monitoring should be performed in order to detect early onset of arrhythmias.

Interpretation of results. Significant diagnostic findings with pulmonary angiography are intraluminal filling defects in the pulmonary arteries and their branches (Fig. 19.3), abrupt cutoff of the radiopaque stream, and a trailing edge of material. Suggestive findings consist of asymmetric filling, lower-zone delay, and prolonged arterial phase.

Evaluation of procedure. Pulmonary angiography is the method of greatest sensitivity and specificity in the diagnosis of pulmonary embolism, precisely identifying the presence, site, and extent of the lesion (Fig. 19.3). Hence, in the presence of an acute severe impairment of circulatory and respiratory function, possibly requiring pulmonary embolectomy, essential anatomic information is supplied by the procedure. It has also been used when the clinical evidence for pulmonary embolism is unquestionably positive, but the perfusion scan appears to be normal or cannot be interpreted because of parenchymal lung disease. It has likewise been suggested as a preliminary step to the institution of thrombolytic therapy.

However, false-negative interpretations have been reported with the method, especially when small emboli and microemboli are present. For this reason, it is advisable in some instances to combine selective pulmonary angiography with pulmonary perfusion scanning (see above), since the latter is useful in determining the status of the arteriolar and capillary beds—portions of the pulmonary vascular tree not visualized by angiography.

Pulmonary angiography is not without adverse reactions. It should never be used in the patient with a known systemic reaction to contrast media. Relative contraindications are primary pulmonary hypertension, ventricular irritability, and left bundle branch block. Also important to point out is that the technique is difficult to perform properly and is costly,

Moreover, it carries an element of risk for the patient. Complications such as arrhythmias, right ventricular perforation, and transient hypotension have been reported.

8. Pulmonary Function Tests

Because of interference with blood flow through the pulmonary arterial bed and the associated bronchoconstriction during the acute phase of pulmonary embolism, the function of the lungs is altered. This manifests itself in a reduction of the maximal expiratory flow rate and in the 1-s vital capacity. There may also be a diminished total vital capacity and an impaired minute ventilation. However, none of these changes can be considered specific for pulmonary embolism; hence, the alterations are not of value in distinguishing this condition from a number of other disorders.

D. Differential Diagnosis

The clinical manifestations of pulmonary embolism may masquerade as those of several different entities associated with symptoms and signs located in the chest. With the advent of selective pulmonary angiography and other diagnostic methods, there has been some resolution of the problem of differential diagnosis.

1. Myocardial Infarction

In the early stage of massive pulmonary embolism, the complaints and physical findings may be confused with those of acute myocardial infarction. However, the evolution of the typical S-T–segment changes and T-wave alterations in the electrocardiogram in the case of the latter and the presence, for the most part, of only nonspecific changes in pulmonary embolism are important distinguishing points. Also, the physical findings and the radiographic changes in the lungs help in the differential diagnosis. Likewise of significance are the alterations in enzyme studies, as noted below.

As already stated, in pulmonary embolism, the LDH is raised but not the SGOT; in myocardial infarction both are increased. Moreover, the MB isoenzyme of serum creatine phosphokinase (CPK) and the LDH isoenzymes are increased in myocardial infarction, while rarely being affected in uncomplicated pulmonary embolism. Usefulness of the creatine kinase MB determination test, however, is limited by the fact that serum levels of this enzyme return to normal fairly quickly after a myocardial infarction, hampering late diagnosis. Lactic dehydrogenase isoenzyme levels, on the other hand, remain elevated for a longer period of time.

Although in both pulmonary embolism and myocardial infarction there may be severe substernal pain and signs of shock, the evolution of the clinical manifestations is different in the two conditions. In pulmonary embolism there is a sudden onset, whereas in myocardial infarction the complaints appear more gradually, with definite premonitory changes frequently preceding the acute stage by several hours or days. For the most part, chest pain in pulmonary embolism is sharp and pleuritic, with no typical localization, whereas in myocardial infarction, it is pressing or constricting, unrelated to respiration and generally located substernally, with radiation to the shoulders, arms, or neck. Pulmonary symptoms, such as dyspnea and tachypnea, are often intense in pulmonary embolism, whereas in myocardial infarction, they may be mild or even absent. Systemic responses, including fever, moderate leukocytosis, and an increased sedimentation rate, are present early in pulmonary embolism; in myocardial infarction they appear later in the clinical picture.

2. Lobar Pneumonia

Pulmonary embolism with infarction is frequently misdiagnosed as lobar pneumonia, since in both conditions there may be such findings as pleural pain, fever, and physical and x-ray signs of consolidation in the lungs. A history of previous attacks of pulmonary embolism or of deep thrombophlebitis in the lower limbs or the existence of the acute stage of the latter would favor the diagnosis of pulmonary infarction. The early appearance of hemoptysis with blood clots in the sputum is also in accord with this diagnosis; in lobar pneumonia, generally

the sputum becomes rusty in color (without the presence of blood clots) later in the clinical course. Abnormalities in the chest film appear more rapidly in pulmonary embolism with infarction than in pneumonia, with multiple bilateral lesions being common; the latter type of change is generally not noted in lobar pneumonia. With regard to enzyme studies, rarely is there an elevation of LDH in lobar pneumonia, whereas in pulmonary embolism with infarction, such an abnormality is frequently noted. Also, in lobar pneumonia there is a consistently high white blood count (generally above 15,000 per cubic millimeter), whereas in nonsuppurative pulmonary infarction, the leukocytosis rarely goes above 15,000 per cubic millimeter. Finally, by means of the pulmonary perfusion scan, the lung ventilation scan, and the gallium-67 lung scan, the distinction can be made between an area of infiltrate and inflammation and one of uncomplicated embolization and infarction.

3. Atypical Pneumonia

Atypical pneumonia may mimic the clinical picture of showers of small pulmonary emboli. With regard to differentiating one from the other, the physical findings and the radiographic changes are of little help. The history of previous attacks of pulmonary embolism or the presence of thrombi in the deep veins of the lower limbs or of the pelvis before or shortly after the appearance of alterations in the lungs helps confirm the existence of small pulmonary emboli.

4. Pulmonary Artery Thrombosis

Pulmonary artery thrombosis is generally diagnosed at autopsy. It is found in such disorders as pulmonary tuberculosis, carcinoma of the lung, chronic bronchitis, coronary artery disease, and valvular heart disease, among others. Generally the clinical manifestations are insidious in their onset, eventually the picture becoming one of progressive right ventricular failure with low output and increasing dyspnea. Rarely is there a sudden appearance of a severe, shocklike state as seen with a massive pulmonary embolism.

The radiographic evidence may be helpful in the differential diagnosis. In pulmonary artery thrombosis, there is enlargement of the right ventricle, of the pulmonary artery, and of its main branches. On fluoroscopy, the occluded main vessel possesses little motion, and it has an elliptic configuration, tapering abruptly below the point of closure.

5. Miscellaneous Disorders Mimicking Pulmonary Embolism

Certain pulmonary disorders, such as spontaneous pneumothorax, chronic lung disease, and pulmonary atelectasis, must also be considered in the differential diagnosis of pulmonary embolism. As has already been stressed, pulmonary perfusion scans and ventilation scans are useful tests in this regard. Recurrent showers of small pulmonary emboli may be mistaken for asthmatic attacks since they are associated with bronchoconstriction which can produce wheezing. The same is true during the early stage of occlusion of larger pulmonary arteries by emboli. It may therefore be necessary to subject suspected asthmatic patients who have elevated serum LDH values or an abnormal pulmonary scan which persists after wheezing has stopped to further investigation, such as the performance of pulmonary function tests, including the determination of the rate of maximum expiratory flow, 1-s forced expiratory volume, and maximum breathing capacity. Information thus obtained may help make the differentiation between the two disorders.

Other conditions which may mimic pulmonary embolism are acute heart failure, paroxysmal tachycardia, and dissecting aneurysm. Such an intraabdominal disorder as subdiaphragmatic abscess may cause symptoms and signs referred to the chest because of irritation of the diaphragm. Idiopathic pleuritis, usually viral in origin, and costochondritis are the most common causes of pleuritic chest pain and hence must be considered in the differential diagnosis of pulmonary embolism. (For differentiation of pulmonary embolism from fat embolism, see E-4, Chapter 16.)

E. Treatment

1. Introduction

Because the prophylactic therapeutic measures for pulmonary embolism are similar in all regard to those for deep venous thrombosis (see Section C, Chapter 17), this section will deal only with the active treatment of the condition.

Therapy for pulmonary embolism has two aims: (1) management of the acute process, in order to restore pulmonary circulation and reverse the altered hemodynamics resulting from occlusion of a portion of the pulmonary vascular tree; and (2) prevention of recurrent embolic episodes. To achieve such goals, both medical and surgical procedures may be required. Treatment is most important for those patients who survive long enough after the embolic episode for the diagnosis to be made in a hospital environment and who would ordinarily have died in the next 24 to 48 h if therapeutic attempts had not been made to control the condition. Others with less marked involvement also require therapy but would probably have lived without it. Nevertheless, such an approach does decrease morbidity from persisting embolic obstruction of the pulmonary bed. The type of treatment program initially instituted, therefore, depends upon the degree to which the pulmonary arterial circulation is compromised and upon the severity of the resulting generalized hypoxia and shock state.

2. Early Medical Therapy for Nonmassive Pulmonary Embolism

Only the medical approach is indicated for patients with 20 to 50 percent involvement of the pulmonary vascular bed in whom blood pressure returns to a fairly normal level and remains stable after a period of transient collapse. Such individuals generally demonstrate either normal P_{O_2} readings or ones that have fallen to 65 mmHg; P_{CO_2} may be below 30 mmHg. The regimen involves complete bed rest with the foot of the bed elevated and no bathroom privileges, symptomatic control of the various complaints, and steps to counteract the abnormal physical or laboratory findings.

Heparin. This drug has several therapeutic effects which are of value in pulmonary embolism. Besides its action on the clotting mechanism, it is a bronchodilator, probably through its ability to lower the level of smooth-muscle–active substances in the blood by inhibiting the platelet-serotonin release reaction. It also produces vasodilatation [1], which may help combat the local inflammatory response.

During the first 24 h following pulmonary embolism, it is advisable to give a much larger dose of heparin than is used in phlebothrombosis (see C-1, Chapter 18), in part, to counteract the direct bronchoconstrictive effect responsible for wheezing frequently found in the early stage of pulmonary embolism and, in part, to deal with the remarkably short half-life of the drug when administered to patients with this difficulty. Hence, initially, with the intermittent route, 10,000 to 15,000 units of the drug are given every 4 to 6 h during the first day, followed by 5000 to 10,000 units every 4 to 6 h subsequently. In the case of the use of the continuous intravenous drip procedure, equivalent amounts of the drug are permitted to enter the vein daily by regulating the delivery of the pump and the concentration of the heparin in the infusion solution. In order to control the dosage at the beginning, the activated partial thromboplastin time (APTT) test should be performed at 6- to 12-h intervals. Regardless of how the drug is given, the purpose of the therapeutic program is to maintain the APTT of the blood at a level about two times the patient's control reading (average normal range of 40 to 43 s). The administration of heparin is continued until there is no clinical or laboratory evidence of venous thrombosis in the original site of origin of the emboli (usually the lower limbs) or of fresh embolization; this usually requires 5 to 7 days from the time of onset of the condition, during which period the patient still remains at complete bed rest. Then in the following week a course of gradual ambulation is instituted. Several days before discharge from the hospital is contemplated, oral anticoagulants are given in conjunction with heparin, in preparation for continuation of the coumarins on an outpatient basis (see E-4, below).

Adjunctive measures. Another therapeutic step is the administration of oxygen by nasal catheter, which, if feasible, is monitored so that the P_{O_2} is maintained between 60 and 120 mmHg. This will relieve or diminish the symptoms of hypoxemia in many patients. Digitalis, intravenously administered diuretics, and various antiarrhythmic agents should be used in appropriate clinical situations. For severe pleuritic pain or marked apprehension, morphine sulfate given slowly intravenously, 1 mg at a time (up to 5 to 10 mg), may be helpful in controlling the symptoms. Codeine sulfate (30 to 60 mg) may be substituted for lesser pain.

3. Therapy for Massive Pulmonary Embolism

Early medical program. For patients suffering from a massive pulmonary embolism and shock or from submassive pulmonary embolism but with signs of significant cardiopulmonary decompensation, heroic medical measures may, in some instances, control the condition, provided that hospitalization had been carried out within 1 or 2 h after development of the episode. Heparin therapy should be instituted immediately and signs of cardiac failure should be treated with the intravenous administration of isoproterenol hydrochloride (parenteral Isuprel) by drip (2 to 4 mg per 500 ml of 5% dextrose in water). If hypotension persists after such a step, levarterenol bitartrate (Levophed) should be given intravenously (2 to 6 ml of 0.2% concentration in 500 ml of 5% dextrose in water). As an adjunctive measure, positive pressure oxygen administration is utilized to control the hypoxemia.

Fibrinolytic agents. If the clinical picture does not improve significantly with the above program, then one of the fibrinolytic (thrombolytic) drugs, streptokinase or urokinase, is given in an attempt to lyse the thrombus, and heparin is discontinued. The action of these agents is particularly marked on fresh clots, whereas those more than 3 to 5 days old are less likely to be so affected.

Streptokinase, which is a bacterial protein elaborated by group C β-hemolytic streptococci, has received more extensive clinical trial in the past several years because of greater availability in the form of a new commercial product, Streptase, a preparation which is not only more potent but also less pyrogenic than the older ones. Another important consideration is the fact that the medication is much less costly than urokinase, the only other effective fibrinolytic agent on the market.

Streptokinase acts with plasminogen to produce an intermediate specific product, an "activator complex," that in turn converts residual plasminogen into the proteolytic enzyme, plasmin. The latter acts on fibrin, fibrinogen, and other plasma proteins to hydrolyze them [9]. Both plasminogen and streptokinase are adsorbed to the thrombus, where, within a self-contained system, the resulting plasmin lyses the fibrin clot. The action occurs within the thrombus as well as on its surface.

Streptokinase is supplied as a lyophilized white powder for reconstitution and dilution, using normal saline or 5% dextrose solution. The activity of the drug is expressed in International Standard Units (IU) of fibrinolytic activity established by the Committee on Thrombolytic Agents of the National Heart and Lung Institute. They are a measure of the ability of the preparation to cause lysis in vitro of a fibrin clot through the development of the plasmin system. The effect of the medication on coagulability may persist for up to 12 h after its discontinuation.

During their lifetime, most people have developed antibodies to streptococci which are capable of neutralizing an equivalent amount of streptokinase, rendering it unavailable for activation of the lytic system. Hence, it is generally necessary to determine the streptokinase resistance (using the streptokinase resistance test reagent [7]), so as to arrive at the appropriate loading amount of streptokinase that would be sufficient to neutralize this state and still deliver an adequate therapeutic quantity of the drug to the patient. In most instances an initial dose of 250,000 IU in 5% glucose solution, administered intravenously over a 30-min period with an infusion pump, has been found to be effective in satisfying such conditions. This is followed by a maintenance dose of 100,000 IU/h for the next 24 to 72 h, the rate of injection being monitored by the thrombin time, a test based on the fact that fibrin-fibrinogen degradation products inhibit the action of thrombin. With such a regimen, the thrombin time is usually prolonged up to three to six times the normal control (up to 60 to 120 s). If this rate of administration of the drug causes

the thrombin time to become less than twice the control, insufficient protection from new thrombus formation exists [16]. A thrombin time that is greater than six times the normal control rate indicates the presence of hyperplasminemia, a situation which is associated with the risk of bleeding. The most precise values during thrombolytic therapy are obtained by the chemical estimation of fibrinogen, but the procedure is time consuming [16].

After termination of streptokinase administration, it is advisable to reinstitute continuous intravenous infusion of heparin to prevent recurrence of thrombosis. However, first the thrombin time must decrease to less than twice the normal control value. In addition to heparin therapy, oral anticoagulants are given, and when the prothrombin time has risen to two times the normal control value, heparin is discontinued.

Urokinase, the other commercially available fibrinolytic agent, acts on the endogenous fibrinolytic system to convert plasminogin directly to the proteolytic enzyme, plasmin, without the production of any intermediary substance. Plasmin, in turn, degrades fibrin clots, as well as fibrinogen and other plasma proteins [9]. Since plasminogen is present in the clot, activation by urokinase occurs within as well as on its surface. Intravenous injection of urokinase produces a shortening of the euglobulin lysis time, a decrease in plasma levels of fibrinogen and plasminogen, and an increase in the amount of circulating fibrin degradation products.

Urokinase most likely originates in the kidneys and is found in the urine. It is extracted in a relatively pure form from human urine or it is prepared from human kidney cells by tissue culture technique (Abbokinase). The drug is nontoxic and nonantigenic, but it is still very costly to produce and the commercial supply is limited. For the most part, it should be reserved for those patients who are allergic to streptokinase.

Since currently Abbokinase is the only preparation commercially available for clinical use in the United States, the following discussion will deal with the administration of this drug. It is supplied as a sterile lyophilized preparation, with each vial containing 250,000 IU of urokinase activity. The material is kept in a deep freeze until it is reconstituted immediately before it is injected by dissolving it in appropriate amounts of sterile water to make the solution isotonic. Since the drug loses potency by adsorption to glass, the solution is administered using a plastic syringe.

A loading dose of Abbokinase is generally 4400 IU per kg body weight, given over a period of 10 min. This is followed by a continuous infusion of 4400 (IU/kg)/h over the next 12 h, using a constant infusion pump. As in the case of streptokinase, the injection is monitored using the thrombin time. Following termination of urokinase therapy, heparin administration and then oral anticoagulants should be instituted to prevent thrombi from subsequently forming.

Both streptokinase and urokinase interfere with the normal coagulation mechanisms through their digestive action on fibrin, fibrinogen, certain blood factors, and other proteins. Hence, a situation is produced in which bleeding may occur. Because of such a possibility, these drugs should only be administered by physicians with wide experience in the treatment of intravenous thrombosis and in hospitals where laboratory monitoring is adequate and readily available.

There is little question that the fibrinolytic drugs produce a greater incidence of bleeding than occurs with heparin or oral coumarin compounds. Moreover, when this complication does develop, it is more severe and more difficult to manage. For these reasons, streptokinase or urokinase should not be given within 10 to 14 days of surgery or of other diagnostic or therapeutic invasive procedures, such as intramuscular injections of drugs, an arterial or lumbar puncture, or liver and kidney biopsies. Since the decreased fibrinogen level in the blood and the fibrinogen degradation products produced by the fibrinolytic agents may cause dissolution of hemostatic plugs and inhibition of coagulation, the drugs should not be used within 6 months of trauma. They are contraindicated if there is a history of gastrointestinal bleeding, severe hypertension, a hemorrhagic diathesis, intracranial bleeding, or hemorrhagic retinopathy.

Because of the potential danger of bleeding, close hematologic control is advisable. Hemorrhage produced by streptokinase is managed by discontinuing the drug and slowly administering ε-aminocaproic acid (ACA; Amicar) in-

travenously in doses of 100 mg per kg body weight. Plasma volume expanders or transfusions may be necessary at times. Because the drug creates a high titer of streptococcal antibodies, another series of treatment is not considered advisable in the following 6-month period.

In the case of serious bleeding produced by urokinase, the drug is immediately discontinued, and if blood loss has been large, packed red blood cells are indicated. Plasma volume expanders (other than dextran) may be helpful to replace the blood volume deficit. Although there is very little proof available for the efficacy of ε-aminocaproic acid in controlling bleeding produced by urokinase, it should be given (see above) if the hemorrhage is unresponsive to blood replacement.

Despite the potential dangers associated with administration of the fibrinolytic drugs, at the same time, they represent one of only a few medical approaches available for the management of massive pulmonary embolism. The alternative effective surgical measure is pulmonary embolectomy, a procedure that has a very high mortality (see below).

In the current evaluation of streptokinase and urokinase, it can be stated that when treatment with them is begun within 5 days after onset of symptoms of pulmonary embolism, a more rapid return toward normal angiographic and hemodynamic measurements can be expected than with heparin [8,15]. After a week of therapy, no difference is noted between the heparin-treated patients and those on streptokinase or urokinase. It would seem at present that in order to determine unequivocally that the fibrinolytic drugs reduce the mortality rate from pulmonary embolism and decrease the incidence and late sequelae of the disorder, more large, controlled clinical studies are required.

Early surgical approach. In some patients with massive pulmonary embolism, it is obvious that the pulmonary circulation must immediately be reestablished if they are to survive. In such individuals, removal of the obstruction by embolectomy may be the only option that is applicable. If time is available, this should be preceded by pulmonary angiography (see C-7, above) to localize the site of occlusion (Fig. 19.3); if not, the operation should be performed without the advantage of such valuable information. To carry out the procedure effectively, cardiopulmonary bypass equipment must be utilized. In recent years, an intraluminal catheter technique (transvenous catheter embolectomy) has been advocated, since such a procedure eliminates the need for cardiopulmonary bypass and open embolectomy. It consists of the insertion of a steerable catheter for extraction of the embolus [6]. The evaluation of such an approach must await more extensive clinical study.

At present the indications for pulmonary embolectomy have not been clearly defined. The reason for this is that the procedure has a very high mortality, as great as 57 percent [3]. A major problem in the evaluation of the operation is that invariably it is performed on seriously ill patients. It is therefore a difficult task to determine which individuals with massive pulmonary embolism are proper candidates for pulmonary embolectomy and which should be treated conservatively. A potential candidate for the operation is, in general terms, one who persists in a state of shock (below systolic levels of 90 mmHg) despite infusion of vasopressor drugs and who demonstrates angiographic proof of involvement of greater than 50 percent of the major pulmonary arteries by surgically accessible pulmonary emboli. The presence of severe hypoxemia (P_{O_2} less than 60 mmHg) supports this decision.

However, some clinical evidence appears to cast some doubt on the practicality and efficacy of pulmonary embolectomy. First, it has been reported that only 25 percent of the patients that might have been considered for the operation survive for 1 h and approximately 22 percent, for 2 h [5]. Also of importance in the evaluation of the procedure is the finding that partial venoarterial pumping, together with infusion of urokinase or streptokinase (see above), has resulted in the survival of patients with massive pulmonary embolism [10]. Another significant point is the fact that individuals who survive this condition for several hours have an excellent chance for recovery with nonoperative management.

4. Control of Recurrent Embolic Episodes

Later medical therapy. In order to prevent subsequent repeated attacks of pulmonary em-

bolism, orally administered anticoagulants, Coumadin or dicumarol, are begun several days before the anticipated date of discharge from the hospital, while the patient is still receiving heparin (see above). As a result, when the latter drug is discontinued, a therapeutic depression of prothrombin activity (approximately doubling of the prothrombin time) will generally have been achieved, and this state is then maintained on an outpatient basis with the continued administration of the coumarins. In most instances, weekly prothrombin times are necessary at the beginning; later the intervals between testing can be lengthened to one reading every 2 weeks but no longer. The patient should remain on such a regimen for from 9 to 18 months. In the presence of prior respiratory or cardiac pathology, an even longer period of treatment is advisable.

When an outpatient anticoagulant program is being considered, it is necessary to weigh very carefully the indications for such a therapeutic approach against the possible hazards of hemorrhage. Only when certain conditions exist should it be implemented. These consist of the following: Laboratory facilities for the determination of prothrombin times should be adequate and readily available and the patient should be oriented, able to comprehend his role in the treatment regimen, and willing to accept the onerous task and financial costs associated with maintenance of the desired prothrombin level in the blood. Moreover, the program must at all times be under the supervision of a physician knowledgeable in the use of anticoagulants.

Later surgical therapy. Since the great majority of pulmonary emboli have their origin in the deep veins of the lower limbs or the pelvic or prostatic vessels, the surgical approach to the prevention of recurrent episodes primarily involves means to block the venous tree, generally, at the level of the inferior vena cava. Technically this is accomplished by either inferior vena caval ligation, clipping or plication of the vessel, or insertion of an intracaval device.

Justification for the use of any one of the above-mentioned procedures exists if one of the following situations is present: (1) authenticated episodes of pulmonary embolism during well-controlled orally administered anticoagulant therapy; (2) the presence of suppurative pelvic or iliofemoral thrombophlebitis, followed by liberation of infected emboli; (3) the coexistence of disorders which contraindicate the use of anticoagulants (see pp. 271 and 273); (4) the performance of a pulmonary embolectomy for a massive pulmonary embolism; and (5) recurrence of pulmonary embolism after discontinuation of an effective anticoagulation program.

Inferior vena caval ligation has declined in popularity in recent years because the procedure is not infrequently associated with the appearance of several serious complications. Among these are the development of intraoperative hypotension; the production of marked alterations of distal venous hemodynamics resulting in venous hypertension and significant edema in both lower limbs (Fig. 19.4); and the formation of large venous collateral channels around the obstructed segment of inferior vena cava which could act as potential routes for recurrent pulmonary emboli. As a consequence, vena caval clipping, plication, and more recently, intracaval devices, such as the Mobin-Uddin umbrella filter, have been substituted.

Partial interruption of the inferior vena cava by means of an external clip applied distal to the renal vein prevents large clots from passing upward in the direction of the right atrium without subjecting the patient to the risk of sudden death from the precipitous fall in venous pressure that may be associated with total ligation of the inferior vena cava. Moreover, patency of the vessel will be maintained in about 75 percent of cases. Consequently, the incidence of disabling postphlebitic syndrome (see Section B, Chapter 20) is significantly decreased, as compared with the results of ligation of the vessel. However, the incidence of nonfatal emboli following the procedure is greater than in the case of ligation, the same objection applying to plication. Moreover, the procedure does not exclude embolization from the upper border of the deformed vena cava.

The Mobin-Uddin umbrella filter, a more recent approach to the problem, is useful in treating patients who are too ill to tolerate an abdominal operation, since it can be inserted into the internal jugular vein under local anesthesia. However, the procedure should be

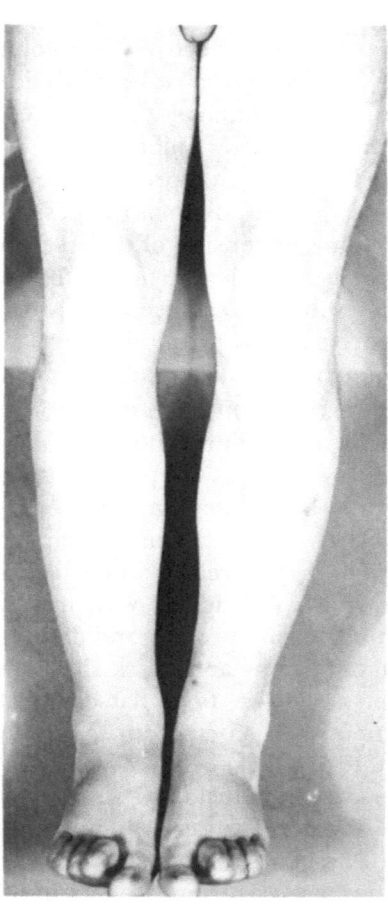

Fig. 19.4. Persistent edema of both lower limbs following inferior vena caval ligation for the prevention of recurrence of pulmonary emboli.

performed by a vascular surgeon, with the help of a radiologist experienced in intracaval catheter manipulation and a surgical assistant. In most instances, the obstruction to caval flow at the level of the third or fourth lumbar vertebra is gradual in development as the fenestrations in the instrument are slowly occluded. As a consequence, sufficient time is available for the formation of a collateral circulation, thus reducing the possibility of the production of venous stasis in the lower limbs. However, there are several serious complications of the procedure, such as retroperitoneal hemorrhage from spokes of the filter protruding through the caval wall, inadequate fixation with secondary embolization of the instrument,[3] its mis-

---

[3] Recently another technique using the Kimray-Greenfield filter has been proposed in order to counteract the possibility of such a complication [6].

placement in iliac, hepatic, or renal veins, and duodenal and ureteral perforations.

F. Prognosis

On the basis of several large series of autopsied patients, the mortality of untreated pulmonary embolism, including massive and submassive episodes, has been found to be about 30 percent. Approximately 10 percent of such individuals die within 1 h after onset of the condition, while of the remainder, the difficulty is not recognized clinically in about two-thirds of the cases.

In those patients in whom the diagnosis is made and proper therapy is instituted early in the condition, the mortality rate falls to about 8 percent [4], thus indicating that the available therapeutic programs are very effective in saving lives.

In the case of those individuals who have fully recovered from pulmonary embolism, there is little subsequent reduction in pulmonary or cardiac reserve. In fact, lung perfusion scans generally demonstrate that normal pulmonary blood flow is reestablished even in large areas of involvement as early as 3 weeks after the acute episode. However, if not prevented, recurrent episodes of pulmonary embolism may cause death, or if not, a permanent reduction in function of the pulmonary and cardiovascular systems as a result of the production of chronic cor pulmonale.

References

1. Abramson DI, Tuck S Jr, Chu LSW, et al: Vascular effects of heparin. Vasc Dis 1:180, 1964
2. Coleman JB, Chang FC: Pulmonary embolism: An unrecognized event in severely burnt patients. Am J Surg 130:697, 1975
3. Cross FS, Mowlem A: A survey of the current status of pulmonary embolectomy for massive pulmonary embolism. In Kittle CF (ed): Cardiovascular Surgery, American Heart Association Monograph 16. Circulation 35 (Suppl 1):86, 1967
4. Dalen JE, Alpert JS: Natural history of pulmonary embolism. Prog Cardiovasc Dis 17:259, 1975
5. Donaldson GA, Williams C, Schnnel JG, et al: A reappraisal of the application of the Trendelenburg operation to massive fatal embolism: Report of a successful pulmonary-artery thrombectomy using a cardiopulmonary bypass. N Engl J Med 268:171, 1963
6. Greenfield LJ: Transvenous pulmonary embolectomy. In Najarian JS, Delaney JP (eds): Vascular Surgery. Miami, Symposia Specialists, 1978, p 545
7. Hirsh J: Dosage regimens for streptokinase treatment: Evaluation of a standard dosage schedule. Aust Ann Med (Suppl) 19:12, 1970
8. Ly B, Arnesen H, Eie H, et al: A controlled clinical trial of streptokinase and heparin in the treatment of major pulmonary embolism. Acta Med Scand 203:465, 1978
9. McNicol GP: The fibrinolytic enzyme system. Postgrad Med J 49 (Suppl 5):10, 1973
10. Sautter RD, Myers WO, Wenzel FJ: Implications of the urokinase study concerning the surgical treatment of pulmonary embolism. J Thorac Cardiovasc Surg 63:54, 1972
11. Sevitt S: Diagnosis and management of massive pulmonary embolism (abridged). Proc R Soc Med 61:143, 1968
12. Shoop JD: Why do a lung scan? JAMA 229:567, 1974
13. Smith GT, Dammin GJ, Dexter L: Postmortem arteriographic studies of the human lung in pulmonary embolization. JAMA 188:143, 1964
14. Smith GT, Hayland JW, Piemme T, et al: Human systemic-pulmonary-arterial collateral circulation after pulmonary thromboembolism. JAMA 188:452, 1964
15. Urokinase-streptokinase embolism trial. Phase 2 results. JAMA 229:1606, 1974
16. Vogel G: Clinical use of streptokinase. In Markwardt F (ed): Fibrinolytics and Antifibrinolytics. New York, Springer-Verlag, 1978, p 185

Chapter 20

Vascular Complications of Musculoskeletal Disorders Produced by Trauma

---

Part 6   Postphlebitic Syndrome

A serious sequela of iliofemoral thrombophlebitis is the development of ambulatory venous hypertension and venous stasis in the affected extremity. This occurs as the result of destruction or incompetency of critical valves in, or permanent occlusion of, the iliofemoral vein. If left unchecked for several years, venous hypertension will eventually be responsible for the appearance of the postphlebitic syndrome, a condition characterized by combinations of pain, dilated and varicose veins, persistent swelling, pigmentation, chronic indurated cellulitis, increased sympathetic tone, stasis dermatitis, and stasis ulceration. The clinical picture resembles that produced by prolonged pooling of blood in the superficial veins of the lower limbs due to primary varicosities, except that the manifestations are much more severe.

A.   Causes and Steps for Prevention of Postphlebitic Syndrome

Before discussing the clinical picture and treatment of the postphlebitic syndrome, it appears advisable first to consider those conditions which have been found conducive to its development and those steps that are effective as prophylactic measures (Table 18.1).

1.   Conditions Leading to an Inadequate Early Treatment Program

The incidence of the postphlebitic syndrome is markedly enhanced if the patient does not seek medical aid for the acute episode of iliofemoral thrombophlebitis during the first 7 to 10 days of his illness. The same situation exists if the physician has not made the correct diagnosis in this period of time and so has delayed instituting the proper therapeutic program. Moreover, if the patient is instructed to begin his ambulation program in the hospital before an adequate collateral venous circulation has been established (as reflected in the reappearance of edema or in an increase in the still existing swelling), he also becomes a good candidate for the postphlebitic syndrome some time in the future. Discharging him from the hospital without emphasizing and explaining the various measures to combat venous stasis (enumerated in A-2, below) will likewise predispose him to the development of the condition.

2.   Posthospital Regimen

On discharge from the hospital following iliofemoral thrombophlebitis, the patient should continue most of the physical practices previously instituted. The foot of his bed should be elevated 12.5 to 17.5 cm (5 to 7 in.) by placing books or blocks of wood of appropriate height under the two distal legs. Each morning, the fabricated elastic stocking with a built-in gradient of pressure should be applied to the involved limb before the patient gets out of bed. He should continue to wear a well-fitting elastic stocking until he determines that its removal for a trial period of time does not result in edema formation. This may occur several months following the acute phase of iliofemoral thrombophlebitis or a number of years afterward, or the patient may have to wear the stocking indefinitely. It is important to emphasize to him that the elasticity of the support is generally lost after 3 or 4 months of usage and that when this is observed, a new stocking, made to order, is required. During the course of the day, he should lie down two or three times and elevate his lower limbs for 10 to 15 min each time.

In order to prevent the development of a stasis ulcer, it is essential to protect the lower portion of the limb (particularly the area around the medial malleolus) from the slightest injury. Scrupulous care must be taken to maintain the local tissues in the best nutritional state. With the appearance of even the slightest break in the continuity of the skin of the ankle, the patient should be put to complete bed rest for several days and the lesion handled very carefully with regard to asepsis. Only mild antiseptics should be applied to the area and dermatophytosis of the feet should be actively treated. Care must be taken to control itching, since scratching may initiate a lesion.

All the above precautions also apply to the patient who has already had a stasis ulcer which healed with intensive therapy. This type of lesion has a great tendency to recur since the underlying agents, ambulatory venous hypertension and venous stasis, still persist even after the skin around the ankle is again intact.

Strict adherence to the described program generally prevents the appearance of the postphlebitic syndrome, except in the relatively rare situation in which initially the thrombotic process responsible for the iliofemoral thrombophlebitis involves not only the main collecting vein, but also the tributaries and collateral vessels which would ordinarily now have to assume the function of draining the blood from the limb. Under such circumstances, all prophylac-

tic measures, including early anticoagulant therapy, are ineffective in preventing the development of a severe degree of venous hypertension.

As a general rule, however, the remaining collateral veins are adequate for the return of blood from the limb and hence the postphlebitic syndrome does not appear. In most instances the occluded portion of the main collecting vein gradually becomes recanalized (over a course of 1 to 2 years),[1] and in the interval the great saphenous vein begins to play a more important role in venous drainage (Fig. 20.1A and B). Also involved in this function are the small saphenous and femoropopliteal veins, with blood passing through them and then into the pelvic veins. Blood in the small saphenous vein may also enter the pudendal plexus by way of superficial vessels located on the medial aspect of the thigh (Fig. 20.1A). Of course, if too great a load is placed on the superficial vessels, their valves may eventually become incompetent, with the subsequent development of secondary varicosities (see B-6, below).

B. Clinical Manifestations of Postphlebitic Syndrome

1. Nocturnal Leg Cramps

A common complaint experienced in the lower extremities in a patient with venous stasis is cramps in the muscles of the calf and foot which occur during the night and awaken him. The symptom may last for several to 20 min or longer and may recur a number of times. The mechanism which precipitates the attack in the leg is evidently the involuntary or voluntary stretching of the Achilles tendon. A similar type of reaction is responsible for cramping in the toes. The basis for the response is not clear, although it appears to be related to an increase in irritability of the neuromuscular junctions, due either to an accumulation of metabolites or to a local alteration in metabolism. The actual cramp results from simultaneous contraction of agonists and antagonists, the position

---

[1] In the remainder, the occlusion persists, but collateral venous channels develop and these bridge the obstructed segment of main collecting vessel.

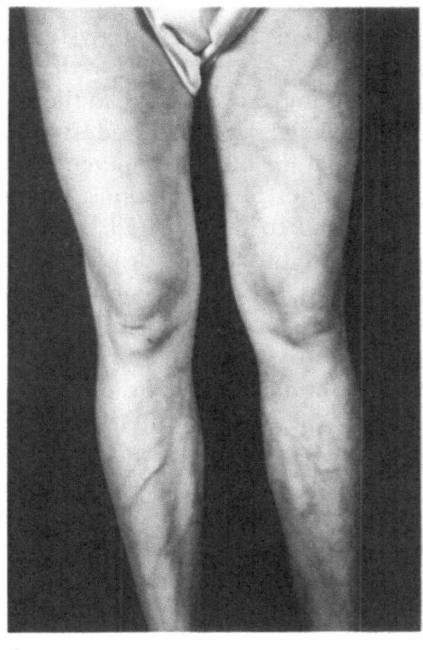 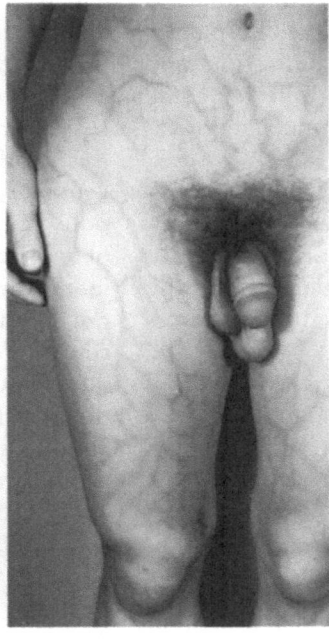

A   B

Fig. 20.1. Development of a superficial venous collateral circulation following iliofemoral thrombophlebitis. **A** Dilated superficial veins on medial and anterior surfaces of the left thigh, as compared with the normal venous pattern present on the right lower limb. **B** Dilated venous collateral network on the outer aspect of the right thigh and lower anterior abdominal wall.

of the limb depending upon which group of muscles is the stronger.[2]

2. Ready Fatigue

A number of vague and nonspecific symptoms may be experienced in the limb suffering from the postphlebitic syndrome. They are initiated and aggravated by prolonged standing or sitting. A bursting sensation in the limb is a rather common complaint.

3. Postphlebitic Neurosis

The patient suffering from acute iliofemoral thrombophlebitis who has no understanding of his difficulty because of poor communication with his physician is a likely candidate for postphlebitic neurosis. Following recovery from the

acute disorder and discharge from the hospital, he may become anxious, tense, and apprehensive and begin to fear that he will soon develop myocardial infarction, pulmonary embolism, or deformity or gangrene of the limb. Locally, he may experience pain on weight bearing, coldness or hypersensitivity, diffuse tenderness, or paresthesias which frequently have no organic basis. Each time edema recurs, generally as a result of excessive standing or sitting, the patient worries that he is again suffering from an acute episode of iliofemoral thrombophlebitis or that he has "chronic thrombophlebitis."

4. Venous Claudication

Following recovery from iliofemoral thrombophlebitis, some patients will begin to develop severe ill-defined aching calf pain on walking. In a sense, this symptom, which may be almost incapacitating, mimics intermittent claudication (see A-1, Chapter 10), but since no associated signs of impaired muscle circulation exist, it cannot be due to local ischemia during the period of physical activity. Another differential point is that the patient does not experience relief on standing for several minutes. In fact, 15 to 20 min of rest are required, and the pain

---

[2] It is necessary to point out that nocturnal cramps may also be present in normal persons in several physiologic states and in a number of abnormal conditions besides venous stasis. Examples of disorders or situations in which they are found are chronic occlusive arterial diseases, hyperphosphatemia, hypocalcemia (as in hypoparathyroid tetany and in pregnancy), hypochloremia (produced in patients on rigidly restricted salt intake who are receiving intensive diuretic therapy), static foot deformities, and peripheral neuropathy.

is most effectively relieved if the patient is seated or in a reclining position. The pain is less severe than intermittent claudication, and the individual can continue to walk for some distance after its onset without much aggravation of the discomfort.

The exact cause for venous claudication has not been determined [10]. However, the finding that successful valvoplasty of incompetent veins in the femoral venous system relieves the symptom [7] may cast some light on the responsible agent.

5. Swelling

The first sign of chronic venous insufficiency is edema, usually most apparent at the end of the day. At first it disappears overnight, but later it will still be present in the morning, the residual swelling gradually increasing in amount on subsequent days if the patient is improperly treated (Fig. 20.2A). If this type of change persists for months and years, it is ultimately replaced by a brawny, nonpitting lymphedema, the extravasated protein in the edema fluid causing a dermal and subcutaneous fibrosis which produces mechanical obstruction of lymphatic channels (Fig. 20.2C).

6. Secondary Varicosities

Prominent, dilated veins demonstrating retrograde flow are common abnormalities in the postphlebitic syndrome. They resemble primary varicosities, also affecting the great saphenous and small saphenous systems (Fig. 20.2B). Associated findings are varicosities in the suprapubic region (Fig. 20.2D) and dilated, enlarged subcutaneous collateral vessels on the outer aspect of the thigh, extending onto the flank and lower portion of the abdominal wall (Fig. 20.1B).

The alterations in the superficial veins are secondary to the ambulatory venous hypertension in the deep venous system following iliofemoral thrombophlebitis. The exact mechanism responsible for the varicosities depends upon the outcome of the opposing processes of organization of the clot in the iliofemoral vein and of fibrinolysis. If the thrombus persists, then permanent anatomic narrowing or occlusion of the lumen of the vein ensues, resulting in an impatent deep venous system. If the fibrinolytic process predominates, the clot is dissolved or becomes recanalized, in the process of which the valves locally are destroyed; this results in a patent but incompetent deep venous system. Under both situations, the venous pressure distal to the affected segments of vein rises because of inability or inefficiency in moving blood in the deep venous system out of the limb in a proximal direction. The resulting increase in venous pressure is transmitted to the communicating veins, distending them and making the valves in them functionally incompetent. As a consequence, there is a retrograde flow of blood from the deep venous system into the superficial venous system via the communicating vessels. Hence, the superficial veins also become distended and, in turn, the valves in them become incompetent. The final result is the production of secondary varicosities.

7. Pigmentation

Typically, brownish pigmentation appears around the medial malleolus (Fig. 20.3A) and, less often, elsewhere on the lower portion of the leg. The change may be due to rupture of delicate venules and capillaries because of the venous hypertension, followed by subcutaneous hemorrhage and alterations in blood pigment deposited in the skin. Or it may result from the accumulation of hemosiderin in the tissues for unknown reasons. There is no apparent correlation between the degree of pigmentation and the severity of the venous hypertension.

8. Vasospasm

In the postphlebitic syndrome, the limb may manifest changes typical of increased sympathetic tone, such as cyanosis, low cutaneous temperature, and increased sweating of the involved foot. In some individuals this type of response may be related to the unnecessarily long period of physical inactivity to which they were subjected while being treated for iliofemoral thrombophlebitis. It is also possible that the reflex arc originally set up by the

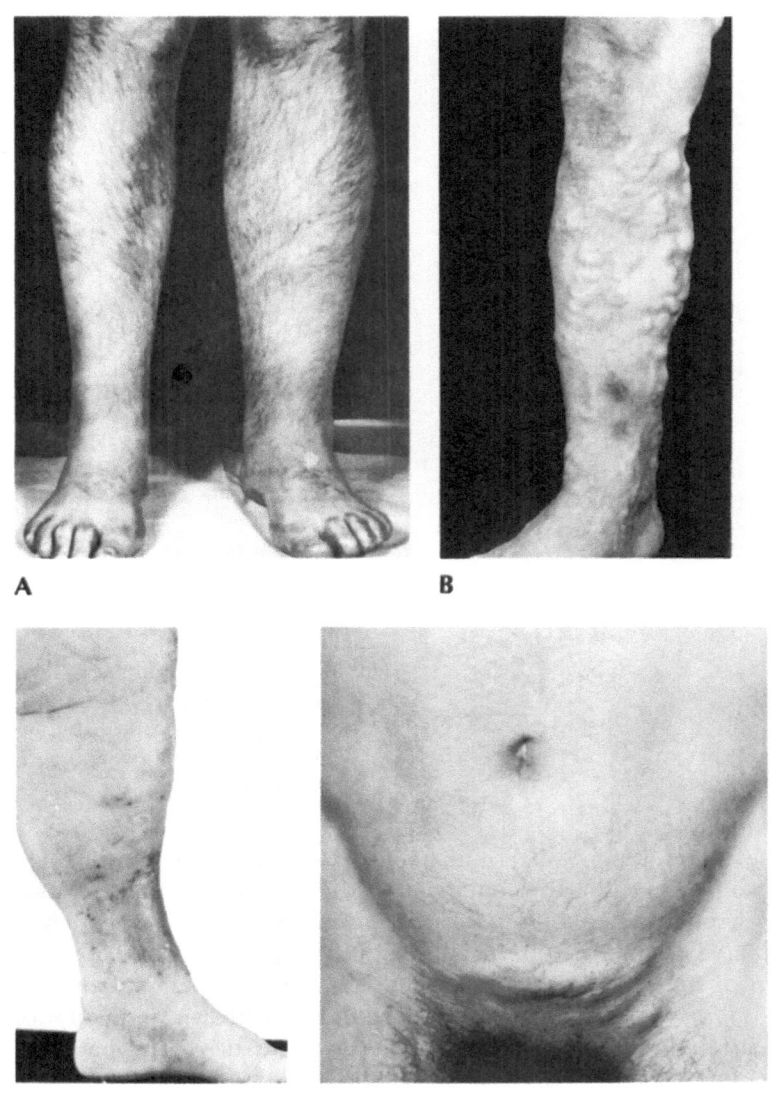

Fig. 20.2. Sequelae of iliofemoral thrombophlebitis (postphlebitic syndrome). **A** Persistent edema of left lower limb. **B** Secondary varicosities. **C** Induration, brawniness, and fibrotic attachment of the skin on the lower portion of the leg. **D** Collateral venous channels (varicosities) in suprapubic region. From Abramson DI: Diagnosis and Treatment of Peripheral Vascular Disorders. New York, Hoeber-Harper, 1956, reproduced with permission.

thrombosed segment of vein during the acute process, which included the peripheral sympathetic nervous system as the efferent arm, persists long into the convalescent period. Likewise of interest in the elucidation of the problem is the histologic finding of irreversible damage of the lumbar paravertebral sympathetic ganglia associated with the postphlebitic syndrome [8].

9. Chronic Indurated Cellulitis

An area of indurated cellulitis is a fairly frequent finding in the postphlebitic syndrome.

It generally takes the form of a hard localized mass on the medial, although occasionally on the lateral, aspect of the leg, in its lower third. Usually the process has a brawny appearance with no signs of activity; however, at times it flares into an acute stage, demonstrating a hard, scalloped, inflamed border, with the skin over the lesion becoming red, hot, and tender. Following treatment or spontaneously, the condition then recedes into a chronic stage. After numerous periods of exacerbation and recession, the area of involvement is infiltrated by fibrous tissue which eventually encircles the limb to form a tight constricting band. Gener-

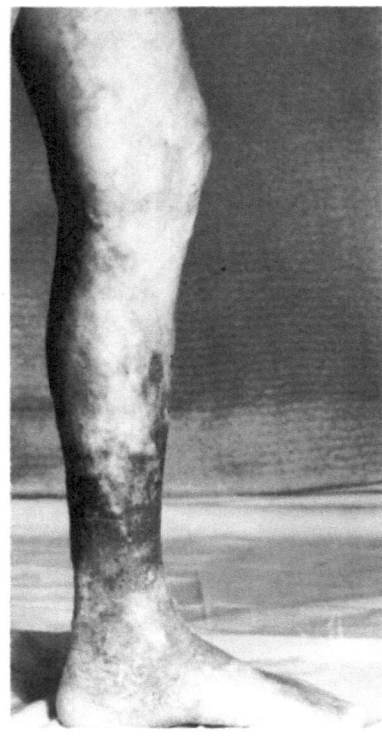

A

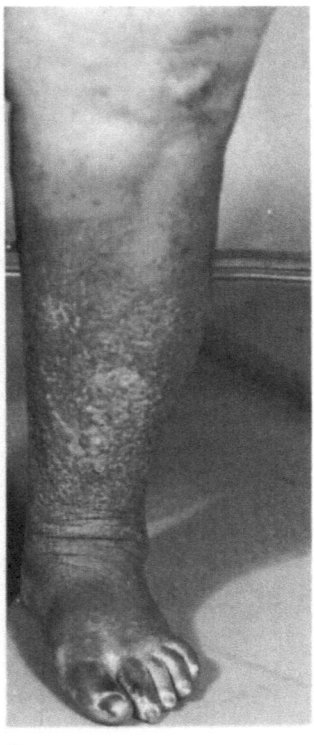

B

Fig. 20.3. Postphlebitic syndrome. **A** Pigment deposited in skin of lower portion of the leg. **B** Stasis dermatitis (weeping eczematous type).

ally, even before this final stage has developed, roentgenography of the area in two planes will reveal calcification in the subcutaneous tissue (at times to the degree of disseminated calcinosis), phleboliths, and calcification of the walls of the superficial veins.

The etiologic factors in chronic indurated cellulitis are persistent venous stasis and chronic edema. Because of the resulting abnormal pooling of poorly oxygenated venous blood, which also interferes with arteriolar circulation, the tissues of the lower part of the limb are deprived of oxygen and nutrient, thus becoming more susceptible to infection, low-grade inflammatory reactions, and superficial thrombophlebitis.

10. Stasis Dermatitis

As one of the more serious results of protracted venous stasis, a weeping eczematous type of dermatitis develops on the lower portion of the leg; at times, an erysipeloid infection is noted instead. A constant associated finding is intense itching, probably due to irritation of terminal sensory nerve endings in the skin, thus aggravating the condition because it initiates persistent scratching. There is generally superficial oozing of serum, or the lesion may be covered by scaly cornified skin surrounded by an area of redness or brown pigmentation (Fig. 20.3B). Stasis dermatitis is probably related to the rise in capillary filtration pressure and an increase in capillary permeability, permitting the movement of protein-rich fluid through the vessel wall into the tissue spaces.

11. Stasis Ulceration

Stasis ulceration is the most serious development of the postphlebitic syndrome. Not only does its treatment require weeks of disability and complete bed rest, but the condition is notorious for recurrences, frequently as often as once or at times even twice a year.

The ulcer is usually located on the medial aspect of the ankle in the area drained by the great saphenous venous system (Figs. 20.4A–D and 20.5A, C–E) and, less often, on the lateral side (Figs. 20.4E and 20.5B); only rarely is it found above the midportion of the leg. The first sign of its presence may be necrosis and separation of the superficial layers of skin, or a portion of the wall of a vein may slough away, together with the overlying tissues. The ulcer generally penetrates the deep fascia and is irregularly shaped, varying in size from a pinhead to a lesion affecting a considerable portion of the lower part of the leg (Fig. 20.5D and E). The base is generally covered by an infected, dirty exudate (Fig. 20.5 E) from which a foul odor frequently emanates. The tissues surrounding the ulcer demonstrate signs of inflammation, edema, induration, dryness and scaliness, and pigmentation.

The appearance of a stasis ulcer of the leg may be associated with pain locally, although this is usually less intense than that observed with the nutritional disturbances resulting from impaired arterial circulation. It is described as a burning, throbbing, or aching sensation, which in most instances becomes much more marked when the individual is sitting, standing, or walking. Occasionally the complaint may be quite disabling, resembling the symptoms associated with major causalgia (see A-1, Chapter 13), probably because of local irritation of the sensory components of the peripheral nerves in the area of the inflammatory process.

The basis for the formation of a stasis ulcer is persistent pooling of blood in the superficial veins (venous stasis), associated with a rise in

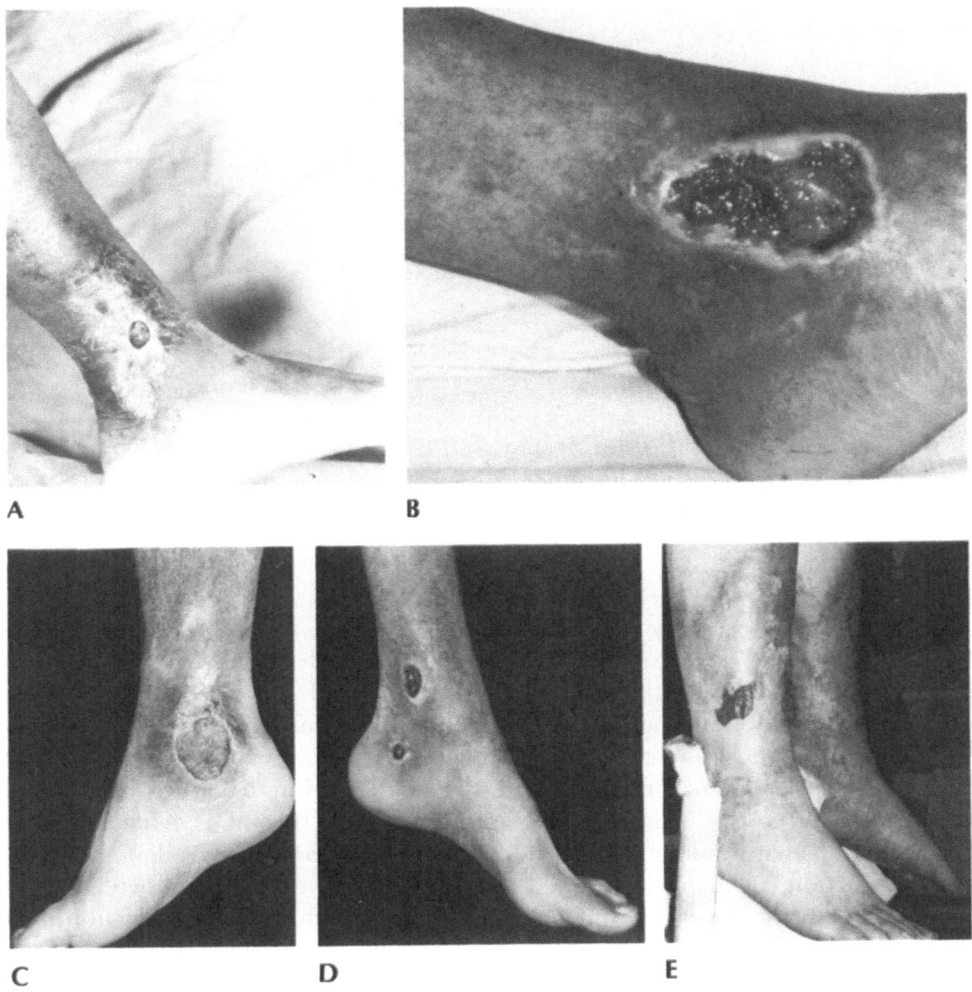

A   B   C   D   E

Fig. 20.4. Venous stasis ulcerations (postphlebitic syndrome) present on the medial (**A–D**) or lateral (**E**) side of the leg, over or above the malleoli.

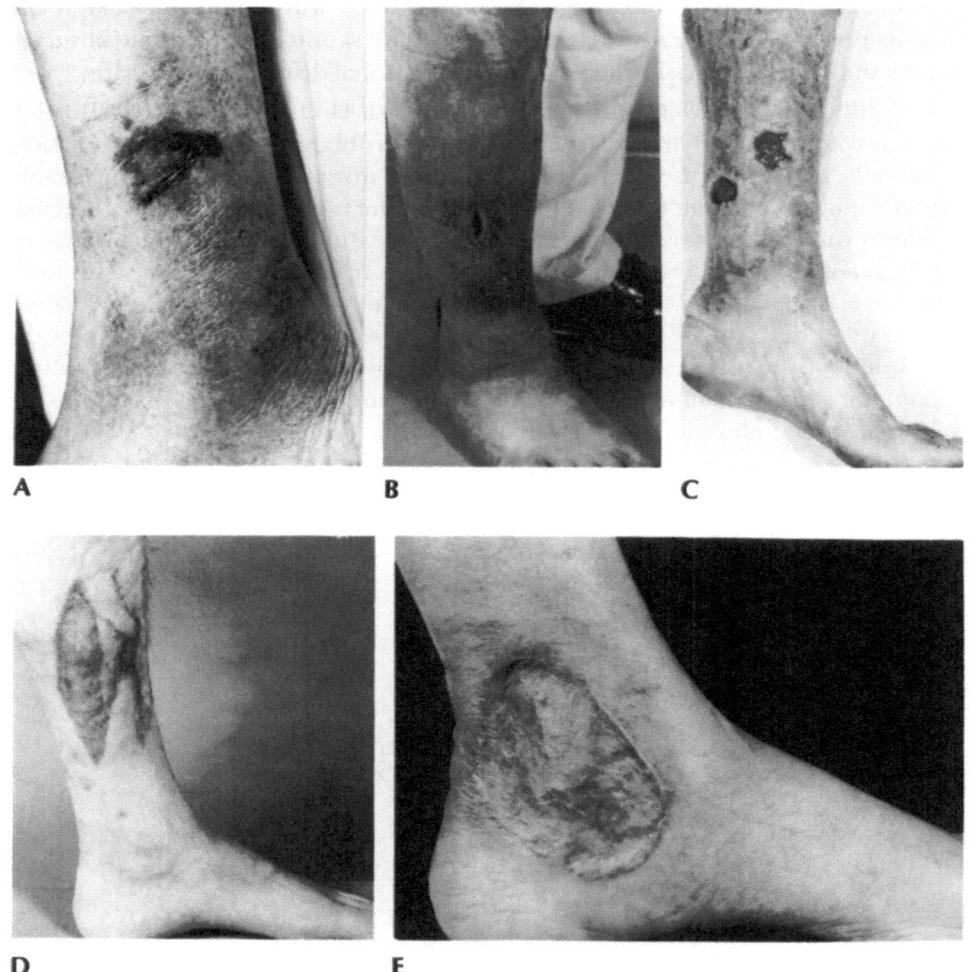

Fig. 20.5. Venous stasis ulcerations (postphlebitic syndrome) of varying sizes on the medial (**A, C–E**) or lateral (**B**) side of the lower portion of the leg. **A** The initial stage of the lesion.

venous pressure which is transmitted back into the microcirculation as a rise in capillary filtration pressure. The latter change is responsible for a greater transudation of fluid into the tissue spaces which, in turn, causes waterlogging, followed by anoxia, impaired nutrition, and accumulation of toxic waste products of metabolism. Such a situation reduces the resistance of the skin, with the result that a minor abrasion, a bruise, or an infection may be responsible for the development of an ulcer, or the lesion may even occur spontaneously.

The reason that the region around the medial malleolus is the site of predilection for venous stasis ulcers is that in this area the protective padding is scanty and the possibility

of exposure to trauma is great. Moreover, the local tissues appear to have a poorer response to infection than elsewhere.

The presence of several poorly supported communicating veins in the vicinity of the medial malleolus may also contribute to the vulnerability of the region to ulcer formation [1,3]. Recanalization of a thrombus in a main collecting vessel like the popliteal or iliofemoral vein is frequently followed by incompetency of the deep venous system due to destruction of the valves in the process (see B-6, above). Such a situation results in a regurgitant flow in the venae comitantes of the posterior tibial artery which causes a rise in local venous pressure in these vessels and also in the ankle perforators. As a consequence, functional incompetency of the valves in the latter is produced, with retrograde flow through them into the superficial veins normally draining the skin in the vicinity of the medial malleolus. An anatomic response to such a situation is the development of a mesh of finely dilated venules around the ankle ("ankle flare").

C. Therapy for Postphlebitic Syndrome

Once the postphlebitic syndrome has developed, the therapeutic approach will depend primarily on which abnormality or abnormalities exist. For the most part they can be managed by medical means, at least during the acute phase of the difficulty. When a surgical procedure is being considered, it is necessary first to establish that an adequate local arterial circulation is present (see Chapters 5 and 6). Then precise venography (see C-2, Chapter 7) should be carried out to determine the exact state of the deep venous system in the involved limb and in the pelvis. Venous pressure measurements at rest and with physical exercise (see C-1, Chapter 7) are also very helpful in determining the extent of functional damage.

1. Nocturnal Leg Cramps

The control of night cramps is palliative, including a reduction in the amount of standing and sitting during the day and efforts to combat venous stasis. It is also advisable to give the patient a clinical trial of oral quinine sulfate, 0.35 g (5 gr) before retiring. If this is not sufficient, another similar dose should be taken before the last meal. Ordinarily such medication will cause a reduction or even elimination of the attacks. However, the relief will only persist so long as the medication is given. One explanation for the therapeutic action of the drug is that it hastens the removal, destruction, or conversion of the waste products in the muscles or at the myoneural junction. Another is that it acts to block neuromuscular transmission by prolonging the refractory period of the nerves. It is necessary to point out that one should be on guard for sensitivity reactions to quinine

and for the possibility of initiating or aggravating tinnitus. If such contraindications exist, then oral diphenhydramine (Benadryl), 50 mg, should be given before retiring. Large doses of calcium lactate or gluconate and dilute hydrochloric acid have also been proposed. The patient should be warned against extending his legs while in bed, since this is the maneuver which frequently precipitates an attack of night cramps.

2. Nonspecific Symptoms

No effective therapy is available for the control of spontaneous pain and venous claudication. However, this does not pose any real problem in treatment, since such symptoms generally disappear with passage of time. Reducing the periods of standing and sitting and wearing a proper compression stocking appear to decrease the severity of the spontaneous pain. Occasionally popliteal vein resection may relieve diffuse bursting pain and aching in the lower portion of the leg, provided venography demonstrates incompetency of the valves in this vessel [2]; ligation of incompetent ankle perforators is carried out at the same time. However, a real question exists as to the efficacy of the procedure [5,9,11].

In the case of the patient who has a postphlebitic neurosis, it is necessary to explain to him in detail that he is suffering from a state of chronic venous insufficiency, which can, to a certain extent, be controlled, and not from "chronic thrombophlebitis." Reassuring him and his relatives on this score will frequently relieve their fears and reduce the severity of the patient's response to his difficulty. Of course, if there is an underlying psychiatric difficulty, treatment of postphlebitic neurosis may prove to be very difficult.

3. Swelling

If, despite rigid adherence to the measures outlined above in A-2, the swelling of the limb is not controlled and, in fact, increases, then more heroic steps are necessary in order to prevent the inevitable consequences of protracted edema. The patient is again placed at complete bed rest, with no bathroom privileges and with the foot of the bed elevated, and given a diet low in salt. At the same time, he receives parenteral furosemide (Lasix) to mobilize the fluid, followed by the same medication given orally. After the swelling has subsided, a heavy one-way stretch elastic stocking is applied to the limb and the patient is cautiously placed on an ambulation program. Repeated measurements of limb circumferences are made following periods of walking to determine whether any edema is reaccumulating. If it is not or if the amount is minimal, physical activity is gradually increased, and the patient is maintained on the medical regimen indefinitely. An elastic stocking with a built-in gradient of pressure is subsequently substituted for the heavy one-way stretch hose.

4. Dilated or Varicose Veins

Prophylactic measures. Therapy for secondary varicosities is, for the most part, preventive. It involves the same measures used to control the edema, namely, the application of a well-fitting elastic stocking, elevation of the foot of the bed, and minimal time spent in the standing or sitting position with the feet in dependency. The first two steps tend to shunt the blood from the superficial veins into those deep vessels which are still patent, at the same time encouraging development of collateral channels in the subcutaneous and deeper tissues. The latter type of vascular tree is able to carry blood more efficiently since it is better supported by surrounding structures and is exposed to a greater pumping action supplied by neighboring muscles. At the same time, the resulting reduced blood flow through the superficial veins causes a decrease in pressure in them, which helps prevent distension and incompetency of these vessels.

Active therapy. The question of how to deal with existing secondary varicosities has not been fully answered. Some vascular surgeons believe that, regardless of the underlying pathogenesis, varicosities are inefficient in the removal of blood from a lower limb and hence should be treated surgically, generally by stripping, followed by ligation of the femoral vein. In practice, however, such a heroic procedure

is rarely carried out for secondary varicosities except possibly if there is an associated treatment-resistant stasis ulceration (see C-7, below).

The more common approach to the management of secondary varicosities is medical, involving the use of compression bandages and elastic stockings. The reason for preferring such measures is the fear that the alternative of stripping varicosities, in the face of pathologic changes in the deep venous system, may have adverse effects, since very few venous channels would now be available for removal of blood from the limb. As a consequence, an even more marked state of venous hypertension would develop. Moreover, it does not necessarily follow that all superficial veins which are dilated as a result of a block in, or incompetency of, the deep venous system are likewise incompetent. It is possible that, instead, they are compensatory and hence useful vessels in the removal of blood from the lower limbs.

On the basis of such reasoning, only very carefully selected cases of varicosities secondary to the postphlebitic syndrome should be stripped. Even in them, if temporary ligation of the veins at the time of operation results in a significant increase in venous pressure in the deep venous system, then surgery should be terminated. Otherwise serious complications may follow [3]. The results of preliminary venography and venous pressure measurements during exercise may help resolve the problem without the need to resort to surgery to obtain the necessary critical information.

5. Chronic Indurated Cellulitis

Although conservative therapy for chronic indurated cellulitis is frequently ineffective, nevertheless, it should be given a clinical trial, especially in the early stage of the condition. This involves a period of bed rest with the foot of the bed elevated, hot, wet soaks to the area, and the use of a wide-spectrum antibiotic. Cultures and sensitivity studies cannot be performed since secretion from the lesion is generally not available.

If medical measures do not produce obvious improvement in a trial period, then surgical treatment is indicated. This includes removal of all abnormal structures in the site, such as involved subcutaneous tissue and fascia and devitalized skin, followed by a split-thickness skin graft applied to well-vascularized muscle so as to cover the defect. During the course of the operation, any incompetent communicating veins encountered should be ligated. If secondary varicosities exist, the great saphenous vein is stripped to just below the level of the knee and ligation of the femoral vein is carried out below the junction with the deep femoral vein. However, first, steps must be performed to demonstrate that a significant rise in deep venous pressure will not occur with such an approach (see C-4, above).

6. Stasis Dermatitis

In most patients stasis dermatitis can only be controlled with complete bed rest, elevation of the foot of the bed, no bathroom privileges, and local therapy. Any type of ambulatory program is generally not effective. First, attempts are made to harden the skin by the continuous application of either Burow's solution, 1:20 concentration, or a dilute solution of silver nitrate (15 ml of a 10% solution in 1 liter of distilled water). The lesion is covered with several layers of gauze which are then soaked with the solution. To prevent evaporation, a piece of oiled silk or plastic is applied over the wet gauze. The lesion is kept moist all during the day, and at night a dry sterile dressing is placed over the area. At the same time, it is necessary to eradicate fungus infections of the feet, since they may act as a portal of entry for bacteria, thus contributing to the dermatitis as well as to subsequent ulceration of the skin. All scaly material and necrotic tissue must be removed by debridement.

7. Stasis Ulceration

Medical therapy. There are numerous approaches to the treatment of stasis ulceration, although, as a general rule, the first attempt should involve some type of medical therapy. This includes measures to eliminate or reduce venous stasis, steps to control secondary infection, and means to stimulate growth of granulation tissue and epithelialization.

Ideally, the control of venous stasis is achieved through a period of bed rest with the foot of the bed elevated. However, in some instances, this program is not feasible or financially possible, and so other less desirable measures have to be substituted which permit the patient to be ambulatory and able to conduct his daily chores. At the same time, such procedures maintain a fairly adequate amount of pressure to the involved limb, so as to cause collapse of the superficial varicose veins. The most common but least effective way to accomplish this goal is through the use of an Ace bandage, a pure gum rubber bandage, or a well-fitting elastic stocking with a built-in gradient of pressure. More efficient means are the compression legging, the vasopneumatic apparatus, and the nonelastic support, like the frequently used Unna boot. When an Ace bandage is applied, first a piece of sterile sponge rubber, cut slightly larger than the general outline and depth of the ulcer, is inserted over the base of the lesion and held in place with the elastic support. The compression legging applies a uniform pressure throughout the limb by means of a rubber bladder incorporated in the outer duck casing and inflated by means of a bicycle pump. An initial pressure of about 35 mmHg appears to be optimal.

The semirigid Unna boot is commercially available in the form of bandages impregnated with a mixture of gelatin, glycerin, and zinc oxide. The bandage is applied to form a boot and left on for 1 or 2 weeks, provided the patient does not experience any symptoms, such as itching or a burning pain. If complaints are elicited or if the secretion from the ulcer softens the overlying portion of the boot, the latter should be removed immediately. At times, the patient becomes sensitive to the ingredients in the boot with the result that a weeping dermatitis develops. If the response to the application of the boot is satisfactory, it is left intact for the desired period of time and then removed. The lesion is cleaned and debrided and if definite signs of improvement are noted, another boot is applied; this sequence is followed until complete healing of the ulcer has occurred. One disadvantage of the method is that no local treatment of the lesion is possible except at infrequent intervals when a boot is removed and a new one applied.

If venous stasis can be controlled, then the next step in healing the postphlebitic ulcer is elimination of secondary infection. This step is most readily accomplished if the patient is at complete bed rest. Under such conditions, all necrotic tissue can be removed by daily debridement after soaking in a whirlpool bath or by some other means of applying lukewarm water containing a mild antiseptic. The use of proteolytic enzymes, such as Elase ointment, may help facilitate softening of the devitalized tissues. Heat, in the form of hot, wet compresses applied to the lesion and kept at the desired temperature with a heating pad or a heat cradle, is helpful in controlling the local infection and removing necrotic tissue, provided that arterial circulation is not impaired. Treatment is given for periods of 3 h, with an hour intervening when all wet bandages are removed and the limb is exposed to the air; the latter step permits the skin to return to its normal state, thus preventing maceration. Such a program is continued during the waking hours. At night a mild local antibiotic is placed on the ulcer and then the latter is covered with a sterile bandage. At no time is adhesive tape permitted to come in contact with the skin.

During the period in which the necrotic tissue is being removed by debridement, appropriate antibiotics are given parenterally or orally. To determine the most effective ones, cultures and sensitivity studies are necessary. However, meaningful information in this regard can only be obtained if these procedures are delayed until most of the necrotic tissue is removed. Then the area is cleansed with a mild antiseptic and covered with sterile gauze. After 24 h, the bandage is removed and the secretion at the base of the ulcer is cultured.

Once venous stasis is controlled, the necrotic tissue has been removed, and the infection in the lesion and the surrounding tissues has been eliminated, frequently the ulcer will heal spontaneously. Granulation tissue will cover the ulcer base and begin to grow upward, soon to be covered by epithelial cells arising from the periphery of the lesion.

If improvement is slow, epithelialization may be facilitated by the use of stimulating ointments, such as 5% crude coal tar applied locally every 24 h. However, patients with chronic ulcers may have become sensitized to such a sub-

stance and hence it is necessary to be careful in its use. If itching or burning occurs soon after application of the medication, it must be removed immediately and discontinued. It is also necessary to point out that coal tar is a photosensitizer. If no ill effects develop, then the daily treatments should be continued for 1 to 2 weeks provided improvement is apparent. Otherwise, the medication should be stopped. Generally no longer than a 2-week period of therapy is warranted, for a folliculitis may develop if it is continued beyond this time. In addition, the restoration process may be inhibited by further treatment.

To increase local circulation and thus facilitate healing of the ulcer, other measures may be of value. Among these are the oral administration of alpha-receptor blocking agents such as phenoxybenzamine hydrochloride (Dibenzyline), 10 mg three times a day, ion transfer with histamine, and, on occasion, even sympathectomy.

Surgical therapy. If a trial of medical therapy has not proved effective in healing a venous stasis ulcer, then it is necessary to utilize more heroic measures. However, before any one of these can be carried out, it is necessary first to control the edema, the inflammation of the surrounding tissues, and the local infection by medical means. Otherwise, the surgical approach has no possibility of being successful.

Among the operative procedures is wide excision of the lesion and the surrounding indurated skin and subcutaneous tissue down to the deep fascia, so as to produce a well-vascularized base, followed by a retiform split-thickness skin graft [9] or dermal overgrafting. At the same time, it is also necessary to ligate incompetent ankle perforators to correct the existing venous stasis [12]. Postoperatively, the limb is immobilized in a large pressure dressing for 6 to 8 days and the patient remains at complete bed rest for 14 to 21 days.

Another operative means of controlling the venous stasis is ligating the femoral vein below its junction with the deep femoral vein, together with ligation and stripping of the great and small saphenous veins. At the same time, care should be taken to remove the portion of the vein underlying the ulcer. However, it is again necessary to point out that the great saphenous vein is ligated only if temporary occlusion of this vessel does not produce a significant rise in venous pressure (30 cm H₂O; 2.2 mmHg).

A number of other surgical procedures have been proposed as treatment for ambulatory venous hypertension which, in part, is responsible for the postphlebitic ulcer, but they have not been exposed to sufficient clinical trial to make it possible to evaluate them properly. Among these are bypass of segmental obliterations of the iliofemoral vein by transposition of the great saphenous vein [4,6], a cross-pubis–saphenous vein bypass procedure, and surgical repair (valvoplasty) of an incompetent femoral vein valve [7]. For the use of bypass procedures, carefully performed venographic studies are essential in order to delineate the site and extent of the deep venous obstruction and to identify a suitable patent deep vein distal to the occlusion for insertion of the graft. Venography, both ascending and reflux, is also required for the diagnosis of incompetent femoral vein valves, as a preliminary to surgical repair of these structures.

References

1. Arnoldi CC: The venous return from the lower leg in health and in chronic venous insufficiency: A synthesis. Acta Orthop Scand (Suppl) 164:1, 1964
2. Bauer G: The long-term effect of popliteal ligation in 136 cases of severe bursting lower leg pain and oedema. J Cardiovasc Surg 6:366, 1965
3. Fischer H, Schneider W: Phlebologie heute. Fortschr Med 87:1001, 1969
4. Frileaux C, Pillot-Bienayme P, Gillot C: Bypass of segmental obliterations of ilio-femoral venous axis by transposition of saphenous vein. J Cardiovasc Surg 13:409, 1972
5. Haeger K, Sandberg I: Zur operativen Behandlung der tiefen Veneninsuffizienz. Zentralbl Phlebol 5:93, 1966
6. Husni EA: Venous reconstruction in postphlebitic disease. Circulation 43(Suppl 1):147, 1971
7. Kistner RL: Surgical repair of the incompetent femoral vein valve. Arch Surg 110:1336, 1975
8. May R, Brinkmann H, Peters D: Lichtmikroskopische Betrachtungen an operativ entfernten Lumbalganglien des menschlichen Grenzstranges beim postthrombotischen Zustandsbild. Zentralbl Phlebol 9:2, 1970
9. May R, Nissl R: The post-thrombotic syndrome. In May R (ed): Surgery of the Veins of the Leg and Pelvis. Philadelphia, Saunders, 1979, Chap 6
10. Negus D: Calf pain in the post-thrombotic syndrome. Br Med J 2:156, 1968
11. Netzer CO: Die Strömungsverhältnisse beim postthrombotischen Zustandsbild. In Kappert A, May R (eds): Das postthrombotische Zustandsbild der Extremitäten. Bern, Huber, 1968
12. Nielubowicz J, Szostek M: Recurrences after Linton flap operation. J Cardiovasc Surg 20:49, 1979

Chapter 21

Vascular and Lymphatic Tumors and Malformations

Tumors and malformations of the blood vessels are subject to wide variation in their nomenclature and even in criteria for their diagnosis. Those which are likely to be encountered in the practice of orthopedics involve both soft and hard tissues of the trunk and extremities.

A. Benign Hemangioma

Hemangiomas, benign lesions of vascular origin, are the most common of all tumors in man. Although generally congenital, they may also develop after local injury. The skin is the usual site, but any organ or tissue may be so involved. As a rule, hemangiomas tend to grow slowly. Thrombosis within the vascular spaces or hemorrhage in the tumor may be either spontaneous, posttraumatic, or the result of treatment; regardless of the underlying mechanism, partial necrosis then occurs. Shrinking of the scar tissue which replaces the dead tissue may cause the mass to decrease in size.

1. Pathology

Gross anatomy. Hemangiomas range in size from a few millimeters to many centimeters. The more vascular parts are soft and compressible, and their color varies from bright red to dark blue. Areas where fibrosis has occurred are pale and firm, while calcified or ossified thrombi appear as small, hard nodules up to 0.5 cm in diameter. The tumors possess no real demarcating "capsule," and hence a boundary with surrounding tissue is not easily identifiable on gross inspection. The only possible exception is a lesion in the skeleton, where vascular spaces may readily be distinguished from normal fatty marrow and cancellous or cortical bone.

Histologic changes. Widely varying types of hemangiomas are identifiable depending upon the size of the predominant vascular spaces. On such a basis, capillary, cavernous, venous, and mixed tumors can be defined. When extensive replacement by poorly demarcated tissue has occurred, the term, sclerosing hemangioma, is appropriate; in this condition the capillaries are small, thin-walled, and collapsed, with a single layer of endothelial cells supported on a recognizable reticulum. Larger spaces of similar structure are present in cavernous hemangiomas. The rarer venous angioma has even thinner walls with no demonstrable reticulum but occasional smooth-muscle cells; red blood cells and thrombi in various stages of lamination and organization are present in the vascular spaces. Calcified or ossified thrombi in soft-tissue tumors present as homogeneous nodules and foci of woven bone. Tissue from a hemangioma in bone through which there has recently been

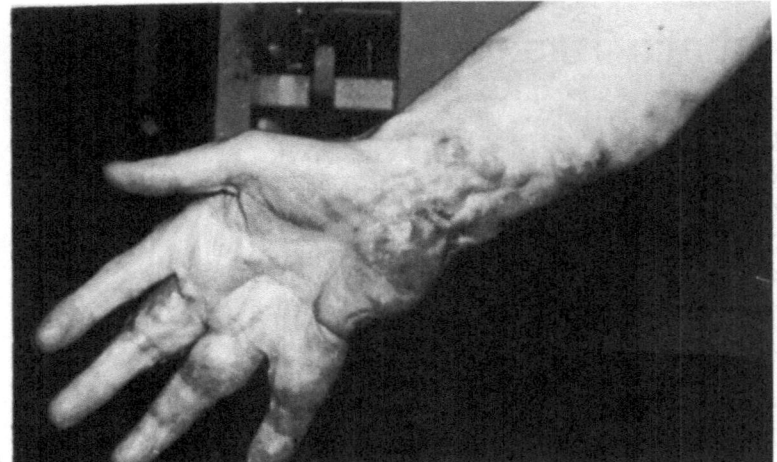

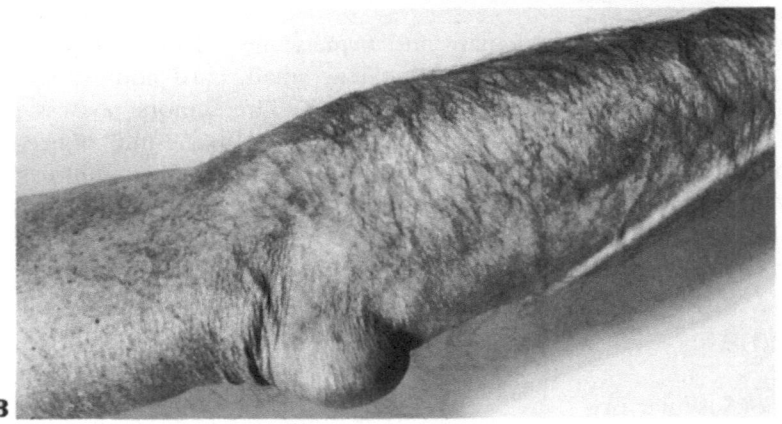

Fig. 21.1. Cavernous hemangiomas. **A** Lesion involving entire hand and distal portion of forearm. **B** Tumor located at elbow.

a fracture shows more extensive hemorrhage and vascular thrombosis, while the reparative callus may appear so active and undifferentiated as to cause confusion with a malignant lesion.

2. Clinical Manifestations

Superficial hemangiomas may be noted as disfiguring lesions at birth, whereas deeper tumors rarely cause psychologic difficulties, except that occasionally diffuse swelling is noted in a muscle or in a segment of a limb. At times the presenting manifestations depend on compression of adjacent structures or result from unequal rate of limb growth. Pain from the tumor itself is an uncommon symptom and does not indicate malignant transformation, for it is generally believed that this does not occur.

Clinical types. The capillary hemangioma can be divided into several categories: the strawberry nevus, the port-wine stain, and the sclerosing hemangioma (dermatofibroma). The strawberry nevus, which is most frequently encountered, is a circumscribed, bright red or purple warty projection of the skin, with delineated margins. It consists of a large number of minute capillaries protruding from the cutaneous surface. The port-wine stain is a flat type of capillary hemangioma, also made up of numerous dilated capillaries, but these are flush with the surface of the skin.

A second group is the cavernous hemangioma, which grossly resembles the capillary hemangioma. It consists of irregular, soft, single or multiple nodules with a cyanotic or purplish-red color (Fig. 21.1). The lesions are either flat, elevated, or warty in appearance.

The mixed hemangioma, falling into a third

group, is made up of the cavernous type, together with an overlying capillary (strawberry or port-wine) component. In its clinical manifestations, it possesses features of both of the others.

Finally, there is the systemic hemangioma, a rare tumor which generally affects a large part of an upper or lower limb but also extends onto the trunk. In most instances, the skin overlying it is marked with a port-wine stain. The involved extremity is usually enlarged and discolored at birth and then progressively increases in size.

Lesions involving bone. Hemangioma is distinctly rare in bones of the limbs. The most common site for the lesion in the skeleton is the vertebral column, usually within the vertebral body; however, there is some question as to whether the changes represent local varicosities rather than real tumors. The second most common site is the adult skull where the hemangioma is likely to be present as a solitary hard swelling a few centimeters in diameter.

The lesion causes swelling at the end of the bone, often interfering with the function of the adjacent joint and compressing vessels and nerves. Even more unusual is the spread of a soft-tissue hemangioma into neighboring bone, presumably by extension rather than by invasion. A tumor located within a bone occasionally leads to a pathologic fracture, producing local pain and dysfunction and, not infrequently, the formation of a large hematoma.

3. Hemangiomas of Special Interest

Disappearing bone disease. This condition, also called massive osteolysis, phantom bone disease, and Gorham's disease, may affect any bone or region of the skeleton in children and young adults. The basic abnormality is cavernous in type and, although the progress of the lesion is unpredictable, the condition is frequently self-limiting.

Maffucci's syndrome. This is a nonfamilial, noncongenital combination of hemangiomatosis and enchondromatosis (Ollier's disease) which appears before puberty. The vascular le-

sions are usually cavernous but they may be capillary or mixed, and they are widespread in many different tissues and body regions.

Benign metastasizing hemangioma. Such an entity is now generally regarded as a misnomer, since it almost certainly represents benign hemangiomas of multicentric origin, appearing at different times in the individual's life. It is not to be confused with metastasizing hemangioma which is another designation for hemangiosarcoma (see Section E, below).

Diffuse skeletal hemangiomatosis. This is an entity in which the tumor tissue is confined to the skeleton. It is a rare condition, usually involving bones of the trunk and limb girdles, which manifests a tendency to be self-limiting.

Hemangioma of synovium. This is a rare cause of recurrent idiopathic hemarthrosis which generally affects the knee. Exploration reveals a well-circumscribed, often pedunculated lesion that may readily be excised. Diffuse synovial involvement has also been reported, under which circumstance total removal is not always feasible and recurrence is likely. The histologic picture is one of mixed cavernous and capillary components.

4. Roentgenography

In long bones the radiographic appearance of a hemangioma is described as resembling a honeycomb. If expansion is a feature, a sunburst effect may be present, produced by the coarse perpendicular trabeculation of subperiosteal reactive new bone. Occasionally osteolysis may predominate, with the process extending to neighboring bones; this may be the result of involvement of the bone by a primarily soft-tissue hemangioma, achieving its most extensive state in the bizarre disappearing bone disease (see above). Hemangiomas of soft tissue possess a single radiographic characteristic which distinguishes them from similar tumors arising in bone. This is the presence of calcified or ossified thrombi (phleboliths) which are so typical as to be pathognomonic. Their presence or absence can help decide whether an intraosseous tumor originated in soft tissue or in the bone itself.

5. Other Diagnostic Procedures

In the presence of a hemangioma of the synovial membrane of the knee joint (see A-3, above), the full size, nature, and position of the lesion must be determined by arteriography and arthrography. For a small-vessel malformation, a localized, small-field angiographic examination with a rapid film changer is useful, since in this manner roentgenograms can be taken well into the capillary and early venous phases. It is also of value to obtain biplane views during angiography so as to achieve more accurate localization of the tumor. Venography is indicated if the arteriogram is normal in a patient suspected of having a vascular malformation.

6. Treatment

Since most soft-tissue hemangiomas cause no symptoms, treatment is not often called for. Also important to consider is the finding that these neoplasms characteristically enlarge rapidly in the first 6 to 9 months of life, to become almost quiescent later or grow at the same rate as the child for the next 6 to 12 months. Then regression begins spontaneously and may continue through puberty. In fact, resolution has been reported as occurring in about 30 percent of cases by age 3 years and in about 70 percent of cases by age 7 years.

Small superficial hemangiomas may be excised or cauterized, but deeper lesions in soft tissue and bone can be difficult to handle, excision and irradiation being the two possible therapeutic methods. However, it is necessary to point out that irradiation therapy carries the possibility of serious consequences, including malignancy in later years or the destruction of growth centers in the involved bone.

With regard to other therapeutic approaches, it has been found that resolution following repeated local applications of carbon dioxide snow occurs no faster than with no treatment. Short-wave diathermy has no role as therapy since it may result in the production of scar tissue.

Treatment may be necessary for some of the secondary effects of hemangiomas, such as unequal growth of long bones of the limb, bleeding, and a pathologic fracture. However, it is necessary to point out that any surgical procedure involving a direct attack on a hemangioma should be undertaken with caution because of the risk of uncontrollable hemorrhage. This also applies to the management of a pathologic fracture through a hemangioma of a long bone. Since healing can be expected to occur at a normal rate, it is customary to handle such a difficulty by closed means whenever possible.

B. Congenital Arteriovenous Fistula

A congenital arteriovenous fistula is a vascular anomaly or malformation in which there are communications of small caliber between the arterial and venous systems locally in the limb, with no intervening capillary bed. It differs from an acquired arteriovenous fistula in that it is unassociated with any antecedent trauma to the vascular tree; moreover, there are generally numerous connections between the arterial and venous trees, instead of one large fistulous tract joining a larger artery and its corresponding vein, as is present in the traumatic type. (For a discussion of acquired arteriovenous fistula, see Section F, Chapter 15.)

1. Pathology

Several different categories of congenital arteriovenous fistulae have been described [3,11]. In one (type I) there is a direct transverse-axis shunt (similar to a patent ductus arteriosus) present in the main peripheral arteries and veins. Such a situation is rarely observed (10 percent). In another category (type II), which represents the most frequent form (60 to 70 percent), there are multiple communications present in the soft tissues and frequently in bone, besides involvement of the main vessels. The lesion resembles a hemangioma (see Section A, above) in vascular pattern and is associated with a progressive increase in circulating blood volume. In type III, the main artery joins the main vein directly through dilated channels, without a capillary bed being present. This arrangement is rarely noted in the limbs and is found most frequently in the brain. The fistulous area resembles a well-defined tumor.

2. Clinical Manifestations

Because of the insidious growth of a congenital arteriovenous fistula, initially very few symptoms are produced. However, if the lesion begins to enlarge rapidly, then pain may be experienced locally, caused by pressure on neighboring peripheral nerves. After many years, there may be complaints associated with the onset of congestive heart failure, due to the protracted load placed on the heart by the persistent increase in venous return.

Examination of the involved limb reveals variable-sized masses under the skin (Fig. 21.2) which represent dilated varicose veins. Over them may be heard systolic and diastolic bruits, associated with thrills, although such findings are not as consistently noted as in the case of the acquired lesion. At times there may be venous pulsations present in the masses. An important differential point from the great majority of acquired arteriovenous fistulae is the finding of an increase in length of the affected limb, thus indicating that the abnormal communications were functioning before the epiphyseal centers were closed (see p. 36). Because of the greater blood flow through the skin proximal to the lesion, the cutaneous temperature in this portion of the extremity is higher than over the corresponding site on the opposite normal limb. Such a finding may be associated with a greater abundance of hair growth. Digital obstruction of the supplying artery causes a rise in blood pressure and a fall in pulse rate (positive Branham's bradycardiac sign), similar to the response observed in an acquired lesion. Below the level of the fistula, the cutaneous temperature is low and signs of venous stasis, such as brawniness and induration of the skin, may be present. Arteriography is very helpful in making the diagnosis of congenital arteriovenous fistula (Fig. 21.3).

3. Treatment

In contrast with an acquired arteriovenous fistula, the surgical treatment of the congenital arteriovenous fistula in the limbs is beset with many problems. However, with the greater use of serial arteriography to outline the extent of the involved vascular bed and the exact number, location, type, and size of the important channels through which most of the blood is passing, it has been possible to develop new surgical methods for coping with the serious situation [11].

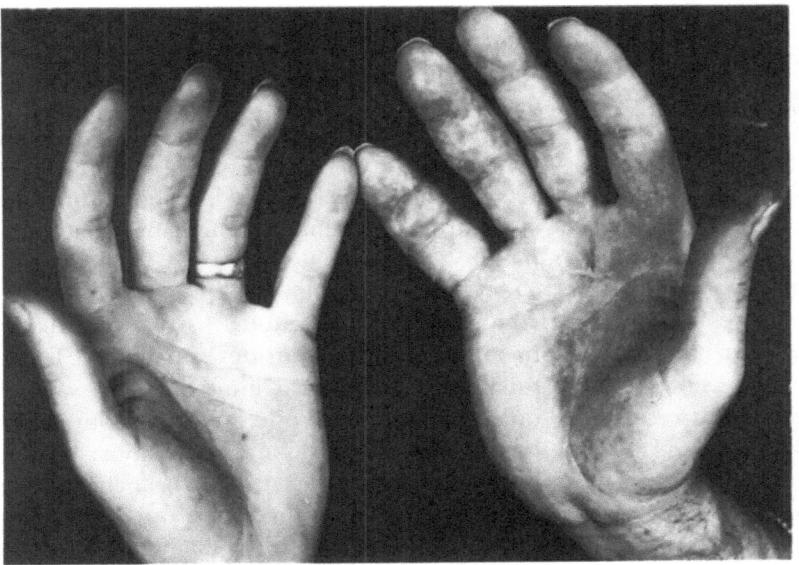
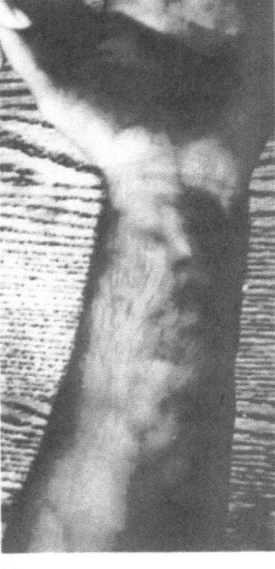

A   **B**

Fig. 21.2. Congenital arteriovenous fistulae. **A** Lesion involving fifth finger of right hand. **B** Lesion involving distal portion of forearm.

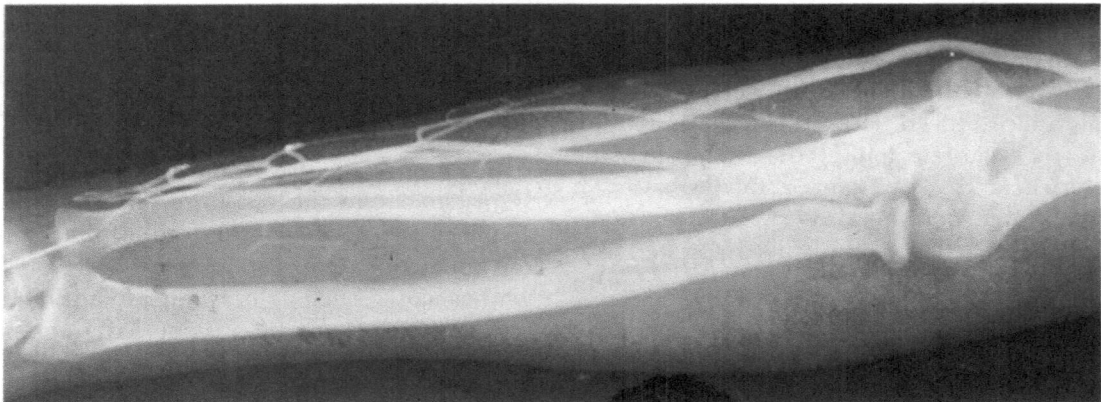

Fig. 21.3. Arteriogram of left forearm in a 19-year-old female patient. Contrast material was injected into the brachial artery in the arm with immediate visualization of the large veins, due to numerous direct communications between arterial and venous systems. Left upper limb was longer and larger in circumference than the opposite normal extremity.

Factors involved in choice of treatment program. The proper therapeutic approach depends mainly upon the anatomic characteristics of the vascular malformation. If the communications are small and not producing systemic changes and if the condition is stationary, a conservative program with regular clinical examinations is justified, at least temporarily. In all other instances, the possibility of surgical intervention should be considered provided there are no contraindications to such a step (see below).

Advantages of early surgery. If an operative approach is considered advisable, then this should be attempted as early as the fourth to the sixth year of life [11]. Such a point of view is based on the findings that spontaneous cure of the lesion is improbable and operative intervention beyond the age of 30 years is associated with a significant increase in the number of surgical complications. Moreover, there is a very good possibility that progression of the untreated lesion will occur, eventually resulting in congestive heart failure. Of course, if this situation already exists, or if bleeding, ulceration, or severe pain is present locally, then immediate surgery is indicated. Another reason for early operative intervention is that such a step may help prevent enlargement of the involved limb to the extent of becoming significantly longer than its normal mate.

Goals of surgical therapy. The purpose of the different operative procedures is the permanent elimination of the major vessels feeding the arteriovenous fistula, with normalization of the hemodynamic state. If this is not achievable, then the goal is to reduce the amount of blood passing into the venous system through the abnormal communications.

Surgical procedures. Operative intervention for the very rare type I and type III congenital arteriovenous fistulae (see above) is frequently successful. In type I, generally found in the arm, simply ligating the few vascular communications between the artery and vein results in a definitive interruption of the shunt. In type III, the entire mass can be excised in toto since structurally it resembles a hemangiomatous tumor.

Attempts to deal with the common type II congenital arteriovenous fistula by surgical means can only be considered palliative. Unfortunately, even such a limited aim is satisfied only after extensive operative procedures, performed on several separate occasions. They involve serial ligations of the branches of the main artery feeding the lesion and of the corresponding tributaries of the main vein. Of prime importance in the execution of such an approach is detailed information regarding the local arterial and venous trees derived from serial arteriograms. The purpose of the procedure is the interruption of all blood flow into and out of the soft tissues and bone. Viability of the limb is maintained by circulation through collateral arterial vessels arising proximal and distal to the fistula. However, despite all precautions, necrosis of the hand or foot may still follow, particularly if the lesion is located in the forearm or leg.

In some patients suffering from a type II lesion, a major amputation may have to be performed [1]. This applies to those in whom the above-described surgical procedure was not followed by a successful outcome, with the subsequent appearance of congestive heart failure, the development of large bleeding cutaneous ulcers overlying the lesion, or the occurrence of gangrene of distal structures.

Other operative approaches. A number of other surgical procedures have been utilized in the treatment of congenital arteriovenous fistula, but for the most part they have produced unsatisfactory results. These include extirpation of varicose veins; ligation of proximal main artery or arteries at the level of the forearm or leg; and extensive ligation of branches of the main artery and vein, followed by injection of sclerosing solution.

C. Glomus Tumor (Subungual Tumor)

The glomus tumor (angiomyoneuroma; glomangioma) is a rare congenital vascular anomaly found in the nail bed of fingers and toes, the palm of the hand, the sole of the foot, and, less often, the forearm. The age incidence is very broad and the distribution between the sexes is about equal. Histologically, the lesion represents an overgrowth of the structures found in the normal glomus, i.e., the arteriovenous anastomosis and its vascular and nervous components. (For the anatomic and physiologic characteristics of the normal glomus, see B-2 and C-4, respectively, Chapter 1.)

1. Anatomic Characteristics

The three major components of the glomus tumor are epithelioid cells, thin-walled vascular spaces, and a collagenous stroma, the proportion of these structures varying widely from lesion to lesion. Although the resemblance to the normal glomus is notable, the mass is many times larger and shows much less organization of form. Usually single, the tumor occurs in the sites of distribution of the glomus itself. It consists of a subcutaneous or, more commonly, a subungual body, varying from 0.8 to 2.5 cm in diameter, which is deep red to purple or blue in color and is sharply demarcated from surrounding tissue by a capsule. Although it primarily affects soft tissue, it can also involve bone, either by eroding it from adjacent structures or, more rarely, by primary intraosseous development. The tuft of a terminal phalanx is the usual location for the abnormality.

2. Clinical Manifestations

Clinically the glomus tumor is identified by intense, sharp, burning pain in the vicinity of the lesion which radiates up the entire limb. The symptom may appear spontaneously or is initiated by exposure to cold or heat or by dependency; elevation of the limb relieves the pain. Patients have been found to go to extremes of bizarre behavior in order to protect the affected limb from contact with any object. Applying pressure to the overlying skin using the head of a pin helps identify the tumor because excruciating pain is experienced when it is compressed. If the lesion is in a subungual location, the involved nail, as well as the phalanx, may be definitely deformed (Fig. 21.4A and B).

The diagnosis of a glomus tumor is often delayed for surprisingly long periods, even several years, probably because of lack of awareness on the part of the physician or because of a slow increase in the severity of the pain or absence of a visible lesion. When differential diagnosis is attempted, first thought is given to melanoma, while angioma and neurofibroma also merit consideration.

3. Therapy

Treatment is provided by complete local excision which generally produces dramatic relief; the sensitivity of the lesion may call for general

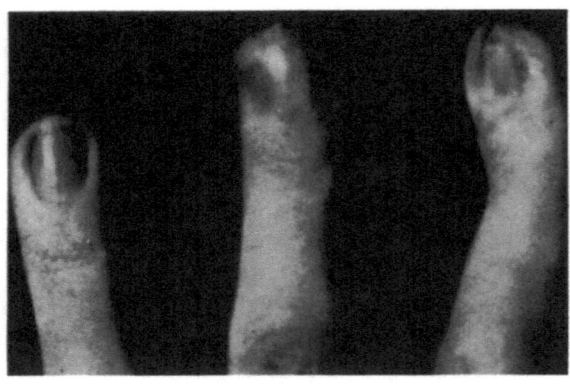
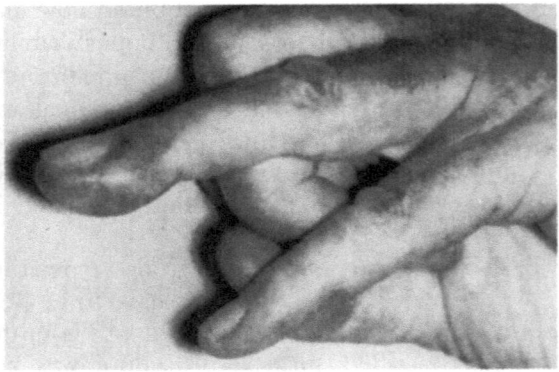

A   **B**

Fig. 21.4. Glomus tumor. **A** Lesion located at tip of left third finger, deforming the digit. From Stout AP: Tumor of the neuromyo-arterial glomus. Am J Cancer 24:255, 1935. Reproduced with the permission of the American Journal of Cancer. **B** Lesion of the fourth finger of long duration, producing bone erosion as detemined by x ray. Excision revealed a small mass, red in color and granular in appearance on section. From Booher RJ: Tumors arising from blood vessels in the hands and feet. Clin Orthop 19:71, 1961. Reproduced with the permission of J.P. Lippincott Co., Philadelphia.

rather than local anesthesia. Those tumors which are the most difficult to locate and eradicate are the small subungual lesions. After incomplete removal, symptoms usually remain. However, the persistence or recurrence of pain following operation may at times also be due to hypersensitivity at the original tumor site or to formation of a neuroma in the scar [9].

D. Hemangiopericytoma

The distinction of hemangiopericytoma as a tumor entity was first proposed by Stout and Murray [10]. It is an uncommon, painless neoplasm of soft tissue, and rarely is it noted in bone. Malignant lesions have been described.

The specific abnormality of hemangiopericytoma is the so-called pericyte of Zimmermann, which is probably a smooth muscle cell possessing no obvious fibrils but capable of contracting. Pericytes normally lie outside the basement membrane of the capillary; upon proliferation, they are separated from the central vascular lumen by reticulin fibers which may be seen with silver staining. The pericyte is probably the precursor of the epithelioid cell found in the glomus tumor (see Section C, above).

1. Pathology

Gross changes. When in an intraosseous location, the tumor is pale, fibrillary, and of soft or rubbery consistency, with no surrounding zone of dense bone. It may be encapsulated, demonstrating no evidence of hemorrhage or necrosis in the tumor tissue.

Histologic changes. Microscopic examination of a hemangiopericytoma reveals a whorled, almost fibromatous pattern, with sheets of cells of uniform appearance surrounding many small clefts. Some of the latter can be positively identified as blood channels (small capillaries), although generally these are obscure or occult and difficult to recognize without using reticulum stains. Clumps of large numbers of tumor cells are found to bulge into the slitlike lumen of a vascular space, but yet they remain outside the basement membrane. Their appearance is distinctly epithelioid. Near the periphery of the lesion, they may be more spindle-shaped, lying in interlacing bundles.

2. Clinical Manifestations

The symptoms and signs of intraosseous hemangiopericytomata are quite variable. Aching discomfort rather than acute pain is the major complaint; swelling is not a regular feature since the tumors are usually too small to produce such an alteration.

3. Roentgenographic Changes

The radiographic findings in hemangiopericytoma are of an intraosseous destructive lesion with an ill-defined margin. There may be expansion of the cortex and even penetration to involve surrounding soft tissues.

4. Treatment

No principles for treatment can logically be proposed since so few cases of hemangiopericytoma have been reported. When unequivocally benign, curettage may be considered, whereas radical excision is advisable for malignant lesions which are accessible, reserving radiotherapy for those in inaccessible sites.

E. Hemangiosarcoma

Hemangiosarcoma, a rare malignant neoplasm originating from blood vessel tissues, has an abnormal endothelial cell as its dominant feature. Since the lesion possesses an intrinsic vasoformative capacity, there is a tendency for the proliferating endothelioblasts to produce recognizable blood channels.

The condition is only occasionally present in bone [2]. When found in such a location, generally direct invasion from adjacent soft tissue or metastasis from a distant primary lesion has taken place. There is no reason to believe that the original tumor is due to malignant change in a benign hemangioma.

1. Pathology

The biologic behavior of hemangiosarcoma is quite variable, being to some extent related to the histologic pattern. At one extreme is the low-grade or doubtfully malignant tumor with many vascular channels and spaces surrounded by reasonably well-differentiated endothelial cells, whereas at the other extreme is the very cellular lesion showing marked pleomorphism, many mitoses, few or no blood-containing spaces, and propensity for early and widespread metastasis.

Gross anatomy. The appearance of the tumor depends upon its vascularity. Very cellular lesions tend to be pale and soft, often with areas of mucoid degeneration or frank necrosis. Those containing more blood vary in color from dark red to blue, with brown areas of pigment deposition. Cavities may be discernible containing blood or recent clot; organized thrombi are unlikely to be present.

Histologic anatomy. Microscopic examination of tissue from a hemangiosarcoma usually reveals findings which vary considerably from lesion to lesion and even within a single location. Anastomosing vascular spaces are of widely differing diameter or may on occasion be absent. When present, they are lined by atypical, heaped-up anaplastic endothelial cells which in solid tumors tend to occur as rosettes, clumps, cords, or sheets. The cells themselves are round, oval, or spindle-shaped, being diagnostic of the condition even in the absence of vascular spaces. However, the latter are frequently found if careful search is made through several sections. There is generally little intercellular stroma, but silver stains will demonstrate the presence of reticular fibers around cords and clumps of cells. It is commonly accepted that the more differentiated tumors, with recognizable vascular spaces enclosing red blood cells and surrounded by layers of endothelial cells, are less malignant than those showing only solid sheets of barely identifiable cells, with few or no vascular spaces.

2. Clinical Manifestations

No particular sex or age predilection has been reported in hemangiosarcoma, and the distribution throughout the skeleton appears to be quite random, with the exception that vertebral involvement is rare and pelvic spread is uncommon. The presenting complaints are pain and tenderness, followed by swelling and, occasionally, the symptoms of a pathologic fracture. Rarely, a bruit may be heard or pulsations detected over the tumor. Because of lack of specificity of the clinical picture, the diagnosis of hemangiosarcoma frequently must rely on histologic examination of biopsy material. Even with such an approach, difficulty may be encountered in differentiating the tumor from hemangioendothelioma and malignant spindle-cell sarcoma.

Like any malignant lesion, hemangiosarcoma can be expected to metastasize. The primary route of dissemination is hematogenous, but this is one of the few bone tumors which can also spread to the regional lymph nodes.

3. Roentgenographic Changes

The diagnosis of a hemangiosarcoma of bone on radiographic evidence alone is to be regarded as virtually impossible. The site of the tumor demonstrates patchy rarefaction due to destruction of cancellous bone; this type of change may extend into and through the cortex in several places to stimulate the formation of reactive subperiosteal bone. Involvement of bone is often extensive, suggesting multiple local lesions. Where tumor growth and accompanying bone destruction are less rapid, an expanding lesion may be seen, with an intact or almost intact shell of subperiosteal new bone and a trabecular pattern not unlike that associated with aneurysmal bone cyst (see Section F, below).

4. Treatment

No single form of treatment has been sufficiently successful to recommend its routine use in hemangiosarcoma. If biopsy shows a mildly malignant tumor in an appropriate site, radical local excision may suffice [4,8], or this approach may be combined with irradiation using large doses (400 rads or more) before or after surgery, or both. For more obviously malignant lesions, amputation is indicated, with or without irradiation; when the tumor site precludes surgery, radiotherapy is the only available course. Hemangiosarcomas are so scarce that reports of the results of adequate treatment with cytotoxic agents are too few for proper evaluation of such an approach.

The results of treatment vary widely. Patients with very cellular undifferentiated tumors fre-

quently die within 3 years of diagnosis, and their 5-year survival rate is about 10 percent. Much better results can be obtained with the less obviously malignant tumors, and the overall outlook is very similar to that which holds for fibrosarcoma of bone, with 30 percent of patients surviving for 5 years.

F. Aneurysmal Bone Cyst

An aneurysmal bone cyst is not truly a vascular tumor since it neither arises from nor contains predominantly vasoformative tissue. Still, this unusual but well-defined entity merits inclusion here because of its similarity to a hemangioma (see Section A, above). Its recognition is attributable to Jaffe and Lichtenstein [5] who separated it from the conglomeration of so-called giant-cell tumor variants.

Aneurysmal bone cysts are benign lytic tumors of bone which are found more often in females than males; usually children or young adults under the age of 30 years are affected. The most common site is the metaphysis of a long bone, with the vertebrae being next in order of frequency; however, almost any bone in the body may be so involved. The lesions tend to enlarge rapidly and bulge out from the cortex.

1. Pathology

Gross changes. When encountered surgically or examined in the rarely available amputation specimen, the gross features of an aneurysmal bone cyst are blood-filled spaces of varying size enclosed within a shell of bone and separated from one another by strands of stromal tissue which may contain trabeculae of bone. Blood in the spaces may be clotted, with subsequent organization into fibrous tissue. Communications exist among the "aneurysmal" spaces so that they share a "pool" of blood which is slowly replaced. Entering a space during operative exploration causes a continuous oozing of blood which is extremely difficult to control, even though the flow is not pulsatile.

Histologic changes. The walls making up the compartments lack the features of blood vessels and have no endothelial lining, but they are separated from one another by solid stromal tissue which is very variable in quantity but of rather constant composition. Spindle cells of fairly uniform size predominate. Scattered among them are hemosiderin-laden phagocytes and multinucleated giant cells. The thicker strands of solid tissue have a central core of osteoid tissue which may be calcified to form a true trabecula of new (tumor) bone. Granulation tissue is found in those areas of tumor where organization of a thrombus is occurring or where there has been extravasation of blood from the spaces into the solid tissue. This may be expected more particularly if there has been a recent fracture in or through the lesion. Under such circumstances, the presence of the later stage of fracture repair by cellular callus can cause great difficulty in interpreting whether the lesion is malignant.

2. Clinical Manifestations

When a long bone in a limb is involved, the presenting findings are swelling near a joint and limitation of motion, associated usually with dull aching pain and tenderness; the symptoms are aggravated and accompanied by dysfunction if a pathologic fracture supervenes. The growth of the tumor is quite variable; occasionally large ones are found by chance on either physical or radiographic examination.

3. Roentgenographic Changes

A typical aneurysmal bone cyst is usually simple to diagnose radiographically. However, when the features are less characteristic, there may be some difficulty differentiating it from a giant-cell tumor, simple bone cyst, enchondroma, and hemangioma. Such a situation exists, as for example, when a fibula contains a central lesion causing fusiform expansion.

At the metaphysis of a long bone, the picture of a lesion is one of a well-circumscribed eccentric rarefaction with marked expansion of the cortex, the latter frequently being less than a millimeter thick. The sparse coarse trabeculae provide a loculated appearance, calling forth the descriptive term "soap bubbles." It is rare for an epiphyseal plate to be crossed and quite

uncommon for the lesion to burst through the limiting shell of subperiosteal bone into the soft tissue or to penetrate a joint cavity.

4. Treatment

Although aneurysmal bone cysts are recognized as being benign, treatment may be required to relieve pain or local pressure and to remove the local swelling. This is best done surgically, but operation is not always feasible. A lesion in a readily accessible bone in a limb may be explored, curetted, and packed with iliac bone chips, using strut grafts for support of articular surfaces where necessary. Since the recurrence rate is about 20 to 25 percent, in the case of tumors which are inaccessible or in sites where uncontrollable bleeding may be a serious hazard, as for example, the sacrum, treatment by irradiation may be employed. As another alternative, limited surgical removal followed by radiotherapy is possible. However, some clinicians are distinctly wary of recommending radiotherapy for aneurysmal bone cysts at any stage, since a few of them have been found later to undergo sarcomatous degeneration. An untreated or poorly treated lesion may eventually become very large, at times resulting in the need for amputation of the limb.

G.   Other Vascular Anomalies

1.   Klippel-Trenaunay Syndrome

Klippel-Trenaunay syndrome (venous dysplasia group) is a congenital vascular malformation which is present at birth. Its manifestations are varicose veins on a single lower limb, associated with cutaneous hemangioma, decreased lymphatic trunks [7], local soft-tissue hypertrophy, and elongation of the extremity with lengthening of the bone. Besides the dilatation of the superficial veins, there is malformation of the deep venous system, the popliteal or femoral vein being compressed by a fibrovascular band or surrounded by a fibrous sheath. At times there may be complete agenesis of the collecting veins in the limb [6].

The differentiation of Klippel-Trenaunay syndrome from primary and secondary varicosities and from congenital arteriovenous fistula (see Section B, above) can be made by laboratory means. Venography reveals the absence or malformations of the deep venous circulation, while arteriography may visualize arteriovenous fistulae at distal ends of small arterial branches which open into typical vascular pools, frequently located within bones.

It is apparent from the above that attempting to treat the varicosities of Klippel-Trenaunay syndrome by multiple ligation or by stripping of the involved vessels, procedures ordinarily utilized in primary varicosities, would make the condition much worse. The only therapeutic approach that could conceivably be of value is some type of reconstruction of the deep venous system.

2. Kaposi's Sarcoma

Kaposi's sarcoma (multiple idiopathic hemorrhagic sarcoma of Kaposi) is a multifocal neoplasm of blood vessel origin with a malignant potential which is located in the skin of the extremities. It is seen most frequently in males, appearing after the age of 40 years. The cause of the condition is not known, although one view holds that it is a dysplasia of the reticuloendothelial system.

The early lesions are composed of bluish-red and reddish-brown macules, varying from a few millimeters to a few centimeters in diameter. They slowly become elevated and then multiply and coalesce to form infiltrated bluish-black hemorrhagic plaques or firm nodules. Telangiectasis may also be noted. Together with the growth of the lesions, definite nonpitting edema of the involved limb occurs. If the neoplasm also affects the viscera, the disease is usually fatal, but when it is limited to the skin, the prognosis is fairly good. However, many patients have a second neoplasm, most frequently a lymphoma or leukemia. Fractional x-ray therapy may be followed by a dramatic improvement in the clinical picture. For extensive involvement, it may be necessary to resort to various forms of local and systemic chemotherapy.

3. Telangiectasis

Telangiectasis has been considered to be a true tumor of blood vessels, although it may also be an acquired alteration of the normal vascular pattern, as in the case of simple telangiectasis. The latter may be found in association with such conditions as acne rosacea, disseminated lupus erythematosus, progressive systemic sclerosis, syphilis, and epithelioma (encircling and covering the lesion). It may also appear after prolonged exposure of the skin to wind and sun or heat from other sources, and it may follow treatment with x-ray or radium. An increased level of estrogen, both absolute and relative to other hormones, may induce the development of spider angiomas at predisposed locations in susceptible individuals. Several clinical types of telangiectasis are presented below.

Cherry angioma (senile vascular nevus). This condition consists of tufts of dilated cutaneous capillaries which give the appearance of bright red or purplish raised papules. The lesions are found on the limbs and trunks of middle-aged or elderly individuals. There is no significance associated with their presence.

Spider angioma (spider nevus). This vascular abnormality has a central, raised, dilated arteriolar feeder vessel communicating directly with radiating venular tributaries running parallel to the skin surface. Surrounding the lesion is an area of erythema. The condition is found on the dorsum of the hand and generally in the skin of the upper half of the body in apparently random fashion. Pressure on the lesion causes blanching. The alterations may be noted shortly after birth or during adolescence. They resemble those of the acquired spider nevi present in pregnant women and in patients with liver disease (hepatic cirrhosis), pulmonary disease, and scleroderma.

Hereditary hemorrhagic telangiectasis (Rendu-Osler-Weber disease). This disorder is an inherited maldevelopment of minute blood vessels of the skin, mucous membranes, and viscera. It is characterized by multiple, slightly raised, small spiderlike telangiectatic lesions. It appears to have a definite familial incidence and is most common among Jews. Because of developmental defects in the vessel wall, hemorrhage from the nose, mouth, and gastrointestinal tract is common.

4. Phlebectasia

Phlebectasia is a congenital vascular anomaly which affects the venous system in a limb. It consists of definite enlargement and fusiform dilatation of venous channels; such changes are associated with an increase in size of capillaries, which results in the formation of capillary lakes, but without any abnormal communications with the arterial circulation. The possibility has been advanced that the condition is a variant of a cavernous hemangioma (see A-2, above).

Clinically, the patient may experience a sensation of heaviness, aching, and fatigue in the affected extremity with mild exertion. Examination reveals numerous superficial, thin-walled channels (the dilated venous sinusoids filled with blood), these vessels giving the limb a cyanotic appearance. The pressure in the prominent veins is normal as demonstrated by their collapse on elevation of the extremity. No abnormal pulsations, thrills, or bruits are present in the vicinity of the lesion. The architecture of the venous network can be visualized by venography.

Phlebectasia may resemble several other conditions. It must be differentiated from a congenital arteriovenous fistula (see Section B, above), in which regard arteriography and oxygen determinations of venous blood are helpful. In primary varicosities, the superficial veins are dilated and tortuous; however, the changes occur in the great or small saphenous vein system, whereas in phlebectasia, the abnormalities do not conform to such a normal anatomic distribution. Moreover, in the latter no regurgitant flow of blood can be demonstrated. Phlebectasia may also be mistaken for livedo reticularis associated with telangiectasis. Finally, it may resemble conditions producing atrophic changes in the skin, such as overexposure to roentgen rays, ultraviolet light, or sunlight.

5. Angiokeratoma Corporis Diffusum

Angiokeratoma corporis diffusum (Fabry's disease) is an inherited systemic disorder of glycolipid metabolism which is associated with swelling of the lower limbs, digital color changes in the fingers (Raynaud's syndrome), articular pain, proteinuria, enlargement of the heart, and hypertension. Also present are cuta-neous lesions on the lower part of the trunk, the proximal segments of the lower limbs, and less frequently the upper extremities. Severe pain may be experienced in the limbs, associated with signs of vasospasm and abnormal sweating.

The characteristic pathologic alteration consists of deposition of glycolipid in the circular smooth-muscle fibers of the vessels, producing large vascular spaces. The lesions are noted in the skin, cardiac muscle and connective tissue, ganglion cells of the central nervous system, and glomerular cells. Death in Fabry's disease is generally due to progressive renal failure.

H. Lymphatic Tumors

Lymphatic tumors are similar in many regards to tumors of blood vessels except that they contain lymph instead of blood. Nonmalignant lymphatic tumors are divided into simple, cavernous, and cystic types. A malignant type of lymphatic tumor is lymphangiosarcoma.

1. Simple Lymphangioma

A simple lymphangioma, which is usually congenital and benign, is made up of a large network of lymphatic spaces fed by lymphatic channels. The lesion is generally found in the skin and mucous membranes and is slow-growing.

2. Cavernous Lymphangioma

A congenital tumor also, cavernous lymphangioma is composed of numerous large dilated lymph sinuses containing lymph and occasionally blood. The masses are generally found in the skin and subcutaneous tissue, although being present elsewhere, too. One type, lymphangioma circumscriptum, is usually located on the upper limb, being made up of a number of thick-walled vesicles filled with clear lymph.

3. Cystic Lymphangioma

A cystic lymphangioma, which is considered to develop from embryonal rests, usually is first noted in early childhood. It consists of several cysts lined with endothelium and containing serous fluid or lymph. Histologically it resembles the cavernous lymphangioma except that the lymph spaces are larger.

4. Lymphangiosarcoma

Lymphangiosarcoma is a rare but very serious complication of long-standing lymphedema, most often noted in patients with postmastectomy swelling of an upper limb. In the case of the latter, generally the lesion develops from 5 to 15 years after operation.

The first sign of tumor is the spontaneous appearance of purplish bruise marks or tender cutaneous nodules on the anterior surface of the involved arm. Then the lesions break down to form crusted ulcers or areas of necrosis. Biopsy study of material from the tumor reveals that the tissue is made up of neoplastic endothelial cells which form poorly defined lymph spaces or solid structures. Neighboring tissues may show signs of infiltration by tumor cells.

References

1. Coursley G, Ivins IC, Barker NW: Congenital arteriovenous fistulas in the extremities: An analysis of 69 cases. Angiology 7:201, 1956

2. Dahlin DC: Bone Tumors. General Aspects and Data on 3987 Cases, 2nd ed. Springfield, Ill, Charles C Thomas, 1967

3. Flynn PJ, Mulder DG: Congenital arteriovenous fistula. West J Surg 67:31, 1959

4. Hartmann WH, Stewart FW: Hemangioendothelioma of bone. Unusual tumor characterized by indolent course. Cancer 15:846, 1962

5. Jaffe HL, Lichtenstein L: Solitary unicameral bone cyst: With emphasis on the roentgen picture, the pathologic appearance, and the pathogenesis. Arch Surg 44:1004, 1942

6. Lindenauer SM: The Klippel-Trenaunay syndrome: Varicosity, hypertrophy, and hemangioma with no arteriovenous fistula. Ann Surg 162:303, 1965

7. O'Donnell TF Jr, Edwards JM, Kinmonth JB: Lymphography in congenital mixed vascular deformities of the lower extremities. J Cardiovasc Surg 17:535, 1976

8. Otis J, Hutter RVP, Foote FW Jr, et al: Hemangioendothelioma of bone. Surg Gynecol Obstet 127:295, 1968

9. Shugart RR, Soule EH, Johnson EW Jr: Glomus tumors. Surg Gynecol Obstet 117:334, 1963

10. Stout AP, Murray MR: Hemangiopericytoma; vascular tumor featuring Zimmermann's pericytes. Ann Surg 116:26, 1942

11. Vollmar JF, Stalker CG: The surgical treatment of congenital arteriovenous fistulas in the extremities. J Cardiovasc Surg 17:340, 1976

Chapter 22

Vascular Complications of Therapy in Musculoskeletal Disorders

---

Part 1   Iatrogenic Vascular Entities

The utilization of appliances and conventional operative procedures for common orthopedic or general surgical difficulties has, on occasion, been responsible for disastrous vascular complications, even gangrene necessitating a major amputation of a limb. Although such situations have most often developed in patients with an underlying impaired local arterial circulation, at times a similar adverse response has been noted in persons with a previously normal local blood flow but subjected to heroic therapy. This chapter deals with various aspects of the problem.

A.   Edema Caused by Protracted Compression of a Limb by a Cast

Not infrequently a properly or tightly applied body or limb cast is responsible for swelling of an extremity, either during the period when it is worn or generally immediately after its removal. In most instances the abnormality becomes less as physical activity is again resumed and then disappears in several days. (For a discussion of pressure necrosis, a much more serious consequence of this type of technique, see B-3, below.)

1.   Pathogenesis

The swelling has been attributed to a number of different mechanisms, among which is the long period of dependency, resulting in loss of vascular tone in the microcirculation of the cutaneous and subcutaneous tissues. Another factor is the continuous pressure on the various vascular structures by the cast, also producing paralysis of the local circulation exposed to this force. Other mechanisms which have been implicated are reduction of muscle tone, absence of muscle contractions, and loss of support to the superficial veins normally provided by the muscle and subcutaneous tissue, the latter structures now suffering from atrophy of disuse produced by the period of immobilization. All such changes result in a rise in venous pressure, which is reflected back into the microcirculation as an increase in capillary filtration pressure. As a consequence, there is a greater transudation of fluid into the tissue spaces, producing edema. An adjunctive factor facilitating this process is an associated increase in capillary permeability resulting from a relative state of ischemia of the cutaneous tissues (including vascular components) produced by the compressive action of the cast. Finally, it is possible that flooding of the paralyzed capillary bed by a large quantity of blood (after elimination of the extrinsic pressure provided by the cast) also contributes to an increase in capillary filtration pressure.

Another etiologic factor in the formation of swelling is destruction of thin-walled lymphatics in the area of the original injury. Since such vessels do not regenerate, signs of lymphatic stasis may appear soon after the external pressure produced by the cast is eliminated. This generally takes the form of hard, nonpitting edema found in the most dependent portion of the limb, as around the ankle and wrist and on the dorsum of the foot and hand. The appearance of permanent lymphedema, however, is highly suggestive of the existence of hypoplastic or aplastic lymph channels and warrants further investigation using lymphangiography. Of importance in this regard is the fact that some patients with chronic congenital lymphedema only develop findings after a sprain, a strain, or a fracture. The explanation is that the trauma to local lymph channels produced by these conditions and by their treatment (including the application of a cast in many cases) causes an overload of the existing inadequate but previously asymptomatic lymphatic system, thus leading to clinical lymphedema.

2.   Differential Diagnosis

It is essential to differentiate the nonspecific swelling which becomes prominent on removal of the cast from iliofemoral or popliteal thrombophlebitis (see A-3, Chapter 18), which might have resulted either from the original injury or from prolonged immobilization of the limb. Of interest in this regard is the fact that when the constricting effect of the cast is removed, generally the swelling resulting from an occlusion of a main collecting vein becomes more marked for a short period of time and then slowly recedes over 2 or 3 weeks if proper therapy is immediately instituted. In fact, in some instances, the tension within the cast built up by the developing edema may produce such severe pain as to require removal of the constriction. On the other hand, this never occurs in the case of the uncomplicated swelling described above. Moreover, at no time is the latter associated with any systemic response, in contrast with iliofemoral thrombophlebitis in which a rise in temperature, pulse rate, and respiration is almost invariably noted.

B.   Vascular Abnormalities following Surgical Therapy

1.   Treatment of Fractures, Dislocations, and Joint Pathology

Aside from the close association that exists between fractures of long bones and coincident injury of main arterial and venous channels (see Chapter 15), surgical treatment of the fracture itself may inadvertently also result in the production of vascular lesions. Some of the more common of these complications are presented below.

Circulatory complications of intervertebral disk operations.   Among the lesions of the vascular system produced by the surgical approach to a herniated disk in the lumbar region is an arteriovenous fistula produced between the aorta or the iliac arteries and the inferior vena cava or iliac veins [2,21]. Operative trauma may also cause a false aneurysm to develop in the abdominal aorta or in the common iliac artery (see Section E, Chapter 15). Serious occult hemorrhage generally occurs if the aorta or an iliac artery is damaged, a situation which requires immediate laparotomy and arrest of bleeding, since otherwise mortality may exceed 50 percent [2].

Injury to vascular structures during intervertebral disk operations is generally due to perforation of the anterior longitudinal ligament by a curette or a pituitary rongeur. The less rigid inferior vena cava and iliac vein are partially immobilized against the vertebral column by the aorta or the iliac artery and hence both venous channels are in a position to be readily traumatized by the instrument.

Complications of internal fixation with screws. The use of Steinmann's pins [22] and of subtrochanteric osteotomy of the femur with internal fixation by a blade plate may be followed by such vascular lesions as false aneurysm [1,5,6] and laceration and thrombosis of the profunda femoris artery (Fig. 22.1) [12], thrombosis of

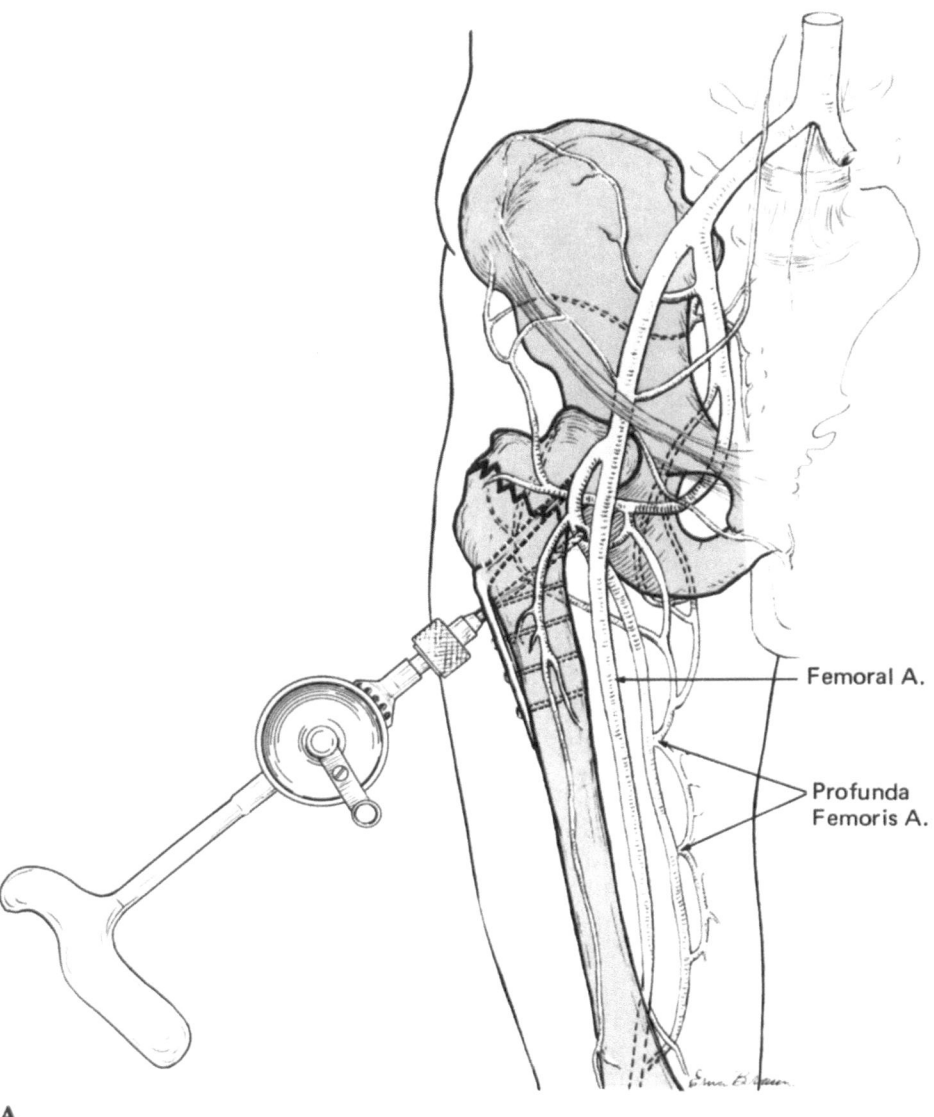

A

— Femoral A.

— Profunda
Femoris A.

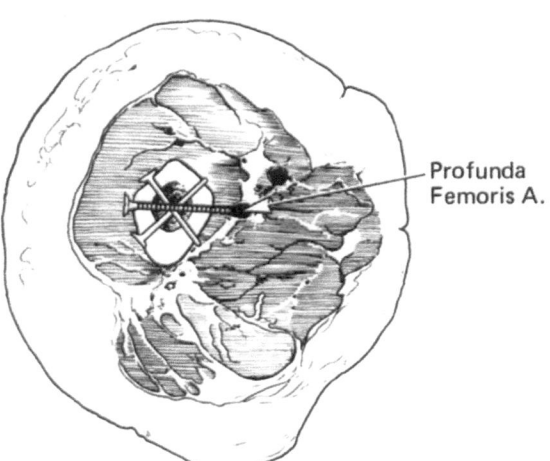

Profunda
Femoris A.

B

Fig. 22.1. Schematic representation of types of iatrogenic injury to the profunda femoris artery. **A** Penetration of vessel by drill point which passed beyond the medial surface of the femur. **B** Protrusion of a pin beyond the medial aspect of the cortex, with penetration of the vessel.

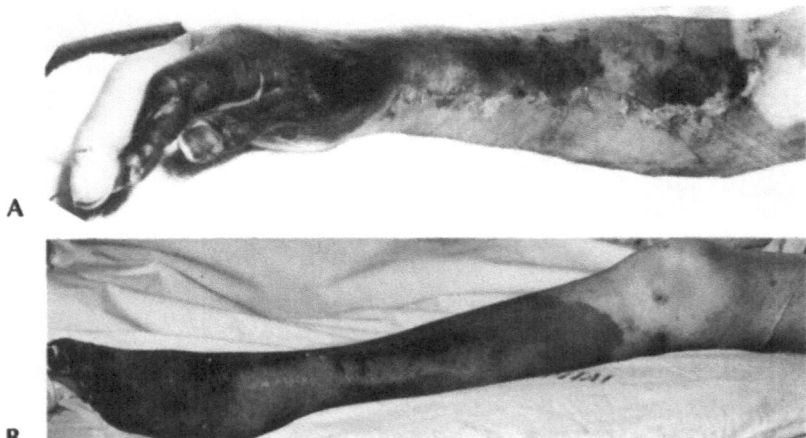

Fig. 22.2. Gangrene of extremities following operative treatment of fractures. **A** Open reduction of fracture of radius with removal of head. Inadvertent trauma to radial artery necessitating ligation of the vessel. Gangrene of thumb and index finger resulted. **B** Open reduction of fracture of the hip and internal fixation in an elderly patient with arteriosclerosis obliterans of the lower limbs. Gangrene produced as a result of trauma to collateral vessels during the course of operation.

the iliac artery, and peripheral arterial emboli arising in a false aneurysm of the iliac artery. In most instances the vascular lesions result from the use of pins or screws which are too long and misplaced, and, as a result, protrude excessively through the medial aspect of the cortex (Fig. 22.1B). The profunda femoris artery is particularly vulnerable to trauma from such a source since this vessel and its branches lie very close to the upper surface of the femur (Fig. 22.1).

Avascular necrosis of the femoral head (see Section F, Chapter 14) may be produced by blade plate fixation for intertrochanteric fractures, due to compromise of the local blood supply to the femoral head proper. As a consequence, secondary arthritis may develop, requiring either total hip replacement, a Moore prosthesis, or some other reconstructive approach.

Other orthopedic measures. Vascular structures have been damaged during reduction of humeral neck fractures and hip fractures (Fig. 22.2B). Avascular necrosis of the femoral head has been reported to occur from reduction of a congenital dislocation of the hip in young children [18]. Iliac arteries have been damaged by prolonged pressure of retractors, and fat embolism (see Chapter 16) has followed correction of contractures of the joints of the lower limbs. Intramedullary nailing may be responsible for vascular complications since collateral vessels may be injured in the process of obtain-

ing sufficient exposure to carry out the procedure. In contrast, closed intramedullary nailing minimizes such a possibility. Removal of cartilages from the knee joint (medial more often than lateral) may, by accidental protrusion of the scalpel, lacerate or transect the popliteal artery (Fig. 22.3). Such a situation requires immediate surgical repair, for otherwise necrosis of the foot may occur or a false aneurysm may develop.

2. Foot Surgery

Currently, the incidence of vascular complications following operations on the foot appears to be increasing (Figs. 22.4, 22.5B, and 22.6A and D). Such a situation may be due to a failure to recognize vascular deficiencies (Fig. 22.4) or to a more heroic approach than is warranted or safe to perform. It is, therefore, imperative to carry out a very careful vascular examination preoperatively (Table 5.2) and record the findings in detail on the progress sheet. Such a practice may at the same time help avoid the ever-threatening malpractice suit (see Section C, Chapter 26).

3. Pressure Necrosis from Adjunctive Measures

The improper application of a rigid cast or an elastic bandage following reduction of a fracture or for some other reason may be responsi-

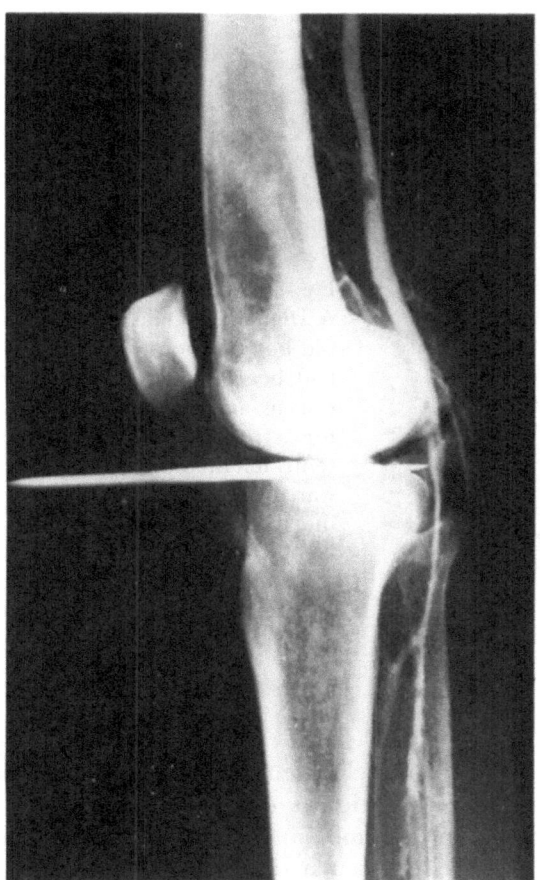

Fig. 22.3. Relationship of the popliteal artery to the medial meniscus of the knee, as noted in a cadaver. The proximity of the point of the scalpel blade (used in performing a meniscectomy) to the vessel is apparent.

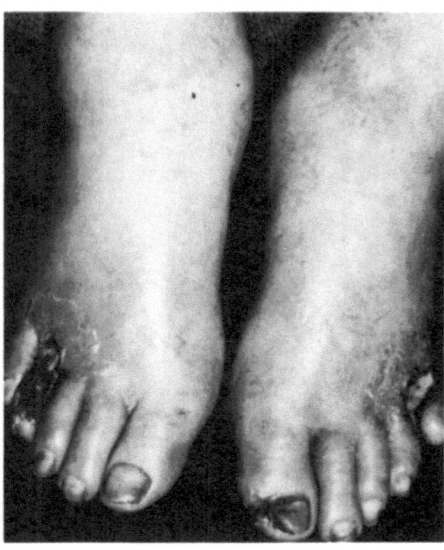

Fig. 22.4. Gangrene of fourth toe of right foot and fifth toe of left foot following operative procedures on hammer toes in an elderly patient with arteriosclerosis obliterans.

ble for the development of nutritional changes that could significantly alter prognosis regarding viability of the affected limb. This is particularly true in the case of fractures in the vicinity of the knee joint, since a tight cast used in such a site may produce spasm and even thrombosis of the popliteal artery, followed by gangrene of the foot in the majority of cases.

Aside from the direct effect upon the vascular tree, much more commonly the tight cast or tight elastic bandage produces protracted pressure ischemia of skin and subcutaneous tissue, particularly in locations overlying bony prominences. As a consequence, eventually the continuity of the skin is destroyed, with the production of an ulcer or localized gangrene, even in the presence of a previously normal local blood flow (Figs. 22.6B and D and 22.7–22.9). In the patient with a compromised arterial circulation, this type of response can be expected much more often, the lesion generally being quite extensive and in most instances resulting in the need for a major amputation.

Because of the dire consequences of faulty technique, every effort should be made to minimize the pressure applied to skin where it is not required, especially in the vicinity of bony prominences. Such a precaution is particularly applicable to the elderly patient who not infrequently is also suffering from arteriosclerosis obliterans.

C. Vascular Abnormalities following Conservative Therapy

1. Bryant Traction

Bryant traction for the treatment of fractures of the femur in children has been reported to be responsible for circulatory complications (Fig. 22.10), including ischemic fibrosis

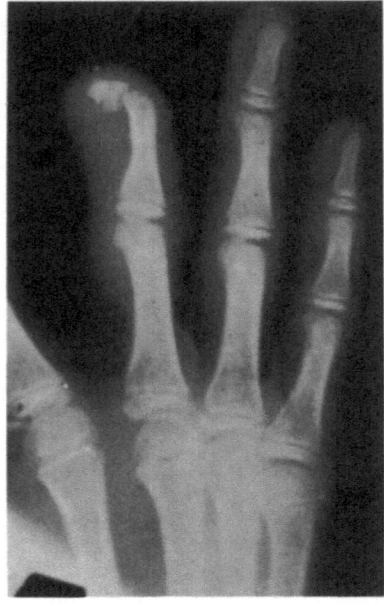
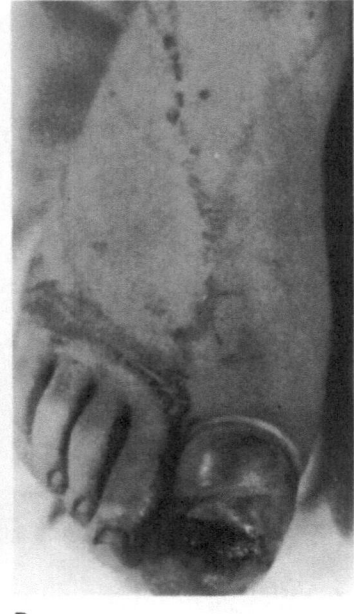

A   **B**

Fig. 22.5. Tourniquet gangrene. **A** Digital ischemia in a 12-year-old boy in whom a rubber band had been applied to the finger during an operative procedure for a paronychia and inadvertently left on for some time afterward. **B** Gangrene of great toe due to failure to remove a rubber band used as a tourniquet in the treatment of an ingrown toenail. Rubber band is noted in place at base of great toe.

[14,16]; the development of a circumferential band of necrosis of skin and underlying muscles in the calf region [16]; gangrene of the foot [16]; growth disturbances and limb shortening; contractural states of the thigh and calf; dysfunction of joints; and flail, shortened limbs (Fig. 22.11). Subsequently, the extremities may become hypersensitive to cold and prone to ulcer formation. Such serious complications are generally noted in children who are over 3 years of age and are obese and in whom Bryant traction may have been applied improperly.

The clinical abnormalities have been attributed to the fact that with the procedure, the limb is held vertically upright for a protracted period of time, with the result that a significant, persistent reduction in blood pressure develops in the leg and foot even when the blood supply was previously normal. Another contributory factor which may further reduce blood pressure and hence local blood flow is full extension of the knee. As a consequence of these mechanisms, there may be sufficient compromise of local arterial circulation to produce a severe degree of ischemia of distal tissues, thus predisposing them to the nutritional changes listed above. Careful medical supervi-sion of young children who are being treated by Bryant traction is therefore imperative, in order to become immediately aware of the presence of vascular difficulties.

2. Moleskin Traction

Moleskin type of traction requires careful application so as to prevent local pressure areas over bony prominences. In the aged, special care must be taken, for otherwise gangrene may be precipitated by the procedure, particularly if an underlying arterial insufficiency exists [13].

D. Adverse Reaction to Parenteral Therapy

1. Intravenous Administration

In premature infants and children who are in very poor physical state due to shock, dehydration, cachexia, or severe general sepsis such as meningococcic septicemia, slight trauma, as for example, that produced by venipuncture or venous cutdown (Fig. 22.12A), may be sufficient to precipitate gangrene in a limb [15].

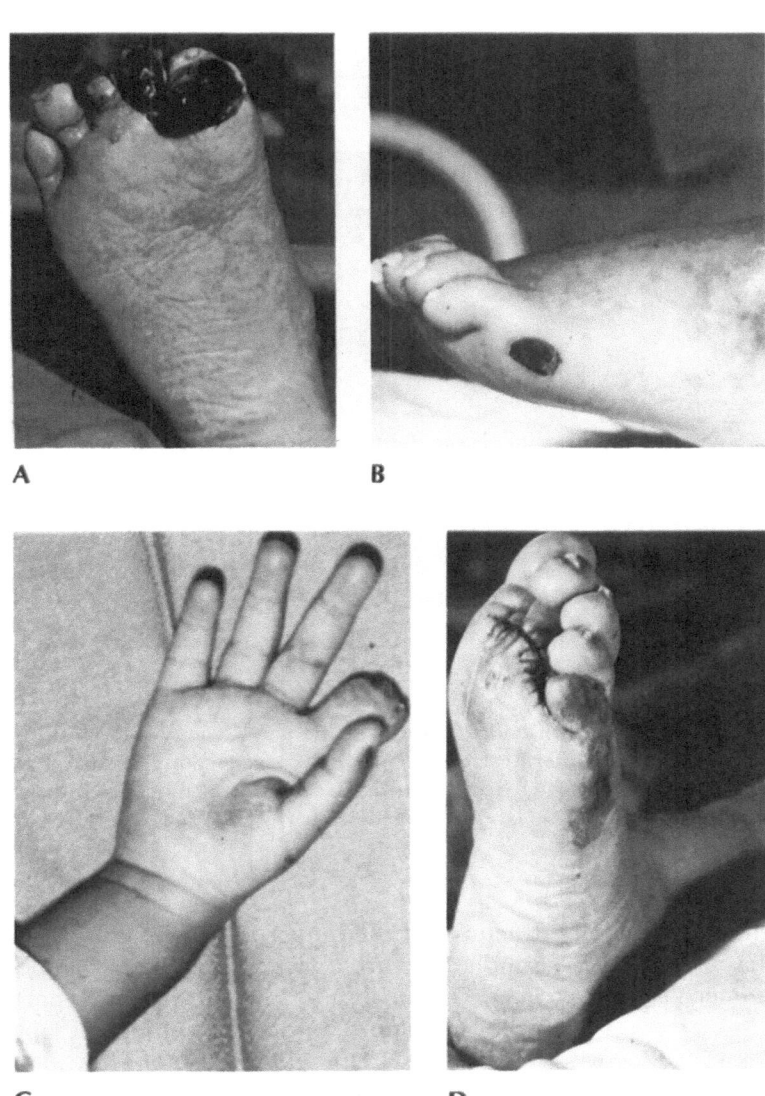

Fig. 22.6. Iatrogenic necrosis due to compression or distension of tissues. **A** Gangrene of great toe and second toe following the subcutaneous injection of a relatively large quantity of procaine as a preliminary step to an operative procedure. **B** Development of a local area of gangrene on the lateral border of the foot following the tight application of an elastic bandage in a patient with a normal local arterial circulation. **C** Gangrene of the distal portion of the index finger, followed by amputation, in a 2-year-old female in whom adhesive tape had been placed around the digit to prevent her from sucking it. **D** Necrosis of fifth toe and adjoining portion of the foot following the tight application of an elastic bandage in a patient who was operated on for removal of a neuroma.

The underlying etiologic factors in the response are hypotension and dehydration which contribute to a rise in blood viscosity and erythrocytic sludging in the capillaries, thus resulting in faulty tissue perfusion and thrombosis [20]. In the case of septicemia, a necrotizing arteritis may also be present. The minor trauma then acts as a trigger mechanism to initiate the gangrenous process. In contradistinction to embolic or thrombotic occlusion of major limb arteries, in this condition, angiography demonstrates complete patency of the arterial tree. However, the rate of filling and the flow through the microcirculation are extremely slow. Because of absence of occluded portions of artery, the disorder is not treated by surgical reconstructive procedures. Careful handling of tissues for venipuncture or incision over a vein in infants is an essential preventive measure.

2. Intraarterial Puncture

Inadvertent puncture of arteries when attempting to give medication intravenously may cause vascular spasm (Fig. 22.12B), thrombosis, or even small aneurysmal dilatations, particularly in newborn infants. In Coumadin-treated patients, arterial puncture for electrolyte studies has been reported to cause compartmental

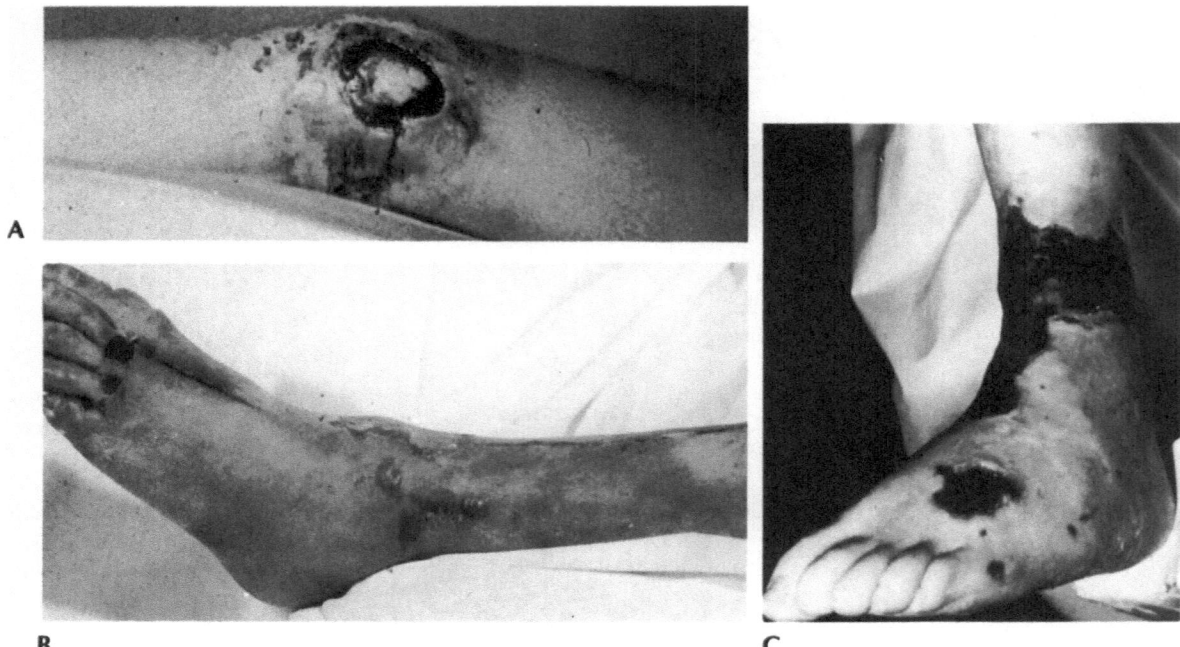

Fig. 22.7. Pressure necrosis from tight casts. **A** Necrotic ulceration over the patella due to application of a cast to a limb of a 19-year-old female patient suffering from a sprained knee. Healing occurred after protracted treatment. **B** Necrosis on outer aspect of left leg due to application of a tight cast. Abrasion of skin on dorsum of foot produced by cast cutter. **C** Gangrene of lower part of the leg and of the foot following application of a cast.

space syndromes, requiring immediate fascial space incisions. Renal dialysis has been associated with arterial embolic phenomena to distal arteries.

3. Injections into Subcutaneous Tissue

Deposition of drugs or solutions in high concentration or of other foreign material in or around the hip joint may result in suppurative arthritis, necrosis of the head of the femur, and joint dysfunction with shortening of the limb (due to epiphyseal involvement). The same type of etiologic agent may produce necrosis in other sites (Fig. 22.6A).

E. Volkmann's Ischemic Contracture

Volkmann's ischemic contracture is most frequently seen after comminuted supracondylar fractures of the humerus and, less often, after simple fractures around the elbow and the knee. This condition has also been reported following improper use of orthopedic appliances, such as the application of tight plaster of Paris casts and constricting bandages and positioning of the elbow in acute flexion in the treatment of a supracondylar fracture. Moreover, forced manipulation during reduction of a fracture or dislocation of the elbow has been found to lead to injury of vascular channels followed by the onset of ischemic paralysis. For such reasons, the subject is included in this chapter rather than elsewhere. The possibility has been raised that Volkmann's ischemic contracture of the forearm is similar to the volar compartmental syndrome of the forearm (see H-5, Chapter 15).

1. Pathogenesis

It is generally accepted that arterial obstruction is necessary for the development of Volk-

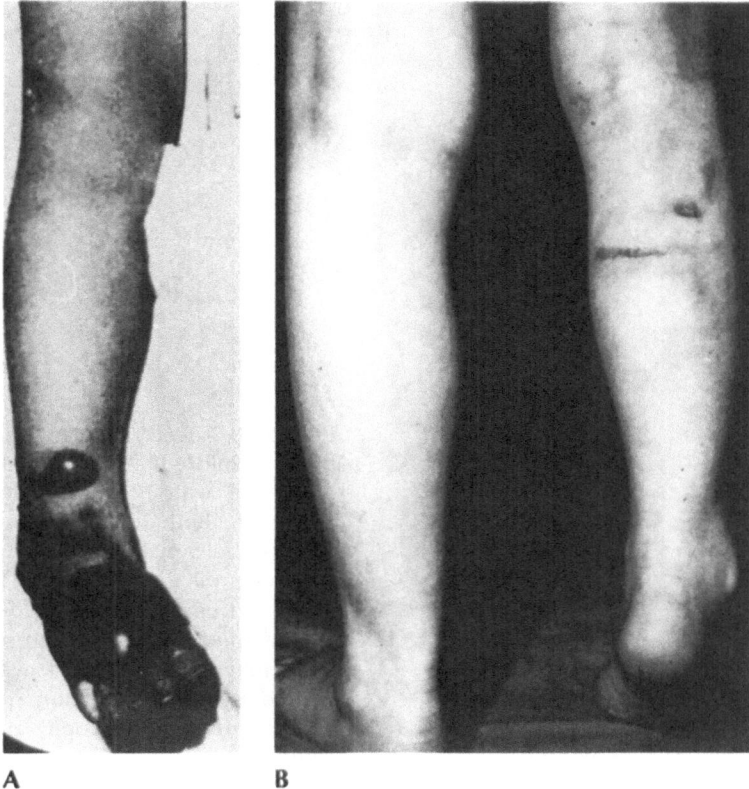

A   **B**

Fig. 22.8. Compression necrosis and fibrosis. **A** Gangrene of foot following application of cast, necessitating a metatarsal-tarsal amputation. **B** Ischemic fibrosis resulting in equinovarus in a 4-year-old male, produced by 3 weeks' application of an elastic bandage for a sprained ankle.

mann's ischemic contracture. Traumatic spasm (see Section C, Chapter 15), traumatic arterial thrombosis (see Section D, Chapter 15), and division of arteries have been implicated as etiologic factors in the production of the condition [8,9]. Generally associated with cessation of flow through main arterial channels is spasm of vessels on which the collateral circulation depends. There may also be severe venous stasis which often coexists with interruption of arterial blood flow and which contributes to the muscular damage. Direct injuries to the bellies of muscles may cause local swelling of these structures within their sheaths, the increasing pressure gradually obstructing venous drainage and contributing to anoxemia of tissues

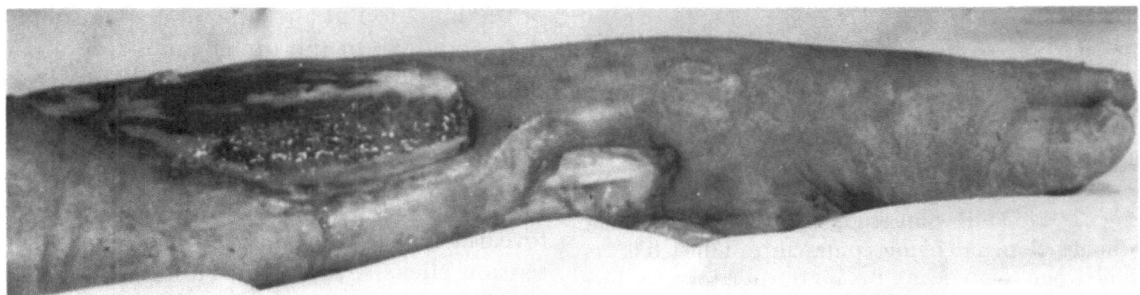

Fig. 22.9. Pressure necrosis. Gangrene of foot and leg with foot drop, followed by a below-knee amputation, due to protracted application of an elastic bandage for the treatment of a sprained ankle in a 62-year-old woman.

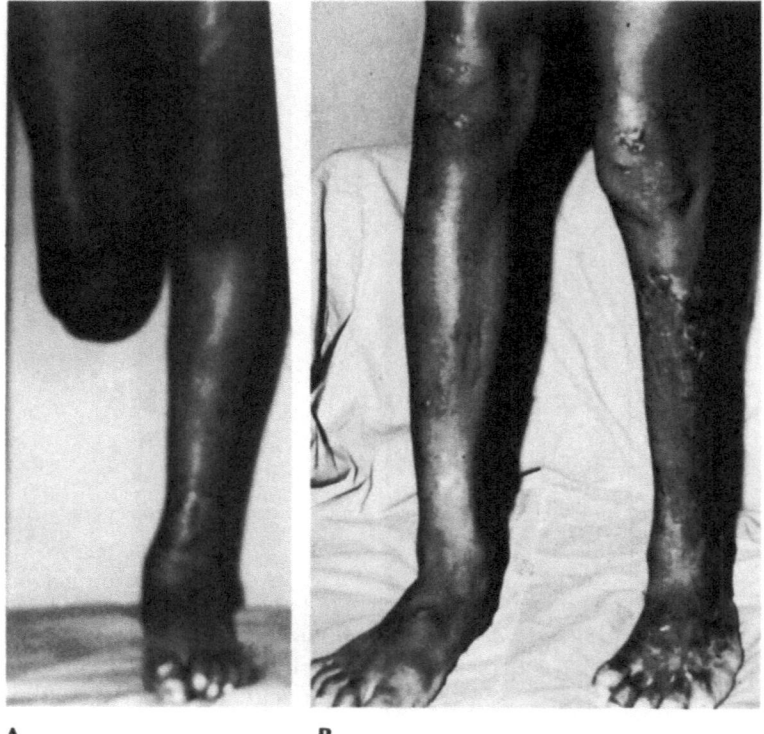

A   **B**

Fig. 22.10. Effects of Bryant traction in children. **A** Fracture of left femur with Bryant traction applied to both lower limbs in an 8-year-old male, resulting in gangrene of the normal right lower extremity and a below-knee amputation. **B** Fracture of left femur in a 4-year-old male treated by Bryant traction, resulting in ischemic atrophy and contracture of the left foot.

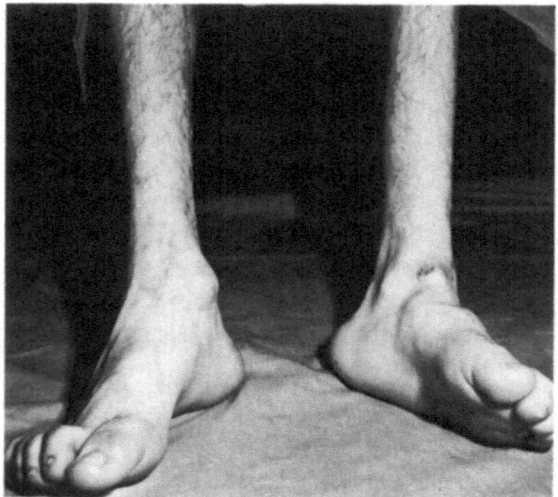

Fig. 22.11. Follow-up study on a 20-year-old male who developed ischemic contracture of the left lower limb when treated with Bryant traction for a fracture of left femur at the age of 2 years. Atrophy of the calf, shortening of the limb, and deformity of the foot are present.

[7]. The fact that certain muscles like the flexor and the pronator muscles in the forearm are more often involved in Volkmann's contracture than others in the upper limb may be related to the characteristics of their intramuscular vascular pattern, making these structures more vulnerable to vascular damage.

2. Clinical Manifestations

The earliest signs of Volkmann's ischemic contracture usually appear 4 to 6 h after the injury or the initiation of a treatment responsible for the condition. In the upper limb, severe pain develops in the flexors of the forearm, associated with swelling, coldness, cyanosis, and flexion contracture of the fingers and absence of pulsations in the radial and ulnar arteries at the wrist. Motor power in the muscles of the forearm is markedly reduced, and passive extension elicits severe pain. However, the muscles do not appear to be completely paralyzed, but instead they are in a state of continuous involuntary tonic contraction, which apparently

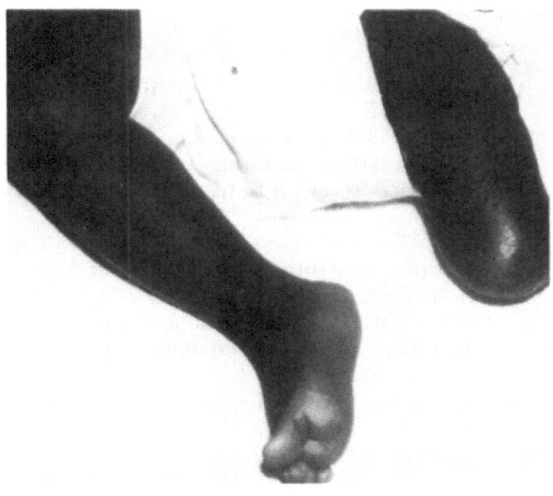

A

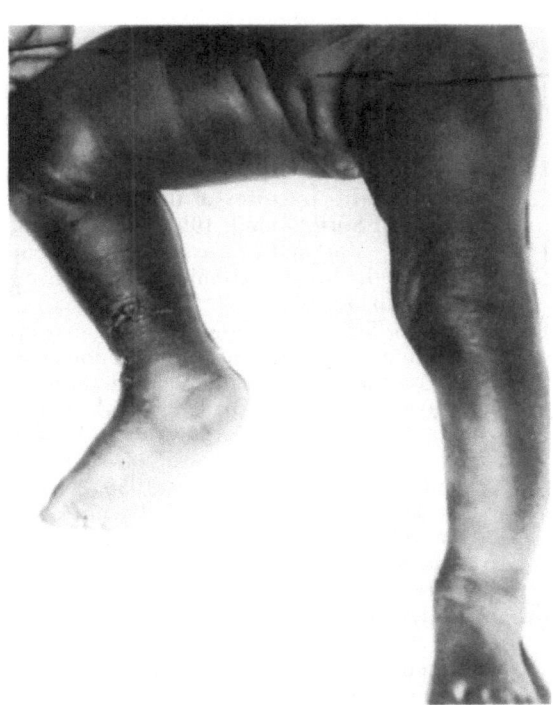

B

Fig. 22.12. Adverse reactions to parenteral therapy in children. **A** Gangrene of left foot, necessitating a below-knee amputation, in a 1½-year-old male, following an attempt to obtain blood from a femoral vein. **B** Gangrene of right lower limb necessitating a below-knee amputation in a 2-year-old female, following an inadvertent puncture of the femoral artery in an attempt to collect a blood sample from the femoral vein.

adds to the state of ischemia. If this situation is not corrected, the muscles become necrotic and eventually are replaced by tough fibrous tissue, with scar formation enveloping the nerves and soft tissues. The early stage of tonic contraction can still be reversed, whereas the later phase of fibrosis is a permanent irreversible state.

In the lower limb, the clinical picture of Volkmann's ischemic contracture consists of a deep boring pain in the central calf area which is difficult to control with sedatives; tenderness in the muscles in which infarcts have developed; a sense of numbness in the toes and remainder of the foot; a stocking-glove type of centripetal anesthesia; and a gradual swelling of the leg and foot. As pulsations in the foot slowly disappear, the skin becomes cold and pale or cyanotic. Paralysis of the muscles of the leg is a constant feature.

3. Treatment

The best therapeutic approach to Volkmann's ischemic contracture is prevention of the condition, which involves vigilant awareness of such a complication. If present, early recognition is essential so as to institute steps which will stop further progression. These consist of immediate measures to release pressure and means to initiate widespread control of vasospasm, including the use of paravertebral sympathetic blocks, stellate ganglion blocks, and high spinal blocks. Cleansing and debridement of the wound, with extension of the incision into the fascial planes so as to release any intrinsic compression of the muscles or nerves, are valuable adjunctive steps. It is essential to expose the involved vessel and if it demonstrates signs of traumatic spasm, attempts should be made to counteract this state (see C-4, Chapter 15). Arterial thrombosis should be treated by resection and reestablishment of circulation using a graft. Immediate arteriectomy has also been proposed [17], together with excision of all irreparably damaged muscle and nerves, followed by such reconstructive procedures as may be required to minimize the deficiency [19].

F. Tourniquet Injuries

Pneumatic tourniquets are frequently utilized during surgical procedures on the limbs, in order to facilitate the required operative approach. However, their use is not without hazard, especially if the pressure sensing devices have not been routinely checked and are incorrect, allowing excessive pressure to enter the cuff [23]. The application of a tourniquet has resulted in acute arterial occlusion and loss of limbs, particularly when there is an underlying arterial insufficiency.

The question as to a specific safe period of time during which a tourniquet can be applied has never been satisfactorily answered. A commonly accepted opinion is that an arterial occlusion pressure should be maintained for less than 2 h because of the possibility of damage from ischemia if prolonged beyond that point. A modification has been proposed, consisting of removal of the pressure for 10 min after 2 h of tourniquet ischemia and then reapplication for the next 1.5 h [4]. Such a schedule, however, has not always been accepted as causing no danger [3,10]. Of interest in this regard is the experimental work on rats indicating that microscopic changes are produced in the muscles when pressures as low as 100 mmHg are applied to the tissues for as little as an hour [11]. These appear about 24 h after the procedure and consist of cellular infiltration, interstitial capillary hemorrhage, and various stages of cellular degeneration. No gross changes are noted with a short period of application of 100 mmHg.

References

1. Bassett FH III, Houck WS Jr: False aneurysm of the profunda femoris artery after subtrochanteric osteotomy and nail-plate fixation. J Bone Joint Surg 46A:583, 1964
2. Boyd DP, Farha GJ: Arteriovenous fistula and isolated vascular injuries secondary to intervertebral disk surgery: Report of four cases and review of the literature. Ann Surg 161:524, 1965
3. Brunner JM: Safety factors in the use of the pneumatic tourniquet for hemostasis in surgery of the hand. J Bone Joint Surg 33A:221, 1951
4. Bunnell S: Surgery of the Hand, 2nd ed. Philadelphia, Lippincott, 1948, p 96
5. Cameron HS, Laird JJ, Carroll SE: False aneurysm complicating closed fractures. J Trauma 12:67, 1972
6. Dameron TB Jr: False aneurysm of femoral profunda artery resulting from internal-fixation device (screw). J Bone Joint Surg 46A:577, 1964
7. Garber JN: Volkmann's contracture as a complication of fractures of the forearm and elbow. J Bone Joint Surg 21:154, 1939
8. Griffiths DL: The management of acute circulatory failure in an injured limb. J Bone Joint Surg 30B:280, 1948
9. Griffiths DL: Volkmann's ischemic contracture: Editorial. J Bone Joint Surg 33B:299, 1951
10. Hinman F Jr: The rational use of tourniquets: Special contribution. Surg Gynecol Obstet 81:357, 1945
11. Husain T: Experimental study of some pressure effects on tissues, with reference to bedsore problem. J Pathol Bacteriol 66:347, 1953
12. Linton RR: Arterial injuries associated with fracture of the extremity. J Bone Joint Surg 46A:575, 1964
13. Miller DS, Harris AJ: Gangrene in the aged associated with fractures of the extremities. J Intern Coll Surg 24:669, 1955
14. Miller DS, Markin L, Grossman E: Ischemic fibrosis of the lower extremity in children. Am J Surg 84:317, 1952
15. Miller DS, Sebeck R: Gangrene of the extremities in infants subsequent to intravenous therapy: Precautions in technique and report of five cases. AMA Am J Dis Child 90:153, 1955
16. Nicholson JT, Foster RM, Heath RD: Bryant's traction: A provocative cause of circulatory complications. JAMA 157:415, 1955
17. Sakor HK: A case of early Volkmann's ischaemia following posterior dislocation of elbow treated successfully by arterectomy. Indian J Surg 14:350, 1952
18. Salter RB, Kostuik J, Dallas S: Avascular necrosis of the femoral head as a complication of treatment for congenital dislocation of the hip in young children: A clinical and experimental investigation. Can J Surg 12:44, 1969
19. Seddon HJ: Volkmann's contracture: Treatment by excision of the infarct. J Bone Joint Surg 38B:152, 1956
20. Shehadi SI, Slim MS, Dabbous IA: Gangrene of lower extremities in infants following acute gastroenteritis. Plast Reconstr Surg 42:530, 1968
21. Spittell JA, Jr, Palumbo PJ, Love JG, et al: Arteriovenous fistula complicating lumbar disk surgery. N Engl J Med 268:1162, 1963
22. Stein AH Jr: Arterial injury in orthopaedic surgery. J Bone Joint Surg 38A:669, 1956
23. Wheeler DK, Lipscomb PR: A safety device for a pneumatic tourniquet. J Bone Joint Surg 46A:870, 1964

Chapter 23

Vascular Complications of Therapy in Musculoskeletal Disorders

Part 2   Untoward Consequences of Protracted Bed Rest or Immobilization of a Limb

Since many orthopedic operative procedures require long periods of bed rest or immobilization of a limb, it is necessary to discuss the sequelae that may result therefrom. This chapter is devoted to such problems and the means to combat them.

A.   Pressure (Decubitus) Ulcers and Gangrene

1.   Pathogenesis

Even in the presence of an adequate circulation through the main arterial channels in the lower limbs, sustained and prolonged pressure over bony prominences (such as the two malleoli, the lateral border of the foot, and the heel) or elsewhere on the skin of the limb may produce ulceration or gangrene (Fig. 23.1). The fact that the sites over the malleoli are covered only by skin and a small amount of subcutaneous tissue and muscle further predisposes them to the development of such a lesion. In the presence of chronic occlusive arterial disease, such as arteriosclerosis obliterans, this tendency to ulcer formation is markedly exaggerated. As a result, even short periods of pressure

may be sufficient to initiate extensive lesions that are frequently unresponsive to conservative or surgical therapy and may eventually require a major amputation (Fig. 23.2A). (For a discussion of pressure necrosis due to application of a tight cast or elastic bandage, see B-3, Chapter 22.)

The initiating factor responsible for the appearance of a pressure ulcer or gangrene of the lower limb may be one or more of a number of different forces: the weight of the extremity against the mattress at the point of contact; the compression of the skin by a tight cast (Fig. 22.7), a brace, or an improperly applied elastic bandage (Fig. 22.8B); and pressure exerted by a contracted limb crossed over the other. All of these mechanisms cause obliteration of the cutaneous microcirculation and hence produce periods of ischemia. In regard to this point, it has been shown that normal cutaneous capillary blood pressure ranges between 13 and 32 mmHg and that external pressures as low as 50 to 60 mmHg completely arrest capillary flow. It can therefore be expected that if a mechanical force of any magnitude is exerted on the skin for a period of time, decubitus ulcers will develop over bony prominences, particularly if minor cracks or abrasions already exist

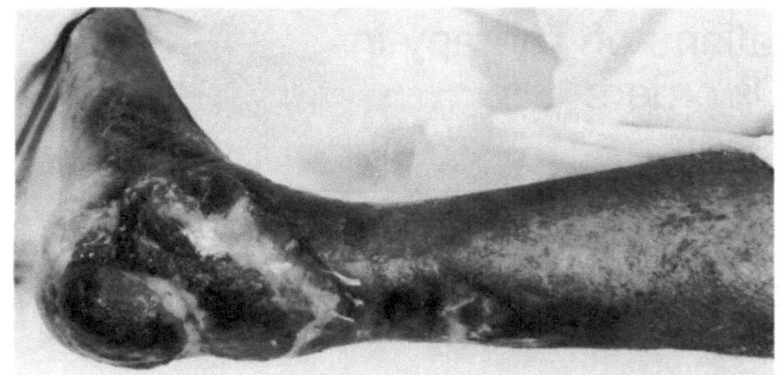

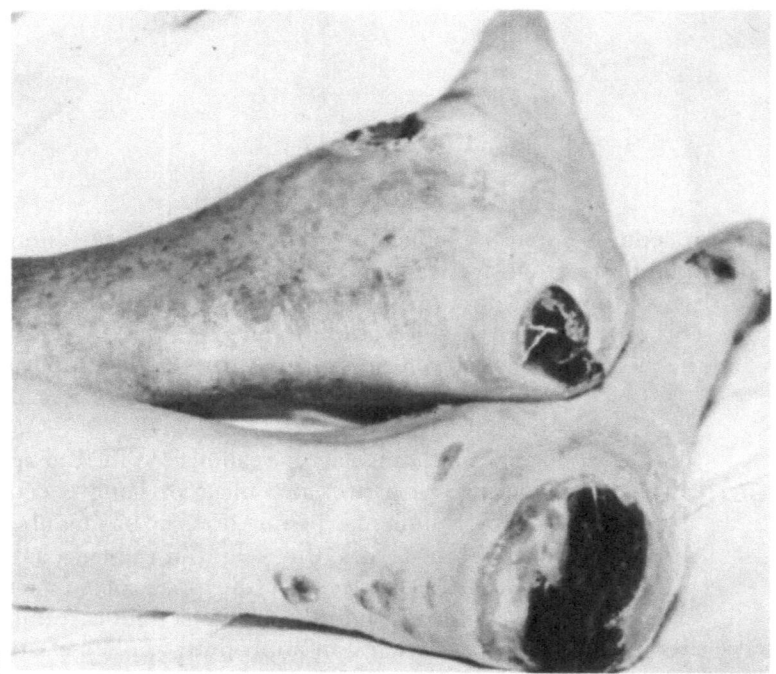

Fig. 23.1. **A** and **B** Pressure gangrene in patients with previously normal local arterial circulation.

in such sites. Moreover, these lesions will generally continue to enlarge because of perpetuation of the state of local ischemia and the introduction of infection.

Although certain contributing factors, alone or in combination, cannot cause pressure ulcers, they do make the patient more vulnerable to the mechanical agents. Among these are such metabolic abnormalities as poorly balanced diets resulting in malnutrition, negative nitrogen and calcium balances, a decrease in the albumin/globulin ratio, avitaminosis, electrolyte disturbances, and anemia. Many of these changes result from deconditioning (see

Section B, below) due to prolonged bed rest, particularly in the case of elderly patients. Other states which predispose to pressure ulcers are disruption of cutaneous vascular reflexes resulting from spinal cord injuries, decreased or absent sensation in the skin of the feet from whatever cause, and an inability to move in bed because of debility. If adequate nursing care is not available, such conditions may result in the maintenance of the same position much beyond a physiologic limit, thus prolonging local pressure to the point of producing irreversible tissue damage, necrosis, and ulceration.

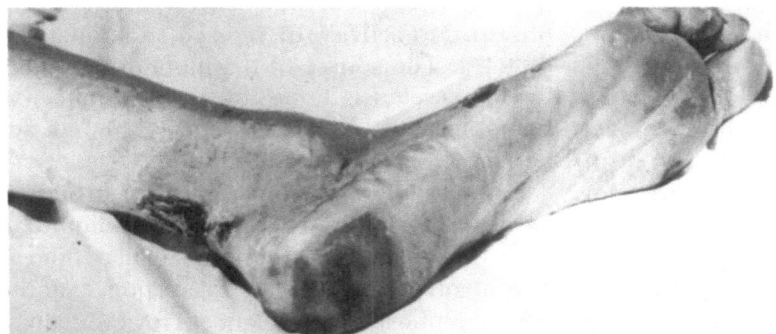
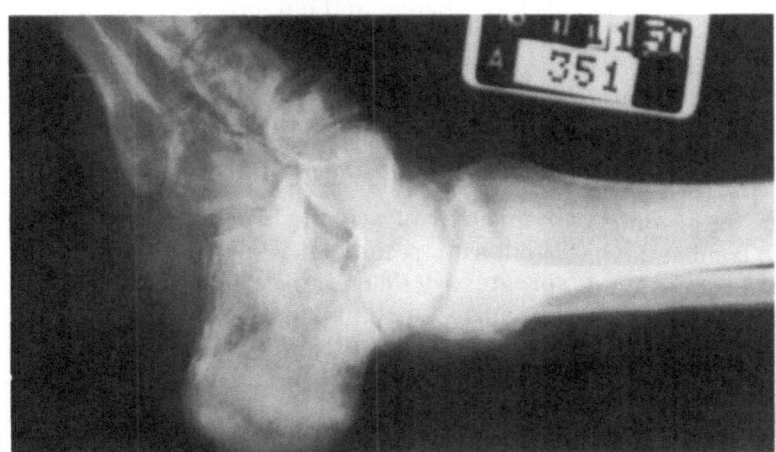

Fig. 23.2. **A** Pressure gangrene of heel and lower portion of leg in an elderly woman with arteriosclerosis obliterans following open hip operation and a protracted period of bed rest. **B** Osteomyelitis of calcaneus following persistent pressure on heel board during Buck's traction for sciatica in an 18-year-old male. Bone infection occurred due to direct contamination from infected cutaneous ulceration.

2. Prophylactic Therapy

The primary goal in the treatment of a pressure ulcer is its prevention. For this purpose, it is necessary to attempt to counteract or eliminate those factors which are responsible for its development. When a cast is being applied, special care must be taken to protect bony prominences from undue and unnecessary pressure. With regard to bed positioning, direct contact with a hard mattress should be minimized by the interposition of appropriate heel pads or by supporting the leg so that the foot is not resting on the bed. Sand bags placed on either side of the limb will maintain it in correct alignment, without eversion of the foot. Also of great importance for the bedridden patient is to turn and reposition him at 2-h intervals, a step requiring an extensive nursing care program. These measures are even more essential if the limb already demonstrates a compromised local circulation, because of the very poor prognosis associated with the presence of a pressure ulcer under such circumstances.

In all of the patients, the various systemic abnormalities mentioned above should be intensively treated.

3. Active Therapy

Once an ulcer has developed, attempts must be made immediately to remove all pressure from the involved site, even to the point of having the patient spend most of the day in a chair if feasible. Then therapy should be directed toward control of any superimposed infection. The lesion should be debrided repeatedly, and when all the necrotic tissue has been removed, attempts to stimulate epithelialization are introduced. All of these measures are similar to those described for the treatment of stasis ulcer (see C-7, Chapter 20). Also proposed for rapid debridement of the lesion is the laser unit, since the beam has been reported to vaporize the necrotic material completely with one application, leaving a sterile base for subsequent conservative treatment. At present, the value of this approach cannot be determined since the available clinical reports are still fragmentary, the cost of the unit contributing to such a situation. Besides local therapy, any existing metabolic disorders (listed above) should be controlled, because otherwise healing of the lesion will be delayed or may not even take place.

B. Deconditioning

Since many of the therapeutic procedures for orthopedic disorders, by necessity, require prolonged periods of partial or complete bed rest or protracted immobilization of the involved limb or limbs, it is important to discuss the deleterious effects on vital processes produced by such a program and means to combat them.

It is generally accepted that the functional capacity of any organ is related, within physiologic limits, to the intensity and frequency of its activity. Hence, it can be assumed that bed rest would be followed by significant deterioration in virtually all organs of the body. The various resulting changes—anatomic, chemical, and physiologic—have collectively been termed deconditioning.

1. Effect of Deconditioning on Metabolic Processes

There is no question that bed rest produces cellular damage and a disturbance of metabolic processes. For example, a negative nitrogen balance, which is a manifestation of catabolism or endogenous tissue breakdown, develops very shortly after the institution of immobilization. In normal persons, losses of 1 to 3.5 g of nitrogen per day are noted, and after 7 weeks on such a regimen, a similar period of physical activity is required to regain an amount of nitrogen comparable to that which was previously excreted [4]. In pathologic states, the loss of nitrogen during immobilization is even greater. Both in normal and in abnormal people, loss of nitrogen takes place primarily in voluntary muscle. (For the vascular changes associated with muscle atrophy, see Section D, below.)

A negative calcium balance also develops during bed rest, 13 g being lost in a 7-week period of immobility [4]. In the first 3 weeks of return to activity, there is an additional loss of 4.4 g. The source of the mobilized calcium being excreted is bone [5]. (For the effect of immobilization on the structure of bone, see Section C, below.)

Among other metabolic changes produced by deconditioning are a negative sodium balance, indicating that the extracellular fluid is also involved in the chemical response, and a negative phosphorus balance. However, there is little change in the potassium content of the body.

2. Effect of Deconditioning on Cardiovascular Mechanisms

Limitation of activity, especially when associated with recumbency, produces significant, progressive deleterious changes in the cardiovascular system. These appear to be due in a large measure to impairment of autonomic control of the heart and the peripheral circulation.

Changes observed under resting conditions. Even at rest, there is some evidence of progressive deterioration in cardiovascular performance. For example, the basal pulse rate shows an increase which averages approximately 0.5 beats/day of bed rest. The heart demonstrates a 17 percent decrease in volume and an 8 percent reduction in transverse diameter. Total blood volume becomes somewhat smaller, while there is a 15 percent decrease in plasma volume. However, resting cardiac output is not significantly changed during the period of immobilization.

Alterations in vasomotor response to standing. Following prolonged recumbency, there is a marked reduction in vasomotor tone, and as a consequence, on standing, stasis of blood takes place in the lower portion of the body, especially in the venous system; this causes a reduced venous return, a lowered cardiac output, and a decrease in cerebral blood flow, the latter not infrequently producing fainting.[1]

---

[1] This is in contrast with the response in the normal person, in whom, on assumption of the upright position, there is immediate vasoconstriction of the peripheral vessels, especially those in the lower extremities and in the splanchnic bed, in order to prevent pooling due to gravity.

Contributing factors are poor muscle tone in the lower extremities, due to bed rest, and malnutrition which frequently results in a decrease in elasticity of the different tissues. Both changes reduce the efficiency of the various mechanisms required to move blood out of the lower limbs against hydrostatic pressure.

Deterioration of vasomotor tone during prolonged bed rest can readily be identified and quantitated by the use of the tilt table. If the deconditioned individual is placed on the table at an angle of 68° for 15 min, there will be an average increase in pulse rate of 38 beats/min over that observed in the supine position; in the pre-bed-rest control period, there is a rise of only 13 beats/min under similar conditions. In the deconditioned person, the systolic blood pressure during tilt falls an average of 14 mmHg below the supine value, compared to no change in the previous control period. The postural adjustment score may remain low for as long as 7 weeks after the initiation of an ambulation program.

Changes observed with exercise. In the deconditioned individual, cardiovascular performance during physical exertion is even more affected than at rest. There is a diminished ability of the heart to do aerobic work, as reflected in a marked rise of the pulse rate during the exercise. For example, after 3 weeks of bed rest, the pulse rate in the last 5 min of a 30-min walk at 3.5 mi/h averages 35 to 40 beats/min faster than that observed during the control period; the exaggerated response requires from 36 to 72 days to return to a normal type of change. There is also a decreased ability to perform intense anaerobic work produced by running for 90 s on a treadmill, at a 15° grade and at a rate of 7 mi/h. The average oxygen uptake during such exercise is reduced by 16 percent, and recovery to the type of response noted during a control period does not occur until 36 days after reconditioning is resumed.

Total inactivity of voluntary muscles results in loss of strength of approximately 3 percent per day. As a consequence, with strenuous exercise, the efficiency of performance decreases 15 percent, thus indicating a marked loss of capacity of the cardiorespiratory system to work under stress.

As strength decreases through disuse, endurance also falls. If the local circulation is impaired for any reason, then recovery of endurance in the performance of muscular activity will be even slower than in normal individuals.

3. Effect of Deconditioning on Joints and Associated Supporting Structures

Normally connective tissue binds the cells and organs together in a structural relationship which is then temporarily altered by the stresses associated with body motion. During a period of rest, this state is again restored by the metabolic activity of the connective tissue. Under such circumstances, the stresses and strains of body motion and the opposing action of the connective tissue are closely enough in balance so that little permanent deformity of the structural relationship exists. Contributing to such a situation is the fact that collagen is laid down as a loose meshwork of randomly oriented areolar fibers in the subcutaneous tissue, around joint capsules, in the muscular planes, and in other moving parts of the body. This arrangement allows for a considerable range of motion to be possible between the moving structures.

When physical activity is limited, as with immobilization of a part, impairment of mobility and of flexibility of the connective tissue of the body quickly results. Dense connective tissue replaces the areolar tissue and as a consequence there is a loss of motion within a few days. Immobilization following trauma leads to an even greater production of fibrosis, which, when once formed, may cause restriction of normal mobility which will persist despite weeks or months of treatment. Particularly difficult to combat are the changes around and in the joints of the lower extremities, which are untowardly affected by the strong muscles and heavy connective tissue in these locations.

Alterations in joint blood flow produced by immobilization have been studied in animals, and the results indicate that after 2 weeks of such a state, the synovial tissue is distinctly paler than that on the control side [20]. Following a longer period of immobilization, there is a generalized reduction in caliber of the microcirculation, with a decrease in the number of capillary plexuses in the innermost synovial tissue layer and a slightly reduced corpuscular flow velocity.

4. Effect of Deconditioning on the Nervous System

Normal function of the nervous system requires a continuous reciprocal action between sensory impulses, received through the various superficial and deep nerve endings, and the subcortical and cortical centers on which they impinge. Limitation of activity by bed rest changes sensory input of all types, and, in particular, it depresses proprioceptive stimuli, which are responsible for regulating neuromuscular performance. As a consequence, when the individual who has been at complete bed rest for a long period of time begins to ambulate, unsteadiness of the lower limbs may be present during the recovery period.

5. Effect of Deconditioning on Mental Processes

Bed rest which deprives the individual of mental stimulation has a stultifying effect on intellectual activity. Lack of sensory stimulation results in progressively decreasing cerebration. However, immobilization does not necessarily have this consequence if intellectual stimulation is maintained.

Emotional responses to diminution of physical activity will vary, depending upon the degree of sensory deprivation and the personality of the individual. The immediate response to limitation of activity is similar to that observed in other situations of stress. Patients may manifest depression, insecurity with anxiety and dependency, aggressiveness with hostility, complaints of discomfort, and changes in sleep patterns. The greater the amount and the more prolonged the limitation of activity, the more marked will be the abnormal emotional responses.

6. Means to Combat Deconditioning

Early institution of a rehabilitation program for the patient requiring immobilization of a limb or limbs or of portions of the body may help prevent the cardiovascular, metabolic, and osseous deterioration, which would otherwise necessitate many months of subsequent controlled ambulation to counteract. While in bed, the patient should routinely exercise the normal limbs and the uninvolved parts of his body to minimize progressive limitation of joints. This is especially true in the case of the hips since they are generally kept in partial flexion by the patient when he is lying on a soft bed, semi-reclining, or sitting. Moreover, since a pillow placed under the knees causes flexion of these joints and also of the hips, such a practice should not be permitted. It is important to point out that both sets of joints must be fully extended while standing or walking, or otherwise, great muscle strength is necessary to support the weight of the body in the upright position. When in bed, the lower limbs should not be maintained in the elevated position for protracted periods of time because the hydrostatic effect will produce a significant reduction in arterial inflow, particularly if underlying local arterial insufficiency exists. Such a situation may result in a state of ischemia of distal structures and possibly the appearance of trophic changes (Fig. 22.10).

As soon as it is feasible, the patient should be permitted out of bed and in a chair. Standing at intervals will help establish the normal stresses on bones and prevent further development of osteoporosis (see C-1 below). At the same time, the deteriorating changes in the vasomotor system and in voluntary muscles will be reduced or eliminated. Controlled ambulation should be instituted as soon as possible.

Besides the above measures, attempts should be made to counteract the abnormal metabolic effects of bed rest. Nourishing diets, including large quantities of protein, are helpful in this regard, as well as medications to treat existing anemia and to stimulate the appetite.

C. Disuse Osteoporosis

Following immobilization of a limb, as in the treatment of a fracture, the involved bone no longer receives stress from the weight of the body or from the pull of contracting muscles (see B-5, Chapter 3). With loss of these stimulating mechanisms, osseous circulation is reduced. Such a situation then causes a decrease in activity of osteoblasts and leads to an increase in bone resorption, associated with a negative calcium balance [18]. As a consequence, the typical findings of disuse atrophy of bone develop [6,7,19,22,24].

1. Pathogenesis

For many years, osteoporosis has been widely assumed to result from a deficiency in matrix formation, with a proportionate reduction in minerals, particularly calcium. The fundamental defect has been considered to be a disorder of protein metabolism rather than a primary disturbance of calcium and phosphorus metabolism [1]. Because of the lack of bone-matrix formation by osteoblasts, normal replacement of bone destroyed by daily physical activity is believed not to occur, with the result that gradual thinning of bone trabeculae takes place. However, this theory of matrix deficiency as the primary cause of osteoporosis has been challenged. Instead, the view has been proposed that the abnormal state is due to prolonged dietary deficiency of calcium, with a resultant decrease in bone formation [21].

Of interest in the elucidation of the cause of disuse osteoporosis are the experimental findings in dogs that this state did not develop in the immobilized limb when prior removal of either one or both parathyroid glands and the thyroid gland had been carried out [3]. The results were considered to indicate that a local factor produced by immobilization may increase the sensitivity of the bone to circulating levels of thyroid and parathyroid hormones. That bone resorption occurs in immobilized limbs is supported by findings of an increased P_{CO_2} and a decreased pH in bone blood.

Another clue regarding the mechanisms responsible for osteoporosis has been derived from the clinical reports that patients on long-term heparin therapy for coronary artery disease (15,000 to 30,000 units daily for 6 months or longer) may develop this state, associated with spontaneous multiple fractures of ribs or vertebrae [9,17]. Smaller doses of the drug do not appear to produce such a result. It has been postulated that heparin has a direct local stimu-

latory effect on the enzyme system responsible for bone resorption [9], a viewpoint which is in accord with the finding of potentiation by this drug of the action of parathyroid hormone in causing resorption of bone from mouse calvaria in tissue culture [8]. It has also been shown that heparin slows bone repair in animals, the possibility being proposed that a substrate competition exists between it and chondroitin sulfate to alter or replace the normal matrix mucopolysaccharides [23]. Another possibility is that heparin decreases lysosomal stability.

2. Bony Changes Associated with Immobilization and Bed Rest

In the case of immobilization, disuse osteoporosis is generally located in the parts of the skeleton which have been enclosed in a cast, being especially marked in sites distal to a fracture. The more prolonged the immobilization, the more obvious is the osteoporosis, the latter process beginning more acutely than that of the postmenopausal or senile types. In the early and acute phase of osteoporosis, there are changes in calcium and phosphorus in the serum; later these are no longer found. With immobilization of a large part of the body, urinary calculi and soft-tissue ossification may develop. In the case of bed rest, bone dissolution appears to occur to a greater extent in weight-bearing bones than in the remainder of the skeleton. Roentgenographic examination of osteoporotic bone shows reduction of density, blurring of trabeculae, and thinning of bone cortex.

3. Treatment

Many programs have been suggested for the treatment of osteoporosis. In the type produced by immobilization, return to full physical activity will usually have some beneficial effect upon the condition. In this regard, it has been found (using gamma-ray transmission scanning) that mineral reaccumulates in the bone following return of ambulation at a rate similar to its loss during bed rest [5]. However, it is important to note that in some instances of extensive osteoporosis, years may be required for restoration of normal structure.

Other therapeutic approaches are the use of fluoride which stimulates bone formation; calcium with vitamin D which produces significant suppression of bone resorption; and estrogen or progesterone which also reduces bone loss. However, fluoride and estrogen may have significant adverse side effects. Furthermore, bone regeneration after fluoride stimulation does not appear entirely normal in structure.

D. Vascular Changes Associated with Muscle Atrophy

1. Immobilization and Tenotomy

It has been found that immobilization of a limb produces atrophy of the affected muscles at a rate almost as great as that which follows nerve denervation (see D-2, below). The degree of change is most marked in the muscles maintained in the shortened position, as compared with those in the stretched or extended position.

The vascular changes associated with disuse atrophy of voluntary muscles have been studied in animals and man, using several experimental approaches. By means of a flowmeter, it has been found that blood flow in the dog's limb immobilized in plaster increases [16]. Similar results have been reported in cats following tenotomy and resulting atrophy of the gastrocnemius, the amount of augmentation being in proportion to the developing atrophy [12]. However, studies using microangiography indicate that no vascular changes occur in muscles after 2 weeks of immobilization [15]. In man, arms immobilized in plaster for 14 days have been found to develop less heat, as determined by calorimetry, than the opposite untreated extremity, such a response being attributed to a paucity in the limb under study of vasodilator substances normally produced by muscle activity [14].

The mechanism responsible for vasodilatation after tenotomy or immobilization is still unknown [13], although a number of possibilities have been offered. Reduction of extramural pressure in tenotomized muscles, in consequence of shortening, has been proposed as a causative factor for a decrease in vascular resistance, resulting in an increase in blood flow [16]. However, it has been found that shortening occurs immediately after section of the tendon, whereas a substantial fall in resistance does not appear until after 13 days [13]. Still a mechanical factor cannot be entirely disregarded, since eventual atrophy of the muscle may have such an effect by decreasing extramural pressure. Another explanation for the vasodilatation is stimulation of afferent nerve fibers by metabolic products released from the atrophied muscles as a result of increased glycolysis [2] and proteolysis [10]. It has also been suggested that arteriolar-capillary systems are converted to arteriovenous shunts or pathways of low resistance as the muscle substance disappears [13]. Under such circumstances, the increased circulation would not necessarily represent an augmentation in nutritive blood flow. Evidence obtained from studies on the gracilis muscle in the anesthetized dog supports the view that the vasodilatation in atrophic tenotomized muscles has its origin in resistance vessels [13].

2. Denervation of Muscles

Section of the peripheral nerve supplying a skeletal muscle causes metabolic changes which result in atrophy of the denervated structure. This is associated with an increase in local blood flow even with reference to the original weight of the muscle [11]. There is little question that immediately after the procedure, the vascular response is primarily due to removal of vasoconstrictor tone by section of the sympathetic nerves in the peripheral mixed nerve. However, the vasodilator effect is also noted in muscles denervated by ventral root section, with vasomotor innervation intact [11]. Therefore, the increase in blood flow which persists in atrophied muscle must be due to some other mechanism. Evidence obtained from a study of the denervated gracilis muscle in the anesthetized dog supports the view that the vasodilatation follows relaxation of both resistance and exchange vessels [13]. The fact that fibrillation is a consequence of denervation may play a role in the vascular response, perhaps as a result of the influence of accumulated metabolites on arterioles and precapillary sphincters.

References

1. Albright F, Reifenstein EC Jr: The Parathyroid Glands and Metabolic Bone Disease: Selected Studies. Baltimore, Williams & Wilkins, 1948, Chap 6, p 145
2. Bass A: In Gutmann E (ed): The Denervated Muscle. Prague, Czech Acad Sciences, 1962, pp 203–272 (quoted in ref. 13)
3. Burkhart JM, Jowsey J: Parathyroid and thyroid hormones in the development of immobilization osteoporosis. Endocrinology 81:1053, 1967
4. Deitrick JE, Whedon GD, Short E: Effects of immobilization upon various metabolic and physiologic functions of normal men. Am J Med 4:3, 1948
5. Donaldson CL, Hulley SB, Vogel JM, et al: Effect of prolonged bed rest on bone mineral. Metabolism 19:1071, 1970
6. Geiser M: Die Rolle der Muskelaktion bei der posttraumatischen Osteoporose. Arch Orthop Unfall Chir 49:268, 1957
7. Geiser M, Trueta J: Muscle action, bone rarefaction and bone formation: An experimental study. J Bone Joint Surg 40B:282, 1958
8. Goldhaber P: Heparin enhancement of factors stimulating bone resorption in tissue culture. Science 147:407, 1965
9. Griffith GC, Nichols G Jr, Asher JD, et al: Heparin osteoporosis. JAMA 193:85, 1965
10. Hájek I, Gutmann E, Syrový I: Proteolytic activity in denervated and reinnervated muscle. Physiol Bohemoslov 13:32, 1964 (quoted in ref. 13)
11. Hudlická O: Blood flow and oxygen consumption in muscle after section of ventral roots. Circ Res 20:570, 1967
12. Hudlická O, Hník P, Štulcová B: Changes in blood circulation in skeletal muscle undergoing atrophy. Physiologist 7:163, 1964
13. Hudlická O, Renkin EM: Blood flow and blood-tissue diffusion of ^{86}Rb in denervated and tenotomized muscles undergoing atrophy. Microvasc Res 1:147, 1968
14. Hultén O: The influence of a fixation bandage on the peripheral blood vessels and the circulation. Acta Chir Scand 101:150, 1951
15. Hulth A, Olerud S: Disuse of extremities. II. A microangiographic study in the rabbit. Acta Chir Scand 120:388, 1961
16. Imig CJ, Randall BF, Hines HM: Effect of immobilization on muscular atrophy and blood flow. Arch Phys Med Rehabil 34:296, 1953
17. Jaffe MD, Willis PW III: Multiple fractures associated with long-term sodium heparin therapy. JAMA 193:152, 1965
18. Jowsey J, Phil D, Kelly PJ, et al: Quantitative microradiographic studies of normal and osteoporotic bone. J Bone Joint Surg 47A:785, 1965
19. Landoff GA: Experimentelle Untersuchungen über die "Knochenatrophie" infolge einer Immobilisation und einer akuten Arthritis. Acta Chir Scand (Suppl) 71:1, 1942
20. Lindström J: Microvascular anatomy of synovial tissue. Acta Rheumatol Scand (Suppl) 7:1, 1963
21. Nordin BE: The pathogenesis of osteoporosis. Lancet 1:1011, 1961
22. Rieder W: Die akute Knochenatrophie. Deutsche Z Chir 248:269, 1936
23. Stinchfield FE, Sankaran B, Samilson R: The effect of anticoagulant therapy on bone repair. J Bone Joint Surg 38A:270, 1956
24. Trueta J: The role of the vessels in osteogenesis. J Bone Joint Surg 45B:402, 1963

Chapter 24

Problems Associated with Minor and Major Amputations of Lower Limbs Suffering from Arterial Insufficiency

At the outset, it is necessary to emphasize that the approach to the removal of a limb with gangrene due to severely compromised local arterial circulation is very different from the guidelines utilized in treating necrosis resulting from trauma or cold injury to a previously normal extremity. In the patient suffering from arteriosclerosis obliterans or thromboangiitis obliterans, there is generally a varying degree of ischemia of tissues proximal to the existing trophic lesion which could be responsible for lack of healing of the operative site; on the other hand, in the case of trauma to a normal limb, blood supply in uninjured structures is usually unaffected, a situation conducive to a subsequent successful outcome.

The contents of this chapter are limited to a discussion of those problems arising from minor or major amputations which are found in patients with chronic or acute occlusive arterial disorders of the lower limbs.

A. Basis for Decision to Operate

If, despite intensive local and systemic therapy (see p. 161), a gangrenous lesion of the toes extends onto either the dorsal or ventral surface of the foot, the likelihood of saving the extremity by continued conservative therapy is poor.[1] Such progression generally indicates that the thrombotic process is no longer limited to the digital arteries but has spread to the larger arcuate vessels of the foot. As a consequence, adjoining toes can be expected to become gangrenous in a short while. Under these circumstances, further delay is not warranted, not only because of the greater expense it will entail but also because it will generally not alter the ultimate outcome. Furthermore, with involvement of larger quantities of tissue, the patient may begin to show signs of absorption of toxic material from the affected site, such as a rise in body temperature, drowsiness, and apathy. Since it is not advisable to permit such a state to persist, he should now be prepared mentally and physically for amputation of the limb.

B. Preoperative Goals

1. Development of Proper Attitude in the Patient

Associated problems. The psychologic preparation of the patient for the removal of one

---

[1] Before carrying out an amputation under such circumstances, however, it is necessary to consider very seriously investigating the possibility of a vascular reconstructive procedure, including a salvage operation, as discussed on p. 165.

of his limbs is frequently a very difficult task. This is especially so if the progression of the nutritional disturbances has been so rapid that there has not been sufficient time for him to become fully aware of the seriousness of his condition. As a result, when faced with a decision which if once consummated is irreversible, frequently his first response is to say that he would rather die than permit the operation. At that moment he is completely overcome by the situation confronting him. It is in such a situation that the orthopedist needs all the tact, patience, and persuasiveness at his command to manage the situation. Considerable pain associated with the gangrene may encourage a more rapid acceptance of a realistic approach to the problem.

Complications of retention of gangrenous limb. If the patient persists in his unwillingness to submit to operation, the possibility of the serious consequences that would inevitably follow should be brought graphically to his attention. First, he must be made to appreciate the fact that his condition will not become better but rather that it will worsen. It should be emphasized that the pain can be expected to become more marked and that the patient will begin to feel sick from absorption of toxic material. It is also necessary to point out that his death will not occur quickly but that the process of becoming more and more of an invalid will be long drawn out. During this period his hospital bills will become a great financial burden on members of his family who will, at the same time, be experiencing mental anguish as they observe his suffering. In almost all instances when the patient is faced with such a sequence of events, he will reluctantly agree to the proper step.

Development of an optimistic viewpoint regarding amputation. Aside from indicating the very unpleasant consequences associated with refusal to be operated upon, it is also necessary to make every effort to encourage the patient to assume a realistic attitude toward the problem and to permit the only therapeutic approach available under the circumstances. It is well to point out that thousands of people who had also believed themselves incapacitated have resumed their daily occupations with the use of a prosthesis in a normal and efficient manner. It should be arranged to have an amputee with a prosthesis discuss the matter of amputation with the patient, at the same time demonstrating how capably he has made an adjustment to his difficulty. Emphasis should be placed on the fact that amputation of one or even both lower limbs should not keep the patient from earning a living and enjoying many pleasures, provided he has the motivation to become rehabilitated.

2. Determination of Proper Time for Amputation

Ideally an extremity should be amputated when it is obvious that continued conservative therapy would be of no avail and reconstructive surgical vascular procedures are not considered applicable. However, there are a number of other factors which influence the decision, either forcing premature amputation or postponing it beyond the propitious time.

Role of infection. In the past, the presence of a spreading superimposed infection that was resistant to available medical therapy necessitated immediate surgery as a life-saving procedure. This was particularly true in the diabetic individual with a nutritional disturbance, prone to ascending lymphangitis, systemic responses, and acidosis. Since the advent of effective antibacterial agents, such a situation arises much less frequently. Still, when an uncontrolled secondary infection does exist, there is no question that this should hasten the decision to amputate. On the other hand, the presence of a dermatitis or an ulcerated area on the upper part of the involved limb, in the vicinity of the contemplated level of amputation, may delay the step until the lesion is controlled.

Physical state of patient. Another factor which interferes with immediate amputation is a poor state of physical fitness. Frequently the candidate for operation is an elderly debilitated individual who is suffering from anemia and inadequate diet. Under these circumstances, if at all possible, it is advisable to delay surgery until the general physical condition of the patient is built up by means of blood transfusions, intravenous fluids and electrolytes, and adequate proteins and vitamins. If removal of the gangrenous limb is imperative because absorption is producing systemic responses, time can be gained for the institution of adequate preoperative treatment through the use of refrigeration of the limb (see "Role of refrigeration," below).

Contribution of associated symptoms. At times excruciating pain will force amputation of an extremity before this is considered necessary on the basis of the severity of the nutritional disturbance alone. Of course, such an approach is adopted only after all means to control the symptom have been futile and there is no alternative for preventing the rapid mental deterioration which would otherwise result. Under such circumstances, continued use of large quantities of narcotics merely accentuates the frequently existing addiction without materially affecting the pain.

Role of refrigeration. This method has been used for many years in the management of patients requiring a major amputation of a lower limb. It was first developed as a means of securing local anesthesia in poor-risk individuals. When it was found that the procedure resulted in delayed wound healing and an increased incidence of local infection, such an approach was discarded.

However, at present refrigeration has a definite but limited role in producing a physiologic amputation and thus obtaining sufficient time to deal adequately with a patient's medical complications. In this manner, the actual amputation could be performed at an elective time with much less risk to the patient. Candidates for refrigeration are those requiring a major amputation but who are also suffering from congestive heart failure, rapid atrial fibrillation, acute myocardial infarction, inflammatory processes in the lungs, or local infections which have not responded to medical therapy.

Refrigeration of a limb has been performed using several different methods. At first the extremity was placed in a plastic bag filled with ice, but this required considerable nursing care as the ice melted and frequent refilling of the container, as well as the need for providing drainage for the water. At present, dry ice is

generally used since it is easy to apply, it facilitates nursing care, and it produces a rapid and prolonged physiologic amputation. A flexible, lightweight compact freezer unit has also been proposed for this purpose [5]. Preceding the initiation of refrigeration, a suitable analgesic, such as meperidine hydrochloride (Demerol), is given intramuscularly in order to obviate the discomfort from cooling. Regardless of the method used, the upper level of refrigeration should not be higher than 7.5 or 10 cm (3 or 4 in.) below the anticipated site of amputation; otherwise the conducted cold may produce vasoconstriction and other adverse changes in the normal tissues and thus interfere with subsequent healing of the stump.

Within a very short time after refrigeration is instituted, the clinical picture changes dramatically. Severe pain from the tissues surrounding the gangrenous structures is relieved, to be replaced by a sense of numbness; signs of absorption from the lesion disappear; the body temperature falls; and the patient's appetite returns. Local infection can now be readily controlled by medical means, thus reducing the possibility of bacteria existing in the lymphatics and veins in the limb proximal to the gangrene. As a result, postoperative infection of the stump is minimized. Refrigeration can be maintained for as long as 2 weeks, during which period any associated medical condition can generally be managed. With the loss of pain and the elimination of absorption from the gangrenous limb, the patient is again able to obtain proper sleep, rest, and nourishment and so becomes a better candidate for the subsequent operative procedure.

3. Steps to Increase Physical Fitness

Once it is clear that amputation of a lower limb must be performed, measures should immediately be instituted to build up the physical state of the patient, provided, of course, that sufficient time is available for such a program.

Controlled exercise. Calisthenic exercises involving the other three limbs and the trunk should be carried out. Such an approach will help counteract the disability and disuse atrophy produced by prolonged bed rest or physical inactivity. As a result, general muscle tone and strength will be regained. At the same time, attempts should be made to prevent or reduce contractures in the joints proximal to the anticipated level of amputation in the involved extremity and to maintain normal range of motion in these structures.

Instruction in transfer and standing. The patient should be trained in transferring from the bed to the chair and then to the standing position with weight bearing only on the uninvolved limb. Moreover, instruction should be given in balancing while the patient stands before a full-length mirror and performs various necessary maneuvers. Such exercises will help in subsequently carrying out gait training.

Instruction in crutch walking. Also of value for future use of a prosthesis is instruction in those exercises which strengthen the muscles of the upper extremities used in crutch walking; the patient should likewise learn to ambulate with crutches and the uninvolved lower limb. Ability to manage by such a means is essential to the amputee even when he has a prosthesis, for there are periods when he must perform physical activities without being in a position to use the latter. At the same time, this type of instruction improves his ability to stand properly and gives him confidence in walking with an artificial leg. Such results will be useful in future gait walking. Moreover, information will be gained regarding the patient's potential as a candidate for a prosthesis.

C. Determination of Optimal Level for Amputation

1. General Considerations

Although a number of objective tests are available to aid in the selection of a proper amputation site, many surgeons still rely mainly on clinical examination to make this decision. However, an error in judgment regarding the adequacy of the circulation at the proposed level may result in lack of wound healing, prolongation of confinement to bed, and a reamputation at a higher level (which increases

morbidity and mortality). All of these factors produce a serious blow to the patient's morale and motivation and result in a considerable increase in hospital costs and medical fees. Hence, it is important to utilize every possible approach to determine the state of the local circulation, so as to be in the most knowledgeable position to make the proper decision at the first attempt.

Of course, if the amputation were performed at a high enough level to ensure unquestioned adequate blood supply, there would be no problem with primary stump healing. But this is not a practical solution to the difficulty since for the patient there are definite advantages in not sacrificing functioning limb length, provided sound healing is still obtainable. Depending upon the level, these include ability to ambulate without a crutch or prosthesis or the possibility of being fitted with a more satisfactory prosthesis, such as one for a below-knee rather than for an above-knee amputation. Preservation of a longer length of limb may also provide greater ease of turning in bed and balancing in the sitting position. Whether the patient is considered a proper candidate for a prosthesis or for a wheelchair existence will also influence the selection of the amputation site.

2. Laboratory and Clinical Means of Evaluating the State of Local Circulation

This section deals with those tests which give information concerning the blood supply to the entire lower limb and hence are of value, in a general way, in the elucidation of the problem of determining the optimal level for amputation.

Oscillometry. This procedure is useful in determining the location and degree of block in the arterial system (see Section B, Chapter 5). Readings of 3 or more units at the lower level of the leg above the ankle indicate that one or both tibial arteries at this site are partially or fully patent. Such findings signify that there is an adequate blood supply to the foot, making possible successful operative procedures on this segment of limb. With absent or markedly reduced figures (0 to 0.5 units), it can be assumed that both tibial arteries at the ankle are either completely or almost completely occluded and that nutritional blood flow to the foot is dependent almost solely on the extent and efficiency of the developing collateral circulation. Under such circumstances, the possibility of obtaining healing of the operative site following either amputation of a toe or toes, a transmetatarsal amputation, or a Syme's procedure is significantly decreased.

If the oscillometric readings obtained from the level of the calf are only somewhat reduced (to approximately 3 units), the likelihood of accomplishing a successful below-knee amputation is very good. With such findings, it can be assumed that the popliteal artery is still partly patent and that there is sufficient local circulation to permit healing of the stump. Very low figures obtained at the calf (0 to 0.75 unit), although indicating that there is almost complete occlusion of the main arteries at this level, do not necessarily rule out a below-knee amputation, inasmuch as the extent and efficiency of the existing collateral circulation cannot be determined through the use of oscillometry. However, if at the same time pulsations are absent in the femoral artery, this type of procedure is definitely contraindicated.

Readings of 1 or more oscillometric units above the knee are generally sufficient to allow for a successful supracondylar and midthigh amputation. Even the absence of oscillometric readings at this level does not negate the possibility of a similar therapeutic response, provided pulsations are still felt in the femoral artery in the groin. With complete occlusion of the latter vessel, the incidence of nonhealing of the operative wound at sites on the thigh significantly increases, particularly in the case of the supracondylar level.

Contrast angiography. This approach provides detailed anatomic data regarding the larger arteries in the limb, information which is essential in determining the amount of blood that can be expected to reach the contemplated level of amputation through main channels. However, if these vessels are occluded and blood supply is dependent solely on circulation through small channels and the collateral arterial bed, contrast angiography is not very helpful in evaluating the physiologic state of perfusion to the tissues themselves. (For a discussion of the technique of contrast angiography, see Section E, Chapter 5.)

Other tests of local arterial blood flow. Certain clinical findings are also of value as supplemental aids in determining the proper site for amputation. Among these are the level of cutaneous temperature demarcation, color changes (particularly dependent rubor of the feet), the presence of rest pain (ischemic neuropathy), and the nutritional state of the skin and subcutaneous tissue of the leg and foot (hair growth, nail growth, dryness and scaliness of the skin, loss of subcutaneous tissue). The results of the reactive hyperemia test are also helpful in determining the state of cutaneous circulation at the contemplated level of amputation. (For the technique of carrying out the reactive hyperemia test, see D-1, Chapter 6.)

Contribution of infection. If infection plays an important role in the progression of the nutritional disturbance, as in the presence of diabetes, the decision with regard to the level of amputation rests on several other factors beside the ones already enumerated. In many such instances the appearance of the foot is misleading, since some of the changes are still reversible if the secondary infection can be halted in time. In other words, part of the destruction of tissue is due to inflammation, while the impairment in local circulation is actually not as marked as physical examination of the limb would lead one to believe. Under such circumstances, a lower level of amputation than previously considered advisable is indicated.

3. Basis for Removal of One or More Toes

The advantage of only removing the ulcerated or gangrenous toe or toes is apparent since normal stance and ambulation are not particularly altered, even when the great toe is so treated. However, great circumspection and care must be employed when utilizing such an approach.

Local vascular states conducive to successful outcome. Unfortunately, amputation of a toe or toes has limited application and should be performed only when certain rigid criteria can be satisfied. First, the gangrenous process must be confined to the distal portion of the digit or digits, with a segment of normal tissue intervening between the lesion and the attachment of the toes to the foot proper. Second, all signs of inflammation of the viable tissues of the digits and the adjoining part of the foot must have subsided. Finally, and most importantly, there must be adequate blood flow to the foot to take care of the markedly increased metabolic needs of the structures at the level of the operative site, so that healing will take place (see below).

Numerous clinical and laboratory tests are available to determine the efficiency of the blood supply to the foot. Besides oscillometry (see above), of equal importance are other means of determining the state of circulation in the two tibial arteries to the foot. Pulsations should be present in at least one of these vessels (preferably the posterior tibial artery) if healing is to be expected. Another very useful procedure is measurement of blood pressure in the arteries at the ankle using the Doppler ultrasonic technique. A reading of 35 to 40 mmHg or higher is support for attempting to remove a toe or toes since the possibility of subsequent healing of the operative site is good. Readings below these levels indicate minimal blood flow through partially occluded arteries in the foot, making a successful operative procedure on toes almost an impossibility. (For a description of the Doppler ultrasonic flowmeter, see D-2, Chapter 5.)

Results in different types of patients. Removal of a toe or toes can most frequently be successfully carried out in the diabetic patient without arteriosclerosis obliterans but with gangrene and ulceration of tips of toes and a superim-

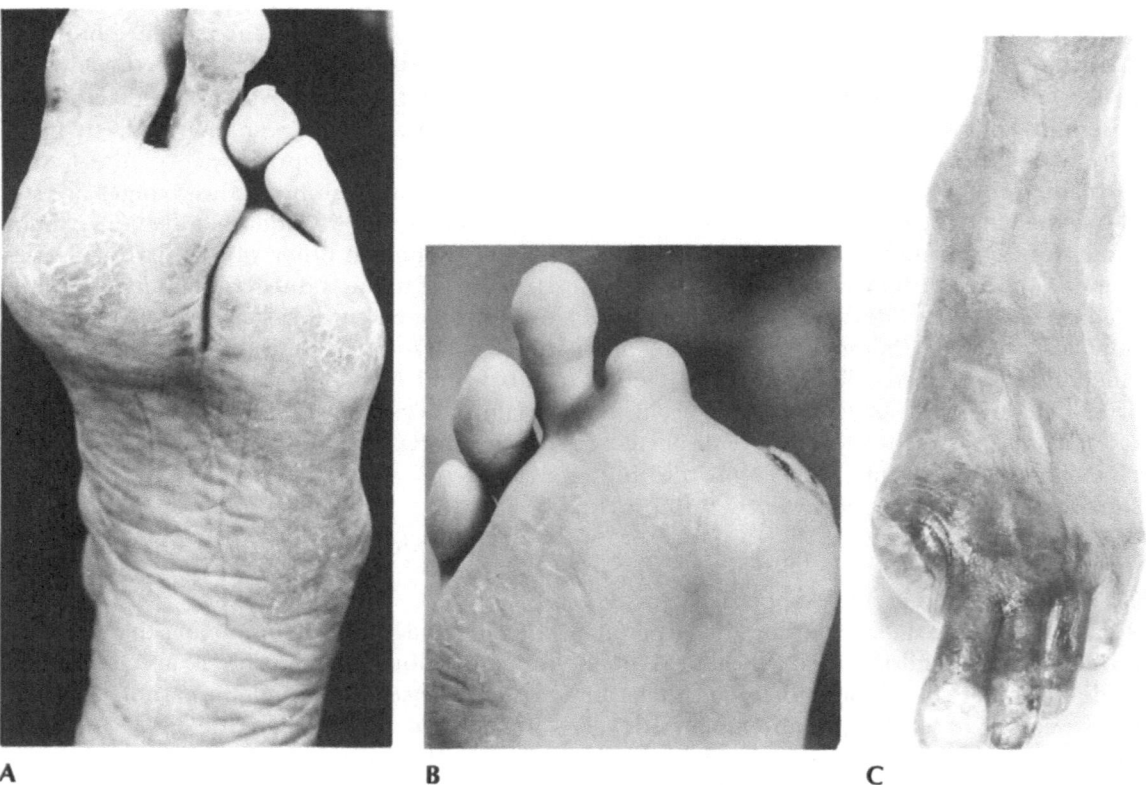

A   B   C

Fig. 24.1. **A–C.** Amputation of a toe or toes in diabetic patients for localized gangrene limited to digits, with complete healing of operative site. In each instance, pulsations were present in one or both tibial arteries in the foot. In **A,** ray resection of third toe was performed.

posed infection (Fig. 24.1). In this type of individual, the occlusive process is generally limited to the microcirculation (in the form of thickening of the basement membrane of arterioles and capillaries) and to the terminal arterial tree (the arcuate and digital arteries), with the main vessels to the foot still demonstrating pulsatile flow. In contrast, the same surgical approach when utilized in a person with senile arteriosclerosis obliterans, in whom the main arterial tree is occluded, will almost invariably result in nonhealing of the operative site and the need for another operation at a much higher level on the limb. Occasionally, a lumbar sympathectomy performed at the same time may increase the possibility of a successful result in the latter type of individual. In patients with thromboangiitis obliterans, this dual approach may be quite effective, provided abstinence from smoking is also carried out. Generally there is a superimposed element of vasospasm in this disorder, which is removed by abolition of sympathetic control over the peripheral cutaneous vessels in the foot (particularly the toes), thus resulting in a significant increase in blood flow locally.

4. Basis for a Transmetatarsal Amputation

Transmetatarsal amputation has certain practical advantages since rehabilitation is simple. All that is needed is the use of a foam rubber insert or a leather-covered steel shank in the toe of the shoe. Moreover, the patient retains an excellent functional lower limb, since removal of the heads of all the metatarsals does not materially affect the three-point bearing surface of the foot. However, although the operation preserves part of the propulsive action of the foot, there is loss of the normal "push-off" which is delivered by the movement of the toes.

Local vascular status conducive to successful outcome. In order for healing to occur following a transmetatarsal amputation, the preoperative state of the circulation in the foot must be fairly normal, as in the case of removal of a toe or toes (see above). There must be pulsations in at least one of the tibial arteries in the foot (preferably the posterior tibial), the oscillometric readings on the leg above the level of the ankle should be 2 or more units, and the ankle blood pressure should be 35 mmHg or more with the Doppler ultrasonic flowmeter.

Involvement of the entire toe or toes by a gangrenous or ulcerative process is no contraindication, provided that the lesion has not extended for any distance onto the adjoining dorsal portion of the foot and infection is controlled by antibacterial therapy. The plantar portion of the foot should be intact so as to supply an adequate flap for covering the operative site.

Results in different types of patients. As in the case of amputation of toes, a transmetatarsal amputation is performed mainly in the diabetic patient who demonstrates an adequate blood supply to the foot (Fig. 24.2). Such a procedure for the patient with senile arteriosclerosis obliterans or thromboangiitis obliterans in whom there are no signs of blood flow through the main arteries in the foot will generally result in failure and the need for a higher

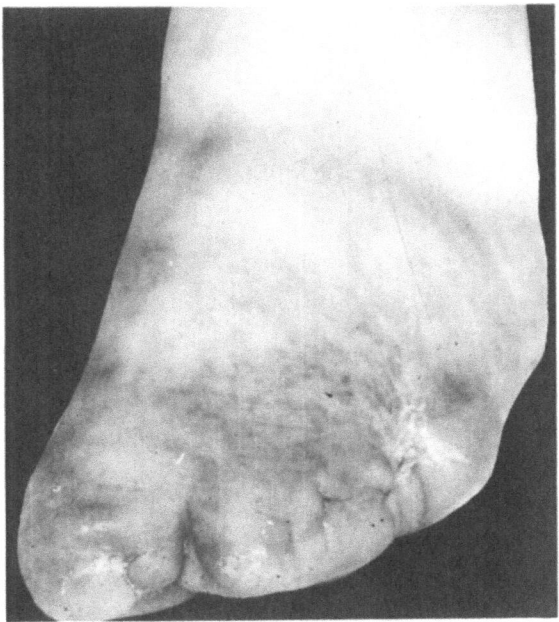

Fig. 24.2. Successful transmetatarsal amputation in a diabetic patient with gangrene limited to the distal portion of three toes. Pulsations were present in the posterior tibial artery at the ankle.

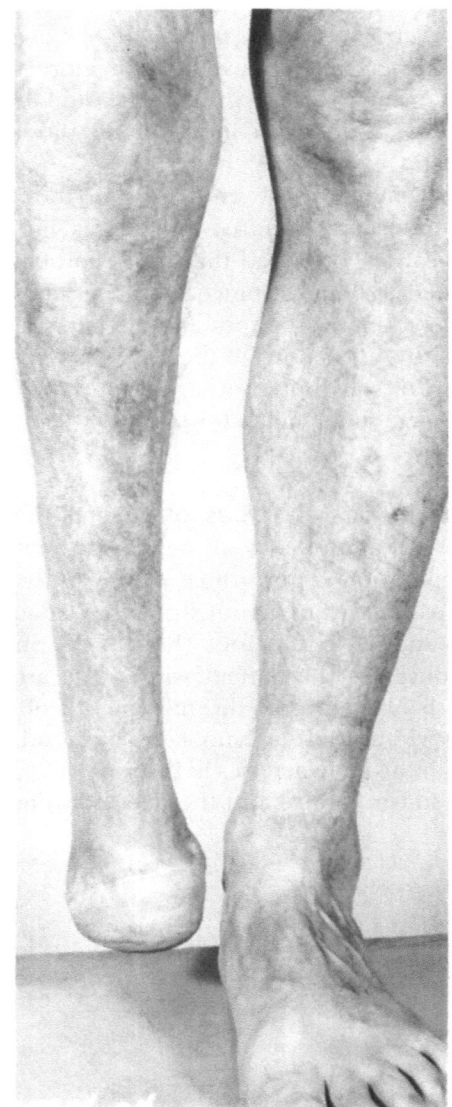

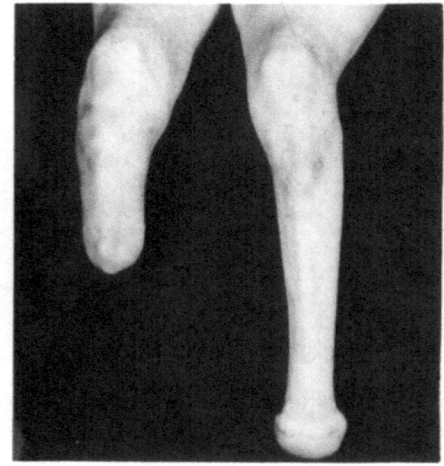

amputation. At times, however, the development of an extensive collateral arterial bed may permit enough blood flow to the operative site to cause healing of the stump.

Even in the presence of adequate blood supply, it is important to keep in mind the possibility that the stump may not heal and that a second, higher amputation may be necessary. Therefore, only the patient who is considered to be in such physical condition that he can undergo two operations if necessary should be subjected to transmetatarsal amputation.

5. Basis for a Supramalleolar Amputation

Since the Syme's procedure, which involves a supramalleolar amputation, retains essentially the full length of the shank, weight-bearing approaches that existing with an intact heel. It has the advantage of enabling the amputee to walk or stand without support using a Syme's prosthesis. The procedure is indicated when the nutritional changes have extended onto a good portion of the foot and hence are too extensive to be dealt with by a transmetatarsal amputation.

Local vascular status conducive to successful outcome. Again, as in the case of removal of a toe or toes and transmetatarsal amputation, healing of the operative site can generally be expected only if pulsations are present in the foot and fairly normal oscillometric readings are obtainable from the leg above the ankle. As already indicated, such a situation exists in the diabetic, with the occlusive process being found only in the terminal arteries and the microcirculation (Fig. 24.3). Even in the presence of adequate local circulation, a common complication of a Syme's amputation is failure of the heel flap to adhere firmly to underlying bone.

Fig. 24.3. **A** Successful Syme's amputation in a diabetic patient with gangrene of the distal portion of the foot and two toes. Pulsations were present in the posterior tibial artery at the ankle. **B** A diabetic patient with gangrene first of the left foot and then the right foot, treated by means of a left Syme's amputation and a right below-knee amputation. Good healing of both operative sites resulted.

6. Basis for a Below-knee Amputation

Indications for procedure. There is complete
agreement that when a major amputation is
contemplated, preservation of the knee joint,
if at all practicable, is highly desirable. The
main reason for such a view is the fact that
this offers better potential for rehabilitation of
the patient than does an operation performed
through the thigh. The increased likelihood of
ambulation using a prosthesis and the greater
capability for self-care make the below-knee
amputee much less disabled than the above-
knee amputee. For one thing, he has better
proprioceptive balance; besides, the below-
knee prosthesis is much lighter than the one
for an above-knee amputation. Even if the patient is not a candidate for a prosthesis, the
increased length of remaining limb and the
presence of an active knee joint permit him
to move about more readily in bed and to get
into a wheelchair with greater ease. Another
very important point to consider is the fact that
the below-knee amputation is attended with a
lower mortality than is one performed above
the knee [6].

Disadvantages of the procedure. Because arteriosclerosis obliterans is a progressive condition, some surgeons are reluctant to perform
a below-knee amputation in patients with this
disorder for fear that healing of the stump will
not take place. Also important in this regard
is the fact that such individuals as a group are
poor operative risks, suffering from atherosclerosis in other vital organs; hence, the need
to subject them to two surgical procedures if
the first attempt is unsuccessful markedly compounds the hazard. Another consideration is
that generally a much longer period of bed rest
is required for stump healing than is the case
for an above-knee site, a situation which is conducive to postoperative complications, particularly in the case of the elderly patient. Among
unquestioned contraindications to a below-
knee amputation is a 15° or more permanent
flexion contracture of the knee;[2] another is

---

[2] In order to prevent such a state, the knee must be
maintained in full extension by means of a posterior plaster
splint during the early period of bed rest; otherwise, the
patient may tend to assume the flexed position of the limb
to avoid discomfort.

poorly viable skin over the extent of the proposed surgical site.

**Local vascular status conducive to successful
outcome.** As already indicated in C-2, above,
oscillometry, contrast angiography, and palpation of the pulses can give pertinent information regarding the state of circulation through
the common femoral artery, the superficial
femoral artery, the deep femoral artery and its
branches, and the popliteal artery and its two
main branches, the anterior and posterior tibial
arteries at their origin. All of these steps are
essential in determining whether a below-knee
amputation will be followed by healing of the
stump. If the results of the tests indicate that
the popliteal artery is even partially patent, the
possibility of a successful outcome is markedly
enhanced. In the absence of blood flow
through this vessel, there is less chance of healing of the stump unless adequate circulation
through the terminal vessels is found during
surgery (see below). Also of importance in this
regard is the existence of a patent deep femoral
artery and its branches, as determined by arteriography. Under such circumstances, an adequate collateral blood flow may have developed
below the level of the knee between these vessels and the twigs of the now occluded popliteal
artery by way of the descending branch of the
lateral femoral circumflex artery and the lowest
perforating artery. If the occlusive process is
present in the superficial and common femoral
arteries, as well as in the popliteal artery, the
incidence of healing of the stump following a
below-knee amputation is markedly reduced.
This is so because the superior genicular artery,
which is an important collateral above the knee,
is commonly obstructed when the vessel from
which it arises, the superficial femoral artery,
is similarly affected. As a result, the circulation
to tissues below the knee is seriously compromised. Nevertheless, on occasion, even in the
absence of a common femoral pulse in the
groin, a successful below-knee amputation can
still be carried out, provided bleeding is sufficiently brisk in the anterolateral compartment
at the time of operation (see below).

Likewise of importance in making a decision
to perform a below-knee amputation is the state
of the cutaneous circulation on the upper part
of the leg. In this regard, the results obtained

with the reactive hyperemia test, skin color, and skin temperature are all helpful in reaching the correct conclusion.

If there still is some question as to whether the knee joint can be preserved, it is advisable first to perform the amputation below the knee, at the same time preparing the patient surgically for the higher amputation if this becomes necessary. As the operation proceeds, if free bleeding and oozing from small vessels in skin and muscles are only minimal, if the main arteries are completely obliterated, and, of greatest importance, if the muscles appear friable and brownish or grayish in color, then it will probably be expedient to change the operative site to above the knee and perform a supracondylar or midthigh amputation without delay. On the other hand, the presence of brisk bleeding, partially patent large arteries through which blood is flowing, and a red, healthy appearance of the muscle structure should all support the belief that the proper site has been selected for amputation.[3] In any event, it is important to explain to the patient preoperatively that whether his knee joint can be saved will depend solely on the vascular status of the tissues in the operative field.

Results in different types of patients. A below-knee amputation is particularly applicable to diabetic patients with extensive necrosis of the foot (Fig. 24.3B), since such individuals frequently have patent or nearly patent popliteal arteries and patent origins of the anterior and posterior tibial branches, despite the fact that at the same time there is severe small vessel obliterative disease in the feet. The patient with thromboangiitis obliterans is usually also a good candidate for a below-knee amputation because the cause for the necrosis of the foot is frequently located in the branches of the popliteal artery and rarely above the level of this vessel.

In the case of the patient with arteriosclerosis obliterans without diabetes, the decision to perform a below-knee amputation will most often depend upon the state of the vascular bed at the time of operation (see above), since in many cases pulsations will not be found in the popliteal artery or even at a higher level. If

the occlusive disease exists in both lower limbs but with gangrene already present in one, it is very important to attempt a below-knee amputation in the latter if at all feasible. Then, if at a subsequent date a thigh amputation is required for the remaining limb, the resulting disability is not as great as would be the case if the patient is left with two high amputations. Only occasionally is an elderly bilateral above-knee amputee able to walk with prostheses [7,17]. However, this is not so if one knee is preserved.

Operative approach. Since the technical aspects of the surgery for a below-knee amputation appear to play a very important role in producing a successful result, it appears necessary to mention some of the factors that may contribute to such an outcome. An optimal level of amputation is one in which the stump consists of 15.0 to 17.5 cm (6 to 7 in.) of the proximal portion of the tibia. A short anterior flap and a long, tapered posterior flap fitted to the anterior flap are generally preferred, although a circular incision is advocated by some surgeons on the basis that the creation of the fish-mouth type of anterior and posterior flaps compromises the skin edges at their apexes [6]. Protection and atraumatic handling of the skin during division of the tibia and fibula are vital. Care must be taken to avoid clamping soft tissue or handling it with forceps. Drains are not used unless the stump is especially vascular and infection is potentially present. A narrow strip of Vaseline gauze should be applied to the suture line of all clean stumps, since this promotes drainage for a few hours (until the Vaseline is absorbed into the dressings) and eliminates crusting and fluid retention. The stump is then covered with a dry dressing which is held in place by an elastic compression bandage so that pressure is evenly distributed. This aids in shrinking the stump, molding it, and eliminating dead space at the same time that the wound is protected. Care should be taken to apply the bandage so that there is no interference with blood flow into the stump or with venous return from the limb. Otherwise, ischemia and edema of the end of the stump will develop.

In recent years attempts have been made to fit the below-knee amputee with a temporary prosthesis at the time of the operation, in order

---

[3] Of course, if tourniquets are utilized during the operation, such pertinent information will not be available to the surgeon.

to reduce or control the edema of the stump and thus permit better local healing and facilitate early permanent fitting [1,2,16]. However, there is a real question as to whether the patient with an ischemic lower limb will benefit from such a procedure since the possibility of necrosis of the stump, due to compromise of the cutaneous circulation by the resulting compression, does exist under such circumstances. One important advantage to the method is that it permits early ambulation with a prosthesis, which has a beneficial psychologic effect on the patient.

In brief, the technique of immediate postoperative rigid dressing is as follows: A graded pressure cast is formed around the stump, the operative site first being covered and protected from pressure with layers of sterile fluffed gauze and a stump sock. A pylon is then incorporated into the cast using plaster.

Role of lumbar sympathectomy. The view has been proposed that removal of vasomotor tone to the lower limb by means of a lumbar ganglionectomy facilitates healing of a below-knee stump because of the resulting increase in cutaneous circulation at the amputation site. However, even in normal individuals, very little experimental evidence is available indicating that blood flow through the skin at the level of the knee and for some distance below this point is enhanced following a sympathectomy. Therefore, in patients with arteriosclerosis obliterans, who frequently demonstrate advanced organic degeneration, loss of elasticity of collateral vessels, and little if any vasospasm, the possibility of a therapeutic vascular response from sympathectomy is even more remote. At the same time, there is an added risk from subjecting individuals who are generally in poor physical condition to another operation which involves entrance into the abdominal cavity. Hence, sympathectomy would appear to be a very questionable therapeutic approach to the extension of the level of safe amputation.

7. Basis for an Above-knee Amputation

An above-knee amputation should be performed only if various tests and associated medical conditions have ruled out the possibil-

ity or practicability of a below-knee amputation. The one great advantage of the procedure is that because of the higher level on the limb utilized, the blood supply can generally be expected to be adequate for rapid healing of the stump, a situation which also results in fewer postoperative complications.

A supracondylar level is the common site of amputation, while a midthigh amputation is indicated when the circulation appears to be severely compromised at the lower site. Even in the absence of pulsations in the common femoral artery in the groin, the collateral circulation in the thigh is generally adequate for healing of the stump following a midthigh amputation. As in the case of a below-knee amputation, the decision whether to perform a supracondylar amputation or to utilize a higher level on the thigh may have to be made at the time of operation, depending upon the state of vascularity observed first in the operative field at the lower site.

Results in different types of patients. An above-knee amputation is generally carried out on patients with arteriosclerosis obliterans. Since most of these individuals are elderly, the loss of the knee joint does not present as much of a problem as it would in a younger age group. In many cases a prosthesis for a supracondylar or midthigh amputee is adequate for the limited activity usually indulged in by the patients. Furthermore, a certain percentage of them, for mental or physical reasons, are not candidates for a prosthesis and the loss of the knee joint does not particularly affect the existing situation to any significant degree. Moreover, an above-knee amputation is much less frequently associated with a second amputation than is the case with a below-knee amputation.

In patients with diabetes demonstrating atherosclerotic changes primarily limited to the terminal arteries in the feet, rarely is an above-knee amputation indicated, since in most instances a below-knee amputation will be followed by healing of the stump. The same situation exists for many patients with thromboangiitis obliterans.[4]

---

[4] Since other types of amputations, such as disarticulation through the knee, guillotine amputation, transcondylar amputation, and the Gritti-Stokes amputation, are rarely utilized for the ischemic limb, they have not been included in the discussion.

D. Complications of a Major Amputation

1. Morbidity and Mortality

Major amputation of lower limbs for ischemic necrosis is associated with high morbidity and mortality rates, mainly because the patients requiring such a heroic measure fall into the fifth to the seventh decades of life and are therefore generally poor surgical risks. It has been reported, for example, that the procedure is followed by a 35 percent 30-day postoperative mortality [12]. Also important are the findings that 22 percent of below-knee amputations fail to heal [9] and that approximately 50 percent of above-knee amputees remain unrehabilitated [8]. Moreover, pulmonary embolism and other thromboembolic phenomena are relatively common after major amputation, particularly in the case of above-knee sites.

2. Nonhealing Stump and Its Management

As in the case of the original lesion, infection and inadequate local circulation are responsible for a very serious complication of a major amputation—nonhealing of the stump.

Local infection.   Although with our present refinements in technique and asepsis and the prophylactic use of antibacterial agents the incidence of wound infection has been markedly reduced, nevertheless at times it is necessary to cope with such a situation. This is particularly true if the ulceration or gangrene of the foot was originally associated with a severe infection leading to lymphangitis and regional lymphadenitis. A rise in body temperature, increased pain in the operative site, purulent discharge from the suture line, edema and redness of the skin of the stump, and leukocytosis all indicate the existence of infection. Rarely, osteomyelitis may result from invasion of organisms through the end of the stump, the process presenting as an abscess or sinus formation.

With regard to prophylactic measures in the control of infection, penicillin or other wide-spectrum antibiotics should be given for at least 1 week before operation in order to help destroy any bacteria which have penetrated the tissues some distance proximal to the gangrenous site. The same medication should then be continued for 10 to 14 days after surgery to prevent infection of the stump from the dressings. Also of use in encouraging healing is a high-protein diet, supplemented by multivitamins, in order to raise the serum protein level above 6 g per 100 ml. At the time of operation, such precautions as care in tying off all bleeding points so as to reduce oozing and accumulation of serum in the wound, elimination of dead space, application of compression dressings, and adequate drainage if indicated will likewise help control infection. Attempts to reduce the amount of tissue subjected to trauma and crushing or made ischemic by ligatures will have a similar effect.

In the active treatment of infection, the measures used will depend upon the degree of involvement. If the process is limited to the edges of the wound (Fig. 24.4A), local application of antibacterial agents and cleansing solutions, together with parenteral use of antibiotics, is generally adequate to control the situation. However, if signs of inflammation are noted over a considerable portion of the stump and marked swelling and pain are present, it can be assumed that the infection is deep and extensive. Under such circumstances it may be necessary to open the entire length of the incision and evacuate the pus and other products resulting from liquefaction of involved tissues. The removal of the necrotic material may then be facilitated by continuous or intermittent irrigation with Dakin's solution. Should a sinus tract develop, antibiotic ointment is applied to a Vaseline gauze wick and inserted at the base of the lesion.

Only when granulating tissues begin to cover the exposed surface of the bone should secondary closure be considered. Until then it is best to keep the lesion open to prevent formation of pockets of pus. In order to remove irritating secretions and necrotic material, the daily use of whirlpool baths with tincture of green soap or Betadine is worthwhile. At all times care should be taken to prevent recontamination of the wound or the introduction of new secondary invaders.

When areas of granulation occur along the

suture line, this generally indicates failure of primary healing or the breakdown of a scar. Unfortunately, with subsequent healing, the suture line may contain dense scar tissue which will not hold up on prolonged contact with a prosthesis. If supervised walking with the prosthesis leads to destruction of the scar, it may be necessary to excise this tissue and carefully reapproximate the wound edges.

Inadequate local circulation. This situation is more frequently responsible for nonhealing of the stump than is infection (Fig. 24.4B). Its presence indicates either that the site of operation was poorly selected, that the surgical procedure was unnecessarily traumatizing resulting in an exaggeration of already existing tissue anoxia, or that the associated fall of blood pressure during the operation was sufficient to produce complete thrombosis of previously partially occluded critical arteries to the limb. Of course, in certain circumstances there may be no alternative but to attempt an incision through structures which are obviously in a precarious state of nutrition.

The treatment of a stump which has failed

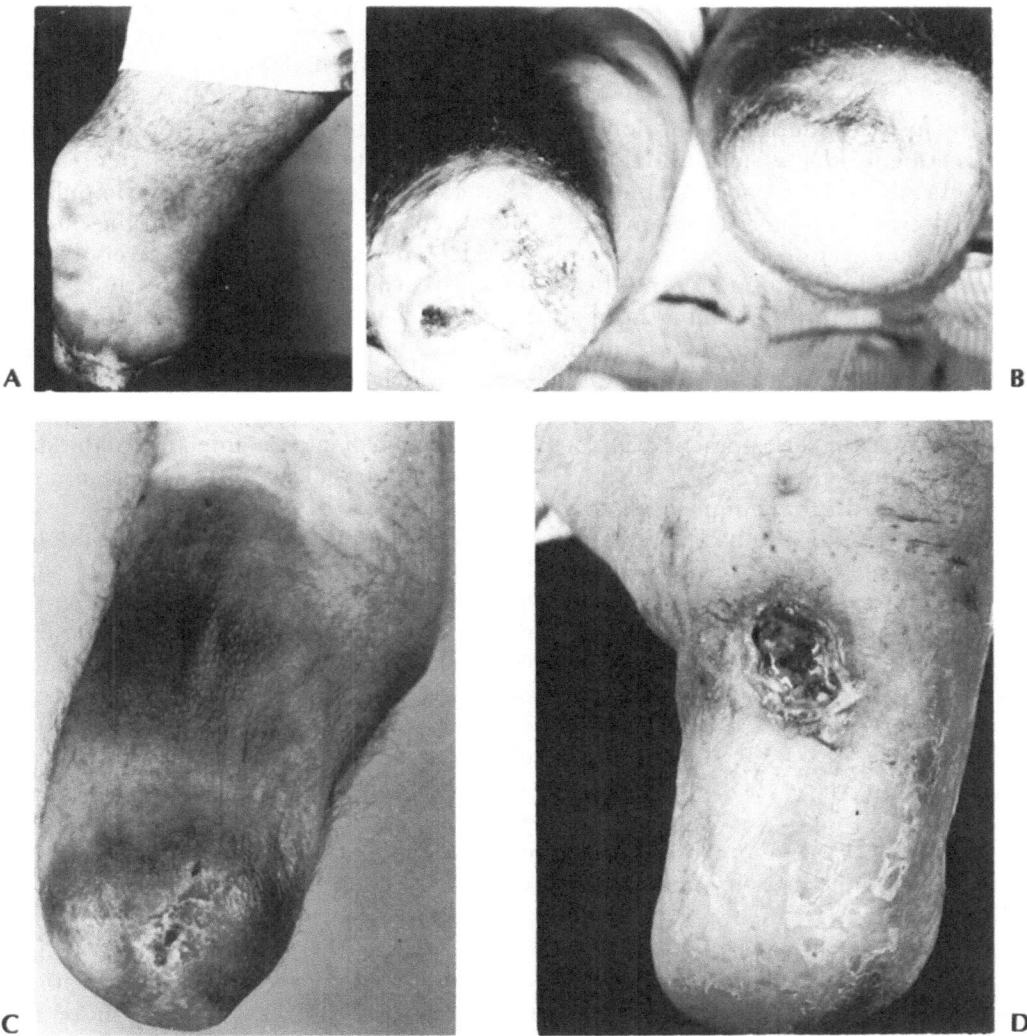

Fig. 24.4. Postoperative complications. **A** Local infection in suture line. **B** Nonhealing of stump due to inadequate local circulation. **C** Edema of stump. **D** Abrasion of skin of stump due to rough spots in socket.

to heal because of inadequate local blood flow will depend upon the degree of tissue destruction. In the presence of extensive gangrene, the best approach is to reamputate as soon as the physical state of the patient will permit. Otherwise there may be absorption of toxic materials from the site, as well as spread of the thrombotic process into vessels of adjoining and proximal structures, thus reducing the chances of a subsequent successful result at a higher level.

If the necrosis is limited to the skin edges or even to part of one of the flaps, without any apparent involvement of deeper tissues, it is best to wait, in order to determine whether the process will become stationary. If this occurs, the gangrenous material can be removed later and perhaps skin grafting performed to facilitate healing, or epithelialization may take place spontaneously. All during the prolonged period of treatment, the wound should be cared for aseptically and the patient should be receiving parenteral antibacterial therapy.

After an adequate period of intensive conservative treatment, if the stump does not heal and there is involvement of adjoining normal tissue, reamputation will have to be performed. Where the original site was below the knee, such a procedure does not pose any particular problem. However, when a supracondylar or midthigh amputation is unsuccessful, difficulty is usually encountered in obtaining a suitable site for reamputation. Certainly under these circumstances, the possibility of being able to use a prosthesis on the resulting stump is slight. In some instances, it may even be necessary to disarticulate the entire lower extremity in order to obtain healing.

3. Phantom Limb

The term, *phantom limb*, refers to the illusion of the presence of a limb after its amputation. In fact, the patient may frequently experience the same pain that was elicited by the previous gangrenous process and is able exactly to localize the symptom to the original site of involvement. The incidence of the condition is higher after proximal than distal amputations. Moreover, phantom limb is practically always present following upper-extremity amputation,

while it is less frequently noted after lower-extremity amputation. Of interest is a study [13] indicating that phantom limb occurs in only 20 percent of children less than 2 years of age following amputation of previously normal limbs; in 25 percent in the 2- to 4-year group; in 61 percent in the 4- to 6-year group; in 75 percent in the 6- to 8-year group; and in 100 percent in children 8 years of age and older.

Pathogenesis. The mechanism of production of the phantom limb has not been clearly elucidated nor universally accepted. The controversy exists between those who believe that the symptom complex is of organic origin and those who propose a psychogenic factor as a cause. According to the first view, painful sensations from an inflamed, compressed, or lacerated stump or from a neuroma due to section of the peripheral mixed nerve produce stimulation of afferent pathways in the latter structure. As a consequence, the incoming impulses establish a reverberating circuit in the internuncial pool of neurons, which travels cephalad until it reaches the thalamus. Such a situation is followed by the development of a vicious circle between the thalamus and the cerebral cortex which is self-perpetuating and not affected by removal of the precipitating factor, such as a neuroma or an infection of the stump. The painful impulses also set off autonomic disturbances in the sympathetic nervous system. The resulting reduction in local blood flow increases the pain by contributing an element of ischemia of the nervous structures in the stump. A weakness in the organic theory is that it fails to account for the fact that the pain of phantom limb does not follow a peripheral nerve distribution and is not an anatomic representation of the missing part [15].

With regard to the view supporting the psychogenic origin of phantom limb, the "body image" concept [11] is used to explain the symptoms. In this regard, it is premised that as a result of various sensations experienced over the years, the individual builds up in his own mind an image of himself in relation to the external world. Because the more distal parts of the body, the fingers and toes, are richly supplied with sensory nerves, they have a proportionately greater representation in the body image than other structures. Hence, their loss following amputation has a marked effect psychologically on the patient. In support of the psychogenic origin is the frequent finding of emotional disturbances in individuals with painful phantoms, which suggests that the pain is maintained by psychic mechanisms arising from the patient's attitude toward his own body. The possibility has also been proposed that the phantom limb is a form of narcissism, rendering the individual incapable of accepting the permanent loss of part of his body [10].

A theory has been advanced that phantom sensation may have origins which are central, peripheral, or a combination of both. It is believed that the sensations resulting from touch or movement and shrinkage are probably central, whereas neuralgic pain and paresthesia are peripheral.

Clinical manifestations. At times the complaints associated with phantom limb may be severe enough to make them incapacitating. They may be experienced as a boring pain in the bone or a sense of tearing, pressing, or burning, perceived in the original site of the amputated toes. The phantom sensation may be continuous or intermittent, and it may be initiated by minor stimuli or impulses, such as slight trauma to the stump, nervous tension, or pain in other parts of the body. Environmental conditions, including cold and change of weather, may aggravate the complaints. Associated findings consist of signs of increased sympathetic tonus in the stump (coldness, cyanosis of the skin, and hyperhidrosis).

Treatment. A large number of therapeutic approaches have been advocated for the control of phantom limb, but none has been found consistently effective in producing permanent relief. Most of the surgical procedures involve interruption of the pain pathways between the periphery and the pain centers in the thalamus and the cerebral cortex. They include injection of alcohol into peripheral nerves; intradural incision of thoracic nerve roots; sympathectomy; and spinothalamic chordotomy. Although some improvement can be expected initially, the late results of surgical treatment are poor. More conservative methods, such as infiltration of the peripheral and sympathetic nervous system with procaine hydrochloride and intensive psychotherapy, appear to be justified in many cases of phantom limb.

4. Other Abnormal Changes in Affected Limb

Symptomatic neuroma formation. Rather commonly the distal end of the severed nerve demonstrates a proliferative mass of Schwann cells and axons in the form of a neuroma. Such an abnormality may be responsible for local pain, tenderness, and hyperesthesia or hypesthesia of the overlying skin, initiated by compression of the mass of nervous structures by forming scar tissue. In some patients the symptoms may be severe enough to preclude the use of a prosthesis. Ultrasound, local injection of alcohol, or even excision of the neuroma may be necessary in order to control the condition.

Joint abnormalities. Contracture of the remaining joints following an amputation may make prosthetic training (see E-2, below) and gait training very difficult. This is especially so if degenerative changes have occurred in the hip and knee on the affected side, causing impairment in extension. Older amputees are prone to these alterations, making them poor candidates for extensive ambulation programs using a prosthesis.

Bony spurs. Another situation which may contribute to inability to utilize a prosthesis is the growth of sharp spurs from the end of the remaining portion of bone. Such structures may cause pain and at times may even penetrate the overlying skin to produce indolent, nonhealing ulcerations. Following a below-knee amputation, a sharp edge may develop on the anterior surface of the stump of the tibia which may produce irritation and abrasion of the skin to the point that surgical revision may be required.

5. Postoperative Depression

As discussed in the section on phantom limb (D-3, above), major amputation of a limb markedly alters the patient's body image and frequently initiates a period of grief for the lost member. In the elderly individual, particularly, this may be followed by a state of depression. He may now consider himself a hopeless, helpless cripple for the remainder of his life, even though he may maintain an optimistic facade. It is therefore essential to discuss this matter in a realistic fashion with the patient in the hope that the mental difficulty can be avoided. A supportive doctor-patient relationship is most important in this regard.

E. Rehabilitative Program

A rehabilitative program is essential for the elderly patient following amputation of an ischemic gangrenous lower limb. It should be started early in the postoperative period, thus reducing the period of bed rest to a minimum. The goal of such an approach is the acquisition of maximum functional capacity in the shortest possible time. This does not necessarily mean total independence in carrying out activities of daily living, since such an objective may be unrealistic if other serious geriatric illnesses coexist. Hence, compromises must be made depending upon the associated difficulties.

1. Early Measures

Bed positioning. The patient, on returning from the operating room, should be placed on a bed with a firm board between the mattress and springs so as to reduce the tendency toward hip and knee flexion when lying supine. At the same time, the pelvis is kept straight to prevent abduction of the stump. The latter should lie flat on the bed; any attempt on the part of nurses and aides to relieve pain by propping it up with pillows should be prevented, for such a measure is probably the most common cause of hip flexion following an above-knee amputation. Several times during the day the patient should assume the prone position, while a pillow is now placed under the anterior surface of the stump to encourage hip extension. In the limb which has been amputated below the knee, it is good practice to apply a plaster splint to the posterior surface to prevent flexion contracture at the knee.

Stump exercises. As soon as the patient has recovered from the anesthetic and is able to comprehend requests, he should be started on a program of supervised active and assistive stump exercises. Such a regimen should help prevent abduction, external rotation, and flexion of the hip, which may otherwise occur in the above-knee stump, and flexion of the knee and hip, in the case of a below-knee stump. As the postoperative pain diminishes, the frequency and intensity of the exercise program are increased; also resistive exercises are introduced to strengthen all muscles involved in moving the stump.

Stump bandaging. Of great importance in preparing the amputee for subsequent application of a prosthesis is proper bandaging of the stump, so as to reduce the swelling (Fig. 24.4C) (which helps tissue healing) and to produce a conical shaping of the stump (so that it can readily be inserted into the socket of the prosthesis).

Stump bandaging is begun 2 to 3 weeks postoperatively depending upon the rate of healing of the wound and the amount of local pain. For a below-knee stump, two 4-in. Ace bandages are sewn together end to end, while two 6-in. Ace bandages are used for an above-knee stump. The greatest tension is utilized distally and then with gradually decreasing pressure as the bandage, applied in a diagonal pattern with some overlapping, approaches the proximal portion of the stump. In the case of a below-knee stump, the upper limit of the applied bandage is the lower part of the thigh, with a figure eight being used across the extended knee. For the above-knee stump, the bandage is applied up to the perineum on the medial side and then is carried around the pelvis and back to the stump with the hip in extension. Circular turns around the limb should never be performed since they may result in a rise in distal venous pressure and produce swelling of the end of the stump. So as to maintain firm pressure on the stump, the bandage should be removed and reapplied with the proper tension four to six times during the day. This measure may require some assistance from medical personnel in the case of the elderly above-knee amputee. For a below-knee stump, it can readily be carried out by the patient.

General conditioning exercises. In order to prevent or counteract the debilitating effects of deconditioning (see Section B, Chapter 23), the patient should be instructed to perform exercises of the trunk and remaining limbs. As soon as feasible, he should be encouraged to stand and balance between parallel bars and, following improvement in these acts, he should progress to the pickup walker or crutch ambulation. In individuals with an above-knee amputation, emphasis is placed on strengthening internal rotators, extensors, and adductors of the hip in the involved side. For those with a below-knee amputation, the extensors of the knee are exercised. All of these measures help prepare the patient for the increased work load associated with gait training with a prosthesis (see below). At the same time, the various conditioning exercises maintain general muscle tone and prevent osteoporosis.

2. Later Measures

Criteria for choice of candidates for prosthesis. Once the amputee has become ambulatory using a pickup walker or crutches and the stump has healed and is properly shaped by bandaging, the decision must be made as to whether to institute prosthetic training, as a preliminary to the use of a permanent prosthesis. Unfortunately, the criteria which have been developed to act as guidelines in determining which individuals are proper candidates for such a program have not been clearly defined. Some of the points which must be taken into consideration are the age and general physical and mental state of the patient, the status of the arterial circulation in the remaining lower limb, the presence or absence of the knee joint, and the interval between surgery and the beginning of prosthetic training. Also of help in arriving at an affirmative decision is the ability of the amputee to perform a "swing through" maneuver on crutches and to climb stairs using crutches and the remaining lower limb. The most significant single factor in the success of the program, however, is motivation—an intense desire and resolve to become ambulatory again. Unfortunately, its strength and durability in the face of severe physical and mental obstacles are difficult to evaluate or predetermine and are not measurable except through clinical judgment. Also, the very important question of whether the patient will continue to use a prosthesis or will lose hope and discard it cannot be answered beforehand.

The factor of age no longer plays such an important role in the selection of candidates for a prosthesis as it did in the past, provided serious cardiac and pulmonary disorders commonly found in the elderly do not coexist. Because of significant advances in the field of biomechanical techniques for prosthetic fitting and in training programs, a much more optimistic attitude now prevails toward prosthetic rehabilitation of the geriatric amputee. However, it is important to keep in mind that such an individual should not be expected to achieve a greater amount of physical activity than he carried out before the amputation. Most of the available evidence supports the view that the use of a prosthesis does not shorten life, even in the presence of cardiac disease [4,14]. Nor does it untowardly affect the prognosis for the remaining lower limb when it is also suffering from a compromised local arterial circulation. In fact, prosthetic ambulation tends to take some of the stress off the latter and to equalize weight bearing [3], as contrasted to the situation that exists with crutch walking. Moreover, it has definite advantages over a wheelchair existence, since the physical load placed on the remaining limb may act to stimulate growth of collateral vessels and counteract the atrophy of muscles and of vascular components that results from disuse.

Prosthetic prescription. Most important in the success of the rehabilitative program for the geriatric amputee is the choice of the type of prosthesis for a major amputation. Besides determining that the artificial limb fits properly and is comfortable, its weight is also a very important consideration.

For the above-knee elderly amputee, the standard prosthesis, consisting of a pelvic band and an articulated external hip joint for stability and suspension of the leg, is the one generally prescribed. It can be used even in the presence of short, irregularly shaped, and scarred stumps and in the patient who has frequent changes in body weight. Moreover, it is readily applied and removed and necessitates few adjustments in fit. Its main disadvantage is that it is quite heavy; also it requires the use of a stump sock which interferes with kinesthetic feedback from the stump. It may need considerable maintenance because of the presence of a metal hip joint and the pelvic band.

Although the suction socket type of prosthesis weighs much less than the standard type, still it requires expenditure of large amounts of energy in its application or removal; hence it is employed only for amputees in good physical shape. Also, the stump socket fit is critical, with the result that changes in weight may cause loss of the necessary negative pressure needed in the socket to suspend it. For all these reasons, suction suspension is ordinarily impractical for the geriatric patient.

For a below-knee geriatric amputee, the patellar tendon-bearing laminated prosthesis has certain advantages over the open-end, so-called standard limb. It is lightweight, allows for complete freedom of the knee joint, and has total contact with the stump. Major weight bearing occurs in the neighborhood of the patellar tendon and around the proximal brim of the socket. The open-end standard limb is rarely prescribed for new geriatric amputees and is generally worn by those who have become accustomed to it and wish to continue using it.

Gait training. The goal of this program is the acquisition of a gait which is as normal as possible under the circumstances and which is carried out with the expenditure of an amount of energy that will not place a great strain on the capacity of the patient's cardiovascular and pulmonary systems. At first, ambulation is limited to short periods so as to prevent abrasions of the stump. The intervals are increased as the skin develops a greater tolerance to weight bearing. Balance on standing is achieved by placing the amputee between parallel bars and having him place all his weight equally on the normal and artificial lower limbs and then on each extremity separately. The procedure is followed by having the patient shift his weight from one side to the other with little or no use of the upper limbs. When he becomes proficient in all these maneuvers, he begins to walk between parallel bars with steps of equal length and with weight bearing of equal duration on

both the prosthesis and the remaining extremity. Having become adept in ambulating between parallel bars, the amputee now begins to walk on level surfaces and up and down stairs. Later he attempts walking on uneven terrain.

Gait deviations are common in geriatric amputees, generally because of existing physical defects and poor habit patterns. In the case of an above-knee amputation, not infrequently the patient has difficulty controlling knee-joint stability; such a problem may require the incorporation of a positive knee-locking mechanism into the prosthesis which allows ambulation with a locked knee. On sitting down, the knee unlocks so that the leg portion of the prosthesis can be flexed.

Local care of stump and prosthesis. The stump should routinely be examined by the patient to determine the state of the overlying skin. It should be washed daily using a mild soap, rinsed well, and carefully dried, followed by the application of talcum powder. Furunculosis, due to excessive sweating from prolonged confinement in a stump sock and socket, and abrasion of the skin (Fig. 24.4D), resulting from rough spots in the socket or from poor fit or alignment, must be diligently treated. The same approach applies to the appearance of eczema of the end of the stump, probably due to constriction of the proximal portion by the socket. All of these conditions may be severe enough to interfere temporarily with the use of the prosthesis. Local treatment of the lesions requires strict attention to sock hygiene, topical application of antibacterial agents and warm compresses, and correction of the causative prosthetic deficiencies. In order to maintain the prosthesis in working order, all parts should be properly lubricated and kept in good repair; the socket should be cleansed frequently.

References

1. Burgess EM: Immediate post-surgical prosthetic fitting. J Bone Joint Surg 48A:1022, 1966
2. Committee on Prosthetic-Orthotic Education, Division of Medical Sciences, National Research Council: The Geriatric Amputee: Princi-

ples of Management, Washington, DC, National Academy of Sciences, 1971

3. Cummings V: Recent concepts in the rehabilitation of the patient with peripheral vascular disease. NY J Med 60:3795, 1960

4. Erdman WJ II, Hettinger T, Saez F: Comparative work stress for above-knee amputees using artificial legs or crutches. Am J Phys Med 39:225, 1960

5. Fuson RL: Hypothermia prior to amputation: New instrument for induction by local refrigeration. Arch Surg 85:158, 1962

6. Lim RC Jr, Blaisdell FW, Hall AD, et al: Below-knee amputation for ischemic gangrene. Surg Gynecol Obstet 125:493, 1967

7. Lowenthal M, Posniak AO, Tobis JS: Rehabilitation of the elderly above-knee amputee. Arch Phys Med Rehabil 39:290, 1958

8. McCollough NC, Jennings JJ, Sarmiento A: Bilateral below-the-knee amputation in patients over fifty years of age: Results in thirty-one patients. J Bone Joint Surg 54A:1217, 1972

9. Mooney V, Harvey JP Jr, McBride, E, et al: Comparison of postoperative stump management: Plaster vs. soft dressings. J Bone Joint Surg 53A:241, 1971

10. Plugge H: Zur Entstehung des Phantomglieds. Dtsch Z Nervenh 154:199, 1943

11. Riddoch G: Phantom limbs and body shape. Brain 64:197, 1941

12. Silverstein MJ, Kadish L: A study of amputations of the lower extremity. Surg Gynecol Obstet 137:579, 1973

13. Simmel ML: Phantom experiences following amputation in childhood. J Neurol Neurosurg Psychiatry 25:69, 1962

14. Simonson E: Changes of physical fitness and cardiovascular functions with aging. Geriatrics 12:28, 1957

15. Weiss AA: The phantom limb. Ann Intern Med 44:668, 1956

16. Weiss M: The prosthesis on the operating table from the neurophysiological point of view. Report of the Workshop Panel on Lower Extremity Prosthetics Fitting, Committee on Prosthetics Research and Development. Washington, DC, National Academy of Sciences, 1966

17. Wolters BJ: Follow-up survey study of a group of elderly above-knee amputees. Arch Phys Med Rehabil 42:68, 1961

Chapter 25

Replantation and Revascularization of Limbs

A. General Considerations

1. Historical Background

Since the pioneer work of Carrel and his associates [4,5] and of Leriche and his associates [18,19] in the early part of this century, great strides have been made in vascular surgery, culminating in the appearance of the new field of replantation of limbs or portions of limbs.

Several basic contributions helped make possible the fairly rapid development of the technique of microvascular anastomosis. In 1960, Edwards [9] published an anatomic study of the fine, terminal arteries in the hand and fingers which supplied fundamental information essential for successful anastomosis of vessels of very small diameter. In the same year, Jacobson and Suarez[13] reported on the techniques of microvascular surgery. Subsequently, many investigations were carried out evaluating microsurgical instruments and methods, all of which were tested on experimental animals. Of greatest importance in the growth of the field was the fact that sophisticated operating microscopes became commercially available, as well as fine suture materials and specially designed surgical instruments capable of being used for the repair of vessels 1 mm or less in diameter.

For a number of years, microvascular techniques were applied to the treatment of almost completely amputated or severely devitalized limbs (revascularization procedures), with successful results being obtained in some individuals in whom it was felt that tissue viability would

otherwise have been lost [15]. However, it was not until 1964 that the first successful replantation of a totally severed human limb was performed by Malt and McKhann [21]. The next year a similar result was reported in two patients in China [6] and in one in England [11], followed by another case from China [25] a year later. In 1968, Komatsu and Tamai [17], from Japan, described a successful replantation of a completely severed thumb. With the development of greater interest in the field, a relatively large number of papers have appeared in the literature recording replantation of digits and larger portions of limbs, associated with a high degree of early success in such endeavors.

2. Goals of the Procedure

The aim of the replantation or the revascularization effort is first to maintain cellular viability of the amputated part through early reestablishment of local circulation; second, to attempt to restore as much function as realistically possible; and third, in the case of the upper limb, to achieve, at least, a prehensile hand. Cosmesis, although not a primary consideration, naturally follows if the attempt is successful.

To accomplish the first goal, it is necessary to solve certain problems in logistics, such as the development of a means of rapid transport of the patient to a hospital with available facilities to fulfill the technical requirements of the microvascular procedure. Also of the greatest importance is the establishment of a team of surgeons and paramedical personnel that can be activated in a short period of time (see B-1, below).

In order to accomplish the goal of restoration of function to the replanted or revascularized part, it is essential to be able to carry out the necessary technical steps with facility and care. Postoperatively, meticulous treatment of the wound is required if good results are to be expected. Finally, of greatest importance in the attempt to bring some degree of function back to the affected part is a long-term rehabilitative program (see B-8, below).

B. Basic Requirements for a Successful Replantation or Revascularization of a Limb

1. Availability of a Vascular Team

One of the most important factors contributing to the success of a replantation procedure is the existence of a surgical team experienced in vascular surgery and trauma and capable of initiating the necessary preliminary steps within an hour or less after arrival of the patient. Its members must be aware of the various pitfalls of, the indications for, and the contraindications to the different surgical approaches, so that decision making does not result in unnecessary delay in determining the correct course to follow. They must also be psychologically prepared to accept with equanimity a situation which frequently is time consuming, physically and emotionally demanding, and often frustrating [23]. At all times, the approach is that of a cooperative effort.

The team is divided into two groups: one which prepares the amputated specimen and the other which prepares the recipient site. Each consists of a hand or vascular surgeon with sufficient experience to perform small-vessel anastomoses, another surgeon who is able to work efficiently under magnification, several residents in surgery, and a scrub nurse who is acquainted with the care of microsurgical instruments. The anesthesiologist is also a very important member of the surgical steam (see B-4, below).

2. Importance of Proper Selection of Candidates for Procedure

A decision as to whether replantation or revascularization should be performed on a specific patient is generally not readily reached. First to be considered in this process are a number of contraindications to the procedure, thus immediately eliminating certain types of patients from the group of potential candidates. Among those objections that are absolute are such factors as extensive crushing injury of the amputated part causing marked destruction of tissues; significant additional wounds of either the specimen or the stump; improper preoperative care of the amputated part producing cellular damage; and the coexistence of serious systemic disorders making the patient a very poor risk for a protracted period of anesthesia [16]. There are several relative contraindications which must also be given some weight in the decision-making process. These include the presence of heavy soil contamination of the specimen and of the stump, as in the case of farm or war wounds; warm ischemic time of the amputated part exceeding 4 to 6 h in the case of a major amputation; distal damage of the specimen; poor motivation of the patient; old age; and previous trauma to the affected segment of limb [16].

If none of the above conditions applies, then it is necessary to consider whether an operation, if successful, has a good possibility of producing long-term improvement in the function of the part. If so, the next step is to weigh the potential advantages of the procedure against the surgical risk to the patient, the expense of treatment, the loss of gainful employment for a protracted period of time, and the cost of a long rehabilitative program [23]. Another factor which enters into the decision making is the emotional reaction of the patient and his family to the loss of a limb or a portion of one. However, this must be objectively evaluated and given emphasis only if there is supporting anatomic evidence that a good functional result can be expected from the operation. At no time is the surgical team justified in carrying out an unwarranted and ill-advised replantation because of the demands of the patient and his family to do so.

Also deserving of consideration are the patient's occupational and avocational demands. Replantation of parts which are unlikely to improve overall function of the limb should be discouraged, especially if work activity can be maintained without such a procedure. In fact, in some instances, hand function may actually be compromised by successful replantation of parts with marginal indications [23].

3. Preoperative Measures

Care of amputated part. One of the most important steps in the success of the procedure is proper care of the specimen from the time of the trauma until replantation is begun. It must immediately be cleansed of gross contamination, covered with sterile saline-soaked dressings, and placed in a plastic bag. The latter is then sealed with rubber bands and enclosed in a chest filled with ice. Immersing the part in a nonphysiologic solution, placing it in dry ice, or exposing it to local heat is contraindicated, since cellular disruption and death of tissue may result.

Care of the patient. At the same time, hemorrhage from the stump must be controlled and other injuries dealt with. The stump should be elevated slightly and maintained in place with loose dressings. Tetanus antitoxin or a toxoid booster injection should be given and antibiotic therapy started. Steps should be taken to control pain, preferably by means other than narcotics.

Transportation of patient. The preliminary emergency measures having been performed with celerity, the patient is transported to a replantation center as rapidly as possible, using whatever means are available and disregarding the cost. The reason for such haste is that unless the replantation procedure is begun within 4 to 6 h from the time of injury, not only will there be less possibility that viability of the part will be maintained, but also signs of toxemia may subsequently develop in the patient due to absorption of breakdown products from the necrotic tissue. This is especially true if the amputated part contains a large bulk of muscle.

Further care of the specimen in the hospital. There is a real difference of opinion regarding the value of preoperative flushing of the vascular tree in the amputated part with a slow infusion of 20,000 units of heparin in saline or low-molecular-weight dextran solution. Such a measure has been advocated to clear the vessels of clotted blood. However, the criticism has been raised that the procedure may instead cause intimal damage which predisposes to thrombosis. Also, there is a belief that spontaneous clotting rarely occurs in the vessels of the amputated part. As a general rule, therefore, it appears advisable to avoid perfusion except when severe crush or muscle injuries are present. Direct clamping of vessels should not be done because of the possibility of increasing the degree of vascular damage.

4. Choice of Anesthetic

The anesthesiologist should try to see the patient in the emergency room where he can determine the type of anesthesia to administer. For upper limb replantation or revascularization, prolonged axillary regional block, using bupivacaine hydrochloride (Marcaine hydrochloride) or lidocaine hydrochloride (Xylocaine), has been found to produce a very effective anesthesia of the hand [16,23,24]. However, when bilateral axillary block is required, the amount injected may be great enough to produce serious side reactions. Therefore, under such circumstances, general anesthesia should be used. In the case of children and uncooperative adults, this procedure is also indicated. Still, it is necessary to point out that prolonged general anesthesia must be administered with great caution, since it may be associated with such complications as pressure ulcerations, pulmonary embolism, and peripheral nerve palsy, among others.

5. Operative Approach

No attempt will be made in this section to describe in detail the exact technical steps involved in microvascular anastomosis, since such information is readily available in the literature [16,24]. Instead, the discussion will be limited to the presentation of some general principles pertinent to the method.

Cleansing, debridement, and tagging of structures.

Preliminary to replantation, the part is surgically cleansed and placed on a separate sterile table containing standard and microscopic instruments. Crushed tissue is excised and generally bone is shortened about 0.5 to 1.0 cm to permit approximation of structures without tension. Some workers [3] are of the opinion, however, that the latter step is not necessary since tension-free repair can be carried out with the use of interpositioned venous grafts (see below), thus preserving functional length. Finally, vessels, cut nerves, and tendons are isolated, identified, and tagged.

Skeletal stabilization.

Before vascular anastomoses are attempted, skeletal immobilization must be accomplished, because this prevents later kinking, trauma, or thrombosis of the vessels and their anastomoses as repair of the wound progresses. The process must be carried out in a manner which is atraumatic to adjacent tissues. Bone fixation may be produced with single pinning, cross pinning, intramedullary Kirschner wires, loop wiring, or the use of an ordinary screw [24].

Treatment of cut tendons.

These structures should also be repaired before the microvascular phase of the operation is begun. The procedure can be performed quickly without prolonging ischemia time unnecessarily, and it has the advantage of obviating the need to attempt tendon repair after the more delicate stages of the operation have been carried out [23]. If the procedure is delayed for a number of days, it may be more difficult to perform because of the development of local scar tissue in the interval.

Vascular anastomoses.

The question as to whether to perform arterial or venous anastomoses first has not been fully answered. Those who initially reestablish arterial circulation claim that such a step is essential in order to revascularize the limb as early as possible [6–8,12,24]. To avoid engorgement of the tissues and stagnation of blood, they advocate removal of the venous clamps for short intervals during the time that the venous anastomosis is still not operative, in order to permit free venous bleeding. The usefulness of such a step has been questioned. If subsequently it is found impossible to carry out venous anastomoses for technical reasons, severe edema will almost invariably develop under such conditions (see B-7, below).

Other microvascular teams [23] believe that venous anastomoses should be performed first to prevent swelling of the part. Also, this step eliminates the excessive bleeding from cut veins that may occur if the arterial anastomosis is performed first. It also precludes the necessity of halting flow for repair of veins, as would be required if this were done as the second procedure.

If practicable, venous grafts should be used instead of Teflon prostheses to bridge arterial and venous defects because of their greater viability and availability [1]. They should not be obtained from the site of injury since donor vessels in this location may also have been damaged by the original trauma. Moreover, by so doing, the already existing compromise of local venous circulation is further exaggerated. Therefore, as a general rule, the grafts should be procured from a normal limb. In the process of inserting the prosthesis, it is necessary to use the proper length of vessel so as to prevent either buckling or excessive tension at the suture line.

At all times, precautions must be taken to minimize the possibility of postoperative thrombosis of the small traumatized arteries. These vessels should be handled gently, their walls must be kept moist with saline solution, and their lumens must continue to be kept free of clots and blood with a dilute heparin-saline solution [10]. Injury to the intima is prevented with the use of atraumatic arterial clamps, and loose tunica adventitia is trimmed and not permitted to fall into the suture line [15]. It is the opinion of some workers that a synthetic vascular suture on an atraumatic needle is preferable to the standard, more irritative silk vascular suture in reducing the incidence of thrombosis [15].

Nerve repair.

Some vascular surgeons [23] believe that all significant nerves should be dealt with as precisely as possible at the time of the initial operation. This approach is based on the view that secondary repairs are technically very difficult, usually require nerve grafts, and give poor functional results. However, for a successful outcome, the original wound must be clean and the nerve stumps must have been divided by a cutting instrument, rather than having been pulled apart by the trauma. If such conditions do not exist, the alternative is a nerve graft, as for example, a substitution for a medial antibrachial cutaneous nerve in the case of the upper limb.

There are other investigators [7,12] who favor delaying nerve suturing for 8 weeks postoperatively, especially if it is impossible to assay the amount of damage sustained by the cut ends. Moreover, they point out that attempts to reestablish nerve continuity further prolong an already lengthy operation.

Application of bandages. The manner in which the dressings are applied at the end of the surgical procedure is of utmost importance. The gauze should avoid direct pressure on the operative site and should not cause circular constriction. At the same time, it should allow for frequent checks of the state of the local circulation. In order to permit some elevation of the limb, nonadhering gauze is applied in longitudinal strips and fluffed gauze is placed around the extremity in a similar manner. The limb is then surrounded with strips of thick sterile foam rubber or sponge secured with a circumferential stretch bandage [16].

6. Postoperative Management

Local measures. The care given to the limb during the first several weeks following surgery may markedly influence the outcome of the operation. Of great importance is frequent examination of the pulsations in the larger arteries and of the nutritional state of the skin (skin color, cutaneous temperature, and turgor and tone of the local cutaneous microcirculation). Skin temperature of the digits, using a thermocouple, is recorded hourly by the nursing staff. A fall below 30°C (86°F) indicates the need for returning the patient to the operating room for reexploration. Oscillometry and the Doppler ultrasonic flowmeter may have to be used

if edema of the limb or its distal segment makes palpation of the pulses difficult or impossible.

When there is any doubt regarding the local circulation in the replanted part, the dressings should be removed and the tissues closely examined. If there are signs of a failing blood flow, the patient must be returned to the operating room and the vessels reexplored. Restoration of circulation if thrombosis exists is essential for maintenance of viability of the replanted part. This generally involves the use of venous grafts, such an approach being successful in salvaging the limb in about 50 percent of the cases [16].

It is important to position the limb properly so as to facilitate maximal venous drainage and thus minimize edema formation. The best position for this purpose is slight elevation of the extremity above heart level, which does not materially affect arterial inflow, at the same time that it accelerates venous outflow somewhat. More marked elevation is contraindicated.

The question as to when the initial dressing change should be carried out has not been answered. Some vascular surgeons are of the opinion that this should be done on the first postoperative day, believing that if the blood-soaked or blood-caked gauze were left on the operative site, it would act to impede local circulation. Others, however, strongly advocate postponing such a step until the tenth to the twelfth postoperative day, since they feel that each early dressing change may have a catastrophic effect on the local circulation by initiating irreversible arterial spasm. Because of such a possibility, the latter program appears to be the proper course to follow.

Systemic measures. To determine whether untoward constitutional responses are developing, it is necessary to monitor urinary output in the first 24 postoperative hours. By this means, early identification of the presence of oliguria or anuria can be made. Several blood pH measurements should be carried out during the same period so as to ascertain whether acidosis exists. Antibiotics should be given prophylactically, based on culture and sensitivity studies of fluid taken from the area of trauma.

In order to help prevent intravascular clotting, low-molecular-weight dextran is given intravenously by microdrip (500 mg daily for 3 or more days) (see C-3, Chapter 17); aspirin, in doses of 2 g (30 gr) daily, is helpful because of its antiplatelet action. Anticoagulant therapy, in the form of administration of intravenous heparin, has also been advocated for 7 to 10 days postoperatively. The dose is 20,000 units daily given continuously [24] and adjusted to produce doubling of the control APTT.

7. Complications of the Procedure

One of the most serious complications of microvascular surgery is infection, since it contributes to thrombosis of the vessels [2]. Even in the absence of this state, occlusion of arteries less than 4 mm in diameter is a frequent possibility [13,26], and when this occurs, the viability of distal tissues is almost invariably placed in jeopardy.

Among other complications is bleeding at the site of the anastomosis, requiring the return of the patient to the operating room to control it or to evacuate a hematoma. Edema is noted not infrequently and when of a severe degree, it may cause compromise of the local arterial circulation. Under such circumstances, complete fasciotomy is necessary, even in such locations as fingers, in order to release the fluid and so decrease tissue pressure. If considerable quantities of plasma and blood are lost through the incisions, replacement therapy should be started.

Most replanted or revascularized structures subsequently demonstrate some signs of heightened vasomotor tone in the form of increased sensitivity to cold, pallor or cyanosis of the skin, and delayed adjustment to warming. Associated symptoms are a subjective sense of coldness and discomfort in the replanted part. With time, the condition appears to decrease in severity. Rarely does an incapacitating posttraumatic painful vascular disorder develop (see Section A, Chapter 13) after replantation.

8. Rehabilitative Program

Rehabilitation of the replanted part should be instituted as early as practicable, including the first postoperative day, and continued for several years if necessary. Of great importance is avoidance of tendon adhesions or development of refractory stiffness of the interphalangeal joints or of the wrist or ankle, since such changes may require secondary reconstruction. One possible untoward response to the early institution of a rehabilitative program, however, is elongation or rerupture of repaired tendons.

At the beginning, very mild passive exercise of replanted fingers is initiated under careful supervision of medical personnel and, later, minimal active exercise. During such measures, the hand is supported by means of a dorsal cast to protect against hyperextension of the digits. After the tenth postoperative day, when the sutures are generally removed, the rehabilitative program is accelerated and moderate active exercises are carried out while the hand is immersed in a warm bath containing a mild antiseptic. By the third postoperative week, active finger flexion exercises are performed using a dynamic splint.

9. Corrective Surgical Procedures

Although ideally primary repair of all injured structures produces the best results, in about 75 percent of patients some type of secondary reconstructive procedure is necessary. The most common repairs are tendolysis, nerve grafts, and capsulectomy. In order to increase functional capacity, such secondary tendon procedures as tendon grafts, staged tendon grafts, and tendon transfer have been performed. These are generally indicated after the osseous framework has healed and adequate skin covering has been obtained. In order to achieve the latter, it may be necessary to use meshed split grafts or pedicle and free flaps if cover of exposed bone, joint, tendon, and nerve is required.

10. Evaluation of Revascularization and Replantation Procedures

As a general rule, the reports in the literature tend to deal principally with the immediate success rate of the operative procedure in maintaining viability of the revascularized or replanted part, while only superficially alluding to the incidence of subsequent return of function of the limb or the degree of persistent neurologic deficits or contracture deformities that develop. With a few exceptions [14,22,27], the results of long-range objective testing of range of motion of joints or of the capacity of the hands or fingers to perform gross or fine movements are not available. Nor has the actual on-the-job use of replanted or revascularized hands or limbs been well documented [22]. In general, revascularization procedures have better results than replantation in regard to total hand function [15,20]. It is apparent, therefore, that only when extensive data on the degree of restoration of useful function of a part have been collected will it be possible to evaluate revascularization and replantation procedures fully.

References

1. Bradham RR, Nunn DB: Autogenous vein grafts and Teflon grafts as small vessel prostheses. AMA Arch Surg 81:136, 1960
2. Breidenbach L, Lord JW Jr: Restoration and preservation of arterial continuity following trauma. Am J Surg 76:578, 1948
3. Buncke HJ, Alpert B, Shaf KG: Microvascular grafting. Clin Plast Surg 5:185, 1978
4. Carrel A: Results of the transplantation of blood vessels, organs and limbs. JAMA 51:1662, 1908
5. Carrel A, Guthrie CC: Complete amputation of the thigh, with replantation. Am J Med Sci 131:297, 1906
6. Ch'en CW, Ch'ien YC, Pao YS, et al: Further experiences in the restoration of amputated limbs: Report of two cases. Chin Med J 84:225, 1965
7. Christeas N, Balas P, Giannikas A: Replantation of amputated extremities: Report of two successful cases. Am J Surg 118:68, 1969
8. Cooney WP III: Revascularization and replantation after upper extremity trauma: Experience with interposition artery and vein grafts. Clin Orthop 137:227, 1978
9. Edwards EA: Organization of the small arteries of the hand and digits. Am J Surg 99:837, 1960
10. Ferguson IA Sr, Byrd WM, McAfee DK: Experiences in the management of arterial injuries. Ann Surg 153:980, 1961
11. Horn JS: Successful reattachment of a completely severed forearm. Lancet 1:1152, 1964
12. Inoue T, Toyoshima Y, Fukusumi H, et al: Factors necessary for successful replantation of upper extremities. Ann Surg 165:225, 1967
13. Jacobson JH II, Suarez EL: Microsurgery in the anastomosis of small vessels. Surg Forum 11:243, 1960
14. Jones JM, Schenck RR, Chesney RB: Digital replantation and amputation—a comparison of function. Reported at the February 1980 meeting of the Am Soc for Surg of the Hand, Atlanta, Georgia
15. Kleinert HE, Kasdan ML, Romero JL: Small blood-vessel anastomosis for salvage of severely injured upper extremity. J Bone Joint Surg 45A:788, 1963
16. Kleinert HE, Tsai T: Microvascular repair in replantation. Clin Orthop 133:205, 1978
17. Komatsu S, Tamai S: Successful replantation of a completely cut-off thumb. Case report. Plast Reconstr Surg 42:374, 1968
18. Leriche, R: De la resection du carrefour aortico-iliaque avec double sympathectomie lombaire pour thrombose artéritique de l'aorte. Le syndrome de l'oblitération terminoaortique par artérite. Presse Med 18:601, 1910
19. Leriche R, Murard J: A propos d'un cas d'artériotomie d l'iliaque externe pour arrêt de circulation dans le membre inférieur, par artérite. Lyon Chir 7:407, 1912
20. Lendvay PG: Replacement of the amputated digit. Br J Plast Surg 26:398, 1973
21. Malt RA, McKhann CF: Replantation of severed arms. JAMA 189:716, 1964
22. Paletta FX: Replantation of the amputated extremity. Ann Surg 168:720, 1968
23. Phelps DB, Lilla JA, Boswick JA Jr: Common problems in clinical replantations and revascularization in the upper limb. Clin Orthop 133:11, 1978
24. Tamai S, Hori Y, Tatsumi Y, et al: Microvascular anastomosis and its application on the replantation of amputated digits and hands. Clin Orthop 133:106, 1978
25. Ts'ui CY, Shih YF, T'ang CY, et al: Successful restoration of a completely amputated arm. Chin Med J 85:536, 1966
26. Urschel HC Jr, Roth EJ: Small arterial anastomoses. II. Suture. Ann Surg 153:611, 1961
27. Weiland AJ, Villarreal-Rios A, Kleinert HE, et al: Replantation of digits and hands: Analysis of surgical techniques and functional results in 71 patients with 86 replantations. J Hand Surg 2:1, 1977

Chapter 26

Medicolegal Aspects of Vascular Difficulties

Since the United States is a highly industrialized country, it can be expected that more and more people will be covered by liability laws, workmen's compensation acts, and disability insurance programs. Therefore, much as they might desire it, orthopedic and general surgeons cannot ignore the medicolegal aspects of their profession. Moreover, the growing incidence of malpractice suits initiated after elective surgery or even following limb- or lifesaving procedures makes the situation more critical.[1] This chapter deals with some of the problems in forensic medicine that have relevance to the vascular complications of musculoskeletal disorders and their treatment.

A. Occupation-related Vascular Syndromes

Because most people employed at manual tasks in industry are covered by workmen's compensation rules and regulations, it frequently becomes necessary to determine whether an existing vascular disorder has its origin in the patient's occupation (a causal relationship) or, if not, whether an underlying circulatory condition has been aggravated by the daily duties

at work. Also of importance is the determination of whether a single traumatic event was responsible for initiating the vascular difficulty or whether it was due to chronic repetitive mechanical stimuli. Several typical examples of occupation-related vascular entities are presented below.

1. Occupation-related Trauma to a Limb with Normal Circulation

Raynaud's syndrome (phenomenon). This state, which clinically resembles Raynaud's disease in all regards, is associated with several occupations. One of these involves the prolonged use of high-frequency vibratory tools, such as a pneumatic hammer (pneumatic hammer disease), riveters, a hand-held pneumatic drill of high frequency and amplitude used by uranium miners [1], or a chain saw. Raynaud's syndrome has also been reported in typists, violinists, and pianists. (For a description of the manifestations of Raynaud's disease or of Raynaud's syndrome, see p. 143.)

The etiologic agent is probably one of gross exaggeration of a normal constrictive vascular response brought on by persistent exposure to violent mechanical vibration [1]. There is some evidence suggesting that vibratory tools induce Raynaud's syndrome only if there is also intermittent cooling of the body and the hands [1,2]. It is of interest that despite the fact that Raynaud's syndrome is transient and entirely reversible, in late stages of the occupation-re-

---

[1] Of interest in this regard is the report of the National Association of Insurance Commissioners, covering the period between July, 1976 and June, 1978, which indicated that fractures and other types of trauma generated more malpractice claims than any other broad category of conditions.

lated condition, organic changes, in the form of subintimal fibrosis, occur in the digital arteries subjected to repeated spasm.

Generally, the color changes first appear in the fingers of the nondominant hand, but ultimately exposure to cold causes all of the digits of both hands to be involved. The condition is relatively benign, spontaneous trophic lesions being rare. However, minor mechanical, chemical, or thermal injuries may be responsible for the production of nonhealing ulcerations of the finger tips. In most instances, early removal of the initiating factor results in abatement of the attacks of Raynaud's syndrome.

Local trauma. If an injury to a limb sustained at work subsequently triggers the development of one of the vascular disorders initiated by trauma, the resulting condition is covered by workmen's compensation or disability insurance programs. Among such clinical entities are major causalgia and posttraumatic vasomotor disorders (see A-1 and A-2, respectively, Chapter 13), neurovascular compression syndromes of the shoulder girdle (see Section B, Chapter 13), palmar artery aneurysm and hypothenar hammer syndromes (see G-1 and G-2, respectively, Chapter 15), superficial thrombophlebitis, and phlebothrombosis and popliteal thrombophlebitis (see A-2 and A-3, respectively, Chapter 18). Extensive trauma to the lower limbs involving superficial and deep lymphatic vessels may also cause permanent secondary lymphedema and some disability if a sufficient number of these channels are severed.

Cold injury. Public servants, like firemen and policemen, and others whose occupation requires prolonged periods of exposure to low environmental temperature may develop frostbite of the hands and feet or trench foot if moisture has also contributed to the production of the condition (see D-1 and D-2, respectively, Chapter 13). Depending upon the duration and severity of the cold, the degree of involvement may vary from the production of erythema or blister formation to extensive destruction of digits and adjoining portions of limbs. It is important to point out that following the acute phase of frostbite or trench foot, the patient may develop Raynaud's syndrome.

2. Occupation-related Trauma to a Limb with Compromised Circulation

Chronic venous insufficiency. In the presence of venous hypertension of the lower limbs, due to primary varicosities or the postphlebitic syndrome (see Chapter 20), a mild abrasion to the lower part of the involved leg sustained at work may be enough to initiate an indolent, nonhealing venous stasis ulcer (see B-11, Chapter 20). At times this type of lesion may develop even with such mild trauma that it does not break the continuity of the skin.

Chronic arterial insufficiency. In the case of the patient suffering from arteriosclerosis obliterans with or without diabetes, thromboangiitis obliterans, or any condition which compromises the arterial circulation to the lower limbs, minor trauma to the foot due to a tool or instrument falling on it may be sufficient to cause an injury that has the potential for initiating gangrene. In the presence of thromboangiitis obliterans, trauma to the hands may have the same result. If the occupation of the patient suffering from a chronic occlusive arterial disease requires him to be outdoors for any period of time during the winter months, he is a good candidate for the development of frostbite even when the environmental temperature has only dropped just below 0°C (32°F).

In the presence of extensive atherosclerotic plaques which also involve the popliteal artery, daily prolonged periods of squatting or acute flexion of knees (positions routinely assumed by such individuals as plumbers during the course of their work) may cause serious aggravation of the existing state. This may take the form of a rapidly developing hemorrhage in a fractured plaque, resulting in acute thrombosis of the popliteal artery and, frequently, gangrene of the foot. Or a weakened portion of the wall of the vessel may develop into an arterial aneurysm with its subsequent serious complications (see E-3, Chapter 15).

In the evaluation of the problem, it must always be kept in mind that sudden occlusions of arteriosclerotic arteries may on occasion also occur spontaneously, without any obvious provocation. Inevitably, therefore, a certain percentage of such episodes will take place while the individuals are at work. They are part of the natural history of arteriosclerosis obliterans and hence are generally not considered compensable if they are first identified clinically while the patient is sitting quietly at a desk with his lower limbs in a normal dependent position. Of importance in arriving at the proper disposition, therefore, is a detailed history, including an exact description of the sequence of events at the time the manifestations of the condition were first noted.

B.   Disability Evaluation in Vascular Disorders

1.   Determination of Presence of Underlying Vascular Disease

For the sake of the record, it is advisable to distinguish occupation-incurred trauma to a limb with a normal vascular tree from that causing aggravation of a preexisting arterial or venous disorder. Pertinent to the problem are the conclusions that can be drawn from the history and the physical findings present not only in the involved limb but also in the others. For example, if it can be elicited that the patient previously complained of intermittent claudication or ischemic neuropathy or if there are symptoms or signs of venous hypertension, such as swelling, night cramps, or pigmentation of the skin of the legs, the inference can be made that he had suffered from a vascular disorder in the past and that the current episode of trauma had contributed to the aggravation of the underlying difficulty. Of course, if a previously recorded preemployment examination is available, listing definite findings of arterial or venous insufficiency, then there is no doubt about the matter. Also of value in this respect is the finding of chronic occlusive arterial disease in an uninjured companion limb.

If an indolent ulcer or gangrene occurs as the result of injury to a limb with a preexisting

arterial or venous insufficiency, the occupation-related trauma that precipitates the lesion must be considered a major aggravating factor, and hence the condition still falls within the guidelines of the workmen's compensation act. Such a view is based on extensive clinical observations that most patients with long-standing arterial or venous disorders of the limbs who avoid injury generally do not suffer from spontaneous local ulceration or gangrene.

2.   Criteria for Establishment of a Causal Relationship

Certain conditions must be met before one can establish a cause-and-effect relationship between trauma and the development of ulcers or gangrene of the limbs. Most importantly the lesion must have been noted within a reasonable time after the involved site was injured. It is also necessary to show that the difficulty was produced by trauma of appropriate magnitude, location, and type. However, the relative importance of these factors in reaching a decision must be judged in the context of whether the preexisting arterial and venous circulations were normal. Another point which is taken into consideration is the superimposition of infection or of other complications of injury which may untowardly affect the outcome, even in the presence of a minor injury and adequate local blood flow.

3.   General Principles in the Evaluation of Permanent Impairment and Permanent Disability

In determining the degree of impairment caused by an occupation-related vascular disorder, certain criteria must be kept in mind [3]. However, no attempt is made in this section to list the various categories and subdivisions of a classification of impairment, since such information is readily available in detailed form from other sources [3]. Instead, only general principles are emphasized.

It is essential for the surgeon involved in any private or public program for the disabled to have an understanding of the various factors to be considered in reaching a conclusion concerning both permanent impairment and permanent disability. Also important but much more difficult to determine is a patient's residual ability to function.

Permanent impairment. This is a state in which there is an anatomic or functional abnormality or loss which is severe enough to interfere with gainful employment. Such a conclusion must be reached only after maximal rehabilitation has been achieved and the condition has reached a stable and nonprogressive level at the time of examination. Following therapeutic surgical procedures, a period of time appropriate for the operation should have elapsed before evaluation of permanent impairment is attempted. Furthermore, all findings should be subject to review at an interval of 6 months to a year, depending upon circumstances, before a final conclusion is reached. Permanent impairment is a very important contributing factor to, but not necessarily an indication of, the extent of permanent disability (see below).

The determination of the severity of the impairment falls completely within the province of the medical examiner. The evaluation of rating of this state is derived from an appraisal of the nature and extent of the patient's difficulty. Unlike permanent disability, permanent impairment can be measured with a reasonable degree of accuracy and uniformity on the basis of impaired function as evidenced by loss of structural integrity, existing pathology, or pain substantiated by clinical findings. Involved in the study are a complete physical examination and accurate objective measurements of function; not considered are subjective impressions and such nonmedical factors as age, sex, and employability.

Permanent disability. This represents a state in which a patient's actual or presumed ability to engage in gainful work is reduced or absent because of physical impairment, with no fundamental or marked change to be expected in the future. Such a conclusion represents an administrative decision, based not only on the medical evaluation of the difficulty, but also on social, psychologic, and vocational factors, including age, sex, education, and economic environment. In a sense, therefore, the conclu-

sion that a patient is permanently disabled is a reflection of his inability to function in all spheres of living.

C. Steps for Avoidance of Malpractice Suits

1. Preliminary Discussions with the Patient

Regarding elective therapeutic procedures. A common complaint among patients in whom the actual beneficial results from an elective operation fell short of expectations is that they had not had a frank and complete preliminary discussion with their doctor concerning the goals that were achievable from the contemplated approach. Generally what also concerns them is that they were not made fully aware of the degree of pain and the possible complications and risks associated with the procedure.

To counteract the development of such an attitude (since false expectation may lead to the initiation of a malpractice suit), it is essential to present the subject to the patient in such detail that there will be no basis for subsequent misunderstanding or disappointment, and this conversation should be so recorded in the hospital chart by the attending surgeon himself and not by a member of the house staff. Also included in the progress notes should be a statement to the effect that the patient is willing to accept the possible risks associated with the procedure and has indicated this by signing the necessary permission and release forms. Of value in helping the patient achieve a realistic view of his problem is the preoperative use of audiovisual aids, such as a short instructional movie.

Regarding limbsaving or lifesaving procedures. Even when the contemplated operation is essential, it is still necessary to present the problem to the patient in a similar fashion, at the same time emphasizing that other less hazardous options are not applicable for apparent reasons. Again, such a conversation should be recorded in detail in the hospital chart.

Regarding diagnostic procedures. In the case of laboratory tests which are essential for the collection of information pertinent to the adoption of the proper therapeutic program but which have an associated element of discomfort and risk, the same approach as the above should also be routinely carried out. For example, the surgeon or the radiologist, whichever one is to perform a contrast angiogram or venogram, must explain the test to the patient; he should also emphasize the great need for the information derived thereby and possible untoward responses that might ensue, at the same time pointing out their rarity. He must personally see to it that the necessary permission forms have been properly signed and he must observe the patient afterward for the appearance of side reactions. To minimize the possibility of serious consequences, certain other steps should be carried out in the arteriographic room, as discussed in E-1 (Preliminary Precautionary Measures), Chapter 5.

Unless all of the above-mentioned or referred-to steps are closely followed each time contrast angiography or venography is performed, the surgeon or radiologist conducting the test is exposing himself to serious medicolegal jeopardy. Of great value in reducing such a possibility is to make a detailed report in the hospital record of all the precautionary steps that were taken. Although time consuming, this may prove very useful if the need to justify the procedure should ever arise.

2. Preoperative or Pretest Measures

A full clinical evaluation of the state of the circulation should be conducted in the limb to be subjected to a surgical procedure or a laboratory test and also in the other limbs. The results should be recorded in detail in the patient's hospital or office chart. Also included should be reports of laboratory tests that are pertinent to the determination of the state of local blood flow.

Together with the above, the full evaluation of the patient's general physical status should be available in the record, as well as a summary of the results of important laboratory tests. Note should be made of the presence of allergic manifestations and past hypersensitivity reactions. If the need arises, the opinions of consultants from other fields should be sought and recorded.

3. Postoperative Measures

Repeated evaluation of circulatory status. Following operation, the limb on which an operative procedure had been performed should be examined daily to determine the state of local circulation (cutaneous temperature, skin color, subpapillary venous plexus filling time, palpation of pulses, oscillometry if feasible, and presence or absence of pitting or nonpitting edema), and the results should be recorded in detail in the progress notes. The other limbs should also be similarly studied. At the same time, systemic responses should be evaluated.

Presence of infection. With the appearance of this complication in the operative site, smears and sensitivity studies should immediately be carried out and appropriate antibacterial therapy instituted. If, after several days of intensive treatment, no signs of improvement are apparent, the sensitivity studies should be repeated, on the basis that the bacterial flora has changed in the interval. All the efforts to control the infection should be clearly recorded in the progress notes. (For the steps necessary to obtain a meaningful sensitivity study, see p. 162.)

Institution of a physical therapeutic program. As soon as feasible, steps should be taken to encourage the patient to use his involved limb in a normal fashion. Such a regimen prevents or minimizes the appearance of superimposed disuse atrophy, vasospasm, and osteoporosis (see C-1, Chapter 23), responses frequently noted in the poorly treated strain or sprain. The decision to initiate an ambulation program should not be influenced by the existence of radiographic evidence of osteoporosis in the bones of the involved limb, a change which may take months and even years to disappear. Actually, an early ambulation program facilitates the reversion to a normal state of consistency of the constituents of the bone. The stance and gait of the patient must be strictly supervised and various types of physical props, such as canes and crutches, should be discarded as soon as possible.

4. Medicolegal Aspects of Trauma to a Limb

After an extremity has sustained an injury, it is very important to perform a vascular examination to determine whether the local arterial and venous trees have also been affected by trauma. The other limbs should be studied in a similar manner and the information recorded in detail in the chart. If vascular problems exist, reconstructive measures should be carried out simultaneously with, or even before, attempting to correct any existing orthopedic condition, since destruction or traumatic thrombosis of a critical artery frequently requires immediate attention by a vascular surgeon in order to maintain viability of the limb (see A-1 to A-4, Chapter 15).

Following application of a cast or of traction in the treatment of fractures, it is essential to make daily vascular examinations of the distal structures of the limb and to document the results in the progress notes. The appearance of abnormal signs is sufficient basis for immediate removal of the compression or traction and for requesting vascular consultative advice.

References

1. Ashe WF, Williams N: Occupational Raynaud's. II. Further studies of this disorder in uranium mine workers. Arch Environ Health 9:425, 1964
2. Davies TAL, Glaser EM, Collins CP: Absence of Raynaud's phenomenon in workers using vibratory tools in a warm climate. Lancet 1:1014, 1957
3. Guide to the Evaluation of Permanent Impairment. Chicago, American Medical Association, 1977, pp 83–85

Index

Page numbers followed by the letter (f) indicate figure; (n) indicate footnote; (t) indicate table.